Down Syndrome Children - An Update

Edited By

Mohammed Al-Biltagi
Associate Professor of Pediatrics
Tanta University
Egypt

Bentham Science Publishers Ltd.
Executive Suite Y - 2
PO Box 7917, Saif Zone
Sharjah, U.A.E.
Email: subscriptions@benthamscience.org

CONTENTS

FOREWORD

English physician John Langdon Down was among the first to describe the disorder now called Down syndrome (DS) about 150 years ago. In 1959, Dr. Jerome Lejeune, a French scientist, reported that Down syndrome results from presence of an extra copy of human chromosome 21. Now we know that Down syndrome is the most common live-compatible human chromosomal abnormality, occurring in 1 in 700-800 newborns. Latest studies have shown that pregnancy termination rates following prenatal diagnoses have decreased the incidence of DS in recent years in some population groups, which may reflect advances in medical interventions for people with Down syndrome and progresses in educational and social support for their families. These advances have also significantly extended the life expectancy for people with Down syndrome. Therefore, Down syndrome will continue to affect a significant size of our population and thus remain as a major public health challenge in the future.

Due to the impacts of presence of an additional copy of the whole chromosome 21, individuals with Down syndrome exhibited a constellation of developmental abnormalities affecting many organ systems. Congenital heart defects, including atrioventricular defects, are discovered in about 50% of kids with Down syndrome. Meanwhile; about 10% of children with Down syndrome develop transient myeloproliferative disorder, and approximately 30% of these patients develop acute megakaryoblastic leukemia, which equates to just about 500-fold greater risk of having acute megakaryoblastic leukemia. Human trisomy 21 is the most frequent genetic cause for developmental cognitive disabilities. The brains of individuals with DS over the age of 40 show the neuropathological changes of Alzheimer's disease.

The landmark discovery of human trisomy 21 as the chromosomal basis for Down syndrome has also positioned this disorder as the most complex human genetic disease compatible with postnatal survival. As a result, progress in Down syndrome research has been slow until 1990s when development of mouse models of Down syndrome, particularly Ts65Dn, enabled scientists to explore the disorder at the molecular, cellular, physiological and organismal levels. The convergence of recent advances in mammalian genome sequencing and chromosome engineering technology has opened up an unprecedented opportunity for unraveling the mechanisms underlying abnormal phenotypes in Down syndrome by generating and analyzing new mouse mutants with precise duplications and deletions of human chromosome 21 orthologous regions. Amidst these remarkable advances related to Down syndrome research, the publication of the e-book "Down syndrome children – an update" edited by Dr. Mohammed Al-Biltagi is welcome news, which will provide the latest information on medically important areas associated with Down syndrome, including the prevalence, genetics, infection in children with Down syndrome, cardiac, skeletal and dental abnormalities, biochemical, respiratory, gastrointestinal and psychological changes, neonatal, neurological, hematological problems, as well as problems with anesthesia. Such a timely update will surely benefit all of us who care so much about

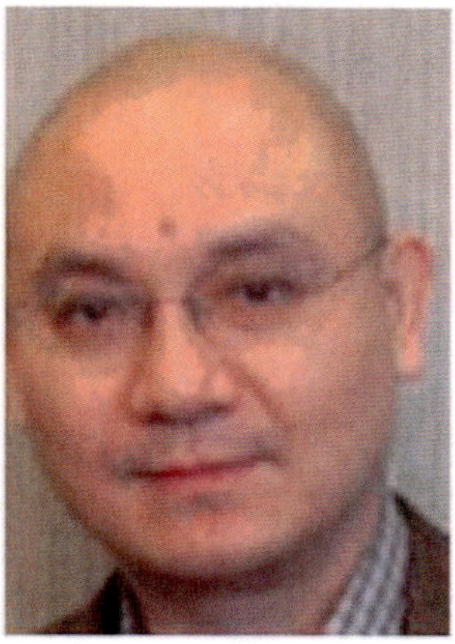

Y. Eugene Yu
The Children's Guild Foundation Down Syndrome Research Program
Genetics Program and Department of Cancer Genetics
Roswell Park Cancer Institute, USA

PREFACE

Down syndrome is the commonest genetic disease in the world; affecting all countries, all races, and both sexes. Since the comprehensive description of clinical features of the syndrome in 1866 by John Langdon Down; and its genetic basis in 1959, researches are still trying to study various aspects of this syndrome to improve the health and the quality of life of the affected people. This book **"Down syndrome children - An update"** is a compilation of Twelve excellent chapters, contributed by established researchers in the field and covering different aspects of the problems that a child with Down syndrome can enface.

In the first chapter; Dr. Al-Biltagi shed some light on the epidemiology of DS, the factors affecting the risk of Down syndrome, and the prevalence of DS in the different parts of the world. In chapter 2; Dr. Solaf discussed the genetic basis of this syndrome together and the role of different genes in development of various syndrome related diseases. Then in the third chapter; Dr. Al-Biltagi and Dr. Hagag discussed the various neonatal problems in DS. After that, Dr. Al-Biltagi and Prof. Osama Tolba shed some light on the various cardiac problems that a child with DS can have.

In the Fifth chapter, Dr. Al-Biltagi discussed the different respiratory disorders that children with Ds have and the prophylaxis against respiratory infections which are relatively common in children with DS. He also explained in the sixth chapter the different anatomical and functional gastrointestinal problems that are common in those children. At the same time, Dr. Saeed discussed in the seventh chapter, reasons for increased incidence of infection in children with DS as well as the different types of infections that children with DS are exposed to and the effect of the infection on DS and how to prevent these infections. Then Dr. El-Shanshory explained the different hematological problems that are frequently encountered in DS children in the eighth chapter. Then Dr. El-Mitwalli described the neuro-anatomic functions of the brain in DS and explained the different neurological disorders that are common in DS children in the Ninth chapter.

In the tenth chapter; Dr. Fu Yong Jiao and his colleagues described the mental development, the behavior phenotypes, the academic achievements in young people with DS as well as the psychology of sex, the various psychosocial problems in children and adolescents with DS and diagnosis, assessment and management of these disorders. In the eleventh chapter, Dr. Alasy and his colleagues described the various aspects of anesthesia related problems and their management in children with DS. Then Dr. Meakkara described the various dental problems and their management in twelfth chapter.

A great effort has been made to accomplish this book. It would not have been possible to complete this book without the sincere efforts of the authors, and especially the staff at Bentham Science Publishers, giving their continuous support. Their patience, enthusiasm and encouragement were a greatly appreciated source of strength during its extended preparation. Perhaps of greater importance, than the book and its many contributions, were the remarkable people that formed a unique collaborative team to make it happen.

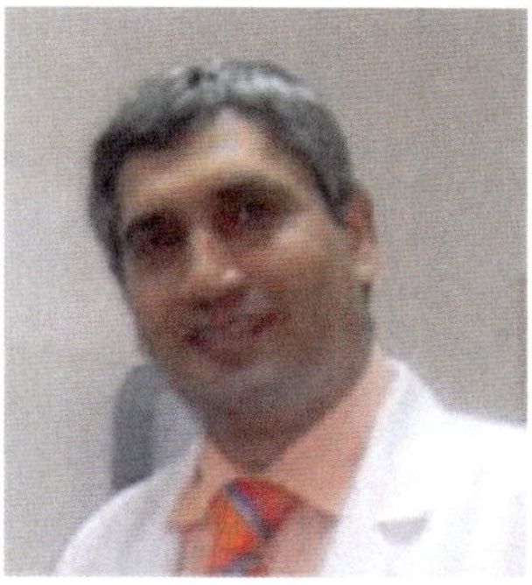

Mohammed Al-Biltagi
Faculty of Medicine
Tanta University
Tanta
Egypt

List of Contributors

Adel A. Hagag	Pediatric Department, Faculty of Medicine, Tanta University, Egypt
Ahmed K. Saeed	Ministry of Health, Kingdom of Bahrain
April Wang	Shaanxi Provincial People's Hospital, China
Ashraf El-Mitwalli	Mansoura University, Egypt
Avijit Gaikwad	American Mission Hospital, Bahrain. M.D, DNB University of Mumbai, India
Feilan Lv	Shaanxi Provincial People's Hospital, China
Fu Yong Jiao	Shaanxi Provincial People's Hospital, China
Guoyan Lee	Pediatricia Shaanxi Provincial People's Hospital, China
Hasan Alasy	Pediatric Department, Faculty of Medicine, Tanta University, Egypt
John Jacob Meakkara	International Hospital of Bahrain, Kingdom of Bahrain
Mohammed Al-Biltagi	Pediatric Department, Faculty of Medicine, Tanta University, Egypt
Mohammed Ramadan El-Shanshory	Hematology Unit, Faculty of Medicine, Tanta University, Egypt
Nermin K. Saeed	Microbiology Section, Pathology Department, Salmaniya Medical Complex, Kingdom of Bahrain
Osama Abd Rab Elrasoul Tolba	Pediatric Department, Faculty of Medicine, Tanta University, Egypt
Solaf M. Elsayed	Genetics Unit, Children's Hospital, Ain Shams University, Cairo, Egypt
Vikas Raj Somarajan	International Hospital of Bahrain, Kingdom of Bahrain,
Vivian Song	Shaanxi Provincial People's Hospital, China

1

2

CHAPTER 1

Epidemiology and Prevalence of Down Syndrome

Mohammed Al-Biltagi*

Pediatric Department, Faculty of Medicine, Tanta University, Egypt

Abstract: Down syndrome (DS) is the commonest chromosomal disorders in the world; affecting all countries, all races, and both sexes. It was identified since premodern art and middle ages. The risk for DS births is multi-factorial and includes both genetic and environmental factors. The prevalence of DS could be affected by different factors including distribution of maternal age in the population, adequacy and completeness of ascertainment, accurateness of diagnosis, level of selective prenatal termination of affected pregnancies, as well as different unrecognized genetic and environmental factors. Incidence of DS is expected to be significantly high in the developing countries, probably due to the higher death rate from comorbidities in DS such as congenital cardiovascular defects. Improving survival of infants with DS because of better care especially of cardiovascular malformations will affect prevalence rather than the incidence of DS. According to World Health Organization; the predictable incidence of DS is between 1 in 1,000 to 1 in 1,100 live births all over the world. The difference in prevalence among populations or countries or in the same population over time will depend on the potential risk factors in common for that community.

Keywords: Africa, America, Arabs area, Asia, Chemical Toxins, Children, Chromosome aberrations, Consanguinity, Cytogenetic, Down syndrome, Environmental factors, Europe, Genetic Factors, Gonadal trisomy mosaicism, Incidence, Ionizing radiation, Maternal age, Paternal age, Prevalence, Smoking, Socioeconomic Status.

1. INTRODUCTION

Down syndrome (DS) is the commonest genetic disease in the world population; affecting all countries, all races, and both sexes. There are some reports that identified paintings of persons with appearance of DS in premodern art and

* **Corresponding Author Dr. Mohammed Al-Biltagi:** Pediatric Department, Faculty of Medicine, Tanta University, Egypt; Tel: (+973)39545472; Fax: (+973) 1759 0495; Email: mbelrem@hotmail.com

paintings and from pictures from the middle ages. In the modern medicine, Jean Etienne Dominique Esquirol (1772-1840) was the first to describe this syndrome followed by Édouard Séguin who described some clinical features of DS after 6 years in 1844. However, John Langdon Down was the first to give a comprehensive description of clinical features of the syndrome in 1866. He was an English physician at the London Hospital, and gave his name to this syndrome. In 1909, Shuttleworth was the first physician who observed the association between the increased maternal age and and the increased risk of DS. However; Jérôme Jean Louis Marie Lejeune (1926-1994); French human geneticist was the first scientist who related this syndrome to trisomic aberration of chromosome 21 in 1959. After that and onward; many researches were done in a try to uncover the role of the extra chromosome 21 in relation to the phenotype of DS. Traditional epidemiological studies concerned with determination of the prevalence of DS have been conducted over the last 100 years. It was of interest for many societies and researches as regard to temporal, racial, geographical, and environmental differences in rates. The prevalence of DS differs from a country to another and sometimes from a district to another within the same country [1 - 3].

2. FACTORS AFFECTING THE RISK OF DOWN SYNDROME

The risk for DS births is multi-factorial and includes both genetic and environmental factors. To understand how a factor can affect the prevalence of DS; it is crucial both to understand the chromosomal imbalance and the genomic content of chromosome 21 and how the expression levels of these genes are altered by the presence of this third copy generally resulting from non-disjunction during the stage of meiosis of either the ovum or the sperm. With development of proper cytogenetic studies, investigators are now able to distinguish the underlying types of chromosomal errors into trisomy 21, translocations, and mosaicism (one normal cell line and one trisomic cell line). The prevalence of DS could be affected by different factors including distribution of maternal age in the population, adequacy and completeness of ascertainment, accurateness of diagnosis, level of selective prenatal termination of affected pregnancies, as well as different unrecognized genetic and environmental factors [4].

2.1. Maternal Age at Birth

Mother age at the time of pregnancy with fetus with DS is one of the most well studied factors that affect the possibility of occurrence of DS since the observation of Shuttlewort in 1909, Van der Scheer in 1927, Thurston and Jenkins 1931 and by Penrose in 1933 [5]. Increased maternal age is considered as one of the most important factors contributing to the increased risk of having DS affected fetus. Many studies described the relationship between mother age over 35 years and the increased risk of DS [6].

Many studies documented that the average maternal age at the time of pregnancy of a fetus with DS is significantly higher than that of mothers with normal euploid fetus in different populations and races [6, 7]. The likelihood of having a baby with DS is less than 1 in 1,400 for a mother under 25 years, and less than 1 in 1,000 for a mother under 30 years. The risk increased to 1 in 350 for mothers who become pregnant at age 35 and continues to increase as the woman get elder, so that by age 42, and by age 49, the chance is 1 in 60 and 1 in 12 correspondingly [8]. However, there are some studies reporting that about eighty percent of children with DS were born to young mothers with age less than 30 years [9].

Many studies showed that there was significant increase in the percent of trisomy in pregnancy losses in women over 40 years than the percent of trisomy in pregnancy losses in women less than 24 years. So, the major fundamental factor accountable for the increased infertility observed with advancing maternal age is the increase in aneuploidy [10 - 12]. Currently, the investigators are able to determine the parental source of the extra chromosome by using chromosome 21-specific DNA markers. They are also able to categorize the stage of error in meiosis whether occurred in meiosis I or meiosis II. Many studies showed that about ninety percent of errors were of maternal origin [13]. Also these studies showed that most of the errors occurred in meiosis I (which begun during the fetal life of the mother and was accomplished many years later at the time of ovulation) than in meiosis II (which is started and completed within 3–4 days at the time of ovulation) with a ratio of 3:1[14].

As a woman is getting elder; the risk for having a baby with trisomy 21 is significantly increased. The increased maternal age increases the risk of aneuploid oocyte formation. Fig. (**1**) showed the different effects of advanced maternal age on oogenesis. The ovum has long duration of oogenesis as meiosis I is initiated in oocytes during fetal life. Interrupted oogenesis with meiotic arrests probably makes the eggs more susceptible to the aging effect than sperms which when associated with damaging changes and toxic environmental effects accumulated over time increases the likelihood of aneuploid oocyte formation. These damaging changes may include diminishing amount of meiotic proteins, or meiotic checkpoints components, or declining of centromere cohesion due to age-related decrease in centromere related proteins MCAK [15 - 18]. Aging also enhances increase of environmentally induced damaging effects to the meiotic mechanism over time or genetic modifications as mitochondrial deletions or cause weakness or loss of centromere cohesion along chromosome arms which may contribute to age related aneuploidy [9]. Maternal aging also contributes to impaired chiasmatic chromosome segregation especially after the age of 35 years. A chiasma is the point where the genetic material can be exchanged between two homologous non-sister chromatids during chromosomal crossover during meiosis. Lack of chiasma, defective configurations of chiasma and decline in chiasma frequency can induce non-dysjunction of chromosome 21 and subsequent DS birth. This impaired chiasma segregation is due to delay regulation of human proteins concerned with segregation of non-exchange chromosome with increasing ovarian age [19].

Advanced maternal age is associated with natural aging of the ovary which is distinguish by a decrease in the entire oocyte pool, a decrease in the number of antral follicles maturing/cycle and in the sex hormonal changes. Decreased oocyte pole may predispose the released oocyte to chromosome malsegregation. Ovarian aging are associated with chromosome non-disjunction, they most likely include other factors than those measured by oocyte or antral follicle pool size and sex hormone levels. Ovarian aging also is associated with inadequate level of hormonal signal and higher rate of meiotic errors [20]. It should be emphasized that advanced maternal age as a risk factor for having a child with DS is restricted to non-disjunction errors that occur in the ovum. Advanced maternal age is not implicated in occurrence of DS due to paternal non-disjunction error in spermatogenesis, postzygotic mitotic error, or translocation either inherited or *de novo* [21]. Maternal age not only affecting the prevalence of occurrence of DS, but also could affect the prevalence of associated anomalies. For example, maternal age above 32 years was more associated with a lesser occurrence of congenital cardiac anomalies in children with DS [22].

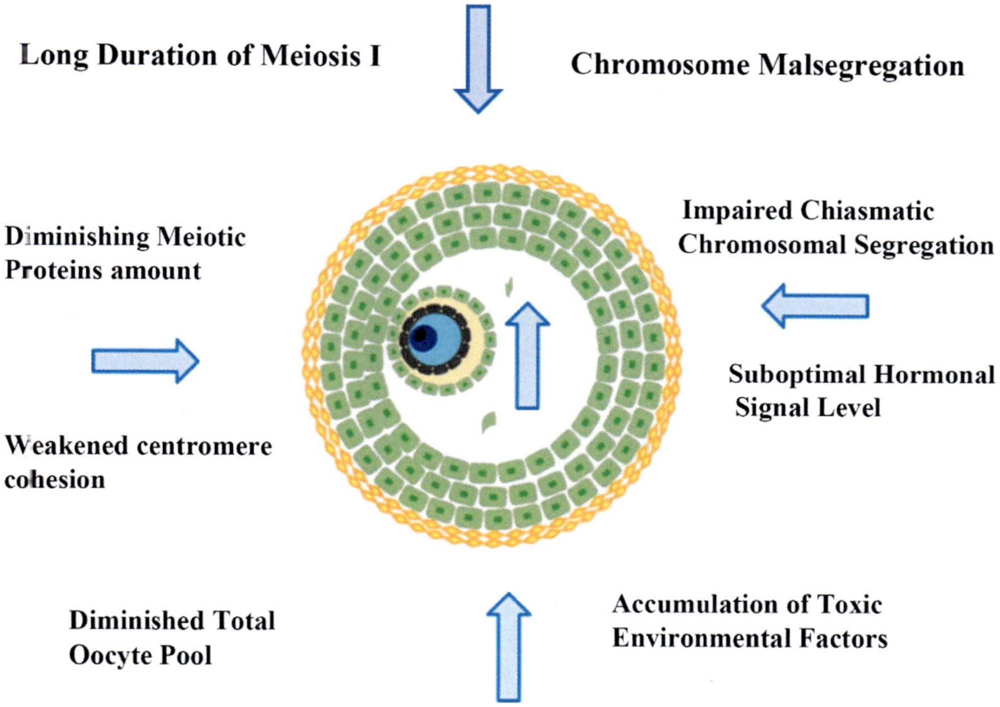

Fig. (1). The different effects of advanced maternal age on oogenesis.

2.2. Altered Recombination Patterns Along Chromosome 21

Exchange of genetic information between two DNA molecules with production of a new combination of alleles is known as genetic recombination. It occurs in both meiosis and mitosis and is mostly natural and a common mechanism for DNA repair. Impaired, reduced or abnormal recombination along chromosome 21 makes chromosome 21 susceptible to malsegregation and is associated with a proportion of maternal non-disjunction errors. This impaired recombination process can take the form of absent exchange or single telomeric exchange; both can result in increased risk of MI errors or in the form of a pericentromeric exchange which leads to an increased risk of MII errors [23].

Properly functioning meiotic mechanisms (*e.g.* spindle function, sister chromatid adhesive proteins, microtubule motor proteins) can correctly segregate all but the most susceptible exchange configurations. In young mothers; this meiotic mechanisms is usually proceeding well; so that presence of a telomeric exchange is the most frequent risk factor for MI non-disjunction. On the other hand, increasing mother age increases the possibility of accumulation of environmental and age-related insults. This affects the integrity of meiotic mechanisms and induces suboptimal exchange patterns and in turn increases the susceptibility to non-disjunction which increases with time and raises the proportion of non-disjunction due to normal exchange configurations. As a result, the most common exchange profile of non-disjoined oocytes changes from susceptible to non-susceptible patterns with increasing oocyte age [24]. The association between advanced mother age and chromosome 21 non-disjunction is limited to abnormalities in the egg and not observed in paternal or in post-zygotic mitotic abnormalities. Most of the abnormalities are MMI abnormalities which are three-fold higher proportion over MMII abnormalities present at all maternal ages. However, this ratio decreases for mothers <19 years and those ≥40 years at the time of their infant's birth [6].

2.3. Maternal Grandmother Age

Increasing mother age is a well-Known risk factor for maternal meiotic non-disjunction. However, there is a significant number of babies with DS born to of young-age mothers. Reports showed that 80% of DS babies are born to young mothers less than 30 years [9]. This observation stimulated the researchers to investigate the effect of the age grand-mothers. They proposed that the grand maternal age can induce disjunction in a grand-mother oocyte producing a trisomic embryo. Losing the extra chromosome in a considerable portion of cells in that embryo would result in a mosaic offspring (the mother) without the DS phenotype, but with the ability to produce a trisomic child, assuming trisomic cells remained in her ovaries. In another way, increasing grandmother age disturbed her daughter meiosis when the grandmother conceived. With advancing age, the grandmother's gonads may not succeed to make the necessary proteins like spindle associated proteins, factors responsible for resting of oocyte, chiasma-binding proteins, DNA repair enzymes, *etc.* which are required for proper meiotic segregation in her daughter germ cells. This consecutively gives rise to non-disjunction of chromosome 21 in the daughter oocyte. This event occurs during the embryogenesis of the mother of the DS child when she was in grandmother's womb. Thus, risk factors associated with non-disjunction would apply to the grandmother of the proband with trisomy as well as to the mother. Therefore, DS does not only depend on the age of the mother, but also on the age of the maternal grandmother which results in non-disjunction of chromosome 21 [8, 25]. However, a recent study done by Kovaleva *et al.* failed to support the suggestion that advanced age of the DS grandmother is responsible for meiotic disturbance in her daughter [26].

2.4. Paternal Age

Specific DNA markers and polymorphic microsatellites have showed that about 90% of trisomy 21 was due to non-disjunction of maternal origin and 10% was of paternal origin [27]. Few studies showed that advanced father age (>49) has been associated with increased risk of DS births which could represent a model for other genetic abnormalities in offspring of older fathers as older men produce more sperms with aneuploidy [28]. However, this risk is considerably low with the appropriate adjustment for maternal age and many studies failed to confirm these effects and relate that risk to the associated advanced maternal age [29].

2.5. Consanguinity

There are conflicting data about the effects of consanguinity on the incidence of DS. Alfi *et al.* indicated that the incidence of DS was more pronounced in the consanguine marriages than non-consanguine [30]. On the other hand; a more recent study done by Rezayat *et al.* showed that the non-consanguine marriages has higher frequency of DS (71.1%) than consanguine marriages (28.9%). This difference may be related to the younger age of the mothers in consanguine marriages (mean = 27.1 ± 6.3) compared with non-consanguine marriages. This could be related to social factors where cultural customs of the communities where consanguine marriage is frequent in adolescence and among younger ages. So, diagnostic tests to detect DS might be done on all pregnancies regardless of the couples' familial relationship [31].

2.6. Parity and Reproductive Function of the Mother

There are contradictory data about the association of DS with multiparity and the relation still remains unclear. This contradiction arises from different factors including the relation of multiparty and the maternal age. Also; several early studies examining the relation between parity and DS used broad (5-year) categories in controlling for maternal age, it has been suggested that at least part of the apparent effect of parity is due to residual confounding. Doria-Rose *et al.* showed a tendency of increasing risk of having baby with DS with increasing number of pregnancy in both younger (age <35 years) and older (age > or =35 years) mothers after results were controlled for maternal age. This association was predominantly strong among older mothers. They explain this association because women with higher parity are less likely to undergo prenatal screening for DS by amniocentesis or chorionic villus sampling with fewer trends to terminate a DS pregnancy than women of lower parity [32, 33]. Clementi *et al.* reported that the higher risk of having a child with DS was limited to only those women with a parity of more than four [34]. Previous studies that depend in diagnosing pregnancies with DS on the second-trimester karyotype analysis in a try to remove the effects of differential pregnancy termination. These studies showed no association between parity and DS after controlling for maternal age [35, 36]. An increased risk of aneuploidy is present in women who have had many spontaneous abortions. DS live birth is more likely for women with a history of repeated spontaneous abortion. For a woman with a priori risk of 1 in 300 for DS, 3 prior spontaneous abortions would increase this risk by 47% to be 1 in 204. So, the risk of recurrence of trisomy-21 is affected by maternal age and parental germline mosaicism [37]. However, there were some old studies which showed that first-born infants may be at higher risk of DS than are those later born, independent of maternal age. However, this had a very small effect if it existed [38, 39].

2.7. Interval Between Pregnancies

Short inter pregnancy interval may increase the risk of having the next child with DS. This is because the periods of anovulatory activity followed by conception appear to correlate with increased occurrence of DS. Pregnancy still has the chance to happen during the transitional period between anovulation and the establishment of regular ovulation after childbirth might be more vulnerable to maternal meiotic non-disjunction [40, 41]. Therefore, a short interval between pregnancies might increase a woman's risk of subsequently bearing a child with DS. However, this observation is still in need for further studies to confirm it.

2.8. Previous Child with Down Syndrome

Moris *et al.* showed that "women who have had a previous DS pregnancy have a constant absolute excess risk above their maternal age-related risk of having a subsequent affected pregnancy. This absolute excess risk is determined by the age at which the affected pregnancy occurred and is higher for younger than for older women. For example; after a DS pregnancy at age 20, this excess is 0.62% at early second trimester, and, after pregnancy with a baby with DS one at age 40, the risk is about 0.04%" [42]. Women who have had a previous trisomic pregnancy, particularly those less than 35 years of age at the time, appear to be at an increased risk of future pregnancies being trisomic [43].The higher recurrence risk for trisomy 21 among younger mothers can be explained if gonadal trisomy mosaicism accounts for a larger proportion of recurrences in women whose maternal age–related risk is low. In these cases; DNA marker analysis does not provide a valuable tool for patient counseling in case of recurrent trisomy 21 [44]. Detection and determination of specific types of chromosomal abnormalities in DS children is of paramount importance as it allows physicians to precisely guide the parent regarding the recurrence risk of DS and available options. Cytogenetic studies should be done to confirm the diagnosis and to determine the risk of recurrence and thus helping genetic counseling. This risk of recurrence varies greatly between the cases as non-disjunction and mosaicism infrequently recur in siblings of people with DS. On the other hand; translocation may be recurrent, depending on the type of translocation. Diagnosis of a chromosome-21 translocation in the fetus or newborn is an indication for karyotype analysis of both parents. If both parents have normal karyotypes, the recurrence risk is 2 to 3 %. If one parent carries a balanced translocation, the recurrence risk depends on the sex of the carrier parent and the specific chromosomes that are fused [45]. There is also increased risk of having a child with DS among second- and third-degree relatives of a proband with trisomy 21. Most families who have had a child with trisomy 21, the risk to second- and third-degree relatives is increased somewhat but still low (less than 1%). Sibs and second-degree relatives in such families should be offered the option of amniocentesis, regardless of maternal age [46].

2.9. Multiple *Versus* Singleton Pregnancies

The risk of DS per fetus/baby is lower in multiple than singleton pregnancies. These approximations can be used for genetic counseling and antenatal screening [47, 48]. This was in contrast to the earlier studies which reported higher frequency of twinning among newborns with DS [49].

2.10. Environmental Factors

2.10.1. Impact of Prenatal Diagnosis on the Prevalence of Down Syndrome and Rate of Pregnancy Termination

The incidence at DS birth is strongly dependent on how many pregnant women are willing to have antenatal screening and diagnosis because of advanced childbearing age (≥35 years), abnormal results of either fetal ultrasound or biochemical screening and subsequent termination of pregnancies with chromosome aberrations. The rate of using these diagnostic tests depends on many factors. The most important factor is the availability of the antenatal diagnostic tests (including chorionic villus sampling, ultrasonographic screening and maternal serum screening) to the community which successively led to the identification of trisomy 21 fetuses mainly in mothers aged less than 35 years. Sensitivity of the implemented antenatal tests will affect the accuracy of diagnosis and hence the decision making. The second important factor is Multidimensional Measure of Informed Choice (MMIC) which includes knowledge, attitude and behavior of the pregnant women towards pregnancy with fetus with DS. According to this measure, women make an informed decision when they have sufficient knowledge about DS and prenatal screening, and when their actual (non-) participation in prenatal screening is consistent with their attitude. This MMIC will depend on the social standards, ethnic factors, economic status and religious factors [50, 51] and in turn will affect the extent of selective prenatal termination of affected pregnancies. In countries where abortion is allowed to terminate pregnancies with DS (as in France and many European countries) the birth prevalence of DS is significantly reduced. However, the situation is not the same among women of other races and from countries which do not allow abortion.

2.10.2. Socioeconomic Status

Hunter *et al.* showed a significant association between low maternal socio-economic status (such as poor nutrition or environmental toxin exposures) and meiosis II chromosome 21 non-disjunction [52]. Babies born to rural mothers are more liable to have increased frequency of congenital malformations and DS than babies of urban mothers. This could be related to inadequate antenatal care and poor medical knowledge in the early stages of pregnancy in the rural areas, prevalence of nutritional deficiency, and other environmental factors that could share in the increased frequency of malformations in rural areas. Educational status of the parents especially of the mother has strong relationship with the use of the health services for antenatal diagnosis. Education appears to be a vital component in improving the parents' knowledge regarding pregnancy care and the health of their progeny [53]. Education also can affect the selective impact of antenatal diagnosis, elective termination, and acceptance of prenatal diagnostic measures among population [54].

2.10.3. Exposure to Chemical Toxins, Drugs and Diseases

Exposure to environmental chemicals, toxins and drugs have the potential for inducing chromosomal non-disjunction including DS. Mothers of DS children are more liable to have significant diseases before conception, particularly psychological diseases, and to use more drugs in the year before pregnancy [55]. Reports showed contradicting results about the effect of autoimmune diseases including gestational diabetes on the risk rate of having a baby with DS. Early reports showed an increased frequency of thyroid autoimmunity among mothers of children with DS [56]. They also reported increased risk of DS among women with either preexisting diabetes or gestational diabetes and supposed presence of bidirectional associations between endocrine dysfunction and chromosome abnormalities as both have common autoimmune pathways [57]. However more recently; Martínez-Frías *et al.* showed that DS is related to maternal age, but does not seem to be related to any type of maternal diabetes [58].

Folic acid plays a vital role in numerous complex metabolic pathways, including of DNA and RNA synthesis and those involved in methylation. Mothers with abnormal folate metabolism and mutation in the methylene tetrahydrofolate reductase (MTHFR) gene or other genes concerned with folate metabolism were reported to have higher incidence of DS children. However, there was no evidence of the beneficial effect of folate supplementation in decreasing incidence of births of children with DS [59]. There are also some evidences of increasing frequency of giving birth to children with DS among mothers using hormonal contraception. Also there was observation of the reversal of sex ratio among those mothers giving birth to more female children with DS than the usual predominance of DS among male children. This observation was noted in mothers of different age group but was more frequent in mothers ≥ 35 years old [58, 60]. It was also observed that the effect was linked to the irregular dose of oral contraceptive that could exacerbate the adverse effect of natural aging-related hormonal imbalance in the ovary and lead to an increased anomaly in follicles. The use of vaginal spermicides was also linked to the occurrence of DS among offspring born to women who used these contraceptive agents during the ten months before conception. However, studies failed to provide substantial precision in estimating the magnitude of the association between reported spermicide use and DS [61].

There are contradicting reports about the effect of cigarette smoking on increasing incidence of DS. Yang *et al.* showed presence of significant positive association between maternal smoking and DS. This effect was restricted to women younger than 35 years of age. They inferred that the habit of periconceptional smoking is associated with meiosis II non-disjunction among women aged <35 years [62]. Rudnicka *et al.* showed no evidence of an association between the birth prevalence of DS and maternal smoking [63]. However, maternal smoking can give rise to increasing nuchal translucency among normal pregnancies and causes significantly decreased free beta- human chorionic gonadotropin values compared to nonsmokers which in turn can affect the accuracy of serum markers for DS screening. However; the mechanism of increasing nuchal translucency is still unclear [64]. A more recent study by Ghosh *et al.* showed a role for smokeless chewing tobacco and oral contraceptive habits as risk factors for DS birth, with smokeless chewing tobacco use primarily was a risk factor in younger women. They related the effect of smoking to disturbances of molecular components common to meiosis I and meiosis II stages that may be the spindle apparatus [60].

Despite ionizing radiation is the only known lifestyle/environmental agent proved to induce non-disjunction in experimental animals but most of studies tried to link exposure of ionizing radiation with increasing incidence of giving birth to children with DS. Laziuk *et al.* found that it was impossible to establish a causal relationship between these clusters of DS and exposure to the Chernobyl fallout, at a geographical level [65]. However, Sperling *et al.* reported the increased incidence of DS births in low-dose irradiation exposed regions in Europe after the Chernobyl reactor accident [66].

3. PREVALENCE OF DOWN SYNDROME

Prevalence of DS is the number of patients diagnosed to have DS in certain population during a specified time period regardless of when the diagnosis of the syndrome was made including the number of both new and old cases. The prevalence is different from the incidence which refers only to the new cases diagnosed during a specified time period among the population and depends on the total birth/year, on the other hand; prevalence is based on real population. Both Prevalence and incidence accuracy depends on the techniques and the methods of evaluating prevalence and incidence rates as well as the size of the survey, and the adequacy of the medical care provided as the survival the rates differ among racial/ethnic groups. For example, the incidence of DS may be significantly lower in developed countries as they have better application and uptake of antenatal diagnostic services that affect the total birth incidence. On the other hand, the incidence of DS could be higher in developing countries, in spite of the higher mortality rate from the associated complications and anomalies with DS such as congenital heart defects. Improving survival of infants with DS is observed because of better care especially of cardiovascular malformations will affect the prevalence rather than the incidence of DS [67]. In countries where abortion is illegal such as Ireland and the Arab countries, both prevalence and incidence are high while incidence is low in countries with high percentage of DS pregnancy terminations as in France [68]. According to WHO; the estimated incidence of DS is between 1 in 1,000 to 1 in 1,100 live births worldwide. The difference in prevalence among populations, countries, or in the same population over time will depend on the potential risk factors in common for that community.

3.1. Prevalence in Africa

Down syndrome cases were not recognized in unmixed African populations on the African continent until 1955 when Luder and Musoke recognized and described the first black African child with DS. The prevalence of DS in African populations is not accurately known because of inaccuracy of most of the studies concerned with the incidence and prevalence of DS in sub Saharan Africa. Most of these studies ignored the influence of important factors such as socioeconomic, cultural, educational, genetic, racial and environmental characteristics of the different African populations on the prevalence of the condition, thus affecting the reliability of the data. The earliest reliable documentation on the incidence of DS was by Adeyokunnu in 1982 when he reported an incidence of 1 in 865 live births (1 - 16 per 1000 live birth s) in Ibadan, South Western Nigeria. He found 95.5% of cases to be the result of regular trisomy 21, and 2.5% of cases to be the result of translocation of trisomy 21. He also reported a high incidence of DS cases among young mothers [69]. However, the real DS incidence may be higher than hat reported due to incomplete ascertainment of cases.

Study done in South Africa over 20 years periods between 1974 and 1993 showed an incidence of DS of about 1 in 500 live births and overall prevalence rate of 1.49 per 1000 with a gradual decline to 1.3 per 1000 in the last 5 years of the study period. They found a higher prevalence (1.88) among the white population compared with the prevalence in colored (1.54) and blacks (1.29). They attributed these differences to the possibility that fewer blacks than whites undergo prenatal screened and diagnosis of the condition and the relative distribution of the number of terminations following prenatal diagnosis, being higher among whites (18.3%), intermediate in colored (5.8%) and lowest in blacks (1.4%). The study showed also a significant decline in rates for the total population and for whites, a downward trend for colored, but no decline for blacks. An increasing risk with advancing maternal age was confirmed, but no maternal age-specific differences in rates by race were demonstrated [70]. However, another studies reported a higher incidence of DS among the African populations. Delport *et al.* reported a higher incidence of DS (1.33 per 1,000 live births) in black South African neonates, born in an urban setting [71]. Venter *et al.* reported incidence of DS of 2.10 per 1,000 live births among in rural black South African neonates while Kromberg *et al.* reported the highest incidence in a previous study to be 1 67 per 1000 live births at an academic hospital in Johannesburg [72, 73]. However, these studies suffer the problem of ascertainment of cases.

3.2. Prevalence in Arab Worlds

The Arab world had rich history, diverse ethnic, cultural and religious makeup. The incidence of DS in the Arab world is generally higher than international figures (Fig. **2**). For example, DS incidence rates were 1:319 live births in Dubai, 1:500 in Oman, 1 in 516 in Libya, 1:546 in Qatar, 1:547 in Arabs in Israel, 1:554 in Saudi Arabia, 1:581 in Kuwait, and 1 in 700 in Egypt [74].

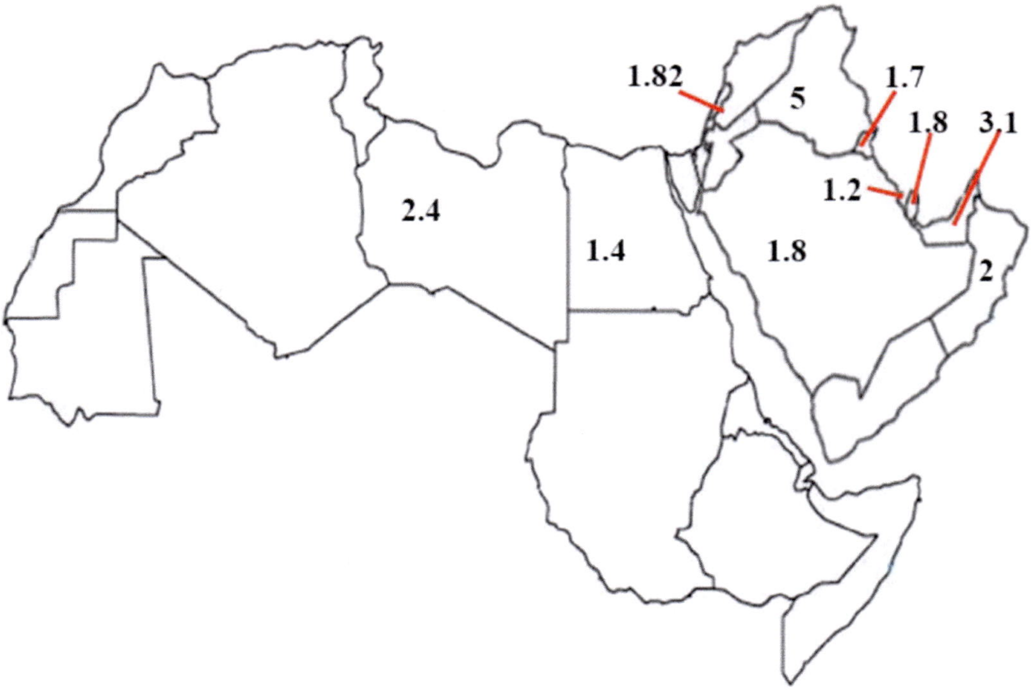

Fig. (2). Shows DS incidence rates/1000 live births in the Arab world according to year 2000 data.

The higher incidence of DS noted in the Arab world is due to its characteristic socioeconomic and religious beliefs and views. There is a common practice of consanguineous marriages, increased maternal age and multiparity. Many of Arabic populations have complete or partial shortage of antenatal screening tests and strategies which can help DS detection and parent decision making to terminate pregnancies with DS fetuses as early as possible. There is a very high rate of consanguinity in Arabs in the last decade; which may reach very high rates particularly in certain Arab countries including Oman (56.3%), Saudi Arabia (42.1-66.7%) and Qatar (22-54%). A study from Kuwait showed the relative risk for closely related parents to have babies with DS was four-fold higher than that for unrelated parents [75].

In Bahrain, the incidence of DS was 0.9/1000 during the period 1989-1993 [76]. This incidence increased to 1.2/1000 during the period 1991-2000. The incidence was 1.1/1000 during 2005 [77]. In Egypt, there was a high prevalence of DS. El-Sobky and Elsayed showed that the incidence of DS was about 1 in 700 live births and overall prevalence rate of 1.42 per 1000 live births. Non-disjunction was present in 93.98% of cases, while translocation was present in 3.5% of cases and mosaicism was present in 1.84% of cases with high prevalence in male (54.13%) than in females (45.87 %). This high prevalence was due to the lack access to prenatal screening and the high incidence of consanguineous marriage which was present in 12% of cases [78]. Another study done between 2000 and 2009 showed that non-disjunction was the most common type of abnormality, followed by translocation and lastly mosaic: 96.1, 3.1, and 0.8%, respectively. Mothers were significantly older at the index pregnancy in the non-disjunction group than in the other two groups; male/female ratio was 1.14:1 and parental consanguinity was reported in 17.3% of the cases [79]. In Upper Egypt; there is a high degree of consanguinity in various areas, along with a high population count provides an excellent opportunity for birth defect investigation. Consanguinity in Egypt is also influenced by population structure and socio-economic, ethnic, and religious factors. There were more children with DS born in rural areas than in urban areas [80].

As regard to Iraq, study done in Fallujah in 2010 showed increased prevalence of children with DS to reach very high level (1/202 Live birth or 5/1000 live births).

The authors related this increase in DS in Iraq to maternal pre-conceptional exposure to environmental pollution specially depleted Uranium which had mutagenic effects. More than 300 tons of depleted uranium in spent shells and aerosolized powder had been used in Iraq in Um-Al-Ma'arik Battle by the United States of America. They found that 56.6% of the samples included were infants of mothers with age less than 35 year-old. This denotes decrease the effect of advanced maternal age as a risk factor for having a DS neonate. This new phenomenon could be due to the effect of exposure to low dose ionizing radiation emitted from the depleted uranium from the weapons used [81, 82].

In Kuwait; the incidence of DS was 1:581 live births with increased maternal age, consanguinity and working in petroleum industry as associated risk factors of having affected children. Karyotyping in Kuwaitis DS with classic trisomy 21, translocation, mosaicism, and non-classical karyotypes showed percentages of 92.9%, 4.3%, 2.2%, and 0.5%, respectively. The male: female ratio was found to be 1.8:1 [74, 83].

In Libya; a study done in 1990 showed that the frequency of DS in Libya was 1 in 516 live births with the mean age of DS mother of 35.62 years; 80% of them were over 30 years of age as compared to 36% of the control Libyan mothers. Cytogenetically; 96% of the cases were of trisomy 21 and male-to-female ratio was 1:1.4 [84, 85]. In Oman, the annual live birth prevalence of trisomy 21 from 2000 to 2004 ranged from 1:423 to 1:358 with an overall prevalence of 1:388 (25.88 per 10.000 live births) with a male/female ratio was 1.31. Interestingly; there were seasonal variations of the DS birth prevalence with the highest prevalence in January followed by December and November [86].

In Palestine; the mean incidence for live birth persons with DS among the Arab citizens of Israel during the period between 1979 and 1997 was 1.24/1.000 (0.8-1.5). The overall incidence rate was 2.43 per 1,000 births (which include live birth and terminated pregnancy) for the same period. There was a tendency to increasing incidence with the increase in maternal age. This reflected higher rate of pregnancy termination when compared with the other Arab countries which reached 36% of the antenatal diagnosed cases and reflected the proper antenatal screening. In 1978 free amniocentesis was offered to women over the age of 37 years, but since 1993 the age limit has been reduced to 35 years. However, utilization amniocentesis by Arab women was 4.2% which is much lower than that of Jewish women (22.2%). On the other hand the incidence in Gaza was significantly higher than that among Arab citizens of Israel which reached 1.6/1.000 live birth which may be due to lack of antenatal screening, poor socioeconomic level and environmental pollutions due to frequent wars [87].

In Qatar; the incidence of DS was 1:546 live birth during 6 years period from 2000 to 2006 (1.95 per 1000 live births). DS was slightly more common in boys (52.7%) than girls (47.3%) and regular trisomy was present in 98%. This high incidence of DS in Qatar may be related to the tendency towards increased maternal age (mean maternal age was 35.4 years, while the mean paternal age was 40 years), absence of antenatal screening measures and the lack of prenatal diagnosis and termination of pregnancy [88, 89]. The incidence of DS in Riyadh was 1 in 554 live births (1.8 per 1,000) during a 9-year period (1982 to 1991) with a trend towards an increased incidence of DS with advanced maternal age or increased maternal parity. In the vast majority of these patients, the type was non-disjunction trisomy 21 with more girls (54%) than boys [90]. The incidence rate of DS in United Arab Emirates (UAE) was 1 in 442 live birth (2.26/1,000 live births) in 1998. This high incidence was due to the pressure on Emirati mothers to have more children and the old maternal age [91]. This incidence increased to be 1 in 319 live births among Emiratis and 1 in 602 live births among non-Emiratis in the Emirate of Dubai in 2007. The mean maternal age was 33.48 years and about 41.66% of the mothers were above 35 years old. The trend of increasing incidence of DS is thought to result from advanced maternal age and high parity [92].

3.3. Prevalence in Asia

Asia is the largest continent in the world and is the most populous. In general the incidence of DS is relatively low in Asia than in other parts of the world (Fig. **3**). China is the first most populous country in the world. A study done in 1991 showed that there were about 154,000 cases of DS in the whole of China with its population of 1,100 million people with a prevalence rate of 0.14/1000 of the total population [93]. In 1998; another study showed no significant different between

Chinese and Caucasian populations in the incidence of DS with overall incidence of 1.28 per 1,000 deliveries in Chinese population [94]. In another study conducted between 1994 and 2007, the most common type was the typical trisomy 21 (86.15%), followed by translocation (8.46%), then mosaic abnormal karyotype (5.39%) in Chinese DS patients. Chinese males are nearly twice affected by trisomy 21 than Chinese females (1.8:1). About 93.08% of DS children were born to younger mothers (<35 yrs.) [95]. A study done in 2012 showed that with the integrated screening for DS in a Chinese population; the overall incidence of DS was 2/1000 [96].

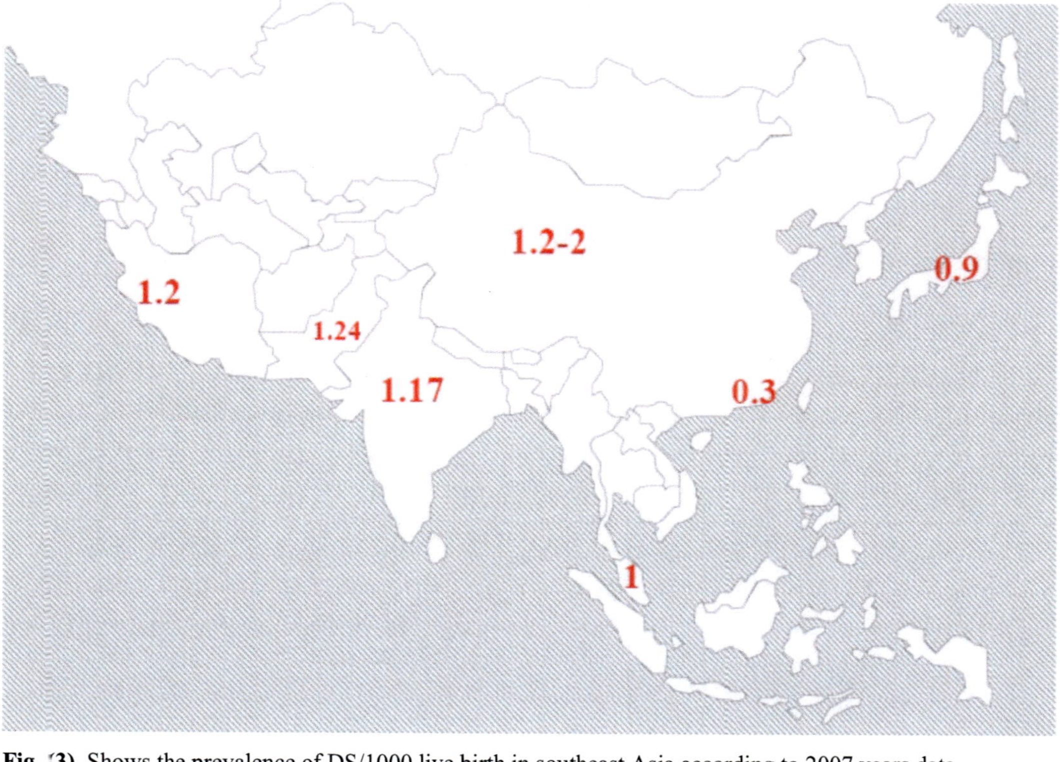

Fig. (3). Shows the prevalence of DS/1000 live birth in southeast Asia according to 2007 years data.

However, overall incidence of DS in Hong Kong during the period from 1962 to 1980 was much lower than the rest of China (1/1114 live births). This lower rate observed among this population was observed along the whole range of maternal age, as compared with the Caucasian counterpart. However, there was a possibility of under diagnosis. The percentage of pregnant women elder than 35 years decreased to nearly half from 16.2% in the period 1962–1970 to 8.6% in the period 1971 to 1980. Of the total DS births; the contribution from those elder than 35 years decreased from 64.7% to 54.7%. An increase in the incidence of DS births however was demonstrable in mothers aged 35 to 39 delivering during that period [97]. In 2010; the Hong Kong Hospital Authority (HA) instituted a universal DS syndrome screening program. This program was effective and achieved expected detection rate and low false positive rates with an estimated first-trimester trisomy 21 term risk lower than 1:250 [98].The overall prevalence of DS in Hong Kong is 0.3 per 1000 population. Prevalence is higher in males with an overall prevalence of 0.34 per 1000 compared with 0.27 per 1000 for females. The difference between genders is most marked in the younger age groups. Prevalence is highest amongst the under 5 years at 0.995 per 1000 population and decreases with age to 0.574 per 1000 in the 20-25 year age group and 0.199 per 1000 population in the 45-50 year age group. The prevalence is 0 per 1000 population by age 80 and over. Almost half (47.5%) of the DS population in Hong Kong is under 20 years of age [99].

In Taiwan; before 2001, the reported incidence of DS was one in 848 live births, or 1.18/1000 live births. After 2001, the widespread use of first-trimester screening augmented with the second-trimester quadruple test resulted in marked reduction in DS live birth rate among Taiwanese population observed between 2001 and 2010 from 2.2/1000 live birth in 2001 to 0.8/1000 in 2010. In the same way, the ratio of live born DS to total DS dropped from 48.74% in 2001 to 25.88% in 2006 due to the wide use of first-trimester screening Taiwan with further reduction to 20.64% in 2008, when the second-trimester quadruple test was implemented [100].

India is the second most populous country in the world with very wide variation in demographics and more than two thousand ethnic groups. This gives rise to different prevalence rates for DS from area to another inside India. Issac *et al.* did a survey of DS in Hyderabad in 1985. They showed an incidence of DS of 1.17 per 1000 or 1 in 853 live births, 96.5% of them were regular trisomy 21 and 3.5% of them had chromosomal mosaicism. The mean maternal age was significantly higher in mothers with DS kids than the controls. Sex ratio was also higher in our sample of DS as compared to the general population [101]. In Baroda region, the overall prevalence of DS was 1.04/1000 in a study conducted in 1998 [102]. On the other hand, a study in Delhi done in 1998 showed much lower prevalence of DS than that recorded in Hyderabad to reach 0.81/1000 [103]. In another relatively recent study done in Mumbai, the prevalence rate was 0.83/1000. There was high frequency of DS in younger couples of first cousin marriages [104]. In other parts of Southeast Asia, the estimated number of people with DS in 2013 were 1,274 cases (out of 1,019,252 people) in Timor Leste, 298,066 (out of 238,452,952 people) in Indonesia, 7,585 (out of 6,068,117 people) in Laos, 29,403 (out of 23,522,482 people) Malaysia, 107,802 (out of 86,241,697 people) in Philippine, 5,442 (out of 4,353,893 people) in Singapore, 81,081 (out of 64,865,523 people) in Thailand and 103,328 (out of 82,662,800 people) in Vietnam.

In Iran, the frequency of this syndrome is one out of 814 live births. A study in Tehran done in 1996 showed that frequency of Trisomy 21 due to non-disjunction was found in 88% of cases. Translocation-trisomy 21 (t21/21) was found in 0.63% and 11.33% of cases were mosaics. Male /female ratio was 1.6/1 [105].

In Japan during an 18-year period between 1980 and 1997, the overall prevalence of DS was 0.58/1000 live births (0.83-0.97/1000 after correction according to the estimated ascertainment ratio: 60-70%). However, the prevalence of DS in Japan failed to decrease despite the use of antenatal screening tests most likely due to the associated increase in pregnancy in mothers with elder age [106]. In a recent study showed increasing number of DS singleton pregnancy to reach 1/392 of singleton pregnancy. The average maternal age of all pregnancies was 32.3 ± 5.5 years old and more than one third of the mothers (35%) were 35 years old or more at the estimated date of delivery. On the other hand; the average maternal age in the cases with trisomy 21 was 38.0 ± 4.7 years old. Advanced maternal age appeared is an important contributing factor to the increased incidence of trisomy 21 in Japan; same as noted in other countries. Consistent with the information obtained from International Clearinghouse for Birth Defects Surveillance and Research (ICBDSR) Annual Report 2011, the highest incidence of DS observed in Japan was at 2008. After that; the rate of DS started to decrease or at least remained stationary from 2009 to 2012. Despite of the fact that the rise of maternal ages would lead to increase of the prevalence of DS, the total number of prenatal diagnosis was stationary or slightly increased, but the rate of mothers over 35 increased two fold from 1998 to 2008 in Japan. Prenatal diagnosis focused on the advanced maternal ages has had the impact on the birth prevalence of DS since 2009 in Japan [107].

Data about DS prevalence in Pakistan are lacking despite being the 6th most populous country in the world. However, the incidence of DS in Pakistan is about 0.9-1.24/1000 of population. A study done in Punjab showed that 95.6% of cases had non-disjunction type of trisomy 21, 3.7% had translocation, and only 0.7% was mosaic. The mean maternal age was 29.8 years. One hundred and sixty (56.7%) cases with trisomy 21 had maternal age> 35 years, whereas 9/11(81.8%) cases of translocation had maternal age < 35 years [108].

In Malaysia, the reported incidence of DS among the Malaysian babies in 1989 was 1:959 live births. According to racial distributions, the incidence among Malay was 1:981 live births, Chinese 1:940 live births, and Indian 1:860 live births. This incidence was lower than those reported from the Western populations. Unlike what is already known, there was also a female preponderance of DS among the Malaysian babies. However, the incidence increased during the period from 2000 to 2007 to be (1:641) in Malay, and (1:758) in Chinese but decreased among Indian Malaysians to be (1:1923). On the other hand; females were nearly twice more affected than male with a ratio of (1.9: 1). The mean maternal age for all cases was 30.5; Malay was 35.5, Chinese 31; and Indian 36 years old. The peak of reported cases with in year 2000 when about (19.2%) of all cases were reported followed by yearly declined to reach more than 50% by 2007 [109, 110].

In Turkey; a sixteen years of survey done between 1994 and 2010 showed that prevalence of DS was 0. 907/1000 live births before the year 2000 and 0.99/1000 live births after 2000. The relatively non changes prevalence during these 16 years is related to the young population in Turkey, high fertility rate in women under 35 years old and the extensive application of prenatal screening programs [111].

3.4. Prevalence in Australia

Data from the Australian registry show that the overall prevalence of DS from 1.1

per 1000 births in 1980 to 2.9 per 1000 births in 2004, which is following the increase in the mean maternal age where the percent of mother elder than 35 years increased from 4.8% in year 1980 to 18.6% in year 2004 with 11.7% being first-time mothers [112]. In 2009, there are over 13.000 population with DS in Australia and more than 270 new baby with DS born every year with a prevalence rate of 1 in every 1,108 live birth babies (0.9/1000 Live birth) which is lower than the worldwide rate of around 1 in 700. This low rate is related to the high termination rates in Australia. In 2010, the overall population rate of people with DS is approximately 1:1,700. This difference between live birth (1/1,108) and the overall population rate (1:1,700) is primarily due to the extremely low life expectancy of people with DS born prior to the mid 1980's. However, note that current life expectancy for people with DS of around 60 years is lower than the general population. However, the health and life expectancy of Australians with DS has improved dramatically over recent decades, resulting in more people living into adulthood and accessing community and hospital based health and social services with noticeable growth of DS population in Australia [113].

3.5. Prevalence in Europe

Although Europe is the second-smallest continents in the world as regard to the surface area; but it has the third ranking of the continents in terms of population after Asia and Africa, with a population of 733-739 million.

Data from the European registries for congenital anomalies showed that DS constitutes about 8% of cases of all the registered anomalies; with over 7000 new pregnancies affected with DS reported in European Union every year. The increased number of affected pregnancies is related to increasing the mean maternal age at the time of conception. However; the effect of increasing maternal age is partially counteracted by the widespread practice of prenatal screening and termination of pregnancy in most of the regions covered by European Surveillance of Congenital Anomalies (EUROCAT). Under the combined effects of maternal age and prenatal screening with the large difference in screening policies between countries in Europe; the pattern of geographic differences in DS live birth prevalence in different parts in Europe has also been altered [114]. These, as well as regulatory and cultural factors, are associated with this wide country differences in antenatal detection rates for DS. The antenatal detection rate of DS ranges between 0-95percent with a mean of 68%. About 88% of these affected pregnancies ended by termination. This resulted in a total prevalence (including terminations of pregnancy) of DS varied from 1 to 3 per 1000 births.

The highest rate of antenatal detection of DS was observed in countries with a first-trimester screening policy while the lowest rate was observed in countries with no official national DS screening or structural anomaly scan policy [115]. An increased prevalence of DS in Europe was observed after Chernobyl fallout. A Study published in 2012 analyzed the prevalence of DS in Bavaria and West Berlin in Germany, Belarus, Hungary, the Lothian Region of Scotland, North West England, and Sweden from 1981 to 1992.

A Study published in 2012 showed an increasing prevalence of DS in Europe associated with Chernobyl fallout. The study analyzed the prevalence of DS in Belarus, Hungary, the Lothian Region of Scotland, North West England, Bavaria and West Berlin in Germany, and Sweden from 1981 to 1992. There were significantly increase in DS births in January 1987 in Belarus and West Berlin when the radioactive clouds with significant amounts of radionuclides with short physical half-lives, especially (131)-iodine, passed over these regions. The study also observed a significant persistent effect in both areas with the peak of reported DS cases was observed in 1987/1988 [66]. Another study done between 2000 and 2006 and published in 2012 showed that the total birth prevalence rate of DS in Europe was 2.3/1000 birth [116].

In Belgium, since the introduction of 'triple screening test' in 1990-1991, the prevalence of DS dropped from 1.26/1000 live birth during the period between 1984 and 1989 to 0.62/1000 live birth during the period between 1993 and 1998. This significant decrease in live birth prevalence of DS in Belgium is mostly due to the wide use of triple test by pregnant women on a large scale as well as the election of termination for most affected pregnancies [117]. In Croatia; a study showed a prevalence rate of DS of 1.4/1000 live birth in region of Primorsko-goranska County between 1996 and 2005. Women aged 35 or more represented 11.6% of all pregnant women. There was no marked decrease in prevalence of live birth DS observed in this region during these 10 years due to too low rate of usage of second-trimester maternal serum screening and amniocentesis with very minimal impact on live birth DS prevalence [118]. In the Czech Republic during the period from 1961 to 2005; the prevalence of DS was 1.07/1000 live birth which remained unchanged during that period [119]. In Denmark the prevalence rate of DS during the period from 1960 to 1970 was 1.14/1000 live birth, 91.4% were regular trisomy 21, 6.2% were cases with translocations and 2.4% were of mosaic nature [120]. The prevalence rate increased to 3.2/1000 live birth during the period between 1990 and 1994; 4.8% were of translocation type and 3.4% were mosaics [121]. The implementation of non-invasive combined antenatal screening of DS in 3 counties in Denmark (Copenhagen, Roskilde and Storstrom) resulted in a reduction in live birth children with DS by 2006 [122].

In England and Wales; with the stationary number of total births in 1989/90 and 2007/8, the the numbers of live births with DS fell by 1% (752 to 743; 1.10 to 1.08/1000 births) due to the increase of antenatal and postnatal diagnoses of DS increased by 71% (from 1075 in 1989/90 to 1843 in 2007/8) and the expansion of and improvements in antenatal screening since 1989 and subsequent terminations. The proportion of antenatal diagnoses has increased most strikingly in younger women, whereas that in older women has stayed relatively constant [123].

Due to the significant increases in the survival of children with DS in the 1950s; there are a large number of people with DS who are currently in their 40s with an average life expectancy for babies with DS born in 2011 of 51 years and median life expectancy of 58 years [124]. Cytogenetic studies showed that classic free trisomy was nearly 97% of all cases, double or triple aneuploidies were 0.3% of all cases, and mosaic cases were about 1% of all cases [125].

On the other hand, the parts of Ireland covered by EUROCAT (Dublin, Kildare, Wicklow and Galway) have a high birth prevalence of DS births as compared with some other countries with crude birth prevalence for the four counties was 18.5/10 000 for all births and 18.3 for live births during the period from 1981 to 1990. Galway had the highest crude birth prevalence of DS (2.35/1000) [126]. This high prevalence rate in County Galway showed further increase in the following decade between 1991-2000 to reach 2.98/1000 live birth despite the falling birth rates and fertility rates. This increase in the prevalence rate is due to the significant increase in the proportion of women in the 30 plus age group [127]. However, the prevalence of DS was much lower in Scotland (1.29/1000 live birth) compared to that observed in Ireland during the same time period from 1980 to 1999. This continued reduction in prevalence rates for DS observed in Scotland achieved through prenatal diagnosis and elective abortion due to the increased use of screening techniques [128].

In Estonia; a study done between 1990 and 2003 showed overall live birth prevalence of DS of 1.17/1000 live births. The prevalence was 1.25/1000 between 1990 and 1994. Then it dropped to 1.09/1000 live births between 1995 and 2003. The period between 1995 and 1998 showed a prevalence rate of 1.22 /1000 live births while was 0.99/1000 live births between 1999 and 2003. Overall, regular trisomy was found in 90.4%, translocation in 6.3% and mosaicism in 2.9%. The overall male to female ratio of DS was 1.09:1 [129]. In France; the mean maternal age has risen from 26 to 30 years during the time period from 1978 to 2005. Total prevalence of DS has increased from 1.4/1000 in 1978 to 2.3/1000 live-births in 2005 and to 2.17/1000 in 2008. Termination of pregnancy after prenatal diagnosis of DS gradually increased reaching 78% in 2005. Live-birth prevalence decreased from 1.4/1000 in 1978 to 0.51/1000 in 2005. Over the last three decades, mean maternal age has increased by 4 years, leading to a two-fold increase in the expected live-birth prevalence of DS infants [130, 131].

In Hungary, a population-based large data set of the Hungarian Congenital Abnormality Registry showed an increase in the recorded total (birth + fetal) prevalence rate of DS. The previous birth prevalence of 1.17 per 100 in the 1970s increased to 1.5/1000 between 1989 and 1999 with a maximum 1.77 in 1992. This increase can be explained by the significantly higher proportion of prenatally diagnosed fetuses with DS and an increasing number of women over 35 years. In addition better ascertainment may also contribute to this increase, but other etiological factors cannot also be excluded [132]. In Netherlands, despite the expansion of antenatal screening, DS live birth prevalence has risen in the last two decades as a result of rising maternal age. DS birth prevalence showed an upward trend from around 1.1/1000 live births in the early 1990s to around 1.4/1000 live births in 2007 [133]. However, a more recent study showed no significant change in overall prevalence of DS births in spite of a significant increase of mean maternal age during the period from year 1997 to year 2007; with a mean prevalence of 1.46/1000 live birth [134]. Participation in prenatal screening in Netherlands varies according to the ethnic groups. Dutch women and women from Surinamese origin had the highest participation rates while women from Turkish, North-African, Aruban/Antillean and other non-Western ethnic origin were less likely to participate in screening [135].

In Norway, data from Medical Birth Registry of Norway (MBRN) showed fixed prevalence rate of DS of 2/1000 of live birth with no significant time trends in prevalence rates from 1967 to 2005. There were some regional differences over time but could probably represent reporting differences. Increasing prevalence rates over time were explained by increasing maternal age [136]. In Russia a study done in Leningrad showed a prevalence of DS of 1.33/1000 during the period from 1982-1989 which was higher than that recorded before during of 1945-1961 with a 1.4- to 2.2-fold increase of birth risks for DS was found in all maternal age groups. The doubling of the risk value occurred by the age of 30-34, in contrast to 35-39 in 1945-1961 [137]. On the other hand; in Gorno-Altaisk, Altai Republic Russia, the frequency of the DS was 0.93/1000 live births during the period from 1983 to 2001. It did not vary significantly during the period studied [138]. In Belarus; where a large part of the population was exposed to ionizing radiation after Chernobyl accident (April 26, 1986); there was a significant peak of DS cases among live births in January 1987 but there was no positive long-term time trends in contaminated or control areas [139].

In Spain, there was a higher prevalence of DS (2.27/1000 live births, stillbirths and induced abortions) compared to the majority of EUROCAT registries during the period from 1991 to 1994 [140]. Also during the period between 1990 and 2004, the prevalence rate of DS showed a further increase from 1.3/1000 in 1990 to 2.91/1000 births in 2004. Sixty three percent of DS births had one or more associated defects. Cardiac and digestive tract anomalies were the most frequent. Changes in maternal age and prenatal screening had influenced DS prevalence and trends in Spain [141]. In Switzerland, study was conducted over 17 years between 1980 and 1996 showed that despite increasing prenatal detection rates of trisomy 21 fetuses and subsequent termination of pregnancies, the number of live born DS children remained constant. The reason was a shift towards a higher mean maternal age from 28 to 30 years between 1980 and 1996 [142].

3.6. Prevalence in North America (Fig. 4)

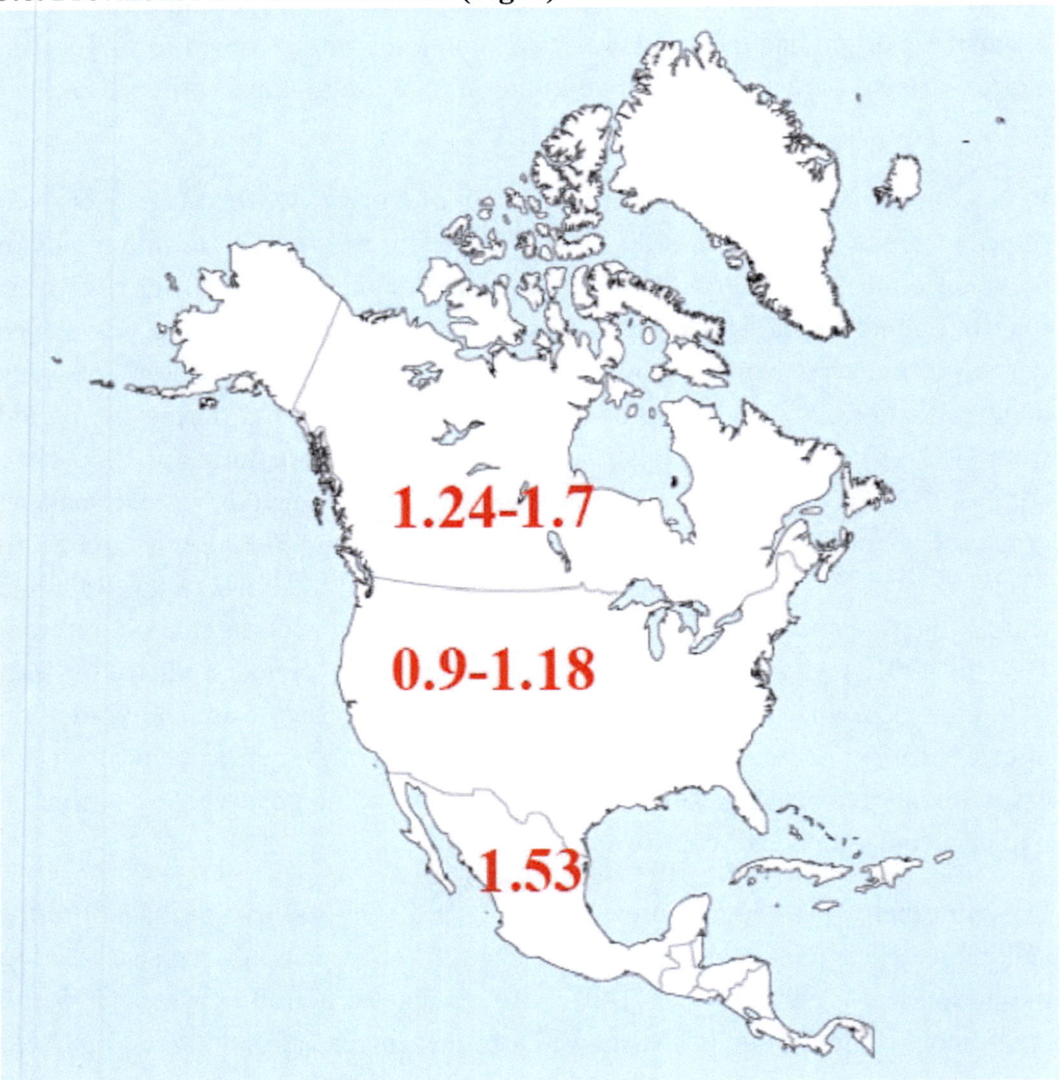

Fig. (4). Shows the birth prevalence of DS/1000 live birth in North America.

In United States of America, the birth prevalence of DS rose by 24.2% from 0.9 to 1.18/1000 live births in 10 representative US regions from 1979 through 2003. There were about 6,000 diagnoses of DS each year in the USA. One in every 691 babies is born with DS which is higher than the previously reported statistic of 1 in every 733. The increase total birth prevalence of DS was largely due to increase number of women conceiving after age 35, portends an ever-growing population of people with DS who may be subject to pathogenic aging and improved longevity in people with DS due to the improved care especially for treatment of congenital heart diseases [143]. The prevalence at birth also varied significantly according to the region, age of the mother, race/ethnicity, infant gender, and presence of CHDs. The lowest prevalence in Arkansas (0.97/1000) and the highest prevalence in Iowa (1.27/1.000) and Utah (1.37/1000) and was significantly higher among males than among females [144]. The prevalence of DS was almost 5 times higher among births to older mothers (3.86/1000) than among births to younger mothers (0.78/1000). The prevalence of DS at birth was significantly lower among non-Hispanic black individuals and was higher among Hispanic individuals compared with the prevalence among non-Hispanic white individuals. The lower prevalence rate among non-Hispanic black individuals may reflect a lower prevalence of DS at birth, under diagnosis of DS prenatally or at birth, differences in access to treatment, and/or lower survival rates among non-Hispanic black individuals [145]. The apparent higher prevalence rate among Hispanic than among non-Hispanic white individuals is due to higher DS prevalence at birth, the higher rates of Hispanic women fertility, late entry to prenatal care, and lower level of insurance coverage among Hispanic [146]. However, these slight racial and ethnic disparities in survival have decreased markedly over time. On the other hand, Presson *et al.* showed that current estimate of DS prevalence is roughly 25%-40% lower than current birth prevalence rate; which corresponds to a prevalence of 0.83 people with DS/1000 population [147].

In Canada; DS remains the most frequently occurring chromosome anomaly. The birth prevalence of DS was relatively constant during the period for 1998–2007 with average 1.41/1000 total births (1.24 and 1.7/1000 for live birth and stillbirth DS respectively). Advanced maternal age is a key risk factor for DS in Canada, though the chromosomal anomaly can also occur in babies born to younger mothers. Despite the rising rates of advanced maternal age at delivery, the national Canadian birth prevalence rates have remained stable over the 1998–2007 time periods. This is most likely due to increased access and utilization of prenatal screening and testing and subsequent termination of pregnancies affected with aneuploidy. Variation exists in the provincial and territorial DS birth prevalence rates in Canada with the lowest birth rate is in Québec (1.12/1000) and the highest rate is Northwest Territories (2.42/1000). A downward trend is noted in Québec that is not seen in Ontario. This difference could be due to the differences in ability to have access to prenatal diagnosis and resulting termination of DS pregnancies which may be higher in Québec compared to Ontario [148]. In Mexico, the incidence of DS is 1/650 newborns. It is higher than that of USA because of poor health care available for most people in Mexico, including prenatal care thus preventing a correct diagnosis. This factor is also augmented by the low rate of pregnancy termination for religious reasons [149].

3.7. Prevalence in South America

According to the Latin American Study of Congenital Malformations (ECLAMC) which was conducted between 1995 and 2008; Chile had the highest rate of DS (2.47/1000 live birth) while Uruguay, had the lowest rate (1.36/1000 live birth). Chile had the highest percentage of women aged 35 years or more giving birth (14%), followed by Uruguay (13%). Despite being the second country with the highest rate in women over 34 years; Uruguay has the lowest rate of DS in Latin America. This could signify the importance of the maternal age as a risk factor for this condition, but it seems not to be the only factor. Other factors should be considered such as ethnicity, for example. It has been reported that mothers of Hispanic origin are at increased risk of having children with DS. The ethnic composition of Chile is mainly of Hispanic and Indian American, while Uruguay has European and African components [150]. This rate of DS live births experienced a significant increase in Chile in the period 1972-2005, bearing a close relationship with the increase in maternal ages. These rates differ in the different Chilean regions, being higher in Santiago and lower in the Southern regions of the country. The mean age of mothers of newborns with or without DS was 36+/-6 and 29+/-6 years, respectively [151]. In general, the high rate of DS among Latin women is also related to the increasing maternal age and their refusal of prenatal screening for DS [152].

CONFLICT OF INTEREST

The authors confirm that this chapter contents have no conflict of interest.

ACKNOWLEDGEMENTS

Declared none.

REFERENCES

[1] Down JL. Observations on an ethnic classification of idiots. 1866. Ment Retard 1995; 33(1): 54-6. [PMID: 7707939]

[2] Patterson D, Costa AC. Down syndrome and genetics - a case of linked histories. Nat Rev Genet 2005; 6(2): 137-47. [http://dx.doi.org/10.1038/nrg1525] [PMID: 15640809]

[3] Shuttleworth GE. Mongolian Imbecility. BMJ 1999; 2: 661-5.

[4] Carothers AD, Hecht CA, Hook EB. International variation in reported livebirth prevalence rates of Down syndrome, adjusted for maternal age. J Med Genet 1999; 36(5): 386-93. [http://dx.doi.org/10.1136/jmg.36.5.386] [PMID: 10353785]

[5] Penrose LS. The relative effect of paternal and maternal age in Mongolism. J Genet 1933; 27: 219-24. [http://dx.doi.org/10.1007/BF02984413]

[6] Allen EG, Freeman SB, Druschel C, *et al.* Maternal age and risk for trisomy 21 assessed by the origin of chromosome nondisjunction: a report from the Atlanta and National Down Syndrome Projects. Hum Genet 2009; 125(1): 41-52. [http://dx.doi.org/10.1007/s00439-008-0603-8] [PMID: 19050929]

[7] Ghosh S, Feingold E, Chakraborty S, Dey SK. Telomere length is associated with types of chromosome 21 nondisjunction: a new insight into the maternal age effect on Down syndrome birth. Hum Genet 2010; 127(4): 403-9. [http://dx.doi.org/10.1007/s00439-009-0785-8] [PMID: 20063167]

[8] Malini SS, Ramachandra NB. Influence of advanced age of maternal grandmothers on Down syndrome. BMC Med Genet 2006; 7(4) [http://dx.doi.org/10.1186/1471-2350-7-4] [PMID: 16412239]

[9] Cooley WC, Graham JM. Down Syndrome: An update and review for the primary physician. Clin Pediatr 1991; 30: 223.

[10] Yusuf RZ, Naeem R. Cytogenetic abnormalities in products of conception: a relationship revisited. Am J Reprod Immunol 2004; 52(1): 88-96. [http://dx.doi.org/10.1111/j.1600-0897.2004.00196.x] [PMID: 15214948]

[11] Pellestor F, Andréo B, Arnal F, Humeau C, Demaille J. Maternal aging and chromosomal abnormalities: new data drawn from *in vitro* unfertilized human oocytes. Hum Genet 2003; 112(2): 195-203. [PMID: 12522562]

[12] Pellestor F, Andréo B, Arnal F, Humeau C, Demaille J. Mechanisms of non-disjunction in human female meiosis: the co-existence of two modes of malsegregation evidenced by the karyotyping of 1397 in-vitro unfertilized oocytes. Hum Reprod 2002; 17(8): 2134-45. [http://dx.doi.org/10.1093/humrep/17.8.2134] [PMID: 12151449]

[13] Muller F, Rebiffé M, Taillandier A, Oury JF, Mornet E. Parental origin of the extra chromosome in prenatally diagnosed fetal trisomy 21. Hum Genet 2000; 106(3): 340-4. [http://dx.doi.org/10.1007/s004390051047] [PMID: 10798364]

[14] Sherman SL, Freeman SB, Allen EG, Lamb NE. Risk factors for nondisjunction of trisomy 21. Cytogenet Genome Res 2005; 111(3-4): 273-80. [http://dx.doi.org/10.1159/000086900] [PMID: 16192705]

[15] Hunt PA, Hassold TJ. Human female meiosis: what makes a good egg go bad? Trends Genet 2008; 24(2): 86-93. [http://dx.doi.org/10.1016/j.tig.2007.11.010] [PMID: 18192063]

[16] Garcia-Cruz R, Brieño MA, Roig I, *et al.* Dynamics of cohesin proteins REC8, STAG3, SMC1 beta and SMC3 are consistent with a role in sister chromatid cohesion during meiosis in human oocytes. Hum Reprod 2010; 25(9): 2316-27. [http://dx.doi.org/10.1093/humrep/deq180] [PMID: 20634189]

[17] Eichenlaub-Ritter U, Staubach N, Trapphoff T. Chromosomal and cytoplasmic context determines predisposition to maternal age-related aneuploidy: brief overview and update on MCAK in mammalian oocytes. Biochem Soc Trans 2010; 38(6): 1681-6. [http://dx.doi.org/10.1042/BST0381681] [PMID: 21118147]

[18] Chiang T, Duncan FE, Schindler K, Schultz RM, Lampson MA. Evidence that weakened centromere cohesion is a leading cause of age-related aneuploidy in oocytes. Curr Biol 2010; 20(17): 1522-8. [http://dx.doi.org/10.1016/j.cub.2010.06.069] [PMID: 20817534]

[19] Steuerwald N, Cohen J, Herrera RJ, Sandalinas M, Brenner CA. Association between spindle assembly checkpoint expression and maternal age in human oocytes. Mol Hum Reprod 2001; 7(1): 49-55. [http://dx.doi.org/10.1093/molehr/7.1.49] [PMID: 11134360]

[20] Warburton D. Biological aging and the etiology of aneuploidy. Cytogenet Genome Res 2005; 111(3-4): 266-72. [http://dx.doi.org/10.1159/000086899] [PMID: 16192704]

[21] Sherman SL, Freeman SB, Allen EG, Lamb NE. Risk factors for nondisjunction of trisomy 21. Cytogenet Genome Res 2005; 111(3-4): 273-80. [http://dx.doi.org/10.1159/000086900] [PMID: 16192705]

[22] Chéhab G, Chokor I, Fakhouri H, Hage G, Saliba Z, El-Rassi I. [Congenital heart disease, maternal age and parental consanguinity in children with Down's syndrome]. J Med Liban 2007; 55(3): 133-7. [PMID: 17966733]

[23] Lamb NE, Sherman SL, Hassold TJ. Effect of meiotic recombination on the production of aneuploid gametes in humans. Cytogenet Genome Res 2005; 111(3-4): 250-5. [http://dx.doi.org/10.1159/000086896] [PMID: 16192701]

[24] Lamb NE, Feingold E, Savage A, *et al.* Characterization of susceptible chiasma configurations that increase the risk for maternal nondisjunction of chromosome 21. Hum Mol Genet 1997; 6(9): 1391-9. [http://dx.doi.org/10.1093/hmg/6.9.1391] [PMID: 9285774]

[25] Papp Z, Varadi E, Szabo Z. Grandmaternal age at birth of parents of children with trisomy. Hum Genet 1977; 39(2): 221-4.
[http://dx.doi.org/10.1007/BF00287015] [PMID: 146021]

[26] Kovaleva NV, Tahmasebi-Hesari M, Verlinskaia DK. [Grandmaternal age in children with Down syndrome in St. Petersburg]. Tsitol Genet 2010; 44(5): 47-53.
[PMID: 21061691]

[27] Ghosh S, Dey SK. DNA diagnosis of DS using polymerase chain reaction and polymorphic microsatellite markers. Int J Hum Genet 2003; 10(3): 17-20.

[28] Fisch H, Hyun G, Golden R, Hensle TW, Olsson CA, Liberson GL. The influence of paternal age on down syndrome. J Urol 2003; 169(6): 2275-8.
[http://dx.doi.org/10.1097/01.ju.0000067958.36077.d8] [PMID: 12771769]

[29] Oliver TR, Bhise A, Feingold E, Tinker S, Masse N, Sherman SL. Investigation of factors associated with paternal nondisjunction of chromosome 21. Am J Med Genet A 2009; 149A(8): 1685-90.
[http://dx.doi.org/10.1002/ajmg.a.32942] [PMID: 19606484]

[30] Alfi OS, Chang R, Azen SP. Evidence for genetic control of nondisjunction in man. Am J Hum Genet 1980; 32(4): 477-83.
[PMID: 6446853]

[31] Rezayat AA, Nazarabadi MH, Andalibi MS, *et al.* Down syndrome and consanguinity. J Res Med Sci 2013; 18(11): 995-7.
[PMID: 24523787]

[32] Doria-Rose VP, Kim HS, Augustine ET, Edwards KL. Parity and the risk of Down's syndrome. Am J Epidemiol 2003; 158(6): 503-8.
[http://dx.doi.org/10.1093/aje/kwg193] [PMID: 12965874]

[33] Haddow JE, Palomaki GE. Multiparity and Down's syndrome. Lancet 1994; 344(8927): 956.
[PMID: 7934367]

[34] Clementi M, Bianca S, Tenconi R. Re: "parity and the risk of Down's syndrome" Am J Epidemiol 2004; 160(6): 610.
[http://dx.doi.org/: 10.1093/aje/kwh241.] [PMID: 15353424]

[35] Chan A, McCaul KA, Keane RJ, Haan EA. Effect of parity, gravidity, previous miscarriage, and age on risk of Down's syndrome: population based study. BMJ 1998; 317(7163): 923-4.
[http://dx.doi.org/10.1136/bmj.317.7163.923] [PMID: 9756811]

[36] Hook EB, Cross PK. Spontaneous abortion and subsequent Down syndrome livebirth. Hum Genet 1983; 64(3): 267-70.
[http://dx.doi.org/10.1007/BF00279407] [PMID: 6224736]

[37] Bianco K, Caughey AB, Shaffer BL, Davis R, Norton ME. History of miscarriage and increased incidence of fetal aneuploidy in subsequent pregnancy. Obstet Gynecol 2006; 107(5): 1098-102.
[http://dx.doi.org/10.1097/01.AOG.0000215560.86673.22] [PMID: 16648416]

[38] Hay S, Barbano H. Independent effects of maternal age and birth order on the incidence of selected congenital malformations. Teratology 1972; 6(3): 271-9. [http://dx.doi.org/10.1002/tera.1420060304] [PMID: 4345335]

[39] Janerich DT, Bracken MB. Epidemiology of trisomy 21: a review and theoretical analysis. J Chronic Dis 1986; 39(12): 1079-93. [http://dx.doi.org/10.1016/0021-9681(86)90141-4] [PMID: 2947908]

[40] Jongbloet PH, Mulder A, Hamers AJ. Seasonality of pre-ovulatory non-disjunction and the aetiology of Down syndrome. A European collaborative study. Hum Genet 1982; 62(2): 134-8. [http://dx.doi.org/10.1007/BF00282301] [PMID: 6219059]

[41] Jongbloet PH, Vrieze OJ. Down syndrome: increased frequency of maternal meiosis I nondisjunction during the transitional stages of the ovulatory seasons. Hum Genet 1985; 71(3): 241-8. [http://dx.doi.org/10.1007/BF00284583] [PMID: 2933319]

[42] Morris JK, Mutton DE, Alberman E. Recurrences of free trisomy 21: analysis of data from the National Down Syndrome Cytogenetic Register. Prenat Diagn 2005; 25(12): 1120-8. [http://dx.doi.org/10.1002/pd.1292] [PMID: 16231400]

[43] De Souza E, Halliday J, Chan A, Bower C, Morris JK. Recurrence risks for trisomies 13, 18, and 21. Am J Med Genet A 2009; 149A(12): 2716-22. [http://dx.doi.org/10.1002/ajmg.a.33099] [PMID: 19921649]

[44] Warburton D, Dallaire L, Thangavelu M, Ross L, Levin M, Kline J. Trisomy Recurrence: A Reconsideration Based on North American Data Am J Hum Genet 2004; 75(3): 376-85. [http://dx.doi.org/10.1086/423331] [PMID: 15248154]

[45] Newberger DS. Down syndrome: prenatal risk assessment and diagnosis. Am Fam Physician 2000; 62(4): 825-32. 837-8 [PMID: 10969860]

[46] Tamaren J, Spuhler K, Sujansky E. Risk of Down syndrome among second- and third-degree relatives of a proband with trisomy 21. Am J Med Genet 1983; 15(3): 393-403. [http://dx.doi.org/10.1002/ajmg.1320150305] [PMID: 6224423]

[47] Boyle B1. Prevalence and risk of Down syndrome in monozygotic and dizygotic multiple pregnancies in Europe: implications for prenatal screening. BJOG 2014; 4 [http://dx.doi.org/10.1111/1471-0528.12574]

[48] Jamar M, Lemarchal C, Lemaire V, Koulischer L, Bours V. A low rate of trisomy 21 in twin-pregnancies: a cytogenetics retrospective study of 278 cases. Genet Couns 2003; 14(4): 395-400. [PMID: 14738112]

[49] Bliumina MG, Lil'in ET, Patiutko RS. [Multiple birth and Down's disease]. Genetika 1975; 11(1): 153-4. [PMID: 131736]

[50] Marteau TM, Dormandy E, Michie S. A measure of informed choice. Health Expect 2001; 4(2): 99-108. [http://dx.doi.org/10.1046/j.1369-6513.2001.00140.x] [PMID: 11359540]

[51] Michie S, Dormandy E, Marteau TM. The multi-dimensional measure of informed choice: a validation study. Patient Educ Couns 2002; 48(1): 87-91.
[http://dx.doi.org/10.1016/S0738-3991(02)00089-7] [PMID: 12220754]

[52] Hunter JE, Allen EG, Shin M, *et al.* The association of low socioeconomic status and the risk of having a child with Down syndrome: a report from the National Down Syndrome Project. Genet Med 2013; 15(9): 698-705.
[http://dx.doi.org/10.1038/gim.2013.34] [PMID: 23558253]

[53] Malini SS, Ramachandra NB. Possible risk factors for Down syndrome and sex chromosomal aneuploidy in Mysore, South India. Indian J Hum Genet 2007; 13(3): 102-8.
[http://dx.doi.org/10.4103/0971-6866.38984] [PMID: 21957357]

[54] Dzurova D, Pikhart H. Down syndrome, paternal age and education: comparison of California and the Czech Republic. BMC Public Health 2005; 5: 69.
[http://dx.doi.org/10.1186/1471-2458-5-69] [PMID: 15963229]

[55] Moore LL, Bradlee ML, Singer MR, Rothman KJ, Milunsky A. Chromosomal anomalies among the offspring of women with gestational diabetes. Am J Epidemiol 2002; 155(8): 719-24.
[http://dx.doi.org/10.1093/aje/155.8.719] [PMID: 11943689.]

[56] Fialkow PJ. Autoimmunity: a predisposing factor to chromosomal aberrations? Lancet 1964; 1(7331): 474-5.
[http://dx.doi.org/10.1016/S0140-6736(64)90803-7] [PMID: 14102254]

[57] Narchi H, Kulaylat N. High incidence of Down's syndrome in infants of diabetic mothers. Arch Dis Child 1997; 77(3): 242-4.
[http://dx.doi.org/10.1136/adc.77.3.242] [PMID: 9370905]

[58] Martínez-Frías ML, Rodríguez-Pinilla E, Bermejo E, Prieto L. Epidemiological evidence that maternal diabetes does not appear to increase the risk for Down syndrome. Am J Med Genet 2002; 114(4): 335-7.
[http://dx.doi.org/10.1002/ajmg.10706] [PMID: 12376933]

[59] Patterson D. Folate metabolism and the risk of Down syndrome. Downs Syndr Res Pract 2008; 12(2): 93-7.
[http://dx.doi.org/10.3104/updates.2051] [PMID: 19026278]

[60] Ghosh S, Hong CS, Feingold E, *et al.* Epidemiology of Down syndrome: new insight into the multidimensional interactions among genetic and environmental risk factors in the oocyte. Am J Epidemiol 2011; 174(9): 1009-16.
[http://dx.doi.org/10.1093/aje/kwr240] [PMID: 21957181]

[61] Rothman KJ. Spermicide use and Down's syndrome. Am J Public Health 1982; 72(4): 399-401.
[http://dx.doi.org/10.2105/AJPH.72.4.399] [PMID: 6461262]

[62] Yang Q, Sherman SL, Hassold TJ, *et al.* Risk factors for trisomy 21: maternal cigarette smoking and oral contraceptive use in a population-based case-control study. Genet Med 1999; 1(3): 80-8.
[http://dx.doi.org/10.1097/00125817-199903000-00004] [PMID: 11336457]

[63] Rudnicka AR, Wald NJ, Huttly W, Hackshaw AK. Influence of maternal smoking on the birth prevalence of Down syndrome and on second trimester screening performance. Prenat Diagn 2002;

22(10): 893-7.
[http://dx.doi.org/10.1002/pd.440] [PMID: 12378572]

[64] Tislarić D, Brajenović-Milić B, Ristić S, *et al.* The influence of smoking and parity on serum markers for Down's syndrome screening. Fetal Diagn Ther 2002; 17(1): 17-21.
[http://dx.doi.org/10.1159/000047999] [PMID: 11803210]

[65] Laziuk GI, Zatsepin IO, Verger P, *et al.* [Down syndrome and ionizing radiation: causal effect or coincidence]. Radiats Biol Radioecol 2002; 42(6): 678-83.
[PMID: 12530149]

[66] Sperling K, Neitzel H, Scherb H. Evidence for an increase in trisomy 21 (Down syndrome) in Europe after the Chernobyl reactor accident. Genet Epidemiol 2012; 36(1): 48-55.
[http://dx.doi.org/10.1002/gepi.20662] [PMID: 22162022]

[67] Olufemi Adebari Oloyede. Subrata D, Ed. Down Syndrome in Nigeria Sub Saharan Africa Prenatal Diagnosis and Screening for Down Syndrome. InTech 2011. ISBN: 978-953-307-355-2

[68] Collins VR, Muggli EE, Riley M, Palma S, Halliday JL. Is Down syndrome a disappearing birth defect? J Pediatr 2008; 152(1): 20-24, 24.e1.
[http://dx.doi.org/10.1016/j.jpeds.2007.07.045] [PMID: 18154892]

[69] Adeyokunno AA. The incidence of Down syndrome in Nigeria. Med Genetik 1982; 19: 277-9.
[http://dx.doi.org/10.1136/jmg.19.4.277]

[70] Molteno C, Smart R, Viljoen D, Sayed R, Roux A. Twenty-year birth prevalence of Down syndrome in Cape Town, South Africa. Paediatr Perinat Epidemiol 1997; 11(4): 428-35.
[http://dx.doi.org/10.1046/j.1365-3016.1997.d01-25.x] [PMID: 9373864]

[71] Delport SD, Christianson AL, van den Berg HJ, Wolmarans L, Gericke GS. Descriptive profile of congenital anomalies in black South African neonates born in an urban hospital. S Afr Med J 1995; 85(1): 11-5.
[PMID: 7784907]

[72] Venter PA, Christianson AL, Hutamo CM, Makhura MP, Gericke GS. Congenital anomalies in rural black South African neonates--a silent epidemic? S Afr Med J 1995; 85(1): 15-20.
[PMID: 7784908]

[73] Kromberg JGR, Christianson AL, Duthie-Nurse G, Zwane E, Jenkins T. Down syndrome in the black population. S Afr Med J 1992; 81(6): 337.
[PMID: 1533293]

[74] Centre for Arab Genomic Studies. Genomic Studies Report on Down syndrome in the Arab world , 2013 [Last accessed on 12 April; 2014]; Avialable at: http://www.cags.org.ae/Down%20Syndrome-English.pdf.

[75] Al-Awadi SA, Farag TI, Teebi AS, Naguib KK, Sundareshan TS, Murthy DS. Down syndrome in Kuwait. Am J Med Genet Suppl 1990; 7: 87-8.
[PMID: 2149982]

[76] Al-Arrayed SS. Review of the spectrum of genetic diseases in Bahrain. East Mediterr Health J 1999; 5(6): 1114-20.
[PMID: 11924098]

[77] Al-Arrayed SS. Personal communication Dubai 2006.

[78] El-Sobky ES, Elsayed SM. Down syndrome in Egypt. Egypt J Med Hum Genet 2004; 5(2): 67-78.

[79] El-Gilany AH, Yahia S, Shoker M, El-Dahtory F. Cytogenetic and comorbidity profile of Down syndrome in Mansoura University Children's Hospital, Egypt. Indian J Hum Genet 2011; 17(3): 157-63.
[http://dx.doi.org/10.4103/0971-6866.92092] [PMID: 22345986]

[80] Shalaby HM. A study of new potential risk factors for Down syndrome in Upper Egypt. Egypt J Med Hum Genet 2011; 12: 15-9.
[http://dx.doi.org/10.1016/j.ejmhg.2011.02.009]

[81] Alaani S, Al-Fallouji MA, Busby C, Hamdan M. Pilot Study of Congenital Anomaly Rates at Birth in Fallujah, Iraq, 2010 2012; 44(1) pii: 44-1-10463
[http://dx.doi.org/10.5915/44-1-10463] [PMID: 23864991]

[82] Alaani S, Savabieasfahani M, Tafash M, Manduca P. Four polygamous families with congenital birth defects from Fallujah, Iraq. Int J Environ Res Public Health 2011; 8(1): 89-96.
[http://dx.doi.org/10.3390/ijerph8010089] [PMID: 21318016]

[83] Naguib K, Al-Awadi S, Moussa M, Mohammed F. Down syndrome in sibs: a study of recessive hypothesis controlling nondisjunction. Bull High Inst Public Health 1992; XXII(1): 125-33.

[84] Verma IC, Mathews AR, Faquih A, el-Zouki AA, Malik GR, Mohammed F. Cytogenetic analysis of Down syndrome in Libya. Indian J Pediatr 1990; 57(2): 245-8.
[http://dx.doi.org/10.1007/BF02722095] [PMID: 2147166]

[85] Elmagrpy Z, Rayani A, Shah A, Habas E, Aburawi EH. Down syndrome and congenital heart disease: why the regional difference as observed in the Libyan experience? Cardiovasc J Afr 2011; 22(6): 306-9.
[http://dx.doi.org/10.5830/CVJA-2010-072] [PMID: 22159317]

[86] Jaiyesimi O, Baichoo V. Cardiovascular malformations in Omani Arab children with Down's syndrome. Cardiol Young 2007; 17(2): 166-71.
[http://dx.doi.org/10.1017/S1047951107000078] [PMID: 17244386]

[87] Merrick J. Down syndrome in Israel. Downs Syndr Res Pract 2001; 6(3): 128-30.
[http://dx.doi.org/10.3104/reports.104] [PMID: 11501215]

[88] Wahab AA, Bener A, Sandridge AL, Hoffmann GF. The pattern of Down syndrome among children in Qatar: a population-based study. Birth Defects Res A Clin Mol Teratol 2006; 76(8): 609-12.
[http://dx.doi.org/10.1002/bdra.20290] [PMID: 16955492]

[89] Wahab AA, Bener A, Teebi AS. The incidence patterns of Down syndrome in Qatar. Clin Genet 2006; 69(4): 360-2.
[http://dx.doi.org/10.1111/j.1399-0004.2006.00593.x] [PMID: 16630172]

[90] Niazi MA, al-Mazyad AS, al-Husain MA, *et al.* Down's syndrome in Saudi Arabia: incidence and cytogenetics. Hum Hered 1995; 45(2): 65-9.
[http://dx.doi.org/10.1159/000154261] [PMID: 7750976]

[91] Hosani HA, Czeizel AE. Congenital abnormalities in the United Arab Emirates. Teratology 2000;

61(2): 161-2.
[http://dx.doi.org/10.1002/(SICI)1096-9926(200003)61:3<161::AID-TERA1>3.0.CO;2-O] [PMID: 10661903]

[92] Murthy SK, Malhotra AK, Mani S, *et al.* Incidence of Down syndrome in Dubai, UAE. Med Princ Pract 2007; 16(1): 25-8.
[http://dx.doi.org/10.1159/000096136] [PMID: 17159360]

[93] Zhang SZ, Xie T, Tang YC, Zhang SL, Xu Y. The prevalence of chromosome diseases in the general population of Sichuan, China. Clin Genet 1991; 39(2): 81-8.
[http://dx.doi.org/10.1111/j.1399-0004.1991.tb02991.x] [PMID: 2015698]

[94] Lau TK, Fung HY, Rogers MS, Cheung KL. Racial variation in incidence of trisomy 21: survey of 57,742 Chinese deliveries. Am J Med Genet 1998; 75(4): 386-8.
[http://dx.doi.org/10.1002/(SICI)1096-8628(19980203)] [PMID: 9482644]

[95] Zheng CG, Qin J, Du J, *et al.* [Cytogenetic study of Down syndrome cases in Nanning, China]. Yi Chuan 2009; 31(3): 261-4.
[http://dx.doi.org/10.3724/SP.J.1005.2009.00261] [PMID: 19273438]

[96] Miao ZY, Liu X, Shi TK, Xu Y, Song QH, Tang SH. First trimester, second trimester, and integrated screening for Down's syndrome in China. J Med Screen 2012; 19(2): 68-71.
[http://dx.doi.org/10.1258/jms.2012.011145] [PMID: 22653574]

[97] Ghosh A, Woo JS, Chan CL, *et al.* Down syndrome and maternal age in Hong Kong Chinese. Asia Oceania J Obstet Gynaecol 1985; 11(1): 93-8.
[http://dx.doi.org/10.1111/j.1447-0756.1985.tb00053.x] [PMID: 3160325]

[98] Sahota DS, Leung WC, Chan WP, To WW, Lau ET, Leung TY. Prospective assessment of the Hong Kong Hospital Authority universal Down syndrome screening programme. Hong Kong Med J 2013; 19(2): 101-8.
[PMID: 23535668]

[99] Gale SC, Ip P, Chow CB, Wong WH, Chung BH, Ip DK. An Estimate of the Prevalence of Down's Syndrome in Hong Kong. HK J Paediatr 2013; 18(4): 230-65. [New Series].

[100] Lin SY, Hsieh CJ, Chen YL, *et al.* The impact of Down syndrome screening on Taiwanese Down syndrome births: a nationwide retrospective study and a screening result from a single medical centre PLos One 2013; 8(9): e75428. eCollection 2013
[http://dx.doi.org/10.1371/journal.pone.0075428] [PMID: 24147155]

[101] Isaac GS, Krishnamurty PS, Reddy YR, Ahuja YR. Down's syndrome in Hyderabad, India. Acta Anthropogenet 1985; 9(4): 256-60.
[PMID: 2967078]

[102] Verma IC, Anand NK, Kabra M, Menon PS, Sharma N. Study of malformations and Down syndrome in India (SOMDI): Delhi Region. Indian J Hum Genet 1998; 4: 84-7.

[103] Modi UJ, Nayak U, Aiyer S, *et al.* Study of malformations and Down syndrome in India (SOMDI): Baroda region. Indian J Hum Genet 1998; 4: 93-8.

[104] Patel ZM, Adhia RA. Birth defects surveillance study. Indian J Pediatr 2005; 72(6): 489-91.
[http://dx.doi.org/10.1007/BF02724426] [PMID: 15985737]

[105] Mehdipour P, Saadat M, Noori-daloii MR. Down's syndrome: cytogenetic studies in 150 cases in tehran. Mjiri 1996; 10(1): 47-52.

[106] Hoshi N, Hattori R, Hanatani K, *et al.* Recent trends in the prevalence of Down syndrome in Japan, 1980-1997 Am J Med Genet 1999; 84(4): 340-5.
[http://dx.doi.org/10.1002/(SICI)1096-8628(19990604)84:4<340::AID-AJMG6>3.0.CO;2-N]

[107] Suzuki S. Recent Incidence of Trisomy 21 in a Japanese Hospital. J Clin Gynecol Obstet 2012; 1(2-3): 56.
[http://dx.doi.org/10.4021/jcgo26w]

[108] Ahmed I, Ghafoor T, Samore NA, Chattha MN. Down syndrome: clinical and cytogenetic analysis. J Coll Physicians Surg Pak 2005; 15(7): 426-9.
[PMID: 16197873]

[109] Hoe TS, Boo NY, Clyde MM. Incidence of Down's syndrome in a large Malaysian maternity hospital over an 18 month period. Singapore Med J 1989; 30(3): 246-8.
[PMID: 2531468]

[110] Azman BZ, Ankathil R, Siti Mariam I, *et al.* Cytogenetic and clinical profile of Down syndrome in Northeast Malaysia. Singapore Med J 2007; 48(6): 550-4.
[PMID: 17538755]

[111] Acikbas I, Tomatir AG, Akdag B, Koksal A. Retrospective analysis of live birth prevalence of children with Down syndrome in Denizli, Turkey Genet Mol Res 2012; 11(4): 4640-5.
[http://dx.doi.org/10.4238/2012] [PMID: 23079965]

[112] Bittles AH, Bower C, Hussain R, Glasson EJ. The four ages of Down syndrome. Eur J Public Health 2007; 17(2): 221-5.
[http://dx.doi.org/10.1093/eurpub/ckl103] [PMID: 16857692]

[113] Tracy J. Australians with Down syndrome--health matters. Aust Fam Physician 2011; 40(4): 202-8.
[PMID: 21597529]

[114] Dolk H, Loane M, Garne E, *et al.* Trends and geographic inequalities in the prevalence of Down syndrome in Europe, 1980-1999 Rev Epidemiol Sante Publique 2005; 53 (Spec No 2): 2S87-95.

[115] Boyd PA, Devigan C, Khoshnood B, Loane M, Garne E, Dolk H. EUROCAT Working Group. Survey of prenatal screening policies in Europe for structural malformations and chromosome anomalies, and their impact on detection and termination rates for neural tube defects and Down's syndrome. BJOG 2008; 115(6): 689-96.
[http://dx.doi.org/10.1111/j.1471-0528.2008.01700.x] [PMID: 18410651]

[116] Wellesley D, Dolk H, Boyd PA, *et al.* Rare chromosome abnormalities, prevalence and prenatal diagnosis rates from population-based congenital anomaly registers in Europe. Eur J Hum Genet 2012; 20(5): 521-6.
[http://dx.doi.org/10.1038/ejhg.2011.246] [PMID: 22234154]

[117] Verloes A, Gillerot Y, Van Maldergem L, *et al.* Major decrease in the incidence of trisomy 21 at birth in south Belgium: mass impact of triple test? Eur J Hum Genet 2001; 9(1): 1-4.
[http://dx.doi.org/10.1038/sj.ejhg.5200575] [PMID: 11175292]

[118] Brajenović-Milić B, Prpić I, Petrović O, Ristić S, Brumini G, Kapović M. The prevalence of live birth Down syndrome in the region of Primorsko-goranska County in Croatia, 1996-2005: the impact of screening and amniocentesis. Matern Child Health J 2008; 12(5): 620-3. [http://dx.doi.org/10.1007/s10995-007-0272-6] [PMID: 17712614]

[119] Sípek A, Gregor V, Horácek J. [Birth defects in the Czech Republic in the period 1961-2005--mean incidences]. Ceska Gynekol 2007; 72(3): 185-91. [PMID: 17616072]

[120] Mikkelsen M, Fischer G, Stene J, Stene E, Petersen E. Incidence study of Down's syndrome in Copenhagen, 1960-1971; with chromosome investigation. wnAnn. Hum Genet 1976; 40(2): 177-82. [http://dx.doi.org/10.1111/j.1469-1809.1976.tb00177.x] [PMID: 1248829]

[121] Mikkelsen M, Hallberg A, Poulsen H, *et al.* Epidemiological study of Down's syndrome in Denmark, including family studies of chromosomes and DNA markers. Dev Brain Dysfunct 1995; 8(1): 4-12.

[122] Kjaergaard S, Hahnemann M, Skibsted L, *et al.* Prenatal diagnosis of chromosome aberrations after implementation of screening for Down's syndrome. Ugeskr Laeger 2008; 170(14): 1152-6. [PMID: 18405480]

[123] Morris JK, Alberman E. Trends in Down's syndrome live births and antenatal diagnoses in England and Wales from 1989 to 2008: analysis of data from the National Down Syndrome Cytogenetic Register. BMJ 2009; 339: b3794. [http://dx.doi.org/ 10.1136/bmj.b3794] [PMID: 19858532]

[124] Wu J, Morris JK. The population prevalence of Down's syndrome in England and Wales in 2011. Eur J Hum Genet 2013; 21(9): 1016-9. [http://dx.doi.org/10.1038/ejhg.2012.294] [PMID: 23321618]

[125] Morris JK, Alberman E, Mutton D, Jacobs P. Cytogenetic and epidemiological findings in Down syndrome: England and Wales 1989-2009. Am J Med Genet A 2012; 158A(5): 1151-7. [http://dx.doi.org/10.1002/ajmg.a.35248] [PMID: 22438132]

[126] Johnson Z, Lillis D, Delany V, Hayes C, Dack P. The epidemiology of Down syndrome in four counties in Ireland 1981-1990. J Public Health Med 1996; 18(1): 78-86. [http://dx.doi.org/10.1093/oxfordjournals.pubmed.a024466] [PMID: 8785080]

[127] O'Nualláin S, Flanagan O, Raffat I, Avalos G, Dineen B. The prevalence of Down syndrome in County Galway. Ir Med J 2007; 100(1): 329-31. [PMID: 17380922]

[128] Huether CA, Haroldson K, Ellis PM, Ramsay CN. Impact of prenatal diagnosis on revised livebirth prevalence estimates of Down syndrome in the Lothian region of Scotland, 1978-1992. Genet Epidemiol 1996; 13(4): 367-75. [http://dx.doi.org/10.1002/(SICI)1098-2272(1996)13:4<367::AID-GEPI5>3.0.CO;2-1] [PMID: 8894639]

[129] Reimand T, Ounap K, Zordania R, *et al.* Descriptive epidemiology of Down's syndrome in Estonia. Paediatr Perinat Epidemiol 2006; 20(6): 512-9. [http://dx.doi.org/10.1111/j.1365-3016.2006.00758.x] [PMID: 17052289]

[130] Rousseau T, Amar E, Ferdynus C, Thauvin-Robinet C, Gouyon JB, Sagot P. [Variations in the

prevalence of Down's syndrome in the French population between 1978 and 2005]. J Gynecol Obstet Biol Reprod (Paris) 2010; 39(4): 290-6.
[http://dx.doi.org/10.1016/j.jgyn.2010.03.008] [PMID: 20430534]

[131] Rousseau T, Ferdynus C, Thauvin-Robinet C, Gouyon JB, Sagot P. [Impact of maternal age distribution on the expected live birth prevalence of Down's syndrome in the metropolitan France between 1965 and 2008]. J Gynecol Obstet Biol Reprod (Paris) 2010; 39(4): 284-9.
[http://dx.doi.org/10.1016/j.jgyn.2010.03.001] [PMID: 20381272]

[132] Métneki J, Czeizel AE. Increasing total prevalence rate of cases with Down syndrome in Hungary. Eur J Epidemiol 2005; 20(6): 525-35.
[http://dx.doi.org/10.1007/s10654-005-4261-z] [PMID: 16121762]

[133] de Graaf G, Haveman M, Hochstenbach R, *et al.* Changes in yearly birth prevalence rates of children with Down syndrome in the period 1986-2007 in The Netherlands. J Intellect Disabil Res 2011; 55(5): 462-73.
[http://dx.doi.org/10.1111/j.1365-2788.2011.01398.x] [PMID: 21375641]

[134] van Gameren-Oosterom HB, Buitendijk SE, Bilardo CM, van der Pal-de Bruin KM, Van Wouwe JP, Mohangoo AD. Unchanged prevalence of Down syndrome in the Netherlands: results from an 11-year nationwide birth cohort. Prenat Diagn 2012; 32(11): 1035-40.
[http://dx.doi.org/10.1002/pd.3951] [PMID: 22865545]

[135] Fransen MP, Schoonen MH, Mackenbach JP, *et al.* Ethnic differences in participation in prenatal screening for Down syndrome: a register-based study. Prenat Diagn 2010; 30(10): 988-94.
[http://dx.doi.org/10.1002/pd.2603] [PMID: 20799374]

[136] Melve KK, Lie RT, Skjaerven R, *et al.* Registration of Down syndrome in the Medical Birth Registry of Norway: validity and time trends. Acta Obstet Gynecol Scand 2008; 87(8): 824-30.
[http://dx.doi.org/10.1080/00016340802217184] [PMID: 18607831]

[137] Kovaleva NV, Butomo IV, Verlinskaia DK, Il'iashenko TN, Davidenkova EF. [Increase in the incidence and risk of birth of children with Down's syndrome in Leningrad (1982-1989)]. Genetika 1994; 30(2): 265-70.
[PMID: 8045388]

[138] Krikunova NI, Minaĭcheva LI, Nazarenko LP, *et al.* [Epidemiology of congenital malformations in Gorno-Altaisk, Altai Republic, Russia]. Genetika 2004; 40(8): 1138-44.
[PMID: 15523853]

[139] Zatsepin I, Verger P, Robert-Gnansia E, *et al.* Down syndrome time-clustering in January 1987 in Belarus: link with the Chernobyl accident? Reprod Toxicol 2007; 24(3-4): 289-95.
[http://dx.doi.org/10.1016/j.reprotox.2007.06.003] [PMID: 17706919]

[140] Gómez D, Solsona E, Guitart M, *et al.* Origin of trisomy 21 in Down syndrome cases from a Spanish population registry. Ann Genet 2000; 43(1): 23-8.
[http://dx.doi.org/10.1016/S0003-3995(00)00017-4] [PMID: 10818217]

[141] Mosquera Tenreiro C, Ariza Hevia F, Rodríguez Dehli C, Fernández Toral J, García López E, Riaño Galán I. Prevalence and secular trend of Down syndrome in Asturias (Spain), 1990-2004. Med Clin (Barc) 2009; 132(15): 580-4.
[http://dx.doi.org/10.1016/j.medcli.2008.10.052.] [PMID: 19327795]

[142] Binkert F, Mutter M, Schinzel A. Impact of prenatal diagnosis on the prevalence of live births with Down syndrome in the eastern half of Switzerland 1980-1996. Swiss Med Wkly 2002; 132(33-34): 478-84.
[PMID: 12458448]

[143] Shin M, Besser LM, Kucik JE, Lu C, Siffel C, Correa A. Congenital Anomaly Multistate Prevalence and Survival Collaborative. Prevalence of Down syndrome among children and adolescents in 10 regions of the United States. Pediatrics 2009; 124(6): 1565-71.
[http://dx.doi.org/10.1542/peds.2009-0745] [PMID: 19948627]

[144] Zigman WB. Atypical aging in Down syndrome. Dev Disabil Res Rev 2013; 18(1): 51-67.
[http://dx.doi.org/10.1002/ddrr.1128] [PMID: 23949829]

[145] Besser LM, Shin M, Kucik JE, Correa A. Prevalence of down syndrome among children and adolescents in metropolitan Atlanta. Birth Defects Res A Clin Mol Teratol 2007; 79(11): 765-74.
[http://dx.doi.org/10.1002/bdra.20404] [PMID: 17990336]

[146] McDonald JA, Suellentrop K, Paulozzi LJ, Morrow B. Reproductive health of the rapidly growing Hispanic population: data from the Pregnancy Risk Assessment Monitoring System, 2002. Matern Child Health J 2008; 12(3): 342-56.
[http://dx.doi.org/10.1007/s10995-007-0244-x] [PMID: 17592761]

[147] Presson AP, Partyka G, Jensen KM, *et al.* Current estimate of Down Syndrome population prevalence in the United States. J Pediatr 2013; 163(4): 1163-8.
[http://dx.doi.org/10.1016/j.jpeds.2013.06.013] [PMID: 23885965]

[148] Public Health Agency of Canada. Congenital Anomalies in Canada 2013: A Perinatal Health Surveillance Report. Ottawa 2013 [Last accessed was on 10th April 2014.]; Available at: http://publications.gc.ca/collections/collection_2014/aspc-phac/HP35-40-2013-eng.pdf.

[149] Ministry of Health. National Center for Gender Equity and Reproductive Health. Comprehensive Care of People with Down Syndrome. Technical Guideline Ministry of Health 2007. Available at: http://www.salud.gob.mx/unidades/cdi/documentos/Sindrome_Down_lin_2007.pdf

[150] Nazer H J, Cifuentes OL. Congenital malformations in Latin America in the period 1995-2008. Rev Med Chil 2011; 139(1): 72-8.
[http://dx.doi.org//S0034-98872011000100010] [PMID: 21526320]

[151] Nazer H J, Aguila R A, Cifuentes O L. [Increasing rates of Down syndrome among newborns in Chile from 1972 to 2005]. Rev Med Chil 2006; 134(12): 1549-57.
[PMID: 17277872]

[152] Press N, Browner CH. Characteristics of women who refuse an offer of prenatal diagnosis: data from the California maternal serum alpha fetoprotein blood test experience. Am J Med Genet 1998; 78(5): 433-45.
[http://dx.doi.org/10.1002/(SICI)1096-8628(19980806)78:5<433::AID-AJMG8>3.0.CO;2-M] [PMID: 9714010]

CHAPTER 2

Genetics of Down Syndrome: An Update

Solaf M. Elsayed*

Genetics Unit, Children's Hospital, Ain Shams University, Cairo, Egypt

Abstract: Since the discovery of the chromosomal basis of Down syndrome (DS) in 1959, researches are still trying to understand the genetic basis of this particular unique common disorder that cannot be simply explained by an additional chromosome 21. Recent advances in molecular genetics had shed the light on several genes peculiar to this disorder like DYRK1A involved in cognitive dysfunctions and GATA1 involved in transient myeloproliferative disease. Some of these genes are actually beneficial when found in excess like COL18A1 which encodes endostatin, a potent angiogenesis inhibitor that inhibit the progression of solid tissue tumors and thus may have a potential therapeutic effect as anticancer therapy, as an anti-inflammatory agent and for protection against diabetic retinopathy. Gene therapy - or better to say chromosome therapy - for patients with DS is a recent break through where scientists were able to silence the extra chromosome and reverse the neuron proliferation dysfunction. This will not only help patients with DS but could be applied to all chromosomal trisomies. By understanding the pathogenetic mechanisms of DS, the near future is holding hope not only for treatment of DS cognitive dysfunction but also cures for solid tumours and certain disorders that will be done through inducing trisomy 21 in affected cells!

Keywords: AIRE, Blessing effect, Chromosomes, Cytogenetics, Down syndrome, DSCR-1, DYRK1A, Endostatin, GATA1, Gene therapy, JAK2, Lucky mothers, Molecular, Mosaicism, Nondisjunction, Overexpression, Polymorphism, Robertsonian translocation, TAM, Trisomy 21.

1. INTRODUCTION: CHROMOSOMAL BASIS OF DOWN SYNDROME

Lejeune *et al.* 1959 are credited with the discovery of the chromosomal basis of Down syndrome (DS) [1]. Shortly thereafter, Polani *et al.* 1960, discovered translocation DS in the daughter of a 21-year-old mother because they had

* **Corresponding Author Dr. Solaf M. Elsayed:** Genetics Unit, Children's Hospital, Ain Shams University, Cairo, Egypt. Medical Genetics Center. 27 A Baghdad St. Korba, Cairo, Egypt; Telephone: 202-24151999; Fax : 202-24150977; E-mail: elsayed683@yahoo.com

Mohammed Al-Biltagi (Ed)

reasoned that some individuals may be affected through a separate, maternal-independent chromosomal mechanism [2]. In the following year, Clark *et al.* 1961 reported mosaic DS, in a 2 year-old girl with physical stigmata of DS but near normal intelligence [3]. The most common chromosomal anomaly in patients with DS is "trisomy" in which there is an additional copy of chromosome 21. This is present in 95% of patients followed by translocation (in 4-5%) in which the extra-copy of chromosome 21 is translocated on one of the acrocentric chromosomes (mostly 14 or 21) [4, 5]. Mosaic DS is least common, found in only 1% of patients [6].

2. ETIOLOGY AND ORIGIN OF EXTRA CHROMOSOME 21

2.1. Nondisjunction Trisomy 21

Finding the origin of the extra copy of chromosome 21 with highly informative DNA markers will not alter the scenario of genetic counseling; it will only confirm the already known fact that the meiotic error in the maternal (not paternal) chromosomes is the origin of the extra copy. Ironically, fetuses with trisomy 21 where the origin of the extra-copy is of maternal origin have an advantage of intrauterine survival. Thus it might be only a scientific interest to determine the origin in spontaneous abortions of trisomy 21 fetuses [7].

Trisomy 21 (also known as chromosome nondisjunction) is caused by failure of the two similar chromosomes (21)s to separate (segregate) properly during meiosis. The vast majority occurs in oocytes [8] specifically during meiosis I (MI) [9]. Causes of this error have been thoroughly investigated and the most significant risk factor found was advanced maternal age in which the error occurs during oogenesis and for chromosome 21, it can occur in both meiosis I and meiosis II [10].

Other risk factors suggested include accumulation of environmental toxic elements which can damage the meiotic machinery of the oocytes causing chromosome nondisjunction. This can occur through different mechanisms; metals acts possibly through epigenetic mechanism while very small particles (nano-sized) might act directly with mitotic and meiotic machinery and with subcellular components. Also, cytotoxic drugs used in different healthcare occupations (causing inhibition of cell growth), continuous exposure to electromagnetic fields (with a limited evidence of causing aneuploidy) have been suggested as other environmental risk factors that may act with aging or genetic predisposition to produce nondisjunction [11, 12]. Some investigators suggested that reactive oxygen species produced by metabolism could diminish the oocyte quality [12].

More than a decade ago, Torfs and Christianson in 2003 suggested an association between low maternal socioeconomic status and the occurrence of non-disjunction of chromosome 21 [13]. Recently, this theory was reinvestigated and confirmed by Hunter *et al.* 2013 but they did not elucidate the actual factors that account for the increased incidence of nondisjunction (whether it is the poor nutrition or the environmental exposure) [14]. Another possible mechanism was investigated by Ghosh *et al.* 2010 who suggested that shorter telomere length contributes by one way or another to the meiosis I or II error and subsequently non disjunction. They found the telomeres of the older mothers of DS are relatively shorter (making them genetically older) compared to the control mothers of the same age with normal euploid babies [15].

2.2. Robertsonian Translocation

The second commonest chromosomal anomalies in DS (4%) is the Robertsonian translocation where the long arm of one of the acrocentric chromosomes (13, 14, 15, 21) is translocated to the long arm of chromosome 21 and so the number of chromosomes will be 46 and not 47 (unbalanced translocation). The advanced maternal age is not a risk factor for this abnormality but if one parent is a carrier for translocation (balanced carrier), the recurrence risk is increased and so cytogenetic analysis for both parents is mandatory to provide accurate genetic counseling [16].

The origin of denovo t (21; 21) DS are usually different from the other reciprocal translocation. For the majority of such chromosomes are not centric fusion or whole arm exchange chromosomes, rather they are isochromosomes (iso 21q) resulting from fusion of sister chromatids [17, 18]. Whether isochromosomes arise during oogenesis is not established, and it is argued that isochromosomes arise post conception in somatic tissues of trisomic conceptus [19].

2.3. Mosaicism

Mosaicism is a condition in which an individual has two or more genetically distinct cell lines that deavelop from a single zygote [16]. Although studies showed that mosaic DS individuals have significantly higher (10 points) mean IQ level than complete trisomy, it is important to note that IQ depends on many factors other than the simple percentage of trisomy cells alone. Nevertheless, these higher IQ scores were inversely correlated to the percentage of trisomy cells in patients' buccal cells and not the lymphocytes. This can be explained by the fact both the brain cells and buccal cells are derived from the ectoderm. On the other hand, the blood cells and heart cells are both derived from the mesoderm and so the presence or absence of CHD was correlated to the number of trisomic cells in lymphocytes and not the buccal cells [20].

3. MOLECULAR GENETICS

Because some patients with DS have partial trisomy but still have DS phenotype, investigators have searched to what is called DS critical region on chromosome 21. A critical region is defined as the smallest chromosomal segment which, when unbalanced, will give rise to the phenotype generally associated with imbalance of a larger chromosomal region that contains it [21]. Delabare *et al.* 1993 reported an area located at band 21q22.3 that is associated with most of the facial features of DS plus the short stature, hypotonia and characteristic dermatoglyphics [22].

3.1. Genes Involved in Cognitive Impairment

Most importantly is dual-specificity tyrosine –(Y) phosphorylation regulated kinase 1 A (DYRK1A) gene. This gene is crucially involved in regulation of cell proliferation and signaling pathways that contributes to normal brain development and function. When this gene is over expressed (when present in trisomy), it can inhibit proliferation of neural progenitor cells in mouse brain [23 - 27] and delay their differentiation and altered their laminar fate *via* attenuation of NFATc signaling pathway (a critical regulator for vertebrate development) *in vivo* [28].

Interestingly, normalization of the over expressed DYRK1A gene in mice was found to improve working memory and restore the differentiation and proliferation of hippocampal cells and the density of the GABAergic synapse markers. This suggests that DYRK1A gene targeted therapy may improve the learning disabilities found in DS [29]. Another potential therapy for the impaired cognitive function and memory in DS is the use of a GABA antagonist (pentylenetetrazol) or inverse agonist which was proved to be very efficient in reversing learning and memory deficits in a DS mouse model. The proposed mechanism for this therapy is that DS brains have excess inhibition of GABA neurotransmitter pathway and imbalance between glutamatergic and GABAergic synapse activity [30].

3.2. Genes Involved in Hematological Malignancies

3.2.1. TAM: A Unique Hematological Finding in DS

The first reported case of DS and acute leukemia (AL) was made in infant in 1930. It was more than thirty years later before a nationwide American survey found more than a casual association between the two conditions [31]. Further studies showed that patients with DS have a 10-30 times more increased risk to develop AL than general population which can be attributed to a gene dosage effect as chromosome 21 is non randomly involved in acquired somatic chromosomal abnormalities in both acute lymphoblastic (ALL) and acute non-lymphoblastic leukemia. It is believed that the additional chromosomal material leads to disruption of the genetic balance and subsequently abnormal response to various genetic and environmental factors and development of leukemia [32].

On the other hand, 10% of DS infants have a unique hematological feature that was even reported prenatally called transient abnormal myelopoiesis (TAM) (transient leukemoid reaction or congenital leukomoid reaction) which spontaneously disappears within several months [33]. About 20% to 30% of babies with TAM subsequently develop myeloid leukemia of DS (ML-DS) [34]. The World Health Organization (WHO) defined TAM as increased peripheral blood blast cells in neonates with DS [35]. Surprisingly, 97.5% of DS neonates in one study had blasts on blood smears (range, 1%-77%) [36].

The GATA binding protein 1 (GATA-1) gene encodes a 50 kDa transcription activation factor that is critical for the normal development of the ontogenesis of the erythroid and the megakaryocytic lineages [37, 38]. Interestingly, GATA 1 exon 2 mutations are described only in children with DS with either TAM or AML and are undetectable when the disease is in remission [39]. It is also not detectable in DS suffering from other types of leukemia nor in patients with acute myeloid leukemia (AML) without DS [40, 41]. Furthermore, if GATA 1 mutation is detected in euoploid individuals with acute megakaryocytic leukemia (AMKL), the expanded blasts also acquire extra-chromosome 21 (somatically) [42]. It is assumed that the presence of the extra copy of chromosome 21 makes the megakaryoblasts more sensitive to GATA1 mutation and if the same mutation occurred in euploid individuals , it will have no deleterious effect unless the cells become trisomy for chromosome 21 [36].

Unfortunately, the type of GATA1 mutation is not prognostic for which patients with TAM will progress to ML-DS, since no difference is seen in types of mutation between patients with TAM and with ML-DS but the somatic mutation of each patient may be used as a stable molecular target for minimal residual disease (MRD) to monitor the resolution of TMD and the therapy response in ML-DS patients [43].

3.2.2. JAK2 Associated ALL in DS

Some children with DS and B- cell ALL were found to have Janus Kinase 2 (JAK2) mutations which is believed to be a gain of function mutation that causes cytokine independent growth. Those patients were younger at diagnosis than those without this specific mutation and the leukemic cells were sensitive to inhibition by a JAK2 inhibitor [44].

3.2.3. CBER1 Gene and Anthracycline- Related Cardiotoxicity in DS

Anthracyclin is one of the chemotherapeutic agents used for treatment of pediatric AML. However, cardiotoxicity is one of its major side effects that may occur especially in DS patients (17.5% of patients) and hinder its use [45]. This increased incidence of toxicity in DS was linked to the over expression of carbonyl reductase 1 (CBR1) gene located on chromosome 21 (21q22.12) in both lymphocytes and hearts of DS individuals [46, 47].

3.3. Genes Involved in Congenital Heart Disease (CHD)

Over expression of both Down syndrome cell adhesion molecule (DSCAM) and collagen type VI alpha 2 (COL6A2) genes located on chromosome 21 cooperatively contributes to atrial septal defects and increased abnormalities of heart rhythm in DS mice models [48]. Further studies suggested the potential contribution of vascular endothelial growth factor (VEGF) [49], ciliome and Hedgehog [50] and folate [51] pathways to the pathogenicity of CHD in DS individuals. Actually, occurrence of CHD is much more complicated. Other factors are involved in the genetic architecture of CHD in DS patients including single nucleotide polymorphisms (SNP) and copy number variations (CNV) in chromosome 21 in addition to a yet-unidentified genetic variation in the rest of the genome [52].

3.4. Genes Involved in Immunological Dysfunctions

It has long been observed that DS individuals are more prone to recurrent infections and increased incidence of autoimmune diseases (immunological dysfunction). Recently, the human autoimmune regulator (AIRE) gene was found to be elevated in DS thymic tissue. This gene is located on chromosome 21 and controls the expression of tissue restricted antigens in medullary thymic epithelial cells through coding for transcription factors [53]. Interestingly, mutations in this gene can also cause autoimmune polyendocrine syndrome type 1. The increased expression of AIRE gene in DS may contribute to the autoimmune diseases in DS through affection of homeostasis and thymic selection processes [54].

4. THE BLESSING EFFECT OF EXTRA CHROMOSOME 21

Surprisingly, the effect of extra chromosome 21 is not always deleterious; a silver lining can be seen in several aspects including:

4.1. Protective Effects Against Solid Malignancy

Unlike hematological malignancies, the frequency of solid tumors in DS children and adults are significantly lower than non-DS population. This observation was reported in large population-based and/or tumor registries. The S-100 b protein was found to be higher in DS patients and may contribute to the lower incidence of neuroblastoma in this population. This S-100 b protein is encoded by a gene located in chromosome 21 and the extra amount produced by the presence of trisomy is capable of inhibition growth and induction of death of neuroblastoma cell line in both humans and murines [55].

The extra chromosome 21 also protects against the progression of tumors. Several genes mapped to chromosome 21 are involved in this process including COL18A1 gene which encodes endostatin, a potent angiogenesis inhibitor for many different types of solid tissue tumors in both human and animal models [56]. A significantly increased amount of endostatin was found in DS individuals and if their serum levels were higher than 20 ng/ml they might be less prone for the development of solid tumors than those with lower levels. And so it might be important to evaluate the use of endostatin levels as a predictive test for development and progression of solid tumour in the future [57].

Endostatin was also found to decrease the levels of vascular endothelial growth factor C (VEGF-C) in tumours and thus inhibiting lymphangiogenesis apparently *via* inhibition of mast cell migration and adhesion [58]. The extra copy of chromosome 21 protects also against tumor progression through another two genes (ironically, the same genes that are involved in cognitive dysfunction (DSCR-1 and DYRK1A)) which play a crucial role in inhibiting the growth of new blood vessels [57, 59]. These two genes encode proteins that disrupt the calcineurin pathway, which is involved in angiogenesis. DSCR1 protein levels were found to be increased in both the tissues of people with DS and in the mouse model of DS.

Both tumor growth and microvessels density were significantly lower in DS mice than in diploid controls. [60]. Other genes involved in inhibition of tumor progression included two putative anti-angiogenic genes [61]: ADAMTS1 which is a protease significantly blocks vascular endothelial growth factor receptor 2 (VEGFR2) phosphorylation with consequent suppression of endothelial cell proliferation [62] and ERG which is a transcription factor implicated in endothelial tube formation and angiogenesis [63]. Reynolds *et al.* also identified another two new genes involved in angiogenesis (JAM-B and PTTG1IP) both are specific to endothelial cells and when over expressed, they inhibit the angiogenesis response to VEGF [61].

4.2. DS and Diabetic Retinopathy

The blessing effect of the extra chromosome 21 is also observed in their lower incidence of diabetic retinopathy and can be explained by the relatively increased amount of endostatin which protects them from this diabetes complication through the same mechanism of reducing angiogenesis [60]. Endostatin inhibits the proliferation and migration of choroid-retinal endothelial cells, suppresses VEGF and fibroblast growth factor (FGF) and the inflammatory mediators (tumour necrosis factor- alpha (TNF-alpha), matrix metalloproteinases (MMPs) and vascular cell adhesion molecule-1 (VCAM-1). Therefore, endostatin can be considered valuable anti-angiogenic agents [64].

4.3. Anticancer Therapy

Endostatin is also a good candidate for cancer therapy in humans. Patients with stage IIIB and IV non-small cell lung cancer were treated- in phase III clinical trial- with Endostar, a recombinant endostatin product in combination with the standard chemotherapeutic regimen. Patients had significant clinical improvement compared to the standard chemotherapeutic regimen alone. This was noted in the rate of response, the progression median time and the clinical benefit rate [65]. Recently, trisomy of the DSCR1 gene was found to suppress early progression of intraepithelial pancreatic cancer caused by oncogenic K-ras [66] and was sufficient to suppress tumor angiogeneis during spontaneous lung tumorigenesis through decreased proliferation and increased apoptosis of lung tumor cells [67].

4.4. Anti-Inflammatory Effect

High levels of endostatatins may also acts as anti-inflammatory. Recombinant human endostatin was effective in reducing proliferation and inducing apoptosis of synovial fibroblasts in rheumatoid arthritis in rats. These findings highlight the potential use of endostatin as a treatment for rheumatoid arthritis [68].

4.5. Vascular Anomalies

As we should expect, individuals with DS have less incidence of vascular anomalies reaching up to 80%. This may be attributed to the protective effect of the increased products of the following genes: VEGF inhibitors, COL18A1, DSCR1 or DYRK1A which are all located on chromosome 21 [69].

4.6. Neuroprotective Effect!!!

Interesting enough, trisomy 21 has a neuroprotective mechanism which improves the outcome following stroke in mice. This could be due to the antinflammatory and anti-apoptotic effects of the over expressed DSCR1 gene product in neurons [70].

4.7. Lucky Mothers??

More than 10 year ago, Zhang *et al*. reported that pregnant mothers of trisomy 21 fetuses do not develop preeclampsia although trisomy21 is associated with pronounced michrochimerism that previously investigated as a possible contributor to the preeclampsia pathophysiology [71].

5. GENE THERAPY IN DS: SILENCING THE EXTRA CHROMOSOME

Jiang *et al*. (2013) actually tested this concept. They inserted a large inducible X inactivation- specific transcript (XIST) into the DYRK1A locus on chromosome 21 in DS pluripotent stem cells which triggered modification of the heterochromatin, silencing for the transcription and methylation of the DNA to form a chromosome 21 Barr body. Interestingly, silencing of chromosome 21 rapidly reversed the neuronal proliferation defect characterizing trisomy 21 [72].

CONFLICT OF INTEREST

The authors confirm that this chapter contents have no conflict of interest.

ACKNOWLEDGEMENTS

Declared none.

REFERENCES

[1] Lejeune J, Gauthier M, Turpin R. Human chromosomes in tissue cultures. C R Hebd Seances Acad Sci 1959; 26:248(4): 602-3.
[PMID: 13629913]

[2] Polani PE, Briggs JH, Ford CE. A mongol girl with 46 chromosomes. Lancet 1960; 2:1(7127): 721-4. [PMID: 14433741]

[3] Clark CM, Edwards JH. Small piece V. 21 trisomy / normal mosaicism in an intelligent child with Mongoloid characteristics. Lancet 1961; 13:1(7185): 1028-30. [PMID: 13693884]

[4] Thuline HC, Pueschel SM. Cytogenetics in Down syndrome. In: Pueschel SM, Rynders JE, Eds. Down Syndrome Advances in Biomedicine and the Behavioral Sciences. Cambridge: Ware Press 1982; p. 133.

[5] Hook EB, Cross PK, Schreinemachers DM. Chromosomal abnormality rates at amniocentesis and in live-born infants. JAMA 1983; 249(15): 2034-8. [http://dx.doi.org/10.1001/jama.1983.03330390038028] [PMID: 6220164]

[6] Mikkelsen M. Down syndrome: cytogenetical epidemiology. Hereditas 1977; 86(1): 45-50. [http://dx.doi.org/10.1111/j.1601-5223.1977.tb01211.x] [PMID: 143464]

[7] Antonarakis SE, Lewis JG, Adelsberger PA, *et al.* Parental origin of the extra chromosome in trisomy 21 using DNA polymorphism analysis. N Engl J Med 1991; 324: 872-6. [http://dx.doi.org/10.1056/NEJM199103283241302] [PMID: 1825697]

[8] Sherman SL, Allen EG, Bean LH, Freeman SB. Epidemiology of Down syndrome. Ment Retard Dev Disabil Res Rev 2007; 13(3): 221-7. [http://dx.doi.org/10.1002/mrdd.20157] [PMID: 17910090]

[9] Antonarakis SE, Petersen MB, McInnis MG, *et al.* The meiotic stage of nondisjunction in trisomy 21: determination by using DNA polymorphisms. Am J Hum Genet 1992; 50(3): 544-50. [PMID: 1347192]

[10] Carpenter AT. Chiasma function. Cell 1994; 1:77(7): 957-62. [PMID: 7766240]

[11] Pacchierotti F, Eichenlaub-Ritter U. Environmental hazard in the aetiology of somatic and germ cell aneuploidy. Cytogenet Genome Res 2011; 133(2-4): 254-68. [http://dx.doi.org/10.1159/000323284] [PMID: 21228560]

[12] Eichenlaub-Ritter U, Wieczorek M, Lüke S, Seidel T. Age related changes in mitochondrial function and new approaches to study redox regulation in mammalian oocytes in response to age or maturation conditions. Mitochondrion 2011; 11(5): 783-96. [http://dx.doi.org/10.1016/j.mito.2010.08.011] [PMID: 20817047]

[13] Torfs CP, Christianson RE. Socioeconomic effects on the risk of having a recognized pregnancy with Down syndrome. Birth Defects Res A Clin Mol Teratol 2003; 67(7): 522-8. [http://dx.doi.org/10.1002/bdra.10071] [PMID: 14565624]

[14] Hunter JE, Allen EG, Shin M, *et al.* The association of low socioeconomic status and the risk of having a child with Down syndrome: a report from the National Down Syndrome Project. Genet Med 2013; 15(9): 698-705. [http://dx.doi.org/10.1038/gim.2013.34] [PMID: 23558253]

[15] Ghosh S, Feingold E, Chakraborty S, Dey SK. Telomere length is associated with types of chromosome 21 nondisjunction: a new insight into the maternal age effect on Down syndrome birth.

Hum Genet 2010; 127(4): 403-9.
[http://dx.doi.org/10.1007/s00439-009-0785-8] [PMID: 20063167]

[16] Nussbam RL, McInnes RR, Willard HF. Thompson & Thompson: Genetics in Medicine. (6th edition.) Philadelphia:: W.B: Saunders Company 2001; pp. 157-62.

[17] Grasso M, Giovannucci Uzielli ML, Pierluigi M, Tavellini F, Perroni L, Dagna Bricarelli F. Isochromosome not translocation in trisomy 21q21q. Hum Genet 1989; 84(1): 63-5.
[http://dx.doi.org/10.1007/BF00210673] [PMID: 2532615]

[18] Shaffer LG, McCaskill C, Haller V. Further characterization of 19 cases of rear (21q21) and delineation as isochromosomes or robertsonian translocation in Down syndrome. Am J Med Genet 1993; 1:47(8): 1218-22.
[PMID: 2532615]

[19] Robinson WP, Bernasconi F, Basaran S, *et al.* A somatic origin of homologous Robertsonian translocations and isochromosomes. Am J Hum Genet 1994; 54(2): 290-302.
[PMID: 8304346]

[20] Papavassiliou P, York TP, Gursoy N, *et al.* The phenotype of persons having mosaicism for trisomy 21/Down syndrome reflects the percentage of trisomic cells present in different tissues. Am J Med Genet A 2009; 15;149A(4): 573-83.
[http://dx.doi.org/10.1002/ajmg.a.32729.] [PMID: 19291777]

[21] Epstein CJ. The consequence of chromosomal imbalance. Am J Med Genet 1990; (Supp 7)31-7.
[PMID: 2149968]

[22] Delabar JM, Theophile D, Rahmani Z, *et al.* Molecular mapping of twenty-four features of Down syndrome on chromosome 21. Eur J Hum Genet 1993; 1(2): 114-24.
[PMID: 8055322]

[23] Becker W, Sippl W. Activation, regulation, and inhibition of DYRK1A. FEBS J 2011; 278(2): 246-56.
[http://dx.doi.org/10.1111/j.1742-4658.2010.07956.x] [PMID: 21126318]

[24] Guedj F, Pereira PL, Najas S, *et al.* DYRK1A: a master regulatory protein controlling brain growth. Neurobiol Dis 2012; 46(1): 190-203.
[http://dx.doi.org/10.1016/j.nbd.2012.01.007] [PMID: 22293606]

[25] Tejedor FJ, Hämmerle B. MNB/DYRK1A as a multiple regulator of neuronal development. FEBS J 2011; 278(2): 223-35.
[http://dx.doi.org/10.1111/j.1742-4658.2010.07954.x] [PMID: 21156027]

[26] Park J, Oh Y, Yoo L, *et al.* Dyrk1A phosphorylates p53 and inhibits proliferation of embryonic neuronal cells. J Biol Chem 2010; 8;285(41): 31895-906.
[http://dx.doi.org/10.1074/jbc.M110.147520] [PMID: 20696760]

[27] Yabut O, Domagauer J, D'Arcangelo G. Dyrk1A overexpression inhibits proliferation and induces premature neuronal differentiation of neural progenitor cells. J Neurosci 2010; 17;30(11): 4004-14.
[http://dx.doi.org/10.1523/JNEUROSCI.4711-09.2010] [PMID: 20237271]

[28] Kurabayashi N, Sanada K. Increased dosage of DYRK1A and DSCR1 delays neuronal differentiation in neocortical progenitor cells. Genes Dev 2013; 15;27(24): 2708-1.
[http://dx.doi.org/10.1101/gad.226381.113] [PMID: 24352425]

[29] García-Cerro S, Martínez P, Vidal V, *et al.* Over expression of Dyrk1A is implicated in several cognitive, electrophysiological and neuromorphological alterations found in a mouse model of Down syndrome. PLoS One 2014; 4;9(9): e106572.
[http://dx.doi.org/10.1371/journal.pone.0106572] [PMID: 25188425]

[30] Martinez-Cue ´C, Delatour B, Potier MC. Treating enhanced GABAergic inhibition in Down syndrome: Use of GABA alfa5-selective inverse agonists. Neurosci Biobehav Rev 2014; 9 pii: S0149-7634(14)00002-5.
[http://dx.doi.org/10.1016/j.neubiorev.2013.12.008] [PMID: 24412222]

[31] Levitt GA, Stiller CA, Chessells JM. Prognosis of Down's syndrome with acute leukaemia. Arch Dis Child 1990; 65(2): 212-6.
[http://dx.doi.org/10.1136/adc.65.2.212] [PMID: 2138446]

[32] Ragab AH, Abdel-Mageed A, Shuster JJ, *et al.* Clinical characteristics and treatment outcome of children with acute lymphatic leukemia and Down syndrome. A Pediatric Oncology Group study. Caner 1990; 67: 1057-63.
[http://dx.doi.org/10.1002/1097-0142(19910215)67:4<1057::AID-CNCR2820670432>3.0.CO;2-K]

[33] Kim GJ, Lee ES. Prenatal diagnosis of transient abnormal myelopoiesis in a Down syndrome fetus. Korean J Radiol 2009; 10(2): 190-3.
[http://dx.doi.org/10.3348/kjr.2009.10.2.190] [PMID: 19270866]

[34] Gamis AS, Alonzo TA, Gerbing RB, *et al.* Natural history of transient myeloproliferative disorder clinically diagnosed in Down syndrome neonates: a report from the Children's Oncology Group Study A2971. Blood 2011; 22;118(26): 6752-9. quiz 6996
[http://dx.doi.org/10.1182/blood-2011-04-350017] [PMID: 21849481]

[35] Vardiman JW, Thiele J, Arber DA, *et al.* The 2008 revision of the World Health Organization (WHO) classification of myeloid neoplasms and acute leukemia: rationale and important changes. Blood 2009; 30;114(5): 937-51.
[http://dx.doi.org/10.1182/blood-2009-03-209262] [PMID: 19357394]

[36] Roper RJ, Reeves RH. Understanding the basis for Down syndrome phenotypes. PLoS Genet 2006; 2:e50: 16596169.
[http://dx.doi.org/10.1371/journal.pgen.0020050] [PMID: 16596169]

[37] Cantor A, Orki S. Transcriptional regulation of erythropoiesis: an affair involving multiple partners. Oncogene 2002; 13;21(21): 3368-76.
[http://dx.doi.org/10.1038/sj/onc/1205326] [PMID: 12032775]

[38] Shivdasani RA. Molecular and transcriptional regulation of megakaryocyte differentiation. Stem Cells 2001; 19(5): 397-407.
[http://dx.doi.org/10.1634/stemcells.19-5-397] [PMID: 11553848]

[39] Wechsler J, Greene M, McDevitt MA, *et al.* Acquired mutations in GATA1 in the megakaryoblastic leukemia of Down syndrome. Nat Genet 2002; 32(1): 148-52.
[http://dx.doi.org/10.1038/ng955] [PMID: 12172547]

[40] Ahmed M, Sternberg A, Hall G, *et al.* Natural history of GATA1 mutations in Down syndrome. Clinical observations, interventions, and therapeutic trials. Blood 2004; 103(7): 2480-9.

[http://dx.doi.org/10.1182/blood-2003-10-3383] [PMID: 14656875]

[41] Groet J, McElwaine S, Spinelli M, *et al.* Acquired mutations in GATA1 in neonates with Down's syndrome with transient myeloid disorder. Lancet 2003; 10;361(9369): 1617-20.
[http://dx.doi.org/10.1016/S0140-6736(03)13266-7] [PMID: 12747884]

[42] Crispino JD. GATA1 mutations in Down syndrome: Implications for biology and diagnosis of children with transient myeloproliferative disorder and acute megakaryoblastic leukemia. Pediatr Blood Cancer 2005; 44(1): 40-.
[http://dx.doi.org/10.1002/pbc] [PMID: 15390312]

[43] Alford KA, Reinhardt K, Garnett C, *et al.* Analysis of GATA1 mutations in Down syndrome transient myeloproliferative disorder and myeloid leukemia. Blood 2011; 25;118(8): 2222-38.
[http://dx.doi.org/10.1182/blood-2011-03-342774] [PMID: 2171530]

[44] Bercovich D, Ganmore I, Scott LM, *et al.* Mutations of JAK2 in acute lymphoblastic leukaemias associated with Down's syndrome. Lancet 2008; 372(9648): 1484-92.
[http://dx.doi.org/10.1016/S0140-6736(08)61341-0] [PMID: 18805579]

[45] O'Brien MM, Taub JW, Chang MN, *et al.* Cardiomyopathy in children with Down syndrome treated for acute myeloid leukemia: a report from the Children's Oncology Group Study POG 9421. J Clin Oncol 2008; 20;26(3): 414-20.
[http://dx.doi.org/10.1200/JCO.2007.13.2209] [PMID: 18202418]

[46] Lemieux N, Malfoy B, Forrest GL. Human carbonyl reductase (CBR) localized to band 21q22.1 by high-resolution fluorescence *in situ* hybridization displays gene dosage effects in trisomy 21 cells. Genomics 1993; 15(1): 169-72.
[http://dx.doi.org/10.1006/geno.1993.1024] [PMID: 8432528]

[47] Kalabus JL, Sanborn CC, Jamil RG, Cheng Q, Blanco JG. Expression of the anthracycline-metabolizing enzyme carbonyl reductase 1 in hearts from donors with Down syndrome. Drug Metab Dispos 2010; 38(12): 2096-9.
[http://dx.doi.org/10.1124/dmd.110.035550] [PMID: 20729274]

[48] Grossman TR, Gamliel A, Wessells RJ, *et al.* Over-expression of DSCAM and COL6A2 cooperatively generates congenital heart defects. PLoS Genet 2011; 7(11): e1002344.
[http://dx.doi.org/10.1371/journal.pgen.1002344] [PMID: 22072978]

[49] Ackerman C, Locke AE, Feingold E, *et al.* An excess of deleterious variants in VEGF-A pathway genes in Down-syndrome-associated atrioventricular septal defects. Am J Hum Genet 2012; 5;91(4): 646-59.
[http://dx.doi.org/10.1016/j.ajhg.2012.08.017] [PMID: 23040494]

[50] Ripoll C, Rivals I, Ait Yahya-Graison E, *et al.* Molecular signatures of cardiac defects in Down syndrome lymphoblastoid cell lines suggest altered ciliome and Hedgehog pathways. PLoS One 2012; 7(8): e41616.
[http://dx.doi.org/10.1371/journal.pone.0041616] [PMID: 22912673]

[51] Locke AE, Dooley KJ, Tinker SW, *et al.* Variation in folate pathway genes contributes to risk of congenital heart defects among individuals with Down syndrome. Genet Epidemiol 2010; 34(6): 613-23.
[http://dx.doi.org/10.1002/gepi.20518] [PMID: 20718043]

[52] Sailani MR, Makrythanasis P, Valsesia A, *et al.* The complex SNP and CNV genetic architecture of the increased risk of congenital heart defects in Down syndrome. Genome Res 2013; 23(9): 1410-21. [http://dx.doi.org/10.1101/gr.147991.112] [PMID: 23783273]

[53] Anderson MS, Venanzi ES, Klein L, *et al.* Projection of an immunological self shadow within the thymus by the aire protein. Science 2002; 298(5597): 1395-401. [http://dx.doi.org/10.1126/science.1075958] [PMID: 12376594]

[54] Skogberg G, Lundberg V, Lindgren S, *et al.* Altered expression of autoimmune regulator in infant down syndrome thymus, a possible contributor to an autoimmune phenotype. J Immunol 2014; 1;193(5): 2187-95. [http://dx.doi.org/10.4049/jimmunol.1400742] [PMID: 25038256]

[55] Satgé D, Sasco AJ, Carlsen NL, *et al.* A lack of neuroblastoma in Down syndrome: a study from 11 European countries. Cancer Res 1998; 58(3): 448-52. [PMID: 9458088]

[56] OÂ Reilly MS, Boehm T, Shing Y, *et al.* Endostatin: an endogenous inhibitor of angiogenesis and tumor growth. Cell 1997; 24; 88(2): 277-85. [http://dx.doi.org/10.1016/S0092-8674(00)81848-6] [PMID: 29008168]

[57] Zorick TS, Mustacchi Z, Bando SY, *et al.* High serum endostatin levels in Down syndrome: implications for improved treatment and prevention of solid tumours. Eur J Hum Genet 2001; 9(11): 811-4. [http://dx.doi.org/10.1038/sj.ejhg.5200721] [PMID: 11781696]

[58] Brideau G, Mäkinen MJ, Elamaa H, *et al.* Endostatin overexpression inhibits lymphangiogenesis and lymph node metastasis in mice. Cancer Res 2007; 67(24): 11528-35. [http://dx.doi.org/10.1158/0008-5472.CAN-07-1458] [PMID: 18089781]

[59] Minami T, Horiuchi K, Miura M, *et al.* Vascular endothelial growth factor- and thrombin-induced termination factor, Down syndrome critical region-1, attenuates endothelial cell proliferation and angiogenesis J Biol Chem 2004; 26;279(48): 50537-4. [http://dx.doi.org/10.1074/jbc.M406454200] [PMID: 15448146]

[60] Ryeom S, Folkman J. Role of endogenous angiogenesis inhibitors in Down syndrome. J Craniofac Surg 2009; 20 (Suppl. 1): 595-6. [http://dx.doi.org/10.1097/SCS.0b013e3181927f47] [PMID: 19795527]

[61] Reynolds LE, Watson AR, Baker M, *et al.* Tumour angiogenesis is reduced in the Tc1 mouse model of Down's syndrome. Nature 2010; 10;465(7299): 813-7. [http://dx.doi.org/10.1038/nature09106] [PMID: 20535211]

[62] Luque A, Carpizo DR, Iruela-Arispe ML. ADAMTS1/METH1 inhibits endothelial cell proliferation by direct binding and sequestration of VEGF165 J Biol Chem 2003; 278(26): 23656-65. [http://dx.doi.org/10.1074/jbc.M212964200] [PMID: 1271691]

[63] Birdsey GM, Dryden NH, Amsellem V, *et al.* Transcription factor Erg regulates angiogenesis and endothelial apoptosis through VE-cadherin. Blood 2008; 111(7): 3498-506. [http://dx.doi.org/10.1182/blood-2007-08-105346] [PMID: 18195090]

[64] Xu W, Ye P, Li Z, Shi J, Wang W, Yao K. Endostar, a recently introduced recombinant human

endostatin, inhibits proliferation and migration through regulating growth factors, adhesion factors and inflammatory mediators in choroid-retinal endothelial cells. Mol Biol (Mosk) 2010; 44(4): 664-70. [http://dx.doi.org/10.1134/S0026893310040138] [PMID: 20873226]

[65] Wang J, Sun Y, Liu Y, *et al.* Results of randomized, multicenter, double-blind phase III trial of rh-endostatin (YH-16) in treatment of advanced non-small cell lung cancer patients. Zhongguo Fei Ai Za Zhi 2005; 20;8(4): 283-90. [http://dx.doi.org/10.3779/j.issn.1009-3419.2005.04.07] [PMID: 21108883]

[66] Lee JC, Shin J, Baek KH. Trisomy of the Dscr1 gene suppresses early progression of pancreatic intraepithelial neoplasia driven by oncogenic Kras. Biochem Biophys Res Commun 2013; 11;440(1): 50-. [http://dx.doi.org/10.1016/j.bbrc.2013.09.033] [PMID: 24041692]

[67] Shin J, Lee JC, Baek KH. A single extra copy of Dscr1 improves survival of mice developing spontaneous lung tumours through suppression of tumour angiogenesis. Cancer Lett 2014; 1;342(1): 70-81. [http://dx.doi.org/10.1016/j.canlet.2013.08.047] [PMID: 24051307]

[68] Huang XY, Zhang XM, Chen FH, *et al.* Anti-proliferative effect of recombinant human endostatin on synovial fibroblasts in rats with adjuvant arthritis. Eur J Pharmacol 2014; 723(723): 7-14. [http://dx.doi.org/10.1016/j.ejphar.2013.10.068] [PMID: 24239715]

[69] Greene AK, Kim S, Rogers GF, Fishman SJ, Olsen BR, Mulliken JB. Risk of vascular anomalies with Down syndrome. Pediatrics 2008; 121(1): e135-40. [http://dx.doi.org/10.1542/peds.2007-1316] [PMID: 18166531]

[70] Brait VH, Martin KR, Corlett A, *et al.* Over-expression of DSCR1 protects against post-ischemic neuronal injury. PLoS One 2012; 7(10): e47841. [http://dx.doi.org/10.1371/journal.pone.0047841] [PMID: 23144708]

[71] Zhang J, Christianson RE, Torfs CP. Fetal trisomy 21 and maternal preeclampsia. Epidemiology 2004; 15(2): 195-201. [http://dx.doi.org/10.1097/01.ede.0000112141.09008.37] [PMID: 15127912]

[72] Jiang J, Jing Y, Cost GJ, *et al.* Translating dosage compensation to trisomy 21. e Nature 2013; 15;500(7462): 296-300. [http://dx.doi.org/10.1038/nature12394] [PMID: 23863942]

CHAPTER 3

Neonates with Down Syndrome

Mohammed Al-Biltagi*, **Adel A. Hagag**

Pediatric Department, Faculty of Medicine, Tanta University, Egypt

Abstract: Neonates with DS have many co morbidities that jeopardize this critical period of life with increased morbidity and mortality. They have more incidences of congenital heart diseases, pulmonary disorders, epilepsies, gastrointestinal anomalies, hematological problems as well as feeding disorders. They need to recognize their problems and for early intervention that could improve their medical conditions as well as their quality of life.

Keywords: Amniocentesis, Airway Abnormalities, Chorionic villus sampling, Congenital heart defects, Cordocentesis, Down syndrome, Endocrine Disorders, Eye, Feeding, Free fetal DNA, Gastrointestinal, Growth, Hematologic Disorders, Neonates, Nuchal translucency, Orthopedic Disorders, Persistent pulmonary hypertension of the neonate, Prenatal screening, Prevention, Quadruple screening, Triple screen, Ultrasonography.

1. INTRODUCTION

Trisomy 21 (Down syndrome) is the most common numerical chromosomal anomalies among live born babies. Down syndrome (DS) is the most common type of developmental disability caused by a microscopically confirmable chromosomal abnormality. It affects more than 5 million people all over the world. It has a well defined characteristic typical and phenotypic features and natural history. The symptoms related to the underlying diagnosis can appear in practically every organ system. Early identification of DS in the newborn is necessary to supply adequate care for the newborns and support for their parents and family; although at times the physical features may be difficult to identify in a

* **Corresponding Author Dr. Mohammed Al-Biltagi:** Pediatric Department, Faculty of Medicine, Tanta University, Egypt; Tel: (+973)39545472; Fax: (+973) 1759 0495; Email: mbelrem@hotmail.com

newborn especially when premature and in mosaic form of DS where there are a wide variation in expression of the disorder according to the percentage of cells that carry the extra chromosome 21, the phenotype may be milder than that of classic trisomy 21 [1]. With the modern advances of the genetic studies of chromosomes, principally chromosome 21, has led to new understanding and awareness on diseases. The capability to recognize and expect the outcome of patients with DS offers the healthcare suppliers the chance to develop individual distinctive approaches to a comprehensive care of neonates with DS [2].

2. DIAGNOSIS OF DOWN SYNDROME

2.1. Antenatal Diagnosis

Antenatal diagnosis of DS helps to achieve an informed decision-making with regard to pregnancy continuation or termination and can help the family to make an appropriate choice. There are two fundamental categories of tests available to detect DS during pregnancy; screening and diagnostic tests.

2.1.1. Prenatal Screening

Pregnancy screening for fetal aneuploidy began in the mid 1960s, using maternal age as the screening tool. Screening programs for DS are well established in many countries with recent advances in prenatal screening tests in the last decades. The pregnant women should be well educated about the benefits, safety and risk of these screening tests. Screening tests help to stratify the baby's risk of having DS and to decide the need of further diagnostic test. These tests do not offer precise and confirmed diagnosis, but they are safer than the diagnostic test for both the mother and the fetus. However, screening tests can occasionally provide false positive and false negative results with sensitivity of multiple marker screening tests for DS is between 61 and 67 % [3]. These tests are recommended for women who are of at more risk to have a pregnancy affected by DS. The benefits and disadvantages of these tests should be discussed before the pregnancy has reached 15 weeks as they are not routinely recommended. It is now achievable to provide all pregnant women with a non-invasive screening test to stratify their risk of having a fetus with aneuploidy and to determine the need for invasive prenatal diagnostic testing. A wide range of interventions has been launched to help the pregnant women to choose the proper prenatal screening. Screening tests usually comprise a combination of a blood test, which estimates the quantity of a variety of materials in the mother's blood (*e.g.* Pregnancy-associated plasma protein A (PAPP-A), beta human chorionic gonadotropin (beta-hCG) and MS-alpha-fetoprotein (AFP) and an ultrasound [4].

There are multiple antenatal screening strategies for DS in the first and second trimesters; and usually done in combination with more than a screening tool. For example; one strategy in Belgium is to combine the nuchal translucency (NT) ultrasound measure at week 12 (weeks 11–14), the level of free-β-human chorionic gonadotropin hormone and pregnancy associated plasma protein-A, in combination with age and medical history [3]. Currently available non-invasive screening choices include maternal age combined with one of the following: (1) first trimester screening (nuchal translucency, maternal age, and maternal serum biochemical markers), (2) second trimester serum screening (maternal age and maternal serum biochemical markers), or (3) 2-step integrated screening, which includes first and second trimester serum screening with or without nuchal translucency (integrated prenatal screen, serum integrated prenatal screening, contingent, and sequential) [5].

2.1.1.1. Prenatal Blood Screening Tests

These tests depend on measuring the levels of various fetal or placental proteins and hormones in the pregnant lady blood. There are two main screening tests used for DS pregnancy; the combined screening test (the preferred approach) and the quadruple test for women who present later during the pregnancy or where combined screening cannot be carried out. The combined screening test combines the result of the nuchal translucency (NT) scan with the result of blood tests for Pregnancy Associated Plasma Protein A (PAPP-A) and Free beta human chorionic gonadotropin (beta-hCG) to stratify the relative risk of having a child with Down syndrome. The blood tests and the scan are frequently done at the same time. The chance estimation depends on the levels of these materials in the maternal blood, maternal age, her weight and the duration of pregnancy. Typically this blood test is done between 10 to 14 weeks of pregnancy. This test is used to screen only for DS and trisomy 18. On the other hand; the maternal serum levels of both alpha-fetoprotein and unconjugated estriol are often lower than normal for maternal and gestational age in women who are carrying a fetus with DS. Combining alpha-fetoprotein and unconjugated estriol and beta-human chorionic gonadotropin is performed in the second trimester and is often referred to as a "triple screen" [6 - 9]. The Quadruple screening test depends on the results of a blood test done between 14 weeks and 2 days and 22 weeks of gestation. It gives most accurate results when done between the 16th and 18th weeks. It is the same like "triple screen" plus Inhibin A which is a hormone released by the placenta. The Quadruple screening test is best indicated when first trimester screening test is not available and even superior to amniocentesis for pregnancies complicated by advanced maternal age. Its results depend on the maternal and the gestational age as well as the ethnicity and maternal weigh. This test is especially indicated for women who are over 35 years old during pregnancy or who on insulin therapy to treat diabetes and for women with a family history of birth defects. Ultrasound scan is not a part of this test [10]. There are certain limitations for these screening tests. For example; first-trimester screening of DS using beta-hCG is not suitable in the case of maternal renal failure [11]. There is also false-positive result that could occur with any of the screening strategies [12]. Taken as a whole, the accuracy and the detection rate for the current screening strategies (the combined first trimester or the quadruple second trimester test) may range between 80% and 85% with a fixed false positive rate of 5% according to the competence of the implemented program with very high sensitivity and specificity [13, 14].

Examination of circulating cell free fetal DNA (CFFDNA) is an efficient and successful screening tool for screening and detection fetal aneuploidy. Detection of this cell-free DNA which released by the fetus into the maternal circulation was first established in 1997. Circulating fetal DNA is therefore obtainable through the collection of a blood sample from the maternal blood without posing any physical harm to the fetus. By examining this source of fetal genetic material, investigators have succeeded in developing DNA-based noninvasive tests for the evaluation of DS and single gene diseases. Since the end of 2011, tests for the noninvasive evaluation of chromosomal aneuploidies have become commercially available in parts of the world. More recently, cell-free circulating fetal DNA analysis have been shown to be applicable to interpreting the fetal molecular karyotype, genome and methylome [15]. The test sensitivity, its success and interpretation reliability depends on and is proportionately related to the amount of circulating cell free (CCF) DNA derived from the feto-placental unit (fetal fraction or FF). Sometimes; the test gives non-useful information such as some fetal disorders are associated with systematically lower FF. With vague results and if the test was done due to presence of ultrasound abnormality; amniocentesis and karyotype/microarray should be considered [16]. On the other hand; false positive CFF-DNA may occurs in certain clinical conditions that necessitates doing diagnostic testing. This needs the practitioners to pay attention and to be able to recognize the limitations of CFF-DNA [17].

2.1.1.2. Prenatal Imaging Screening

Ultrasonography is used for DS screening for the first time since about 25 years ago. Genetic sonogram is a term used to describe various mixtures of markers that could be detectable at second-trimester. The recent and numerous improvements in developments in first-trimester screening and the latest introduction of noninvasive prenatal testing for aneuploidy screening greatly affect the prevalence of these conditions in the second-trimester and the efficiency of the screening accuracy of the genetic sonogram [18]. One of the important sonographic markers that are usually done in the first trimester is measuring the nuchal translucency. This marker may be augmented with nasal bone assessment or other measures. Presence or absence of major anomalies and other soft markers are also used in prenatal screening in the second trimester [19]. There are numerous second-trimester sonographic markers for DS that can be searched for. These include presence of mild ventriculomegaly, increased nuchal fold, hyperechoic bowel, and absent or hypoplastic nasal bone. The genetic sonogram will continue to have a place in prenatal screening despite it has many limitations. It is particularly important in twin and higher-order multiple pregnancies, in countries with limited access to the most recent genetic screening tests, in cases with borderline results at maternal serum screening tests, and as noninvasive supplementary test for high-risk women reluctant to undergo invasive diagnostic testing [18]. Higher detection rates and lower false-positive rates can be achieved by combining first- and second-trimester screening tests than that observed by using maternal age and first- or second-trimester screening alone [19].

A nuchal thickness scan (NT Procedure) is a sonographic prenatal measuring of the size of the nuchal pad at the nape of the fetal neck using high-resolution ultrasound. The ideal timing for this scan is between the 11th and 14th weeks because the accurateness is best during that time. It is used to recognize increased risks for chromosomal conditions like DS in a fetus, particularly with old maternal age. It results from accumulation of fluid under the skin in the clear space in the folds of soft tissue at the back of the developing baby's neck forming what is called nuchal fold observed in the early stage of fetal development. More fluid tends to accumulate in this area in fetuses with heart failure, serious anomaly of the heart and great arteries, and genetic or chromosomal abnormalities. The higher the degree of fetal nuchal translucency (FNT), the more is the risk of presence of such abnormalities [20, 21].

The nuchal fold area is measured it in the longitudinal midline plane of the fetus, using a very standardized technique. There are two different ways of measurements – the nuchal translucency and the nuchal fold. Nuchal translucency is measured earlier in pregnancy at the end of the first trimester, and for which there is a lower threshold for increased diameter, while the nuchal fold is measured towards the end of the second trimester. There is an increased tendency to have more amount of fluid around the neck in fetuses with DS than non-DS syndrome fetuses. The scan may also help to verify both the correctness of the pregnancy dates and the fetal viability. It also can detect other less common chromosomal abnormalities due to its high definition imaging [22, 23]. Some difficulties may interfere with measuring NT as unusual position of the baby or overweight mother. This test has about 20% false positive rate (FPR) and sensitivity of 85%. The risk stratification can be assessed using especial computer program taking into consideration also; the age of pregnant woman, maternal weight, the gestational age, the size of the fetus, and maternal smocking and ethnicity. Combined prenatal screening is always positive for DS when NT thickness exceeded 4.0 mm. The upper NT threshold value depends on 2 factors, the maternal age and the gestational age. In women aged 35 to 37 years, combined prenatal screening is always positive when NT exceeded 2.8 mm, 3.0 mm, and 3.4 mm at 11, 12, and 13 weeks of gestation, respectively. In women over 42 years of age, the upper threshold value for NT was 1.8 mm, 2.4 mm, and 2.7 mm at 11, 12, and 13 weeks of gestation, respectively. In women less than 35 years of age, there are lower threshold values below which combined prenatal screening for DS is always negative. Adding nasal bone screening during the same examination may increase sensitivity further and reduce the false positive results [24].

The nasal bone length normally grows in a linear pattern during pregnancy and the growth pattern is well correlated with the gestational age. Nasal hypoplasia is present both in postnatal and in prenatal life in many cases with trisomy 21. About 65% of trisomy 21 fetuses have absent or short nasal bone discovered by sonographic studies dine at 11–24 weeks of gestation. The absence of fetal nasal bone has a high positive likelihood ratio for DS in the first trimester screening, and the presence of nasal bone may potentially lower the need for invasive testing [25]. Assessment of the fetal nasal bone improves the performance of first-trimester screening for DS [26]. Fetal nasal bone hypoplasia at the second and third trimester scan is associated with a high risk for DS and it can be used as a screening marker for this chromosomal abnormality [27].

The incidence and frequency of shorter femur is increased in DS fetus with a risk of 1/31 pregnancies. However, shorter femur is a poor marker for DS [28, 29]. In the same way; the intracardiac hyperechogenic focus is a controversial marker for DS. It is a common finding among the normal population during the second trimester. However, DS is present in about 10% to 18% of cases present with intracardiac hyperechogenic focus especially when compound with other ultrasound markers. Thus; it has a statistically significant tendency towards an association with increased risk of DS, but when present separately, this marker did not present any significant association with the syndrome. The prevalence of aberrant right subclavian artery (ARSA) seems close to 1% which increases to 8–37% in DS fetuses. Aberrant right subclavian artery in combination with other ultrasound signs increased the risk for trisomy 21, but the independent ability of ARSA as an isolated marker to predict fetal trisomy 21 is unclear [30]. Prenatal diagnosis of ARSA should prompt meticulous anatomic survey, and karyotype analysis might be offered even in the absence of associated findings [31, 32]. Evaluation of the cerebral lateral ventricles is an essential part of the standard sonographic examination of the fetus. Ventricles of normal size provide reassurance of the normal development of the cerebrum. Mild lateral cerebral ventriculomegaly (between 10 to 15 mm between 15 and 40 weeks' gestation) is present in 1/1000 babies [33]. Persistent ventriculomegaly may indicate chromosomal abnormalities [34].

Fetal echogenic bowel is present in 0-6% to 1-4% of all second trimester fetuses and is detectable at the time of routine antenatal ultrasound scanning. Fetal small bowel becomes progressively more visible by ultrasound scan during the second trimester as relatively 'bright' meconium accumulates within its lumen from about 16 weeks' of gestation. There is a higher incidence of echogenic bowel in fetal aneuploidy, especially Trisomy 21 and less frequently trisomy 18 or 13, Turner's syndrome and triploidy. The cause of echogenic bowel in aneuploidy is less clear. It is thought to be due to decreased bowel motility with increased water absorption from the meconium. There appears to be decreased microvillar enzymes activity in the amniotic fluid of aneuploid fetuses [35]. The accuracy of ultrasound as DS screening examination has been improved by combining its findings in the first trimester of pregnancy with biochemical screening in the first and second trimester especially among pregnant women with advanced maternal age [36].

2.1.2. Invasive Prenatal Diagnosis

Invasive diagnostic tests can confirm or to exclude that child will be affected by DS. However, these tests carry more hazards to both mother and fetus. At the same time both screening and diagnostic tests cannot predict the full impact of DS on a baby. Diagnostic tests are usually indicated with a positive screening test in order to confirm DS diagnosis when screening test is above a set risk cut-off level on non-invasive screening or to pregnant women with personal, obstetrical, or family history places them at increased risk [6]. Then an invasive diagnostic test such as chorionic villus sampling or amniocentesis is offered to the high risk mother for definitive diagnosis of affected baby with DS. However; these invasive tests carry a risk of fetal loss of around 1% and cannot be performed until 11 weeks of pregnancy. The risk of miscarriage associated with invasive testing is an important psychological barrier to these diagnostic testing for DS. However, this risk can be avoided using cell-free fetal DNA analysis [37].

2.1.2.1. Amniocentesis

Amniocentesis is an accepted and effective prenatal diagnostic test for chromosomal disorders. It is one of the most common procedures for detecting abnormalities before birth. It is done by a needle aspiration of the amniotic fluid through inserting a needle with ultrasound guidance through the overlying skin into the uterus and amniotic cavity followed by withdrawing a sample through the abdomen for biochemical, cytological and genetic analysis as well as for chromosomal variations. Comparatively big amounts of amniotic fluid (up to 20 ml) could be aspirated without significant technical difficulties. It is frequently applied to women over 35 years of age as they have a greater risk of having a fetus with chromosomal abnormalities than younger women. This test is done between the 16th and 20th weeks of pregnancy. The fluid contains cells that have been shed by the fetus. These cells will be cultured in the laboratory so that the chromosomes in them can be analyzed. However; the amniotic fluid (AF) supernatant contains cell-free fetal DNA (cffDNA) fragments. Trisomy 21 can be prenatally diagnosed by the quantitative fluorescent polymerase chain reaction (QF-PCR) method in AF supernatant. This karyotype analysis method greatly reduces the requirement for the specimen size. It will be a benefit for early amniocentesis and could avoid pregnancy complications. The method may become an ancillary method for prenatal diagnosis of DS [38]. Fluorescence *in situ* hybridization (FISH) kit can be used to rapidly and accurately detect the most common chromosome aneuploidies by using less sample volume with relatively low cost. FISH can be a reliable and rapid prenatal diagnostic tool as an adjunct to classical cytogenetic study. It can be used for rapid and accurate prenatal diagnosis of women with high risk of maternal serum screening [39].

The age of the mother of 35 year and above is an anchor for the pre-determination regarding performing or avoiding amniocentesis. Advanced maternal age (AMA) is the main reason to have amniocentesis and is considered an independent risk factor [40]. The advantage of genetic amniocentesis for the sole indication of AMA is much more benefiting than the potential amniocentesis-related fetal loss rate [41]. Performing amniocentesis prior to 14 weeks leads to higher pregnancy loss rates, increase in talipes and an increase in amniotic fluid leakage [42]. An important side effect of early amniocentesis is that aspiration of large amounts of amniotic fluid earlier in gestation can cause neonatal orthopaedic (talipes) and respiratory complications (respiratory distress syndrome). Analysis of cell-free fetal DNA needs small specimen size and hence allows early amniocentesis. A major drawback of second trimester amniocentesis is that a final result is usually obtainable only after 17 weeks' of pregnancy which may not a suitable time to allow for surgical termination of pregnancy. Second-trimester genetic amniocentesis can result in 0.2% of total pregnancy loss within 4 weeks of testing. This significant risk should be informed to the pregnant ladies as a part of patient counseling before amniocentesis. Specific standards should be followed in order to ensure that damage to the pregnancy is limited [43].

2.1.2.2. Chorionic Villus Sampling

Chorionic villus sampling (CVS) was described for the first time in China in 1975; then passed into further development in the Western world during the 1980s. It is done through ultrasound guided aspiration of placental tissue rather than amniotic fluid. Chorionic villus sampling could be done earlier than the amniocentesis (between 10th and 13th week of pregnancy) and could be done as early as 6 weeks' gestation. Early chorionic villus sampling may be associated with somewhat more risk of failed tissue culture and maternal cell contamination than amniocentesis. If CVS will be done early; much less amniotic fluid is removed than that could be removed in late sampling [44].

There are two methods of CVS, transcervical and transabdominal. The transcervical CVS has a significantly greater risk of pregnancy loss and spontaneous miscarriage. At the same time, transcervical CVS has more difficult technique and has more failure rate to obtain the sample than transabdominal CVS. Transabdominal CVS is preferred over either early amniocentesis or transcervical CVS when earlier diagnosis is indicated. However, with difficult transabdominal CVS, transcervical CVS in the first trimester or second trimester amniocentesis may be indicated [45]. It should be noted that even with normal CVS or amniocentesis result, does confirm that the baby has no abnormalities. Chromosomal mosaicism may increase the chance of false negative results.

2.1.2.3. Cordocentesis [Percutaneous Umbilical Blood Sampling (PUBS)]

Cordocentesis is a diagnostic procedure that checks the fetal umbilical cord blood to detect presence of fetal abnormalities; done after 17 week of gestation. It is the only procedure that provides direct access to the fetal circulation. It is indicated when the diagnosis cannot be confirmed using amniocentesis; CVS; ultrasound or the results of these tests were inconclusive. Ultrasound imaging is used first to identify the insertion of umbilical cord into the placenta is first identified using; then a thin needle is introduced through the abdomen and uterine walls to the umbilical cord where the fetal blood is collected and sent for analysis. The length of the procedure should be shortened as much as possible. Cordocentesis can detect chromosomal abnormalities and certain hematological abnormalities with high levels of accuracy. However; despite being relatively safe, cordocentesis carries the potential risk of miscarriage with a rate between 0.1-0.2/1000 procedures. Bleeding at the puncture site, or infection can occur. Transmission of hepatitis or human immunodeficiency virus may complicate the procedure. Fetal bradycardia and premature rupture of membranes may also occur [46, 47].

2.2. Postnatal Diagnosis

Diagnosis of Down syndrome can be easily done at birth or shortly thereafter by its unique dysmorphic characteristics which may vary from patient to another according to the physical expression of the syndrome and should be confirmed by genetic karyotyping. Diagnosis of DS in the neonatal period can be very challenging. Systematic examination can assess the presence of external clinical features and can help in recognizing neonates with DS and the need for mores investigations to detect presence of associated abnormalities. However, the diagnosis may be overlooked if too much dependence is placed on finding the classic faces.

2.2.1. Physical Examination

A thorough systematic examination should involve all the body parts of the newborn from the head to the toes. The syndrome is usually diagnosed by presence of a triad of hypotonia, the distinctive features and presence of mental retardation. Hypotonia is often the first observed characteristic feature of DS and its presence should raise the index of suspicion and prompt further assessment. Neonates with DS have a poor Moro reflex. The distinctive features of DS predominantly affect the head, neck and extremities. Each characteristic dysmorphic is present in 47 to 82 percent of cases [48]. The head may show many features such as mild microcephaly, brachycephaly with a short and round skull with a flat occiput, large anterior fontanel or a third fontanel along the sagittal suture line. The hair may be silky, fine and soft. They usually have oblique palpebral fissures with upward and outward slanting and prominent epicanthal folds. They may have hypertelorism due to wide nasal bridge. The iris may show grayish white spots of depigmentation seen in a ring around the pupil called Brushfield spots. Presence of cataract or glaucoma should be excluded [49]. The ears may be low set, smaller and may appear posteriorly rotated, folded, with stenotic meatus. They also have a flat face profile with hypoplasia of the midface, small nose and a flat nasal bridge (Fig. **1**). The oral cavity is small with high arched palate. The tongue is of normal size but is protruded due to the small mouth cavity as well as low muscle tone allowing the jaw to hang slack and the tongue to protrude. Babies with DS usually have short neck with loose skin at the nape [50].

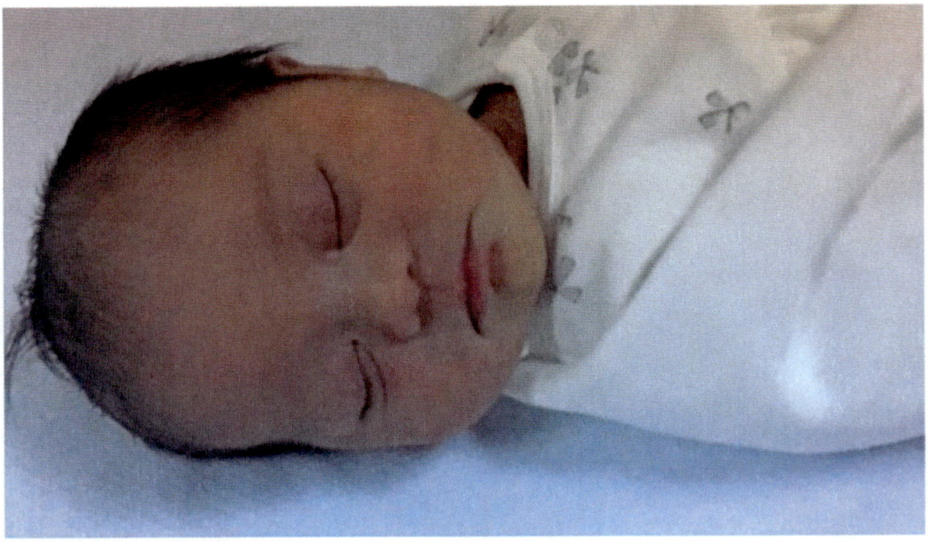

Fig. (1). Showed facial features of Down syndrome in 4 days old baby girl with DS who presented with neonatal jaundice. It showed hypertelorism, oblique palpebral fissures with upward and outward slanting.

The extremities are the second most affected organ after the head in DS neonates. There is generalized muscular hypotonia in approximately 80% of DS newborns with hyperextensible large joints. In general, there is a short stature with broad, square hands and short fingers. There are low-set thumbs that are separated more than usual from the second finger and clinodactyly of the fifth finger. The fifth finger may have only one joint. Simian crease is a single deep transverse crease on the palm of the hand may present on one or both hands (Fig. **2A**). Ectrodactyly is reported in some cases of DS. It is characterized by a deep median cleft of the hand and/or foot due to failure of apical ectodermal ridge while developing limbs [51]. There may be a dysplasia of the pelvis with a narrow acetabular angle and dislocation of knee joint may be observed. Examination of the feet may reveal a wide space with a plantar crease between the first and second toes (sandal sign) (Fig. **2B**). The skin is soft and velvety with cutis marmorata (marbling of skin) is common [52].

(A) **(B)**

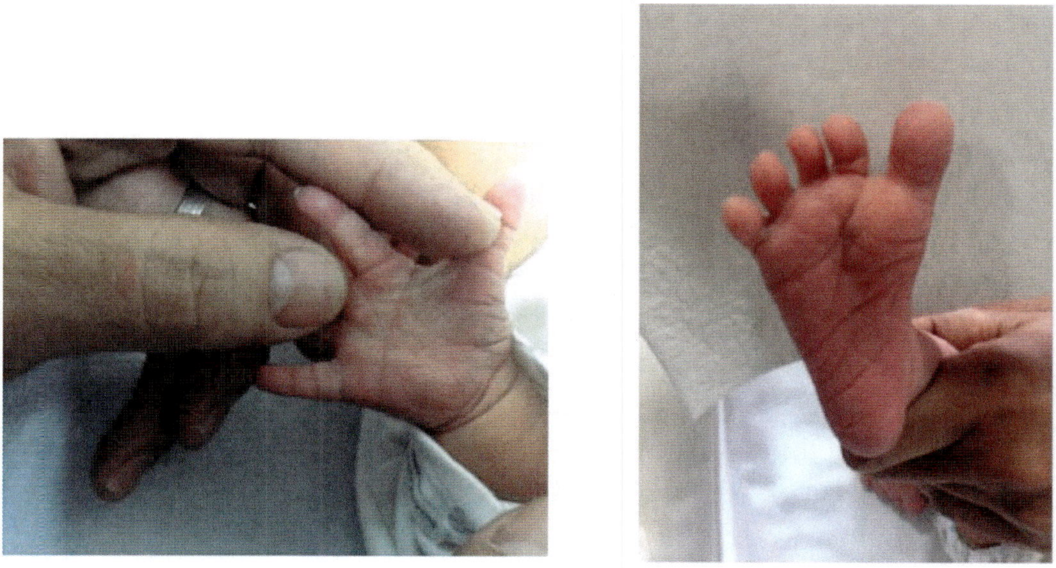

Fig. (2). **(A)** showed presence of Simian crease while **(B)** showed wide space with a plantar crease between the between first and second toes (sandal sign).

The chest should be checked for signs of respiratory distress as there is a high incidence of persistent fetal circulation in neonates with DS. Presence of any cardiac murmur or abnormal heart sounds may indicate presence of congenital heart defects that are seen in approximately 40-60% of infants with DS. Peripheral pulses and oxygen saturation should be checked in 4 limbs to exclude aortic coarctation and ductal-dependant lesions. The abdomen may be distended and should be checked for presence of bowel sounds, masses, and organomegaly. Presence of bilious emesis may indicate a bowel obstruction. The patency of the anus should be checked for imperforate anus [2].

2.2.2. Investigations

Karyotyping of a newborn should be done when DS is suspected. It is necessary to confirm the diagnosis, provide a basis for genetic counseling, and determine the recurrence risk of having another baby with DS. Referral to a medical geneticist for counseling is appropriate, because the risk of having a second child with DS varies with karyotype and maternal age. There are three main genetic types of DS: nondisjunction, translocation, and mosaic. Ninety five % of all patients with DS result from meiotic non-disjunction of the chromosome 21 pair. The underlying meiotic error is of maternal origin in 90% of cases and is of paternal origin in 10% of cases. The risk of DS in a future pregnancy is determined by the genetic type of DS, and by considering maternal age at the time of a future pregnancy and by family history. The risk is relatively low is non-disjunction type but the risk is significant in translocation type. Positive family history raised the index of suspicion for an inherited unbalanced translocation. In general, the expected recurrence risk for mothers who have had an infant with "classic" nondisjunction DS is about 1%. This risk will further increases if maternal age is greater than 40. The recurrence risk for mosaic DS is 1-2%. The recurrence risk of the unbalanced translocation will depend on whether one of the parents has a balanced translocation. The recurrence risk is 12% if the mother is the carrier; and 1% if the father is the carrier [53].

Detection of associated complications can be done with different diagnostic tools. Cardiac assessment can be done by chest radiograph, ECG and referral to Pediatric cardiologist when indicated to do echocardiographic examination as about 50% of infants will have congenital cardiac disease. Full blood count is necessary to assess presence of different haematological problems that are common in DS as thrombocytopenia, transient polycythaemia or even leukaemia. Thyroid function tests are very important investigation to exclude presence of congenital hypothyroidism as congenital hypothyroidism is present in about 1% of infants with DS. Newborn Metabolic Screening card is sufficient. Presence of clinical signs suggestive of hypothyroidism *e.g.* prolonged jaundice; is indication for thyroid function testing as T4 and TSH [54].

2.3. Informing the Parents

Having a baby with DS is real unexpected difficult news to the parents in the newborn setting. Healthcare professionals are the first people to see a baby during the ultrasound or in the delivery room and therefore the first to recognize that the baby may have DS. The parents' happiness of having birth of a new baby is spoiled when they know that he/she has DS. The parents usually respond with distress, anger and/or grief before they accept their child condition. So; it is very important that the professionals take care when making the announcement and to provide support to parents. There were two schools of ways of how to inform the parents of their baby's condition. One school, is that the family should be informed once or as soon as the stage of shock of the mother and as soon as she recovered from the immediate effects of delivery while the other school is to delay informing the parents to give the mother a time to have normal loving bonding to her baby and to give her a time to recover after delivery. Therefore, distressing news should be withheld from her decreasing the possibility of postpartum depression. However, there is no standard consensus and guidelines for physicians till now [55]. Not all the parents react in the same way in response for this breaking news. Some will consider it as a crisis while others are not. So, it is important to build strategies to help the parents to cope with this news including family support during their early contact with the infant and explanations with accurate information of the infant's condition and plan of care.

All newborns with DS - whether diagnosed prenatally or postnatally - should be examined by a neonatologist. The obstetricians and pediatricians jointly should be the persons responsible to convey the news, to the new parents in a private situation as soon as a physician suspects a diagnosis of DS. The parents should be informed at the same time and together, if feasible. However, sometimes, it is wise to inform the father first then discuss the situation and the how to inform the mother. Presenting the diagnosis to families must be accomplished in a supportive, positive, caring, and honest manner. Conversations should start with positive words. Language should be clear, and straightforward. Language that conveys pity or sorrow should be avoided. A balanced point of view of the condition with accurate, up-to-date information and explanation of its genetic nature should be offered. Unsolicited personal opinions should be avoided. The parents should be given the time they need to realize and digest the news. They also should have enough times to ask questions. Repeated visits may be essential to deal with queries and distress. Referral to genetic service is recommended for discussion of recurrence risk, particularly if the trisomy is due to a chromosome translocation or if other chromosomal abnormalities are found on karyotype examination [55].

3. GROWTH AND DEVELOPMENTAL CHARACTERISTICS OF NEONATES WITH DS

Neonates with DS may have normal growth parameters at birth. Then the growth rate starts to reduce with the nadir of growth velocity is most reduced between 6 months and 3 years of age. They have lower percentiles as regard to neonatal length, weight, and head circumference than in the control infants except for weight/length percentiles denoting that growth deceleration of children with DS begun prenatally; and overweight begins after birth [56]. Short stature is a principal feature in most children with DS. Average height at most ages is around the 2nd percentile for the general population. Presence of additional medical conditions (*e.g.* congenital cardiac, sleep related upper airway obstruction, coeliac disease, nutritional inadequacy due to feeding problem; and thyroid hormone deficiency) may additionally impair the growth. Growth charts are very useful for early detection of additional growth impairment. So; using growth charts specific for children with DS is required [57].

Normal neonates have a weight loss of 5% in the first week of life in bottle fed infant and of 7-10% in the first week for the breastfed infant. This early weight loss may exceed 10% of the weight in newborns with DS and usually needs more than two weeks to reach their birth weight. However, in absence of serious medical problem, most of those babies reach a centile close to their birth centile by the fourth week of their postnatal life. If the early weight loss which is greater than 10% failed to be recovered quickly or if there is a delay in regaining birth weight more than 4 weeks; careful clinical evaluation for presence of associated complications as feeding difficulties or major underlying pathology should be done. Breast feeding should be promoted and maintained.

Most babies with DS are born prematurely usually at 38 weeks of gestation. The centile lines on the UK-WHO Neonatal and Infant Close Monitoring (NICM) chart are very comparable to those for babies with DS. So, it is recommended to plot measurements of preterm babies with DS using this chart. At the same time, modification for prematurity should be done in any case till the end of the first year (corrected age) for infants who were born between 32-36 week of gestation and p to 2 corrected age years for those who were born before 32 weeks. After, the age of 4 weeks; the baby's weight may not track a certain centile line but usually tracks within one centile space. Because of the increased incidence of poor growth patterns at any age in infants with DS; it is always essential to evaluate the child's general health condition and put into consideration the need for additional assessment and investigation as many systemic health disorders can affect growth and causing feeding difficulties are more common in DS [58]. Growth retardation (as noted in both height and head circumference references) was also observed in otherwise healthy children with DS especially during 3 critical periods of growth (during pregnancy, during the first three years of life, and during puberty). This growth retardation results in shorter final stature and smaller head circumference when compared to the general population [59].

In general, there is no typical pattern of development in children with DS. However, they have characteristic developmental delays. There may also be other differences in the way children with DS develop when compared with children who do not have DS. At the same time; children with the syndrome are as different from each other as are all children. They usually have delayed motor skills; generally due to the generalized hypotonia observed in DS kids. They can support head between 3-5 months instead of 3 months for the typical developed infants. They start to rolls over at approximately 8 months rather than 5 months in the typically developed infants. They usually can sit alone between 6 and 16 months of age (average 9 months) compared to 5 to 9 months in the typically developed infants. They will be able to stand alone at approximately age 18 months compared to 11 months in the typically developed infants. They can walk alone at the age of 2 years compared to 1 year for the normal children. Because of this expected delay; they should not be compared in their development with other children. It was noted that there is greater difference in age between typical healthy infants and those with DS in the more complex skills [60]. However, the progression of motor development of the DS is following the same course as that observed in the typical infants except that they need more time to acquire skills, mainly antigravitational ones, among them in the standing position [61].

The verbal development in children with DS showed definitive delay. On the other hand; the social skill showed developmental lag only in reciprocal smile. However, they are social and with good visuo-spatial skills which is considered as relative strengths in the syndrome but they have weak verbal skills and motor planning. Interestingly; some studies showed that children with translocation and mosaicism have better mean age of achievement of developmental milestones than that of children with trisomy. However; some studies rejected these differences [62, 63].

4. MEDICAL PROBLEMS COMMON IN NEONATES WITH DS

4.1. Congenital Heart Diseases

Congenital cardiac defects are present in about half of infants with DS (40 - 60 %). They also are more liable to have pulmonary hypertension, mitral valve prolapse, aortic regurgitation and many other acquired cardiac conditions. The most common anomalies are complete atrioventricular canal defects (60 %), ventricular septal defects (32 %), followed by tetralogy of Fallot (6 %), ostium secundum atrial septal defect (1 %) and isolated mitral cleft (1 %) [64]. Neonates with DS have an increased prevalence of persistent pulmonary hypertension of the neonate (PPHN). They have an increased risk of developing PPHN even in the absence of structural heart disease and should be followed until resolution of the pulmonary hypertension [65]. Hypertrophic cardiomyopathy with complete atrioventricular canal defect was reported in an infant with trisomy 21 [66]. There is also a report for development of biventricular hypertrophic cardiomyopathy and pericardial effusion as a complication of transient neonatal myeloproliferative disorder [67]. Accordingly, all newborn babies with DS should be examined with an electrocardiogram and if possible with a screening echocardiogram in the first postnatal month, even if there is no audible murmur.

4.2. Gastrointestinal Abnormalities

Higher incidence of various gastrointestinal abnormalities is observed in neonates with DS (4-10%) compared to the non-syndromic neonates. These anomalies are important cause of morbidity during the first year of life. These anomalies include oesophageal atresia/trachea-esophageal fistula (0.3-0.8%), pyloric stenosis (0.3%), duodenal stenosis/atresia (1-5%), Hirschsprung disease (1-3%) and anal stenosis/atresia (<1-4%).These defects are more frequent in the DS population, as much as 25–30% of all cases of duodenal defects are in children with DS [68]. Coexistence of imperforate anus without a fistula, and Hirschsprung disease, was reported in a female neonate with DS [69]. It was observed that DS neonates who presented with gastrointestinal abnormalities are more liable to have a relatively high prevalence rate of congenital hypothyroidism [70]. There is also a higher incidence of cardiac malformations among neonates and children who have gastrointestinal anomalies. So, it is wise to do cardiac evaluation as early as possible for all patients with gastrointestinal system malformations [71].

Gastro-esophageal reflux and swallowing dysfunction are common in neonates with DS. It can be asymptomatic or presented with respiratory distress and tachypnea secondary to aspiration [72]. Dysphagia can occur in some neonates with DS who have an aberrant right subclavian artery which is relatively common in DS neonates (19-36%) compared to non-syndromic neonates. It may cause impairment to the passage of solid food through the esophagus and induce feeding difficulties. Impaired oral motor function, gastro-esophageal reflux and other congenital disorders are other causes of feeding problems in children with DS [73]. Constipation is a real health trouble in children with DS and occurs mainly as a consequence of the hypotonia. However, in serious cases, Hirschprung disease should be excluded. Congenital hypothyroidism may be another reason for abdominal distension and constipation. Constipation may also be a manifestation of food allergy in DS children but not in neonates [1]. Compared to Non-DS children, children with DS who were subjected to surgical correction of Hirschprung disease are more prone to an increased rate of postoperative complications and longer hospital stay. During long-term follow-up; most patients with DS are severely constipated and have an increased incidence of enterocolitis [74].

4.3. Upper Airway Abnormalities

Otorhinolaryngological disorders are common in neonates with DS due to their facial anatomy, narrow ear canals and often weaker immune system. Otorhinolaryngological disorders have special importance in neonates and children with DS because of their high incidence and severity and their role in increasing the DS-related morbidity. Midface hypoplasia is a constant finding in children with DS. It impairs the nasopharyngeal function and induces Eustachian tube dysfunction. Bony borders of the nasopharynx are narrow in DS children which cause relative narrowing airways by the normal sized soft tissue of the nasopharynx and induction of Eustachian tube dysfunction. Chronic middle ear disease and chronic rhinorrhoea are caused by mid-face problems, together with hypotonia and macroglossia (children with DS have a relatively large tongue compared to the oral cavity) [75]. Laryngomalacia is one of the most common disorders seen in neonates with DS [50]. Systemic co-morbid conditions are present in 93% of cases. Gastroesophageal reflux disease is the most common co morbidity. Infants with DS have increased risk of hearing loss (HL). Normal and adequate hearing capabilities at one year of age have an important role in language development. Implementation of newborn hearing screening program is important for early detection and diagnosis of hearing loss during first year of life [76]. Early detection and proper management of hearing loss is more likely to improve language abilities that may indirectly influence educational vocational costs and may increase lifetime productivity. Evaluation of hearing loss using auditory brainstem response testing should be done at the age of 6 months in infants with DS (if such testing was not done earlier) [77].

4.4. Respiratory Abnormalities

Respiratory problems are a major reason of sickness and death in neonates with DS. Exacerbation of the respiratory problems in neonates occurs due to existence of airway abnormalities (*e.g.* tracheolaryngomalacia, pulmonary anatomical changes like abnormal lung growth, pulmonary hypoplasia, and subpleural cysts); presence of congenital heart diseases (CHD) with haemodynamic instability; and as a result of hypotonia [78]. Infection with respiratory syncytial virus (RSV) is more frequent and is associated with increased risk of hospitalization in children with DS. Recurrent wheeze is very common among children with DS (it is found in up to 36%) and is related to previous RSV infection and to other factors such as tracheomalacia [79]. Neonate with DS have also higher incidence of persistent pulmonary hypertension of the newborn (PPHN) compared with the general population [80, 81].

4.5. Endocrine Disorders

Thyroid gland disorders are the most common endocrinopathies associated with DS. Thyroid disorders occur in up to 28–40% of children with DS, and their frequency increases up to 54%, with increasing age. These disorders could be overt producing symptoms and signs that can be detected or can be subclinical and missed unless being in mind. Clinically manifest disorder can either due to hyper function (hyperthyroidism) or hypo function (overt hypothyroidism) of the gland. Subclinical hypothyroidism (SH) is usually presented with by hyperthyrotropinemia, elevated TSH and normal T4 levels. About 50% of all children with DS may have an increased levels of TSH with normal levels of T3 and T4, which suggest presence of subclinical hypothyroidism [82]. DS Infants particularly male infants had high levels of TSH at neonatal screening, indicating the presence of mild hypothyroidism already in early life. However; TSH levels could not predict development of obvious thyroid disease later in childhood [83]. The decreased T4 concentration and mildly elevated TSH concentrations point to a mild hypothyroid state in newborns with DS and support the existence of a DS-specific thyroid (regulation) disorder [84]. Symptoms of hypothyroidism are non-specific and can be missed with manifestations of DS. Due to the importance of thyroid hormones to the brain development and functions; early detection and treatment of hypothyroidism is warranted to avoid jeopardizing the already jeopardized brain functions. Since the symptoms of thyroid disease often simulate the general symptoms present in DS, a sensitive thyroid-stimulating hormone test should be performed at least yearly [85].

Primary hypogonadism commonly occurs in male patients with an extra sex chromosome or autosome at the time of puberty due to meiotic germ-cell failure. Primary hypogonadism may involve a combined dysfunction of Sertoli and Leydig cells, which can present independently of presence or absence of cryptorchidism soon after birth [86]. Interestingly, diabetes mellitus is more frequent in children with DS (occurs in about 1%). Congenital diabetes is an extremely rare form of diabetes and differs from type I or type II diabetes. It was reported in a neonate with DS and later it was proved to be permanent diabetes. It seems to be due to a selective beta cell defect with undetectable C-peptide but normal alpha-cell function [87].

4.6. Ophthalmic Disorders

Ocular abnormalities occur in more than half of children with DS. Most of these ocular malformations in DS are generally of a minor nature, and comprise a variety of nonspecific hyperplasia or hamartomata, hypoplasia, tissue defects and heterotopias. These involve virtually every portion of the globe [88]. The most frequent ocular characteristics in DS according to the order of incidence are: slanting palpebral fissures, epicanthus, refractive errors (myopia, astigmatism), iris abnormalities (Brushfield spots), strabismus, blepharitis, lacrimal obstruction, retinal changes (increased retinal vasculature), amblyopia, nystagmus and cataracts. Lacrimal system dysfunction is relatively common in neonates with DS. The most frequent cause of congenital epiphora in DS is due to functional block of the lacrimal pump. Eyelid muscle hypotonia and eyelid changes, common in DS, are the main hypothesis of lacrimal dysfunction [89]. Children with DS are more prone to both congenital and acquired cataracts than other children. DS are present in about 3–5% of cases presented with congenital or infantile cataract. This necessitates that the red (fundus) reflexes should be checked at birth [90]. Keratoconus is rare in childhood but develops later in life in individuals with DS. Visual screening is essential for detecting defects that can be treated. An early start is especially important in finding congenital cataract. It was recommended that infants with DS should have an ophthalmic evaluation in within the first 6 months of life, with subsequent follow up examinations to be performed every 1–2 years during childhood and adolescence [1].

4.7. Hematologic Disorders

Newborns with DS may have thrombocytopenia (up to 66%) and polycythaemia (up to 33%). Polycythemia may be asymptomatic or symptomatic and results in hypoglycemia or respiratory problems. There is no relationship between thrombocytopenia and polycythemia. Neonates with DS showed significantly higher incidence of presence of circulating blasts than in the reference group. However, thrombocytopenia occur significantly more frequently in DS neonates with presence of circulating blasts than in those with no circulating blasts. So; thrombocytopenia should be differentiated from pre-leukaemia. Complete blood count screening should be performed routinely in DS neonates [91].

About 10 % of newborns with DS develop transient myeloproliferative disorder (leukemoid reaction; TMD) which is extremely rare in other infants. It is a self-limiting disease distinguished by leukocytosis and the presence of megakaryoblasts in the peripheral blood and bone marrow, anaemia, thrombocytopenia, and organomegaly. DS cases with severe form of TMD may present with hepatic fibrosis which is characterized by diffuse intralobular sinusoidal fibrosis and extramedullary haematopoiesis [92]. Children with DS have an increased risk of developing both acute myeloid as well as lymphoblastic leukaemia. These leukaemias have specific presenting additional characteristics cytogenetic changes besides the constitutional trisomy 21, and underlying biologies. Myeloid leukaemia in children with DS may be preceded by a preleukaemic clone (transient myeloproliferative disorder, TMD), which may disappear spontaneously but may need treatment when symptoms are severe. Twenty percent of children with transient leukaemia subsequently develop myeloid leukaemia, usually with an onset before the age of 5 [92].

The treatment of leukemia in children with DS is the same as in other children. However, the toxicity of some chemotherapeutic agents is increased in patients with Down syndrome [93]. Phenotypically normal infants who exhibit leukemoid reactions within the first two months of life should be evaluated by karyotyping for mosaic DS [94]. Children with DS have lowered T- and B-lymphocyte counts and functions which may explain part of their susceptibility to infections. On the other hand, there is a lower allergy risk in children with DS. There is no specific clinical picture in relation to disturbances of the immune system, which means that screening is not useful [95].

4.8. Orthopedic Disorders

The skeletal system of children with DS is distinguished by presence of generalized hypotonia which causes ligamentous laxity, and joint hypermobility presenting in a variety of ways. Children with DS may have occipitocervical, atlantoaxial instability, hyperflexibility, scoliosis, late hip dislocation (after two years of age), slipped capital femoral epiphysis, patellar subluxation or dislocation, and various forms of foot deformities. Previously, X-ray imaging of the flexed and extended cervical spine are recommended as screening tests for atlantoaxial instability when those children reach the age of two years or before they undergo general anesthesia. Although screening radiographs are controversial, 13 % of children with DS have asymptomatic atlantoaxial instability that should be monitored and may prevent them from participation in contact sports [96]. Due to the relative immune deficiency in DS; a case of neonatal osteomyelitis was reported in neonate with DS. It was caused by non-encapsulated *Haemophilus influenzae* biotype I, which was isolated from pus at the site of infection [97].

Coexistence of Marfan syndrome in neonates with DS may mask the usual phenotypic features of DS which suggests the possible interaction of the two syndromes. Co-occurrence of achondroplasia and DS was also described in 6 cases. The appearance has some features from both conditions and the diagnosis can be done by physical examination, radiography, cytogenetic study, and mutation analysis. Radiographic examination may show typical findings of achondroplasia, such as disproportionately large skull, shortening of limb segments, and lumbar lordosis. Genetic studies may show the underlying defect *e.g.* G1138A mutation. This co-occurrence may be due to interaction of these two distinct genetic disorders in the same patient produces a phenotype typical of each syndrome with some overlapping signs [98 - 100].

4.9. Urinary Tract Disorders

Children with DS have significantly increased risk of urinary tract anomalies (3.2%). They also have significantly elevated risks of anterior urethral obstruction, cystic dysplastic kidney, hydronephrosis, hydroureter, hypospadias, posterior urethral valves, prune belly syndrome, and renal agenesis. On the other hand; there is no significantly increased risk of ectopic kidney or ureteropelvic junction obstruction in the DS population [101]. Severe obstructive uropathy may result in Potter's sequence and an early perinatal death. So; a chromosomal analysis is recommended in any case of obstructive uropathy in the fetal or neonatal period [102].

Children with DS frequently have associated neurogenic or functional bladder dysfunction, which can lead to upper urinary tract deterioration. Symptoms of urinary tract anomalies may be missed as many of these symptoms (*e.g.* voiding disorders and delayed toilet training) are usually perceived as a consequence of delayed psychomotor development. Urinary tract anomalies such as hydronephrosis, hydroureter, renal agenesis and hypospadias must be considered in children with DS. For early detection of these anomalies; it is mandatory to do early and regular sonographic and urodynamic evaluation of the bladder function [103]. Unfortunately, there are no available specific guidelines towards the attitude in delay in daytime and nighttime continence in children with DS. Besides the standard treatment, visual instruction is helpful as well as showing them how to do. The advice is to start training at the moment the child can sit properly and understand the items stool, urine and toilet. Improved understanding and identification of the various urological anomalies associated with DS will aid in the care of these patients [104].

4.10. Dermatological Disorders

Skin is one of the organs that are affected by the chromosomal aberration in DS. There are certain dermatoglyphic manifestations more common in DS than in normal population. There are reduced frequency of digital whorls; presence of a high (*i.e.* distally placed) palmar axial triradius associated with a large hypothenar pattern, transverse arrangement of ridges over the distal palm; and over the hallucal area of the sole (which consists of the first interdigital and thenar distal areas combined). A tibial arch or open field is characteristic. The latter configuration is rare in normal individuals, in whom a true pattern in the form of a loop or whorl is usual. Although the above findings occur occasionally in normal people, they are common in people with DS [105].

DS is associated with rare dermatological disorders and increased frequency of some common dermatoses. The skin findings such as xerosis and Mongolian spots are the most frequently seen in the neonates with DS. Seborrheic dermatitis, cheilitis and fissured tongue are seen frequently, as well. Other skin conditions observed in DS include; plantar hyperkeratosis, alopecia areata, geographic tongue, café-au-lait macula, livedo reticularis, cutaneous infections, pityriasis capitis simplex, cutis marmorata, neurotic excoriation, trichotillomania, keratosis pilaris and diaper dermatitis. The prevalence of the skin disorders including Mongolian spot, seborrheic dermatitis, cheilitis, and fissured tongue are significantly higher in patients with DS than normal individuals [106]. If there is palmoplantar hyperkeratosis, the serum vitamin A levels should be evaluated as it may be a result of vitamin A deficiency [107]. Other rare but DS-specific problems are elastosis perforans serpiginosa and milia-like idiopathic calcinosis cutis [108]. Atopic dermatitis has lower prevalence in DS than in non-syndromic children [109].

4.11. Neurological Disorders

Neurological disorders in children with DS, (excluding cognitive delay and hypotonia) are common problems and its prevalence can reach 40% of them. Motor ocular disorders and epilepsy are the predominant disorders detected. There is a wide diversity in clinical expression of neurological manifestations in DS, which requires a high index of suspicion and a systematic search by the clinician caring for children with DS [110]. The prevalence of epilepsy in DS population is approximately 1-13%. It increases to 8% in children with DS; about 40% of these cases started in infancy and often presenting as infantile spasm or West syndrome. Infantile spasms occur in 0.6-13% of children with DS, representing 4.5-47% of seizures in these children. Curiously, these patients have electroencephalographic (EEG) characteristics of idiopathic rather than symptomatic infantile spasm. It appears that DS patients have better seizure control compared to other patients with symptomatic infantile spasms, and early initiation of appropriate treatment may contribute to the prevention of late seizure development and better developmental outcome. Lennox-Gastaut syndrome exhibits also some distinctive features in children with DS including later onset and high incidence of reflex seizures. Other seizure types including partial and generalized tonic clonic seizures have also been described in children with DS. There is a high rate of EEG abnormalities in children with DS, even among children without epilepsy, however, no patterns specific to DS have been identified and EEG does not correlate with outcome. Various cellular and molecular mechanisms contribute to epileptogenesis in DS and offer an interesting field of study [111]. It is likely that the increased seizure susceptibility is due to a combination of medical risk factors and inherent neurologic abnormalities characteristic of DS. It is recommended that all DS children with seizures undergo investigations to determine the etiology of the seizure [112].

4.12. Dental Disorders

Different forms of oro-facial anomalies and problems are present in children with DS including skeletal anomalies and neonatal teeth. Skeletal anomalies include mid-face hypoplasia, with depressed bridge of the nose, and relatively small in size of the bones of the mid-face and maxilla. Narrow palate due to abnormally thick sides of the palate is relatively common in children with DS. This narrow palate may occasionally give the impression of a high arched palatal. However, the height is generally not significantly greater than normal. Cleft lip and/or palate are reported in 3%-5% of DS patients [113]. Natal teeth may present in the upper or lower jaws. These teeth may cause anxiety of the parents that may need immediate removal [114].

5. FEEDING NEONATE AND INFANT WITH DS

Care of neurologically impaired infants usually is complex and challenging. Feeding a baby with DS can be a real challenge. Mothers of these infants who want to breastfeed should be supported, given sound information, and assisted to set realistic expectations [115].

5.1. Breastfeeding

Breastfeeding is the ideal type of feeding for a neonate with DS. It is easier to digest than other formulas and is associated with decreased rates of both upper and lower f respiratory infections, as well as a lower rate of otitis media, respiratory allergy, and atopic diseases than bottle feeding. Breastfeeding has in addition more stimulating effect on the oral motor development, which help proper development of speech. At the same time, breast feeding enhances maternal-infant bonding which is a critical process; starts in early infancy and continues over the next few years. The psychological benefit derived from this maternal-infant attachment is extremely important, because of the infant's disability, so the mother may not trust her own competence. If the baby has difficulty in direct breastfeeding (*e.g.* due to hypotonia, cardiac defects, or prematurity); expression of the breastmilk may be beneficial in improving the child health as well as the mother's emotional well-being [116]. In this condition, it is better to encourage the mother to feed the infant expressed milk by various methods, such as a nursing supplementer or a bottle, or, occasionally, by gavage feeding. After numerous weeks, the infant will have better sucking ability, and becomes capable of nursing effectively [117].

Down syndrome babies are less likely to breastfed compared with normal children. The main reasons are increased incidence of the infants' illness, being sleepy in the early postnatal weeks, presence of sucking and swallowing abnormalities, and coincidence of maternal frustration or depression due to having a handicapped newborn. Adequacy of breastfeeding can be judged by the weight gain. If the breast-feeding infant is not achieving adequate weight, sufficient concern should be directed to partial supplementation with formula or additional expressed breast milk. A nursing supplementer may also help to supply extra caloric intake while the infant continues to breast feed [118]. If the baby is too much sleepy, the infant should get up to feed at least every three hours, or every two hours if only on-demand breast feeding is being used and is inadequate to provide both the caloric and nutritional needs of the infant and for encouragement of the mother's milk supply. The mother may need to pump her breasts to enhance the production of a sufficient supply of milk. To avoid gastro-esophageal reflux which is relatively more common in infants with DS; the feeding infant can be held in a semi sitting position and keeping the bottle correctly angled to prevent swallowing of air with numerous burping of the child [117]. Support in breastfeeding should become a significant tip of health supervision for children with DS. A lactation consultant may help the mother to choice the proper way of lactation, and assess the adequacy of nursing [116].

5.2. Bottle Feeding

Bottle feeding can be tried if the baby has poor weight gain with the breast feeding, has a problem with latching, has a hard time to suck or if the mother prefers to use formula feeding. The mother should also be supported and asked to awaken her infant at least every 3 hours to guarantee enough caloric and nutritional intakes. No specific formula is currently recommended except if there is a particular medical disorder, or if there is failure to gain adequate weight gain. Formula additives or gavage feeding may be needed in infants with very reduced weight gain. However, bottle feeding still has many problems as the same latching and swallowing problems as nursing. The mother may need to try different bottle nipple types, including some that slow the flow of liquids, before finding the one that works best for the infant. If the baby has a lot of difficulty swallowing and regurge, the mother can use special anti-reflux formula or adding a thickening agent to the formula [120, 121].

5.3. Weaning

The diet of an infant with DS should be introduced gradually according to the usual scheme for the food groups. However, there are many factors that can delay the introduction of solids to them and interfere with developing efficient oral and feeding skills such as delayed teething, small size mouth cavity, hypotonia of the facial and tongue muscles, large tongue, and high arched palate. Many DS children suffer from mouth breathing due to narrow nasal passages, and may have problems with coordinating sucking, swallowing and breathing whilst feeding [122].

When the baby is physical and emotionally ready to try solid foods such as rice cereal or pureed fruits and vegetables, an adaptive feeding chair can help to support the head, neck, and body upright while feeding. All babies are messy eaters when they first try solid foods; it is normal for them to spit out the food as they get familiar with the texture and taste and figure out the chewing and swallowing process. But because babies with DS have thicker tongues with low muscle tone, it may take them longer to learn how to coordinate the tongue and jaw movements necessary to consume solid foods. This means feeding times may go on for a while. If the baby starts to tire in the middle of a feeding, the mother may need to shorten the sessions and feed the baby more frequently (six to eight times a day) until more food is taken in than spit out. The parents should know that they need more patience to train a child with DS to feed from a spoon and to drink from a cup. Sometimes parents prefer delaying the weaning process, depending on their child's feeding skills. Some infants with DS may require the help of a Pediatric Dietitian for feeding difficulties, poor weight gain, weaning advice, and oral sensitivity [116].

5.4. Feeding Problems for Neonates and Infants

Babies with DS have a lot of systemic health problems. About 40-60% of them have congenital heart defects which interfere with proper weight gain and they usually undernourished. They may need high caloric intake and nutritional support before and after corrective cardiac surgery [123]. Abnormal increase in child weight is one of the classic features of congenital hypothyroidism. Thyroid function should always be evaluated in those with rapid weight gain. Proper thyroid hormone treatment will help to control weight gain. Diet supplementation with Zinc was found to briefly improve thymic function. In addition; thymic functions were found to be related to the pituitary-thyroid axis. Children with low zinc levels may show improvement of thyroid function with zinc supplementation, thus reducing the incidence of subclinical hypothyroidism [124].

The incidence of coeliac disease in DS is more common than in non-syndromic children. A gluten-free diet is required to manage coeliac disease for life. Constipation is a common trouble in infants and children with DS due to generalized low muscle tone and delayed walking. High fiber diet and adequate fluid intake may help in constipation management. Laxatives may be needed as well. Structural disorders of the gastrointestinal tract are more prevalent in infants and children with DS. These anomalies need nutritional support either before or after the surgical correction. Assistance from a specialist dietitian is needed. Infants and children with DS are liable for repeated infections. These infections as well as prescribed medications including the antibiotics with affect the child appetite as well as increase the metabolic state. Daily intake and inclusion of probiotic yoghurt or probiotic yoghurt drink may stimulate the growth of beneficial healthy bacteria in the intestines following antibiotic use. The child's nutritional status, his growth and well-being can be affected by food refusal and loss of his as a result of associated of illness. High caloric diet may be needed after recovery according to the tolerance of the child [125].

Many children with DS are intolerant to lactose, and can het benefit and fell better with the use of a milk-free diet. Low-lactose or lactose-free milk can be use. However some milk products like yoghurt can be well tolerated. Other types of food intolerance including food allergies may be encountered in children with DS. Some parents of children with DS may prefer to eliminate cow's milk from their child's diet due to symptoms related to allergy as blocked or runny nose, and wheeze, irritability, colic, or crying. However, use of other milk formula should be used with cautions. Goat's milk as well as rice milk is not advised for children. The goat's milk protein is less nutritious than that in cow's milk, while rice milk should be avoided before the age of four and half years. At the same, soya infant formula should be avoided before the age of 6 months and preferable not to be used before the age of 2 years. Dietary restriction should be avoided as possible and used only when extremely indicated as it can lead to nutritional deficiency and failure to thrive. It should be done under complete dietary supervision [126, 127].

5.5. Nutritional Intervention in Neonates and Infants with DS

There is marked oxidant stress in DS population as evidenced by the increased activity of some important antioxidant enzymes, together with decreased glutathione levels in whole blood and elevated uric acid levels in plasma, probably as an antioxidant compensation related to the redox imbalance in DS individuals and cause profound disturbance of the antioxidant defense system. These reactive oxygen radicals are generated due to encoding gene mutation, which disproportionately elevates the activity of superoxide dismutase [128, 129]. The heart is one of the affected organs by this oxidative stress. The most important antioxidants available in the diet are vitamins (A, C and E), beta-carotene, co-enzyme Q and the minerals (zinc and selenium). Antioxidant supplement can reduce the risk of leukemia in DS. Antioxidant intervention with vitamins E and C attenuated the systemic oxidative damage present in DS patients [130].

Dietary vitamin supplements have been recommended for children with DS with the assumption of improving of the cognitive capabilities, or immune or thyroid function. Vitamins A, C and E, zinc and selenium; all are well known to help to improve the resistance to infection. There are lower blood levels of vitamins B in DS children which are essential to preserve adequate and healthy function of the nervous system. Night time supplementation with vitamin B6 together as well as the essential amino acids is intended to stimulate the growth hormone during sleep, which in turn improves growth. However, certain vitamin supplements when taken in high doses are likely to be toxic and may impair liver function. Excess vitamin A in excess may result in neurologic and dermatologic abnormalities; while excess vitamin C can induce urinary tract irritation and increased frequency. However; the long-term side effects of megavitamin therapy are not identified. At the same time, study done in 2008 showed an increased risk for AML associated with regular multivitamin use during the first year of life or for an extended duration [131].

DHA (Docosahexaenoic acid, a fatty acid) is a vital fatty acid for proper correction and maintenance of the cell walls of the nerves of the brain and retina protecting them from the damage induced by the free radicals and helps to recover the induced damage. The availability of DHA is the main reason for the higher I.Q. and lower rate of schizophrenia in breast-fed children than non-breast-fed. So, it is imperative for breast-feeding mothers to make sure that they have a high and adequate supply of DHA. DHA is also adequately available in oily fish, and to a lesser degree in some meats and eggs. It is also present in many well known products of fish oils. Flax seed oil (linseed oil) is one of the best sources of omega

3 fatty acids. The body can produce a certain amount of DHA from flaxseed oil and other oils high in linolenic acid [132].

One study confirmed that constant shortage of serine and excess of cysteine and lysine can be caused by over expression of certain genes on the 21st chromosome. However, another study failed to confirm such abnormalities in serum or urinary amino acid levels. Some supporters asserted that over expression of the cystathione beta-synthase gene can induce a "functional" folic acid deficiency in which serum levels are normal but the body can't use all of it and is unable to repair the damaged DNA. Supplementation is supposed to alleviate this assumed problem. This theory needs to be confirmed by further scientific studies. Amino acid supplements can induce unpleasant odor in the user's urine and sweat [133, 134]. The amino acid tryptophan is needed and used by the body to synthesize serotonin. People with DS have low serum serotonin levels [135]. However, low serotonin levels in the brain cannot be confirmed in people with DS due to inability to study it in the current time. Oral intake of 5-hydroxytryptophan, a compound the body uses to make serotonin, failed to produce noticeable benefits [136].

6. IMMUNIZATION OF NEONATE AND INFANT WITH DS

Immunodeficiency associated with DS is not a contraindication for vaccination. Vaccinations can prevent a good number of infectious diseases that children with DS could be exposed to. Appropriate vaccinations are tremendously essential, due to increased frequency of and susceptibility to upper respiratory, ear, nose and throat infections as a result of frequent association of structural anomalies in DS infants. All infants with DS should be given the ordinary recommended sequence of vaccination: diphtheria-tetanus toxoids- pertussis vaccine, intramuscular and live oral poliovirus vaccines, *Hemophilus influenzae* type b polysaccharide vaccine, pneumococcal vaccine, meningococcal vaccine and measles-mumps-rubella combination vaccine. The hepatitis B vaccine series should be started at birth, whether the child will be living in an institutional setting or at home. This vaccine series is necessary because persons with DS are more liable to develop a carrier state if they are infected with hepatitis B virus. Annual influenza vaccination has been recommended as another way to reduce the rate of otitis media in infants and children with DS. Varicella vaccine should be given when children with DS reach the age of one year. When these children are two years old, the administration of polyvalent pneumo- coccal vaccine should be considered [137 - 139].

7. PREVENTION OF DS

7.1. Primary Prevention

Down syndrome cannot be prevented. However, some preventative measures (such as avoiding late reproduction, pre-implantation genetic diagnosis and folic acid supplementation) could be considered. To make further progress there is an urgent need to refocus etiological research so as to build on recent findings [140].

7.2. Secondary Prevention

Recently; significant interest has been directed to the so-called 'secondary' prevention of DS through prenatal screening followed by invasive prenatal diagnosis and termination of affected pregnancies. In the past; women were selected for prenatal diagnosis on the basis of high risk – largely advanced maternal age or family history. However, this had non-significant effect on the birth prevalence since most cases occur without any specific indication. Moreover, the advanced age group includes a disproportionate number who would not accept pregnancy termination for religious reasons and many who would not accept the hazards of invasive prenatal diagnosis after an extended period of infertility. Today the situation is very different. Antenatal screening using multiple biochemical and ultrasound markers is routine in developed countries. The best techniques are now capable of detecting more than 90% of affected pregnancies and this approach appears to be generally acceptable to pregnant women. These successes with so-called 'secondary' prevention have not been matched with progress in primary prevention [141, 142].

CONFLICT OF INTEREST

The authors confirm that this chapter contents have no conflict of interest.

ACKNOWLEDGEMENTS

Declared none.

REFERENCES

[1] American Academy of Pediatrics. Committee on Genetics. American Academy of Pediatrics: Health supervision for children with Down syndrome. Pediatrics 2001; 107(2): 442-9.

[2] Ranweiler R. Assessment and care of the newborn with Down syndrome. Adv Neonatal Care 2009; 9(1): 17-24.
[http://dx.doi.org/10.1097/01.ANC.0000346090.05240.ab] [PMID: 19212160]

[3] Neyt M, Hulstaert F, Gyselaers W. Introducing the non-invasive prenatal test for trisomy 21 in Belgium: a cost-consequences analysis. BMJ Open 2014 Nov 7; 4(11): e005922.
[http://dx.doi.org/10.1136/bmjopen-2014-005922] [PMID: 25380810]

[4] Wax JR, Cartin A, Chard R, Lucas FL, Pinette MG. Noninvasive prenatal testing: impact on genetic counseling, invasive prenatal diagnosis, and trisomy 21 detection. J Clin Ultrasound 2015; 43(1): 1-6.
[http://dx.doi.org/10.1002/jcu.22243] [PMID: 25303161]

[5] Chitayat D, Langlois S, Wilson RD. Prenatal screening for fetal aneuploidy in singleton pregnancies. J Obstet Gynaecol Can 2011; 33(7): 736-50.
[PMID: 21749752]

[6] Powell KJ, Grudzinskas JG. Screening for Down syndrome in the first trimester. Reprod Fertil Dev 1995; 7(6): 1413-7.
[http://dx.doi.org/10.1071/RD9951413] [PMID: 8743140]

[7] Grandjean H, Sarramon MF. Sonographic measurement of nuchal skinfold thickness for detection of Down syndrome in the second-trimester fetus: a multicenter prospective study. The AFDPHE Study Group. Association Francaise pour le Depistage et la Prevention des Handicaps de l'Enfant. Obstet Gynecol. Obstet Gynecol 1995; 85(1): 103-6.
[http://dx.doi.org/10.1016/0029-7844(94)00327-A] [PMID: 7800304]

[8] Vintzileos AM, Egan JF, Smulian JC, Campbell WA, Guzman ER, Rodis JF. Adjusting the risk for trisomy 21 by a simple ultrasound method using fetal long-bone biometry. Obstet Gynecol 1996; 87(6): 953-8.
[http://dx.doi.org/10.1016/0029-7844(96)00058-0] [PMID: 8649705]

[9] DeVore GR, Alfi O. The use of color Doppler ultrasound to identify fetuses at increased risk for trisomy 21: an alternative for high-risk patients who decline genetic amniocentesis. Obstet Gynecol 1995; 85(3): 378-86.
[http://dx.doi.org/10.1016/0029-7844(94)00384-P] [PMID: 7862376]

[10] Kwon JY, Park IY, Kwon SM, Kim CJ, Shin JC. The quadruple test for Down syndrome screening in pregnant women of advanced maternal age. Arch Gynecol Obstet 2012; 285(3): 629-33.
[http://dx.doi.org/10.1007/s00404-011-2052-1] [PMID: 21837420]

[11] Rozenberg P, BussiA"res L, Senat MV. [Down syndrome screening in France: the worst consensus]. J Gynecol Obstet Biol Reprod (Paris) 2007; 36(2): 95-103.

[http://dx.doi.org/10.1016/j.jgyn.2006.12.021] [PMID: 17289296]

[12] Valentin M, Muller F, Beaujard MP, *et al.* First-trimester combined screening for trisomy 21 in women with renal disease. Prenat Diagn 2014; 14
[http://dx.doi.org/10.1002/pd.4528]

[13] Benn PA, Ying J, Beazoglou T, Egan JF. Estimates for the sensitivity and false-positive rates for second trimester serum screening for Down syndrome and trisomy 18 with adjustment for cross-identification and double-positive results. Prenat Diagn 2001; 21(1): 46-51.
[http://dx.doi.org/10.1002/1097-0223(200101)21:1<46::AID-PD984>3.0.CO;2-C] [PMID: 11180240]

[14] Shaw SW, Chen CP, Cheng PJ. From Down syndrome screening to noninvasive prenatal testing: 20 years ?(tm) experience in Taiwan. Taiwan J Obstet Gynecol 2013; 52(4): 470-4.
[http://dx.doi.org/10.1016/j.tjog.2013.10.003] [PMID: 24411028]

[15] Chiu RW. Noninvasive prenatal testing by maternal plasma DNA analysis: current practice and future applications. Scand J Clin Lab Invest Suppl 2014; 244: 48-53.
[http://dx.doi.org/10.3109/00365513.2014.936681] [PMID: 25083893]

[16] Palomaki G, Kloza E, Lambert-Messerlian G. Circulating cell free DNA testing: are some test failures informative? Prenat Diagn 2015 Mar; 35(3): 289-93.
[http://dx.doi.org/10.1016/j.tjog.2013.10.003] [PMID: 24411028]

[17] Clark-Ganheart CA, Iqbal SN, Brown DL, Black S, Fries MH. Understanding the Limitations of Circulating Cell Free Fetal DNA: An Example of Two Unique Cases. J Clin Gynecol Obstet 2014; 3(2): 38-70.
[http://dx.doi.org/10.14740/jcgo229w] [PMID: 25298847]

[18] Odibo AO, Ghidini A. Role of the second-trimester ?~genetic sonogram ?(tm) for Down syndrome screen in the era of first-trimester screening and noninvasive prenatal testing. Prenat Diagn 2014; 34(6): 511-7.
[http://dx.doi.org/10.1002/pd.4329] [PMID: 24436177]

[19] Shamshirsaz AA, Ravangard SF, Turner G, *et al.* Efficacy of the genetic sonogram in a stepwise sequential protocol for down syndrome screening. J Ultrasound Med 2013; 32(9): 1607-13.
[http://dx.doi.org/10.7863/ultra.32.9.1607] [PMID: 23980222]

[20] Bijok J, Ziora-Jakutowicz K, Ilnicka A, Dangel J, Jakiel G, Roszkowski T. [Increased nuchal translucency in chromosomally normal fetuses and pregnancy outcomes--a retrospective study]. Ginekol Pol 2013; 84(3): 172-9.
[PMID: 23700843]

[21] Pandya PP, Brizot ML, Kuhn P, Snijders RJ, Nicolaides KH. First-trimester fetal nuchal translucency thickness and risk for trisomies. Obstet Gynecol 1994; 84(3): 420-3.
[PMID: 8058241]

[22] Renna MD, Pisani P, Conversano F, *et al.* Sonographic markers for early diagnosis of fetal malformations World J Radiol 2013 Oct; 5(10): 356-71.
[http://dx.doi.org/10.4329/wjr.v5.i10.356] [PMID: 24179631]

[23] Czuba B, Borowski D, Cnota W, *et al.* Ultrasonographic assessment of fetal nuchal translucency (NT) at 11th and 14th week of gestation--Polish multicentre study. Neuroendocrinol Lett 2007; 28(2): 175-81.

[PMID: 17435666]

[24] Miron P, CÔté YP, Lambert J. Nuchal translucency thresholds in prenatal screening for Down syndrome and trisomy 18. J Obstet Gynaecol Can 2009; 31(3): 227-35.
[PMID: 19416569]

[25] Has R, Kalelioglu I, Yuksel A, Ibrahimoglu L, Ermis H, Yildirim A. Fetal nasal bone assessment in first trimester down syndrome screening. Fetal Diagn Ther 2008; 24(1): 61-6.
[http://dx.doi.org/10.1159/000132409] [PMID: 18504384]

[26] Kagan KO, Cicero S, Staboulidou I, Wright D, Nicolaides KH. Fetal nasal bone in screening for trisomies 21, 18 and 13 and Turner syndrome at 11-13 weeks of gestation. Ultrasound Obstet Gynecol 2009; 33(3): 259-64.
[http://dx.doi.org/10.1002/uog.6318] [PMID: 19248005]

[27] Xie HN, Zhu YX, Li LJ, He H. [Ultrasonographic fetal nasal bone assessment in prenatal screening for Down syndrome]. Zhonghua Fu Chan Ke Za Zhi 2008; 43(3): 171-4.
[PMID: 18788563]

[28] Shipp TD, Bromley B, Mascola M, Benacerraf B. Variation in fetal femur length with respect to maternal race. J Ultrasound Med 2001; 20(2): 141-4.
[PMID: 11211134]

[29] Kovac CM, Brown JA, Apodaca CC, *et al.* Maternal ethnicity and variation of fetal femur length calculations when screening for Down syndrome. J Ultrasound Med 2002; 21(7): 719-22.
[PMID: 12099558]

[30] De León-Luis J, Gámez F, Bravo C, *et al.* Second-trimester fetal aberrant right subclavian artery: original study, systematic review and meta-analysis of performance in detection of Down syndrome. Ultrasound Obstet Gynecol 2014; 44(2): 147-53.
[http://dx.doi.org/10.1002/uog.13336] [PMID: 24585513]

[31] Fehmi Yazıcıoglu H, Sevket O, Akin H, Aygün M, A-zyurt ON, Karahasanoglu A. Aberrant right subclavian artery in Down syndrome fetuses. Prenat Diagn 2013; 33(3): 209-13.
[http://dx.doi.org/10.1002/pd.4042] [PMID: 23319208]

[32] Esmer AC, Gul A, Nehir A, *et al.* Detection rate of trisomy 21 in fetuses with isolated and non-isolated aberrant right subclavian artery. Fetal Diagn Ther 2013; 34(3): 140-5.
[http://dx.doi.org/10.1159/000354650] [PMID: 24051543]

[33] Pilu G, Falco P, Gabrielli S, Perolo A, Sandri F, Bovicelli L. The clinical significance of fetal isolated cerebral borderline ventriculomegaly: report of 31 cases and review of the literature. Ultrasound Obstet Gynecol 1999; 14(5): 320-6.
[http://dx.doi.org/10.1046/j.1469-0705.1999.14050320.x] [PMID: 10623991]

[34] Mercier A, Eurin D, Mercier PY, Verspyck E, Marpeau L, Marret S. Isolated mild fetal cerebral ventriculomegaly: a retrospective analysis of 26 cases. Prenat Diagn 2001; 21(7): 589-95.
[http://dx.doi.org/10.1002/pd.88] [PMID: 11494298]

[35] De Oronzo MA. Hyperechogenic fetal bowel: an ultrasonographic marker for adverse fetal and neonatal outcome? J Prenat Med 2011; 5(1): 9-13.
[PMID: 22439068]

[36] Rumi Kataguiri M, Araujo Junior E, Silva Bussamra LC, Nardozza LM, Fernandes Moron A. Influence of second-trimester ultrasound markers for Down syndrome in pregnant women of advanced maternal age. J Pregnancy 2014; 785730.
[http://dx.doi.org/10.1155/2014/785730] [PMID: 24795825]

[37] Hill M, Fisher J, Chitty LS, Morris S. Women's and health professionals' preferences for prenatal tests for Down syndrome: a discrete choice experiment to contrast noninvasive prenatal diagnosis with current invasive tests. Genet Med 2012; 14(11): 905-13.
[http://dx.doi.org/10.1038/gim.2012.68] [PMID: 22935718]

[38] Wu D, Chi H, Shao M, *et al.* Prenatal diagnosis of Down syndrome using cell-free fetal DNA in amniotic fluid by quantitative fluorescent polymersase chain reaction. Chin Med J (Engl) 2014; 127(10): 1897-901.
[PMID: 24824252]

[39] Liu H, Liao C, Huang YN, *et al.* [Application of fluorescence *in situ* hybridization to prenatal diagnosis of aneuploidy in 110 uncultured amniotic fluid samples]. Zhonghua Yi Xue Yi Chuan Xue Za Zhi 2010; 27(4): 453-6.
[http://dx.doi.org/10.3760/cma.j.issn.1003-9406.2010.04.021] [PMID: 20677157]

[40] Grinshpun-Cohen J, Miron-Shatz T, Ries-Levavi L, Pras E. Factors that affect the decision to undergo amniocentesis in women with normal Down syndrome screening results: it is all about the age. Health Expect 2014; 12
[http://dx.doi.org/10.1111/hex.12200] [PMID: 24816429]

[41] Bornstein E, Lenchner E, Donnenfeld A, Barnhard Y, Seubert D, Divon MY. Advanced maternal age as a sole indication for genetic amniocentesis; risk-benefit analysis based on a large database reflecting the current common practice. J Perinat Med 2009; 37(2): 99-102.
[http://dx.doi.org/10.1515/JPM.2009.032] [PMID: 18999912]

[42] Daniilidis A, Karydas H, Zournatzi V, Tantanasis T, Giannoulis C, Tzafettas J. A four-year retrospective study of amniocentesis: one centre experience. Hippokratia 2008; 12(2): 113-5.
[PMID: 18923654]

[43] Anuwutnavin S, Chanprapaph P, Ruangvutilert P, Eammatta M, Tontisirin P. Short-term outcomes after second-trimester genetic amniocentesis in Siriraj Hospital. Int J Gynaecol Obstet 2014; 124(3): 222-5.
[http://dx.doi.org/10.1016/j.ijgo.2013.09.019] [PMID: 24380612]

[44] Rueangchainikhom W, Sarapak S, Orungrote N. Chorionic villus sampling for early prenatal diagnosis at Bhumibol Adulyadej Hospital. J Med Assoc Thai 2008; 91(1): 1-6.
[PMID: 18386536]

[45] Alfirevic Z, Sundberg K, Brigham S. Amniocentesis and chorionic villus sampling for prenatal diagnosis. Cochrane Database Syst Rev 2003; (3): CD003252.
[http://dx.doi.org/10.1002/14651858.CD003252] [PMID: 12917956]

[46] Berry SM, Stone J, Norton ME, Johnson D, Berghella V. Fetal blood sampling. Am J Obstet Gynecol 2013; 209(3): 170-80.
[http://dx.doi.org/10.1016/j.ajog.2013.07.014] [PMID: 23978246]

[47] De Jesus I, Simon E, Potin J, Arlicot C, Perrotin F. [Predictive factors for fetal tolerance to cordocentesis: a monocentric retrospective study]. Gynecol Obstet Fertil 2012; 40(12): 734-40. [http://dx.doi.org/10.1016/j.gyobfe.2012.07.036] [PMID: 22981975]

[48] Fried K. A score based on eight signs in the diagnosis of Down syndrome in the newborn. J Ment Defic Res 1980; 24(3): 181-5.
[PMID: 6448299]

[49] Karlica D, Skelin S, Culic V, Znaor L, Karlica H. The ophthalmic anomalies in children with Down syndrome in Split-Dalmatian County. Coll Antropol 2011; 35(4): 1115-8.
[PMID: 22397246]

[50] Mitchell RB, Call E, Kelly J. Ear, nose and throat disorders in children with Down syndrome. Laryngoscope 2003; 113(2): 259-63.
[http://dx.doi.org/10.1097/00005537-200302000-00012] [PMID: 12567079]

[51] Kavurt S, Celik IH, Ada BS, Bas AY, Demirel N. Isolated ectrodactyly in a newborn with Down syndrome. Genet Couns 2014; 25(2): 209-14.
[PMID: 25059021]

[52] Willich E, Fuhr U, Kroll W. Skeletal changes in Down's syndrome. A correlation between radiological and cytogenetic findings (author's transl). Rofo 1977; 127(2): 135-42.
[PMID: 198345]

[53] Ahmed I, Ghafoor T, Samore NA, Chattha MN. Down syndrome: clinical and cytogenetic analysis. J Coll Physicians Surg Pak 2005; 15(7): 426-9.
[PMID: 16197873]

[54] de Groot-van der Mooren MD, Gemke RJ, Cornel MC, Weijerman ME. Neonatal diagnosis of Down syndrome in The Netherlands: suspicion and communication with parents. J Intellect Disabil Res 2014; 58(10): 953-61.
[http://dx.doi.org/10.1111/jir.12125] [PMID: 24628769]

[55] Lantrès A. [Notifying parents of Down's syndrome: the experiences of parents]. Soins Pediatr Pueric 2011; (263): 36-8.
[PMID: 22288264]

[56] Clementi M, Calzolari E, Turolla L, Volpato S, Tenconi R. Neonatal growth patterns in a population of consecutively born Down syndrome children. Am J Med Genet Suppl 1990; 7: 71-4.
[PMID: 2149978]

[57] Myrelid A, Gustafsson J, Ollars B, Annerén G. Growth charts for Down's syndrome from birth to 18 years of age. Arch Dis Child 2002; 87(2): 97-103.
[http://dx.doi.org/10.1136/adc.87.2.97] [PMID: 12138052]

[58] Down Syndrome Medical Interest Group. THE 2011 DSMIG / RCPCH GROWTH CHARTS FOR CHILDREN WITH DOWN SYNDROME. http://www.dsmig.org.uk/pdf/Chart%20Fact%20Sheet%20A4%204pp.pdf , 2015 [Accessed on: Janurary 2015];

[59] Van Gameren-Oosterom HB, Van Dommelen P, Oudesluys-Murphy AM, Buitendijk SE, Van Buuren S, Van Wouwe JP. Healthy growth in children with Down syndrome. PLoS One 2012; 7(2): e31079.

[http://dx.doi.org/10.1371/journal.pone.0031079] [PMID: 22363551]

[60] Pereira K, Basso RP, Lindquist AR, da Silva LG, Tudella E. Infants with Down syndrome: percentage and age for acquisition of gross motor skills. Res Dev Disabil 2013; 34(3): 894-901. [http://dx.doi.org/10.1016/j.ridd.2012.11.021] [PMID: 23291506]

[61] Tudella E, Pereira K, Basso RP, Savelsbergh GJ. Description of the motor development of 3-12 month old infants with Down syndrome: the influence of the postural body position. Res Dev Disabil 2011; 32(5): 1514-20. [http://dx.doi.org/10.1016/j.ridd.2011.01.046] [PMID: 21367575]

[62] Koshy B, Navamani K, Oommen SP, Srivastava VM. Growth and development profile of Indian children with Down syndrome. Indian Pediatr 2012; 49(8): 676-7. [PMID: 22962246]

[63] Menon PS, Sachdev HP, Verma IC, Ghai OP. Developmental milestones of Down's syndrome patients in north India. Indian J Med Res 1981; 73: 369-73. [PMID: 6456224]

[64] Al-Biltagi M. Echocardiography in children with Down syndrome. World J Clin Pediatr 2013 Nov 8; 2(4): 36-45. [http://dx.doi.org/10.5409/wjcp.v2.i4.36] [PMID: 25254173]

[65] Shah PS, Hellmann J, Adatia I. Clinical characteristics and follow up of Down syndrome infants without congenital heart disease who presented with persistent pulmonary hypertension of newborn. J Perinat Med 2004; 32(2): 168-70. [http://dx.doi.org/10.1515/JPM.2004.030] [PMID: 15085894]

[66] Benjamin W. Eidem, Carolyn Jones, Frank Cetta. Unusual Association of Hypertrophic Cardiomyopathy with Complete Atrioventricular Canal Defect and Down Syndrome. Tex Heart Inst J 2000; 27(3): 289-91. [PMID: 11093415]

[67] Wacker A, Scheel-Walter HG, Neunhoeffer F. [Biventricular hypertrophic non-obstructive cardiomyopathy as a symptom of transient myeloproliferative disorder in a newborn with Down syndrome]. Z Geburtshilfe Neonatol 2009; 213(2): 64-6. [http://dx.doi.org/10.1055/s-0029-1214406] [PMID: 19319796]

[68] Weijerman ME, de Winter JP. Clinical practice. The care of children with Down syndrome. Eur J Pediatr 2010; 169(12): 1445-52. [http://dx.doi.org/10.1007/s00431-010-1253-0] [PMID: 20632187]

[69] Flageole H, Fecteau A, Laberge JM, Guttman FM. Hirschsprung's disease, imperforate anus, and Down's syndrome: a case report. J Pediatr Surg 1996 Jun; 31(6): 759-60. [PMID: 8783095]

[70] Jaruratanasirikul S, Patarakijvanich N, Patanapisarnsak C. The association of congenital hypothyroidism and congenital gastrointestinal anomalies in Down's syndrome infants. J Pediatr Endocrinol Metab 1998; 11(2): 241-6. [http://dx.doi.org/10.1515/JPEM.1998.11.2.241] [PMID: 9642639]

[71] Orün UA, Bilici M, Demirceken FG, *et al.* Gastrointestinal system malformations in children are

associated with congenital heart defects. Anadolu Kardiyol Derg 2011; 11(2): 146-9. [http://dx.doi.org/10.5152/akd.2011.034] [PMID: 21342865]

[72] Marin J, Lopoo J. An infant with trisomy 21 and tachypnea. Pediatr Emerg Care 2006; 22(3): 170-2. [http://dx.doi.org/10.1097/01.pec.0000202457.64978.3d] [PMID: 16628100]

[73] Roofthooft MT, van Meer H, Rietman WG, Ebels T, Berger RM. Down syndrome and aberrant right subclavian artery. Eur J Pediatr 2008; 167(9): 1033-6. [http://dx.doi.org/10.1007/s00431-007-0637-2] [PMID: 18172685]

[74] Travassos D, van Herwaarden-Lindeboom M, van der Zee DC. Hirschsprung's disease in children with Down syndrome: a comparative study. Eur J Pediatr Surg 2011; 21(4): 220-3. [http://dx.doi.org/10.1055/s-0031-1271735] [PMID: 21351043]

[75] Lyons M, Vlastarakos PV, Nikolopoulos TP. Congenital and acquired developmental problems of the upper airway in newborns and infants. Early Hum Dev 2012; 88(12): 951-5. [http://dx.doi.org/10.1016/j.earlhumdev.2012.09.001] [PMID: 23017879]

[76] Raut P, Sriram B, Yeoh A, Hee KY, Lim SB, Daniel ML. High prevalence of hearing loss in Down syndrome at first year of life. Ann Acad Med Singapore 2011; 40(11): 493-8. [PMID: 22206065]

[77] Colozza P, Anastasio AR. Screening, diagnosing and treating deafness: the knowledge and conduct of doctors serving in neonatology and/or pediatrics in a tertiary teaching hospital. Sao Paulo Med J 2009; 127(2): 61-5. [http://dx.doi.org/10.1590/S1516-31802009000200002] [PMID: 19597679]

[78] Biko DM, Schwartz M, Anupindi SA, Altes TA. Subpleural lung cysts in Down syndrome: prevalence and association with coexisting diagnoses. Pediatr Radiol 2008; 38(3): 280-4. [http://dx.doi.org/10.1007/s00247-007-0699-3] [PMID: 18097658]

[79] Bertrand P, Navarro H, Caussade S, Holmgren N, Sanchez I. Airway anomalies in children with Down syndrome: endoscopic findings. Pediatr Pulmonol 2003; 38(2): 137-41. [PMID: 12833493]

[80] Bloemers BL, van Furth AM, Weijerman ME, *et al.* Down syndrome: a novel risk factor for respiratory syncytial virus bronchiolitis--a prospective birth-cohort study. Pediatrics 2007; 120(4): e1076-81. [http://dx.doi.org/10.1542/peds.2007-0788] [PMID: 17908728]

[81] Cua CL, Blankenship A, North AL, Hayes J, Nelin LD. Increased incidence of idiopathic persistent pulmonary hypertension in Down syndrome neonates. Pediatr Cardiol 2007; 28(4): 250-4. [http://dx.doi.org/10.1007/s00246-006-0011-6] [PMID: 17486396]

[82] Tüysüz B, Beker DB. Thyroid dysfunction in children with Down's syndrome. Acta Paediatr 2001; 90(12): 1389-93. [http://dx.doi.org/10.1111/j.1651-2227.2001.tb01601.x] [PMID: 11853334]

[83] Myrelid A, Jonsson B, Guthenberg C, von Dobeln U, Anneren G, Gustafsson J. Increased neonatal thyrotropin in Down syndrome. Acta Paediatr 2009; 98(6): 1010-3. [http://dx.doi.org/10.1111/j.1651-2227.2009.01245.x] [PMID: 19239410]

[84] van Trotsenburg AS, Vulsma T, van Santen HM, Cheung W, de Vijlder JJ. Lower neonatal screening

thyroxine concentrations in down syndrome newborns. J Clin Endocrinol Metab 2003; 88(4): 1512-5. [http://dx.doi.org/10.1210/jc.2002-021303] [PMID: 12679431]

[85] Sarici D, Akin MA, Kurtoglu S, Gunes T, Ozturk MA, Akcakus M. Thyroid functions of neonates with Down syndrome. Ital J Pediatr 2012 Sep; 17: 38-44. [http://dx.doi.org/] [http://dx.doi.org/10.1186/1824-7288-38-44]

[86] Grinspon RP, Bedecarras P, Ballerini MG, *et al.* Early onset of primary hypogonadism revealed by serum anti-Mulerian hormone determination during infancy and childhood in trisomy 21. Int J Androl 2011; 34(5 Pt 2): e487-98. [http://dx.doi.org/10.1111/j.1365-2605.2011.01210.x] [PMID: 21831236]

[87] Shehadeh N, Gershoni-Baruch R, Etzioni A. Congenital diabetes in an infant with trisomy 21. J Pediatr Endocrinol Metab 1998; 11(4): 575-6. [http://dx.doi.org/10.1515/JPEM.1998.11.4.575] [PMID: 9777580]

[88] Ginsberg J, Ballard ET, Buchino JJ, Kinkler AK. Further observations of ocular pathology in Down ?(tm)s syndrome. J Pediatr Ophthalmol Strabismus 1980; 17(3): 166-71. [PMID: 6446600]

[89] Salvio CC, Hida WT, Filho JV, Cunha M, dos Santos Araujo J. [Congenital epiphora in patients with Down syndrome]. Arq Bras Oftalmol 2007; 70(3): 423-7. [http://dx.doi.org/10.1590/S0004-27492007000300007] [PMID: 17768547]

[90] Haargaard B, Fledelius HC. Down's syndrome and early cataract. Br J Ophthalmol 2006 Aug; 90(8): 1024-7. [http://dx.doi.org/10.1136/bjo.2006.090639] [PMID: 16672328]

[91] Jackson GL, Sendelbach DM, Rambally B, Manning MD, Engle WD. Circulating blasts and associated hematologic disorders in neonates with Down syndrome. Am J Perinatol 2012; 29(4): 259-66. [http://dx.doi.org/10.1055/s-0031-1285103] [PMID: 21809264]

[92] Hon KL, Leung TY. Transient myeloproliferative disorder and non-immune hydrops fetalis in a neonate with trisomy 21. Hong Kong Med J 2014; 20(1): 78.e3-e4. [http://dx.doi.org/10.12809/hkmj133750] [PMID: 24473698]

[93] Zwaan MC, Reinhardt D, Hitzler J, Vyas P. Acute leukemias in children with Down syndrome. Pediatr Clin North Am 2008 Feb; 55(1): 53-70. [http://dx.doi.org/10.1016/j.pcl.2007.11.001] [PMID: 18242315]

[94] Saenz RB. Primary care of infants and young children with Down syndrome Am Fam Physician 1999 Jan 15; 59(2): 381-90. [PMID: 9930130]

[95] Ram G, Chinen J. Infections and immunodeficiency in Down syndrome. Clin Exp Immunol 2011; 164(1): 9-16. [http://dx.doi.org/10.1111/j.1365-2249.2011.04335.x] [PMID: 21352207]

[96] Caird MS, Wills BP, Dormans JP. Down syndrome in children: the role of the orthopaedic surgeon. J Am Acad Orthop Surg 2006; 14(11): 610-9. [PMID: 17030594]

[97] Hankinson TC, Anderson RC. Craniovertebral junction abnormalities in Down syndrome. Neurosurgery 2010; 66(3) (Suppl.): 32-8. [http://dx.doi.org/10.1227/01.NEU.0000365803.22786.F0] [PMID: 20173525]

[98] Williams R, Kirkbride V, Corcoran GD. Neonatal osteomyelitis in Down's syndrome due to non-encapsulated Haemophilus influenzae. J Infect 1994; 29(2): 203-5. [http://dx.doi.org/10.1016/S0163-4453(94)90794-3] [PMID: 7806884]

[99] Eayrs K, Shettihalli N, Adwani S. Down syndrome masked by Marfan syndrome in a neonate. BMJ Case Rep 2013 Mar 11; pii-bcr2013008807. [http://dx.doi.org/10.1136/bcr-2013-008807]

[100] de Azevedo Moreira LM, Matos MA, Schiper PP. Co-occurrence of achondroplasia and Down syndrome: Genotype/phenotype association. Birth Defects Res A Clin Mol Teratol. Birth Defects Res A Clin Mol Teratol 2010; 88(4): 228-31.

[101] Kupferman JC, Druschel CM, Kupchik GS. Increased prevalence of renal and urinary tract anomalies in children with Down syndrome. Pediatrics 2009; 124(4): 615-21. [http://dx.doi.org/10.1542/peds.2009-0181] [PMID: 19752083]

[102] Ariel I, Wells TR, Landing BH, Singer DB. The urinary system in Down syndrome: a study of 124 autopsy cases. Pediatr Pathol 1991; 11(6): 879-88. [http://dx.doi.org/10.3109/15513819109065484] [PMID: 1837925]

[103] Ebert AK, Brookman-Amissah S, Rosch WH. [Urological manifestations of Down syndrome: significance and long-term complications -- our own patient cohort with an overview]. Urologe A 2008; 47(3): 337-41. [http://dx.doi.org/10.1007/s00120-007-1614-0] [PMID: 18210071]

[104] Mercer ES, Broecker B, Smith EA, Kirsch AJ, Scherz HC, A Massad C. Urological manifestations of Down syndrome. J Urol 2004; 171(3): 1250-3. [http://dx.doi.org/10.1097/01.ju.0000112915.69436.91] [PMID: 14767322]

[105] Verbov J. Anomalies in dermal ridge arrangement in Down's syndrome. Clin Exp Dermatol 2007; 32(1): 116. [http://dx.doi.org/10.1111/j.1365-2230.2006.02280.x] [PMID: 17034421]

[106] Bilgili SG, Akdeniz N, Karadag AS, Akbayram S, Calka O, Ozkol HU. Mucocutaneous disorders in children with down syndrome: case-controlled study. Genet Couns 2011; 22(4): 385-92. [PMID: 22303799]

[107] Ercis M, Balci S, Atakan N. Dermatological manifestations of 71 Down syndrome children admitted to a clinical genetics unit. Clin Genet 1996; 50(5): 317-20. [PMID: 9007317]

[108] Madan V, Williams J, Lear JT. Dermatological manifestations of Down's syndrome. Clin Exp Dermatol 2006; 31(5): 623-9. [http://dx.doi.org/10.1111/j.1365-2230.2006.02164.x] [PMID: 16901300]

[109] Mannan SE, Yousef E, Hossain J. Prevalence of positive skin prick test results in children with Down syndrome: a case-control study. Ann Allergy Asthma Immunol 2009; 102(3): 205-9. [http://dx.doi.org/10.1016/S1081-1206(10)60082-8] [PMID: 19354066]

[110] Gaete B, Mellado C, Hernandez M. [Prevalence of neurological disorders among children with Down syndrome]. Rev Med Chil 2012; 140(2): 214-8.
[http://dx.doi.org/10.4067/S0034-98872012000200010] [PMID: 22739951]

[111] Arya R, Kabra M, Gulati S. Epilepsy in children with Down syndrome. Epileptic Disord 2011; 13(1): 1-7.
[http://dx.doi.org/10.1684/epd.2011.0415] [PMID: 21398208]

[112] Stafstrom CE. Epilepsy in Down syndrome: clinical aspects and possible mechanisms. Am J Ment Retard 1993; 98 (Suppl.): 12-26.
[PMID: 8102531]

[113] Shore S, Lightfoot T, Ansell P. Oral disease in children with Down syndrome: causes and prevention. Community Pract 2010; 83(2): 18-21.
[PMID: 20222361]

[114] Ndiokwelu E, Adimora GN, Ibeziako N. Neonatal teeth association with Down ?(tm)s syndrome. A case report. Odontostomatol Trop 2004; 27(107): 4-6.
[PMID: 15900817]

[115] Danner SC. Breastfeeding the neurologically impaired infant. NAACOGS Clin Issu Perinat Womens Health Nurs 1992; 3(4): 640-6.
[PMID: 1476843]

[116] Atanassova K, Dilova P, Popova T, Angelova Z. [Nutrition specification for babies with Down syndrome]. Akush Ginekol (Sofiia) 2009; 48 (Suppl. 2): 53-5.
[PMID: 20380104]

[117] McBride MC, Danner SC. Sucking disorders in neurologically impaired infants: assessment and facilitation of breastfeeding. Clin Perinatol 1987; 14(1): 109-30.
[PMID: 3549110]

[118] Pisacane A, Toscano E, Pirri I, *et al.* Down syndrome and breastfeeding. Acta Paediatr 2003; 92(12): 1479-81.
[http://dx.doi.org/10.1111/j.1651-2227.2003.tb00835.x] [PMID: 14971802]

[119] Aumonier ME, Cunningham CC. Breast feeding in infants with Down‘s syndrome. Child Care Health Dev 1983; 9(5): 247-55.
[http://dx.doi.org/10.1111/j.1365-2214.1983.tb00323.x] [PMID: 6227426]

[120] Lee N. Inquiries regarding Kassing‘s bottle-feeding article. J Hum Lact 2003; 19(1): 19.
[PMID: 12587639]

[121] Kassing D. Bottle-feeding as a tool to reinforce breastfeeding. J Hum Lact 2002; 18(1): 56-60.
[http://dx.doi.org/10.1177/089033440201800110] [PMID: 11845739]

[122] Faulks D, Mazille MN, Collado V, Veyrune JL, Hennequin M. Masticatory dysfunction in persons with Down ?(tm)s syndrome. Part 2: management. J Oral Rehabil 2008; 35(11): 863-9.
[http://dx.doi.org/10.1111/j.1365-2842.2008.01878.x] [PMID: 18793251]

[123] Unger R, DeKleermaeker M, Gidding SS, Christoffel KK. Calories count. Improved weight gain with dietary intervention in congenital heart disease. Am J Dis Child 1992; 146(9): 1078-84.
[http://dx.doi.org/10.1001/archpedi.1992.02160210080026] [PMID: 1514555]

[124] Napolitano G, Palka G, Lio S, *et al.* Is zinc deficiency a cause of subclinical hypothyroidism in Down syndrome? Ann Genet 1990; 33(1): 9-15.
[PMID: 2142391]

[125] Lisch W, Pitz S, Geerling G. [Therapy for systemic metabolic disorders based on the detection of basic corneal landmarks in childhood]. Klin Monatsbl Augenheilkd 2013; 230(6): 575-81.
[http://dx.doi.org/10.1055/s-0032-1328524] [PMID: 23794426]

[126] Reading CM. Down‘s syndrome: nutritional intervention. Nutr Health 1984; 3(1-2): 91-111.
[http://dx.doi.org/10.1177/026010608400300208] [PMID: 6242480]

[127] Turck D. Cow‘s milk and goat‘s milk. World Rev Nutr Diet 2013; 108: 56-62.
[http://dx.doi.org/10.1159/000351485] [PMID: 24029787]

[128] Carratelli M, Porcaro L, Ruscica M, De Simone E, Bertelli AA, Corsi MM. Reactive oxygen metabolites and prooxidant status in children with Down ?(tm)s syndrome. Int J Clin Pharmacol Res 2001; 21(2): 79-84.
[PMID: 11824651]

[129] Garlet TR, Parisotto EB, de Medeiros Gda S. Systemic oxidative stress in children and teenagers with Down syndrome 2013; 11;93: 558-63.
[http://dx.doi.org/10.1016/j.lfs.2013.08.017]

[130] Parisotto EB, Garlet TR, Cavalli VL, *et al.* Antioxidant intervention attenuates oxidative stress in children and teenagers with Down syndrome. Res Dev Disabil 2014; 35(6): 1228-36.
[http://dx.doi.org/10.1016/j.ridd.2014.03.013] [PMID: 24685938]

[131] Blair CK, Roesler M, Xie Y, *et al.* Vitamin supplement use among children with Down‘s syndrome and risk of leukaemia: a Children‘s Oncology Group (COG) study. Paediatr Perinat Epidemiol 2008; 22(3): 288-95.
[http://dx.doi.org/10.1111/j.1365-3016.2008.00928.x] [PMID: 18426524]

[132] Chen YJ, Chen CC, Li TK, *et al.* Docosahexaenoic acid suppresses the expression of FoxO and its target genes. J Nutr Biochem 2012; 23(12): 1609-16.
[http://dx.doi.org/10.1016/j.jnutbio.2011.11.003] [PMID: 22444500]

[133] Lejeune J, Rethoré MO, de Blois MC, *et al.* [Amino acids and trisomy 21]. Ann Genet 1992; 35(1): 8-13.
[PMID: 1535189]

[134] Heggarty HJ, Ball R, Smith M, Henderson MJ. Amino acid profile in Down‘s syndrome. Arch Dis Child 1996; 74(4): 347-9.
[http://dx.doi.org/10.1136/adc.74.4.347] [PMID: 8669939]

[135] Pueschel SM, Reed RB, Cronk CE, Goldstein BI. 5-hydroxytryptophan and pyridoxine. Their effects in young children with Down‘s syndrome. Am J Dis Child 1980; 134(9): 838-44.
[http://dx.doi.org/10.1001/archpedi.1980.02130210022007] [PMID: 6447999]

[136] Weise P, Koch R, Shaw KN, Rosenfeld MJ. The use of 5-HTP in the treatment of Down‘s syndrome. Pediatrics 1974; 54(2): 165-8.
[PMID: 4277102]

[137] Hedari CP, Khinkarly RW, Dbaibo GS. Meningococcal serogroups A, C, W-135, and Y tetanus toxoid conjugate vaccine: a new conjugate vaccine against invasive meningococcal disease. Infect Drug Resist. 2014 Apr 3;7:85-99. eCollection 2014. RE:view [http://dx.doi.org/10.2147/IDR.S36243]

[138] Thomas CA, Shwe T, Bixler D, *et al.* Two-dose varicella vaccine effectiveness and rash severity in outbreaks of varicella among public school students. Pediatr Infect Dis J 2014; 33(11): 1164-8. [http://dx.doi.org/10.1097/INF.0000000000000444] [PMID: 24911894]

[139] Costa-Carvalho BT, Martinez RM, Dias AT, *et al.* Antibody response to pneumococcal capsular polysaccharide vaccine in Down syndrome patients. Braz J Med Biol Res 2006; 39(12): 1587-92. [http://dx.doi.org/10.1590/S0100-879X2006001200010] [PMID: 17160268]

[140] Cuckle HS. Primary prevention of Down ?(tm)s syndrome. Int J Med Sci 2005; 2(3): 93-9. [http://dx.doi.org/10.7150/ijms.2.93] [PMID: 16007260]

[141] Gu EZ, Gu Q, Han P, Tian D, Chen YY. [Influencing factors of utilization of prenatal screening for Down‘s syndrome]. Zhonghua Yu Fang Yi Xue Za Zhi 2012; 46(4): 307-10. [PMID: 22800626]

[142] Miao ZY, Liu X, Shi TK, Ge JM, Xu Y. First trimester and second-trimester integrated screening for Down‘s syndrome. Zhonghua Yi Xue Za Zhi 2011 Jan 18; 91(3): 185-8. [PMID: 21418900]

CHAPTER 4

Cardiovascular Disorders in Children with Down Syndrome

Mohammed Al-Biltagi[1,*], Osama Abd Rab Elrasoul Tolba[2]

[1] *Pediatric Department, Faculty of Medicine, Tanta University, Egypt*

[2] *Pediatric Department, Faculty of Medicine, Tanta University, Egypt*

Abstract: Down syndrome (DS) is commonly associated with cardiovascular disorders either congenital or acquired. Congenital cardiac diseases (CHDs) occur in about half of children with DS. They also are more liable to have pulmonary hypertension, mitral valve prolapse, aortic regurgitation and many other acquired cardiac conditions. Meanwhile, they are also of a higher risk for developing obesity than the control children which predisposes them to an increased risk of atherosclerosis. Antenatal detection of DS as well as CHDs can be detected by presence of some soft signs during routine antenatal 4-chamber view. Children with this syndrome should have echocardiographic examination in the first month of life for all neonates, before any cardiac surgery, as follow-up after cardiac surgery, for serial evaluation of pulmonary hypertension, before involvement in major non-cardiac surgery and before involvement in physical exercise as well as serial follow up for early detection of any cardiac disorder. In this chapter, prevalence, pathomechanism and methods of detection of cardiac disorders in children with DS as well as their management are discussed.

Keywords: Aberrant right subclavian artery, Atrioventricular septal defects, Cardiac functions, Children, Congenital Cardiac Diseases, DSCR1 gene, Down syndrome, Echogenic intracardiac foci, Fallout Tetralogy, Fetal echocardiography, Hypothyroidism, Mitral Valve prolapse, Nuchal translucency, Over-expression, Patent ductus arteriosus, Pathomechanism, Pericardial Effusion, Single umbilical artery, Soft signs, Ventricular septal defects.

* **Corresponding Author Dr. Mohammed Al-Biltagi:** Pediatric Department, Faculty of Medicine, Tanta University, Egypt; Tel: (+973)39545472; Fax: (+973) 1759 0495; Email: mbelrem@hotmail.com

1. INTRODUCTION

Down syndrome is commonly associated with cardiovascular disorders either congenital or acquired. Congenital heart diseases occur in approximately half of children with DS. At the same time; children with DS who were born with normal heart at birth may furthermore develop cardiac problems in the future like pericardial effusion, pulmonary vascular disease and right cardiac failure due to airway/respiratory anomalies. Meanwhile, they are also of a higher risk for developing obesity than control children which predisposes them to an increased risk of atherosclerosis [1]. Adolescents with DS are also at increasing risk to develop mitral valve prolapse and aortic regurgitation [2]. So; the aim of this chapter is to highlight the different aspects of cardiovascular diseases in children with DS.

2. CONGENITAL HEART DISEASES (CHD)

2.1. Prevalence of Congenital Heart Diseases in Children With Down Syndrome

The incidence of CHD showed marked increase from 0.8% in normal population to reach 40-60% in DS cases and they form about one tenth of all children with congenital heart diseases. These CHDs may be simple or complex which could have deleterious effects on the affected children and their families. They may have congestive heart failure, pulmonary vascular disease, pneumonia, or failure to thrive. CHDs are the most common cause of death among those children in the first 2 years of life [3, 4].

The most common CHD observed in children with DS are Atrioventricular septal defects (AVSD; with or without other CHD) (Fig. **1**). It forms approximately 45% of all CHDs observed in DS children. The second most common CHD was ventricular septal defects (VSD; with or without other CHD) which forms approximately 35% of all CHDs observed in DS children. Isolated secundum atrial septal defect (ASD) forms 8%, isolated persistent patent ductus arteriosus (PDA) forms 7% and an isolated Fallout Tetralogy (TOF) forms 4%. Arch abnormalities (aortic coarctation, right aortic arch, aberrant right subclavian artery) constitute the remaining 1% of CHDs [5]. On the other hand, there is less frequency of certain cardiac malformation in children with DS than non-DS children *e.g.*, heterotaxy, aortic coarctation or transposition of the great arteries which could reflect the effects of presence of 3 copies of certain a gene or genes on chromosome 21 on only specific developmental points [6].

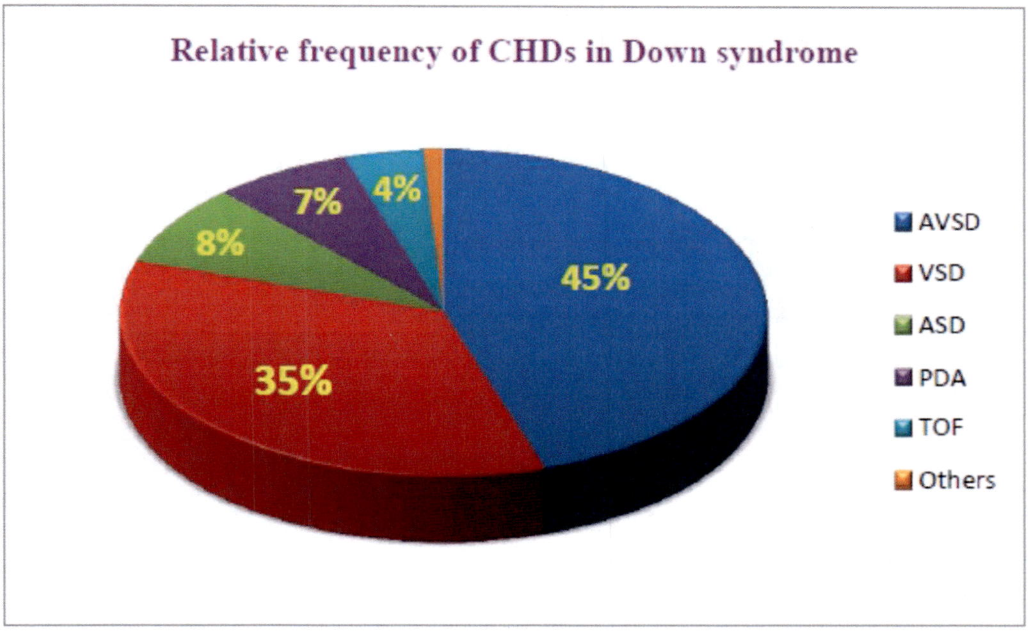

Fig. (1). Showed the relative frequency of CHDs in children with Down syndrome.

2.1.1. Factors Affecting the Rate of Congenital Cardiac Diseases in Children with Down Syndrome

Despite AVSD is the most common cardiac anomalies in children with DS, however; the relative frequency of each CHD will vary by different factors. Table **1** showed the different factors that could affect the frequency of CHDs in DS populations.

2.2. Pathomechanism of CHD in Children with DS

Development of human heart is very complex and starts very early by the 3rd week of pregnancy and develops progressively till the 8th week of pregnancy. The primitive tube develops and begins to beats at 25 days of gestation and ends in the four-chamber heart through many steps including looping, cell migration, cell transition, and septation [17]. This development depends on many factors and can be affected by a series of molecular signaling pathways and morphological events that when deviated from normal can lead to CHDs. This series of molecular signaling pathways and morphological events is under the control of genes some of them are located on chromosome 21 or affected by other genes located outside that chromosome but under the control of genes present on chromosome 21. In DS children, presence of extra copy of chromosome 21 with variations in gene dosage, environmental factors and genetic modifications not linked to chromosome 21 contribute to the development of CHD [18].

Table 1. Different factors affecting the rate of congenital cardiac diseases in children with Down syndrome.

Factor	Associated CHD
Consanguinity [7]	In consanguineous marriage - VSD is the most frequently CHD encountered. - There is predominance of left-right shunt lesions. - There is relative rarity of cyanotic and complex CHD in this DS population
Maternal age [8]	Mother older than 32 years had lesser incidence of occurrence of CHD in children with DS
Ethnicity [9 - 13]	- AVSD is twice as many blacks and half as many Hispanics affected compared to whites. - In Saudi; VSD was the most prevalent (33.3%) followed by AVSD (22.8%), ASD (21.1%), patent ductus arteriosus (14%) and tetralogy of Fallout. - In Turkish sample, the most common single defect was AVSD (34.2%), followed by secondm ASD (16.7%) and VSD (16.5%). - In Guatemalans; patent ductus arteriosus (PDA) was the most prevalent cardiac anomalies followed by VSD, ASD and then AVSD. - In Mexican, ASD, VSD and PDA were most common cardiac malformation while AVSDs were less common.
Sex [6]	AVSD is twice in females than in males
Maternal smoking [14]	associated with ASVD, TOF, and ASD but not with VSD
Maternal Alcoholism [15]	Increases incidence of VSD
Folic acid deficiency [16]	Increases incidence of AVSD or ASD but not VSD

The basic mechanism of DS is the presence of an extra copy of all or part of human chromosome 21 (Hsa21) in most cases. Triplication of Hsa21 lead to presence of an extra set of the approximately 200–300 genes on the chromosome with 1.5-fold increase in the expression of some, if not all, of these genes which lead to the many abnormalities associated with this condition. Nevertheless, all of these genes do not inevitably exhibit a basic 1.5-fold increase in expression, but only 30% of HSA21 genes have this 1.5-fold expression. This results from gene regulation by dosage compensation, which means that only a subset of these genes will exhibit the expected 50% increase in expression [19, 20]. The end result is presence of genetic imbalance which leads to abnormal interaction between Hsa21 genes and other disomic genes with production of either relatively subtle or massively disruptive effects on genes present on chromosomes other than 21 and seriously disrupt one or more of cardiac developmental pathways [21]. This genetic imbalance induces modulation of transcription factors, chromatin remodeling proteins, and related molecules or other targets which causes of pathways concerned in cardiac development and may cause various cardiac anomalies noted in DS [22].

Down syndrome critical region (DSCR) is present on the long (q) arm of chromosome 21 and contains a number of genes that might be responsible for the different phenotypes that characterize DS. These genes may includes genes present in different critical regions as Down syndrome critical region 1 gene, or DSCR1, on chromosome 21q22.12; DSCR2 on chromosome 21q22.3; DSCR3 on chromosome 21q22.2; DSCR4 on chromosome 21q22.2; and DSCR5 in the chromosome region 21q22.1-q22.2 [23]. Down syndrome critical region 1 gene is the most well studied and known also as Calcipressin-1, Adapt78, MCIP1 (myocyte-enriched calcineurin-interacting protein 1) or regulator of calcineurin 1, which is a 252 amino acid protein that belongs to the RCAN family (Regulators of Calcineurin) and exists as 4 alternatively spliced isoforms. DSCR1 gene is abundantly expressed in skeletal muscle, as well as in the brain and heart, and is thought to influence cardiac and nervous system development as it is possibly part of a signal transduction pathway involving both the heart and brain and is implicated in cardiac valve formation and in the inhibition of cardiac hypertrophy [24]. Over-expression of DSCR1 gene is involved in the pathogenesis of DS, especially mental retardation and cardiac defects [25]. It is suggested that patients with DS are less liable to certain cancers is due to the effects of this gene in reducing blood supply to the tumour cells [26].

Over expression of other genes of chromosome 21 in different cell types including fibroblast and fetal hearts leads to hyperactive interferon signaling which is a possible candidate pathway for cell senescence and autoimmune disorders in DS, and abnormal purine metabolism that may have a potential role in cardiac defects [27]. The trisomic genes present in Hsa21 may change the expression of some disomic genes present on chromosomes other than Hsa21, leading to a cellular manifestation and a DS phenotype and may affect heart development and further increase the vulnerability to cardiac defects in children with DS. At the same time; about 50% of people with trisomy 21 have CHD, whereas the rest have a structurally normal heart, indicating that trisomy 21 is a significant risk factor but is not causal for abnormal heart development suggestive of other factors may have a role in developing CHD in people with DS like genetic modifiers and environmental factors. Such genetic modifiers interact with dosage-sensitive gene(s) on Hsa21 to result in CHD. For example, missense mutations in genetic modifier CRELD1 (cysteine-rich with Epidermal Growth Factor (EGF)-like domains) have been found in DS patients with AVSD. CRELD1 (3p25.1) is one of the well-studied non-chromosome 21 loci variations that may predispose to a heart defect. It is referred as a candidate for the AVSD2 locus. CRELD1 belongs to an epidermal growth factor-like family and encodes a cell surface protein that likely acts as a cell adhesion molecule. CRELD1 encodes a novel cell adhesion molecule that is expressed during cardiac cushion development. Another example of genetic modifiers that can affect heart development is the somatic mutations in basic helix-loop-helix (bHLH) transcription factor HEY2 (gridlock) that has been identified in CHD in people with DS but not in euploid populations with heart defects [27 - 29]. Missense mutations in *GATA4* (MIM 600576) have also been shown to cause cardiac septal defects in humans, including AVSD especially in population with DS [30].

Other genetic factors may also play a part in development of CHD in people with DS. The nuclear factors of activated T cells (NF-ATs) are member of a group of transcription factors that transduce calcium signals in the immune, cardiac, muscular, and nervous systems. These factors can assist to organize and regulate the early activation of inducible genes while in some tissues can regulate cell differentiation and adaptation with a role in controlling the chondrocytes, myocytes, adipocytes and keratinocytes, and in the development of cardiac valves and cardiac muscle cells [31].

Environmental factors can adjust the action and interact with the trisomic genome and may modify the development of associated CHD in children with DS. For example; maternal cigarette smoking, is associated with ASVD, TOF, and ASD but not with VSD [14]. Another example is the maternal alcohol use which increases the incidence of VSD in children with DS and maternal folic acid supplementation may reduce risk for CHD. Deficiency of folic acid supplementation in the mothers during pregnancy was more frequent among infants with DS and AVSD or ASD than among infants with DS and no heart defect or with VSD [15,16]. Summary of patho-mechanism of congenital heart diseases in DS is demonstrated in Fig. (**2**).

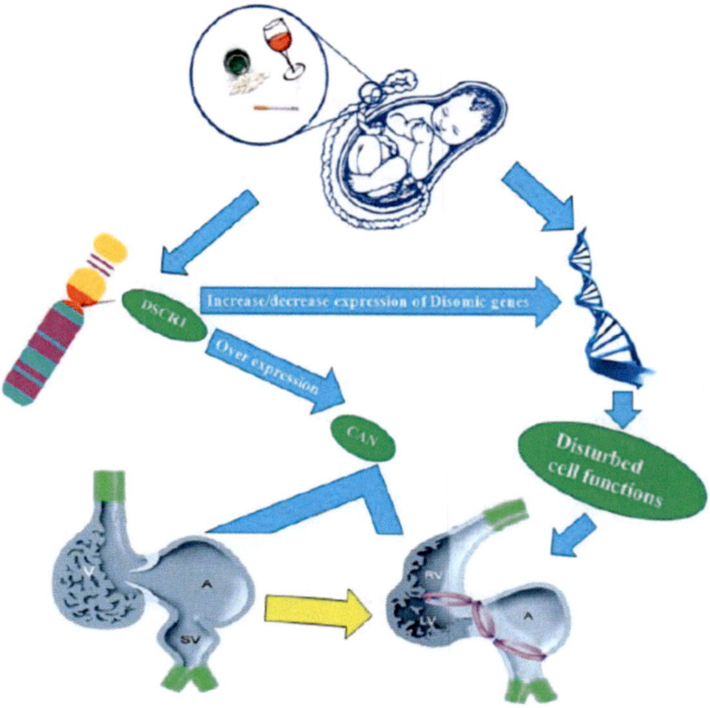

Fig. (2). Showed the patho-mechanisms of congenital heart diseases in DS. There is over expression of the genes present in DSCR, which directly affect cellular function in a fully differentiated cell to cause a functional phenotype of DS or in an immature cell to produce a developmental phenotype through different mechanisms. One of them is through Calcinurin 1 (CAN). Also; these trisomic genes may alter expression of other disomic genes, altering their cellular expression which leading to a cellular manifestation and a DS phenotype. Gene modifiers and environmental factors can also play a role.

2.3. Antenatal Anticipation of CHD in Children with DS

Antenatal screening for CHD is cases suspected to have DS aims to help both the parents and the treating physician for the best possible preparation, and to make the most informed decisions. This gives the parents a chance to decide for the possibility of pregnancy termination in cases of severe malformations as legal age of pregnancy termination is less than 24 weeks. It also helps for in utero treatment of the potentially treatable and less severe disorders, *e.g.* treatable fetal arrhythmias and allows treatment of malformations of the complications that may occur, preventing or attenuating their evolution through surgical correction in utero [32]. This also will help for preparation of emotional and psychological support for parents and to identify babies with complex CHDs that need delivery in a special tertiary care level center equipped with a Neonatal Intensive Care Unit so that during the transition from pre- to post-natal life, the baby does not face periods of hypoxia or acidosis and can be given immediate care. Antenatal diagnosis and appropriate treatment of CHDs may prevent the devastating consequences of early circulatory collapse, such as brain damage [33].

Antenatal ultrasound examinations for routine anomaly scanning are an integral role of usual antenatal care almost everywhere especially in the well developed countries. Fetal ultrasound examinations are usually done at three different stages of pregnancy - around week 9 - 12 (mostly transvaginal), week 19 - 22 and week 29 - 32. These examinations usually include a four chamber heart view that could detect 67% of all CHDs when done by will trained professionals especially when these anomalies are accompanied with change in chamber size such as the hypoplastic left heart syndrome. Anomalies associated with little changes in chamber size as transposition or coarctations are less likely to be detected. According to previous studies, only twenty to thirty percent of all CHDs are discovered during the routine antenatal care. In specialized centers, however, this percent increases to about 60–95% [34].

Being a fetus with DS is a significant risk factor for CHDs. However, presence of certain "soft markers" increases the risk of CHDs in such fetuses. Presence of single umbilical artery (SUA); abnormal nuchal translucency; intracardiac echogenic foci; unsatisfactory or abnormal 4-chamber cardiac views; extracardiac malformations and/or fetal arrhythmia; increase the risk of CHDs. However, most of these soft signs are non-specific and could also present in fetuses without abnormalities [35]. At the same time; any fetus with a structural malformation should be considered as at high risk for CHDs.

2.3.1. Single Umbilical Artery (SUA)

Single umbilical artery (Fig. **3**) is present in 0.5% and 7% of all pregnancies and 1 in 100 live births. Normally, umbilical cord contains 2 arteries and 1 vein. SUA results from atrophy or agenesis of one of the arteries. It can be detected during the routine gray-scale, second-trimester ultrasound examination usually after 18 weeks of gestation but can be diagnosed as early as 14 weeks of pregnancy using color-flow Doppler [36].

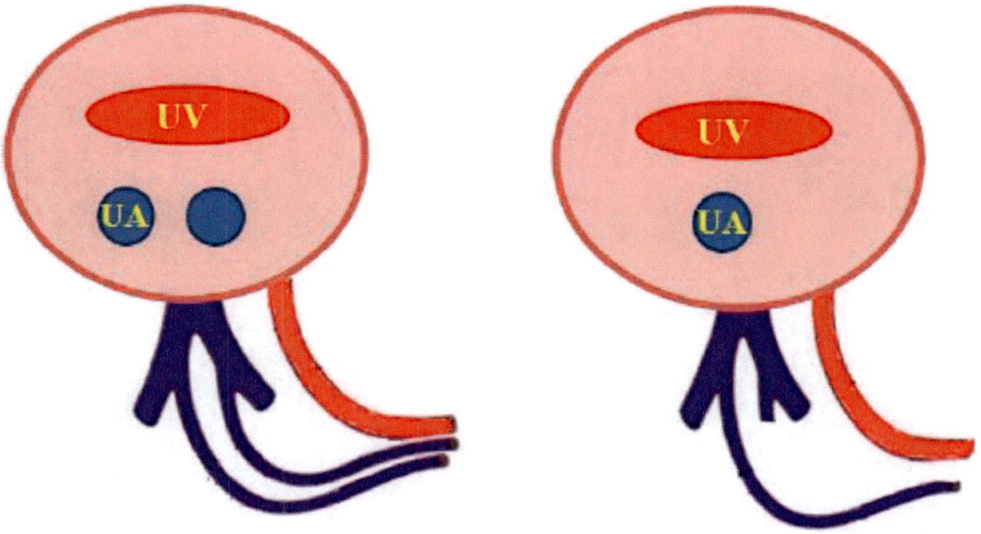

Fig. (3). Shows the umbilical cord which normally contains Wharton's jelly surrounding three blood vessels ; a single vein and 2 arteries (a 3 vessel cord) [left side] . Occasionally, one artery wastes away or fails to develop leaving only a single umbilical artery (a two vessel umbilical cord) [Right side].

SUA has been associated with fetal chromosomal, gastrointestinal tract abnormalities, renal and cardiac abnormalities (especially AVSD), and problems with the central nervous system as well as low birth weight and constituted about 5–6% of referrals for fetal echocardiography. Strong justification to do fetal echocardiography is present if SUA is associated with extracardiac abnormalities or with abnormal four-chamber and outflow tract views [37]. However, fetal echocardiography most likely will not provide additional diagnostic data to the prenatal assessment of the fetus with isolated single umbilical artery when normal four-chamber and outflow tract views of the heart have previously been done [38].

2.3.2. Echogenic Intracardiac Foci (EICF)

Echogenic intracardiac foci (Fig. **4**) are related to CHDs through their strong association with DS, as well as with trisomy 13 (Patau syndrome). They are detected in about 4% of obstetric sonograms, and their incidence can vary according to the race; with the highest rates occur among Asian populations and lowest rates of EICF are seen in the Black populations. Also, detection of EICF is inversely related to maternal body mass index (BMI). Low maternal BMI is an independent risk factor for the detection EICF [39].

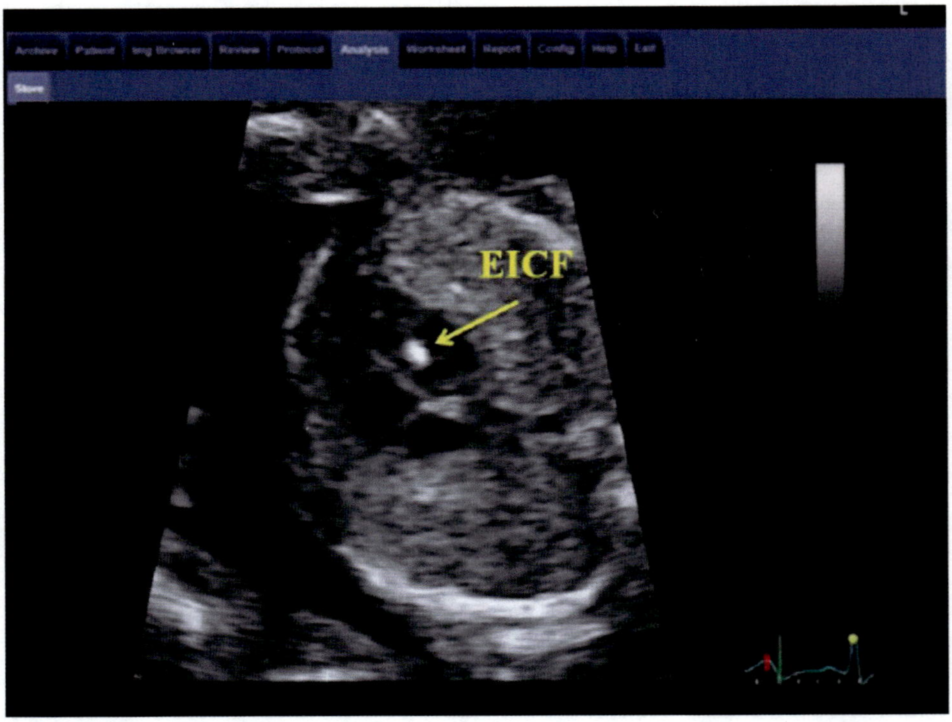

Fig. (4). Four-chamber view showed isolated Echogenic Intracardiac Focus (EICF) in left ventricle.

These foci are discrete areas of increased echogenicity in the region of papillary muscles. Their origin remains unclear. These foci may result from the aggregation of chordal tissues that have failed to fenestrate completely, the enhancement of abnormal tissue, or from a collection of fibrous tissue with increased echogenicity. They may also represent true microcalcifications within the cardiac muscle [40]. They are considered as a normal developmental variation, but either inflammatory or hypoxic conditions could be implicated in its look [41].

Detection of EICF is subjective and depends on many conditions like the resolution of the sonographic machine, technique, completeness of the examination, the size and echogenicity of EICF and the sonographer's experience. The larger the size of the left ventricular papillary muscle and the larger the masses of chordae tissue, the more likely is detection of the echogenic foci in this area [42]. For proper visualization and grading of EICF, an appropriate transducer frequency ($\leq$ 5 MHz) and an appropriate gain setting should be used. These foci can be diagnosed on the standard 4-chamber view of the fetal heart. Fetal position is also essential because intracardiac foci are best visualized when the cardiac apex is oriented toward the transducer [43]. EICF are classified according to their echogenicity, laterality and number as shown in Table **2**.

Table 2. Showed the different classifications of Echogenic intracardiac foci.

Parameters	**Classification**	**Clinical Importance**
Echogenicity [44]: Relating foci echogenicity to echogenicity of thoracic spine	**Grade 1:** less echogenicity than that of the thoracic spine (Hypo-echogenic)	
	Grade 2: has the same echogenicity of bone (Iso-echogenic)	
	Grade 3: more echogenicity than that of the thoracic spine (Hyper-echogenic)	
Laterality [45]: according to which ventricle is affected	Left ventricle (88% of cases)	associated with a lesser risk for fetal aneuploidy
	Right ventricular (5%)	associated with a higher risk for fetal aneuploidy
	Biventricular (7%)	associated with a higher risk for fetal aneuploidy

(Table 2) contd.....

Parameters	Classification	Clinical Importance
Number [46]	Single	associated with a lesser risk for fetal aneuploidy
	Multiple (more than 1)	associated with a higher risk for fetal aneuploidy

These foci are of no hemodynamic or other short or long term clinical or functional significance, but their importance arises from being a possible marker of a chromosomal abnormality [47]. A single EICF should be regarded as an incidental finding in pregnant mothers less than 35 years and in those without abnormal serum aneuploidy screening results [48]. In low-risk people for aneuploidy, the presence of an EICF is not an indication to do invasive procedures. In high-risk people; this depends on the previous calculated risk. In euploid fetuses, cardiac function is not significantly impaired but more researches in particular populations may be reasonable. Fetuses with diffuse myocardial calcification or several foci may need additional studies [41]. Color Doppler twinkling artifacts from isolated EICF occur in some fetuses and may be regarded as an additional echocardiographic feature of EICF. Care should be given to the recognition and interpretation of these artifacts so that they may be precisely differentiated from real color flow generated by atrioventricular valvular regurgitation jets [49]. Other importance for EICF is that these foci cam be misdiagnosed with other cardiac conditions. These conditions include intra-cardiac tumors (rhabdomyomas, teratomas, fibromas, hemangiomas), ventricular thrombi (especially if adherent to the papillary muscles in the left ventricle), dystrophic valves, air in the chambers from fetal demise, endocardial fibroelastosis that is usually multiple and along the endocardial surface, idiopathic infantile arterial calcification, viral infections or metabolic disorders [50].

2.3.3. Abnormal Nuchal Translucency During Nuchal-fold Scan

Nuchal-fold scan is a specialized ultrasound examination that is done between 11 and 14 weeks of gestation especially when fetal abnormalities are suspected. It can be simply included in the regular pregnancy scan. Nuchal translucency results from increase the amount of liquids in the obvious space in the folds of soft tissue at the back of the developing baby's neck forming what is called nuchal fold observed in the early stage of fetal development. During nuchal scanning, the thickness of this nuchal fold area is measured it in the longitudinal midline plane of the fetus, using a very consistent and classic method [51]. Strict criteria should be followed to obtain an adequate ultrasound image for the evaluation of nuchal translucency and the normal upper values of measurement are dependent upon pregnancy duration and fetal age [52]. Fully automatic approach for computing nuchal translucency measurement was recently introduced in the ultrasound scans of the mid-sagittal plane of a fetal head. The nuchal translucency measurement is computed from the segmented region. Experiments show that the algorithm efficiently and effectively detects the nuchal translucency region and provides accurate measurement which suggests suitability for clinical use [53].

There is increased evidence that an increased nuchal-fold thickness (Fig. **5**) can indicate denote existence of some anomalies such as chromosomal abnormalities especially DS.

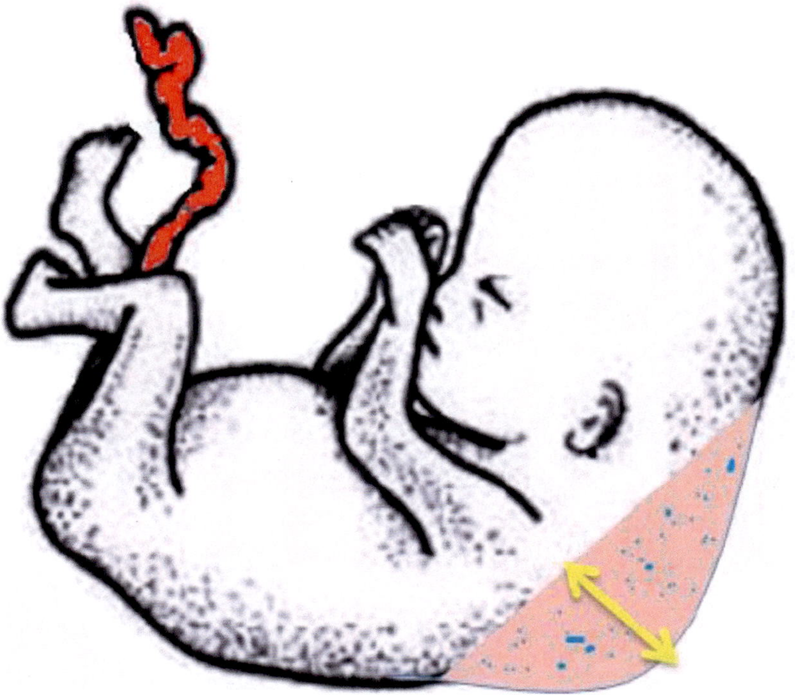

Fig. (5). A demonstration of 13 week fetus with markedly increased nuchal translucency (arrow) bulging the fetal skin (Trisomy 21).

Many studies have proved that an increased nuchal-fold thickness (fetal nuchal translucency measurement of 3.5 mm or greater in the first trimester) can also be accompanied with an increased risk of a congenital heart defect in approximately 4–7% of cases. However, there is no specific relationship between nuchal-fold thickness and certain types of heart malformation. The exact underlying pathophysiologic mechanism of increased nuchal translucency is not clearly determined. Increased nuchal translucency in cases with CHDs may be related to venous congestion in the head and neck of the fetus, abnormalities of lymphatic drainage, altered distribution of subcutaneous tissue, glycosaminoglycan and proteoglycan accumulation, fetal anemia and/or decreased fetal movement [54,55]. Nuchal edema due to fluid accumulation as a result of cardiac failure is another potential reason [56].

Nuchal-fold scan is a screening examination and a positive result of the nuchal-fold measurement can be a key sign for the need of additional tests such as complete fetal echocardiographic examination or an amniocentesis. Its sensitivity to detect trisomy 21 pregnancies in the first trimester reaches 83% which increases to 94% when combined with maternal age and bi-test pregnancy-associated plasma protein (PAPP-A) with second-trimester free chorionic gonadotropin (β-hCG) or tri-test alpha-fetoprotein (AFP), estriol and free β-hCG with a 5% false-positive rate [57]. However, even in chromosomally normal fetuses, presence of increased nuchal translucency is related to poor fetal outcomes. About 20% of chromosomally normal fetuses with increased nuchal translucency are more prone to have poor outcome, as miscarriage, intrauterine death, parental choice to terminate the pregnancy, or one or more anatomic or genetic fetal anomalies. The chance of an uneventful pregnancy outcome depends on the initial degree of increase in nuchal translucency. However, if the detailed ultrasound examination at around 20 weeks is normal, a favorable outcome can be expected with confidence, irrespective of initially increased nuchal translucency [58, 59].

Some studies showed an increased incidence of general risk of cardiac defect of 2% when the nuchal translucency is above the 95th centile and a significantly higher risk (6%) when the nuchal translucency is above the 99th centile even without chromosomal aberration. They also showed that 56% of all fetuses with serious cardiac defects had nuchal translucency measurements above the 95th centile [60, 61]. However, other studies failed to demonstrate any strong association between increased nuchal translucency and cardiac defects, although demonstrating some association [62, 63]. Measurement of nuchal translucency thickness cannot be utilized as a diagnostic tool of congenital heart disease but it shows enormous guarantee to identify fetuses at increased risk of CHD, and therefore may help direct resource-efficient use of fetal echocardiography. However, by itself, increased nuchal translucency does not predict presence of certain type of cardiac defect in the fetus [64]. The combination of an increased nuchal translucency, tricuspid regurgitation and an abnormal ductus venosus (DV) Doppler flow profile is a strong marker for CHDs. A fetal echocardiogram should be done at 20 weeks' gestation in fetuses when the nuchal translucency is equal or more than 95th percentile but less than 99th percentile. When the measurement is equal or more than 99th percentile, or when tricuspid regurgitation and/or an abnormal DV flow pattern are found along with the increased nuchal translucency, an earlier echocardiogram is indicated, followed by a repeat scan at around 20 weeks' gestation [65].

2.3.4. Abnormal Four-Chamber View During Antenatal Ultrasound Examination

Abnormal four-chamber view during the antenatal ultrasound examination increases risk of DS as well as presence of CHDs in the affected fetus. The characteristic cardiac features related to the increased risk of DS are mainly asymmetric ventricular sizes and the possible presence of septal defects. In addition, the phenomenon of tricuspid regurgitation is strongly linked to and its prevalence increases with the nuchal translucency. Tricuspid regurgitation is considered to be a transient and physiological finding in the second half of pregnancy and in postnatal life. It is observed in about 30-50% of fetuses with trisomy 21 and in only approximately 1-5 % of the euploid fetuses at 11–13 weeks of gestation [66, 67]. Other findings proved that the mitral valve-tricuspid valve distance could be useful finding as an additional marker at the time of the second trimester sonogram. Normally, the tricuspid valve inserts into the atrioventricular septum closer to the cardiac apex than does the mitral valve. Lack of this apical offset causes arrangement and appearance of the mitral and tricuspid valves within the fetal heart that can be indicative of AVSD. Classically; this finding can be assessed subjectively during the fetal anatomic survey at 20 or 22 weeks of pregnancy [65].

Presence of tricuspid regurgitation detected by pulsed Doppler together with increased nuchal translucency, and abnormal flow pattern in the 'a' wave of the ductus venosus increases the risk of associated CHDs. The combination of all 3 markers might increase the detection rates. So, in high-risk group and in fetuses with tricuspid regurgitation and/or an abnormal ductus venosus flow pattern along with an increased nuchal translucency, first or early second trimester echocardiography performed by experts is warranted. The early examination of the fetal heart should be completed by a detailed echocardiogram at around 20 weeks of gestation [68]. However, presence of isolated tricuspid regurgitation is always insignificant. After CHDs are excluded; this tricuspid regurgitation in the fetus does not significantly affect haemodynamics and does not predict any pathology [69]. The presence of an aberrant right subclavian artery (ARSA) is another potential new soft marker that is more commonly seen in fetuses with trisomy 21 and other chromosomal defects than in normal fetuses. An ARSA has been found postnatally in 1–2% of normal individuals (from neonates to adulthood) at autopsy, but its incidence is increased in cases of DS, with figures ranging between 2.9% and 37%. Although it can be considered a weak marker, the second trimester diagnosis of an ARSA should prompt a detailed search for additional "soft markers" and potential structural defects including CHDs [70 - 72].

2.3.4. Detection of Associated Non-Cardiac Anomalies During Antenatal Ultrasound Examination

In general; extra-cardiac anomalies occur in 15-45% of cases with CHDs. Presence of either CHDs or extra-cardiac anomalies requires excluding of other associated anomalies. The presence of an extra-cardiac anomaly significantly increases the mortality in infants with CHDs. One study done by Güçer *et al.* showed that the most commonly encountered extra-cardiac malformations are craniofacial malformations followed by malformations of genitourinary, musculoskeletal, respiratory, gastrointestinal, spleen anomalies and other central nervous systems. They showed also that ventricular septal defect, atrial septal defect (ASD), aortic coarctation, single ventricle, pulmonary stenosis, hypoplastic right heart syndrome, double outlet right ventricle, ASD+VSD, aortic arcus anomalies, and right and left atrial isomerism cases were often (>50%) accompanied by extracardiac malformations. On the other hand they found no extra-cardiac malformations were associated with pulmonary atresia with intact interventricular septum, Ebstein malformation, or mitral stenosis (MS) [73]. Table **3** showed some of the commonly associated extra-cardiac malformations in fetuses with DS who have CHDs.

Table 3. Commonly associated extra-cardiac malformations in fetuses with DS who have CHDs.

Congenital Heart Diseases [74]	Associated extra-cardiac malformations
VSD	Dandy-Walker, clubfoot, SUA
AVSD	Agenesis of the corpus callosum, SUA, Hydrocephalus, Hydrops, Unilateral renal dysplasia
COA	Transient mild cystic hygroma, Hydrocephalus, Hydrops
Single ventricle	Spleen malformation
Conotruncal heart defects	Gastrointestinal & genitourinary systems anomalies

AVSD . atrio-ventricular septal defect; CHD . congenital heart defect; COA . coarctation of the aorta; SUA . single umbilical artery; VSD . ventricular septal defect.

2.4. Antenatal Detection of CHD in Children with DS

2.4.1. Fetal Echocardiography

When CHDs are suspected in cases with DS; fetal echocardiography should be considered. Fetal echocardiography is able to define fetal cardiac structures as early as 10 - 12 weeks of pregnancy using high-resolution vaginal probe transducers but conventional trans-abdominal echocardiography can detect fetal cardiac anomalies by 16 - 18 weeks of gestation. However, the ideal time for fetal echocardiographic examination is between 20 and 22 weeks of gestation. At this period, the cardiac structures of the fetus can be easily identified more obviously with ultrasound screening in more than 90% of cases because the heart is big enough to visualize the detail, ribs are not as dense and the fetus has various positions. However a lot of difficulties enface because of unique fetal physiology, the aliasing effect of the flow across defects and valves, the incapability to distinguish the fetus for orientation reference, and failure to check the fetus for clinical findings. Other factors may include maternal Obesity, presence of polyhydramnios or oligohydramnios, previous abdominal surgery and the fetal Position. Evaluation of detailed cardiac structures during the third trimester is more difficult because of acoustic shadowing by dense ribs, maternal obesity or prone fetal position [75].

Knowing the fetal embryology, circulatory physiology and the changes that occur at birth is of paramount importance to perform adequate fetal echocardiography. In the embryo; the heart starts beating at day 21 post conception. It starts development as a straight solitary median cardiac tube with ineffective contractions and grows more rapidly than any other organ in the chest cavity and consequently loops to form atrium at 5 weeks with beginning of the circulation. Over the following 3-4 weeks, the atria, ventricles, and truncus arteriosus septate and develop. The primitive double aortic arch is distinguished into the typical left 4th arch and the left 6th arch is preserved as the ductus. The pulmonary veins combine and connect to the heart through the common pulmonary vein. So when the embryo is 7-8 weeks old; the heart is completely septated and the intracardiac structures are well defined with 4 chambers heart [76].

Fetal circulation (Fig. **6**) has its own specific features which differ from the postnatal heart. The oxygenated blood coming from the placenta enters the fetus *via* the umbilical vein. Then, the umbilical vein drains blood into the IVC and then into the right atrium; so that the major part of this blood then flows across the Foramen Ovale into the left atrium then to LV and through the ascending aorta to head, neck, arms and some to the rest of the body. The blood coming from the Superior Vena Cava (SVC) returns to the right atrium and mainly flows through the tricuspid valve, enters RV, and is then pumped out to the pulmonary artery. Because of the quite high pulmonary vascular resistance in the fetus, very little blood flow passes through the pulmonary artery branches and crosses the lung. Because of that; the majority of blood entering the pulmonary artery is shunted through the ductus arteriosus and down the descending aorta to the lower body, umbilical artery, and low resistance placental bed [77]. When the baby is born and starts breathing; its own pulmonary vascular resistance decreases. The oxygen saturation of the blood increases. When the umbilical cord is clamped, the low resistance placental bed vanishes and the systemic vascular resistance begins to increase. With these changes, ductus arteriosus starts to close and the flow across the Foramen Ovale diminishes and may even change its direction with declining of pulmonary vascular resistance [78].

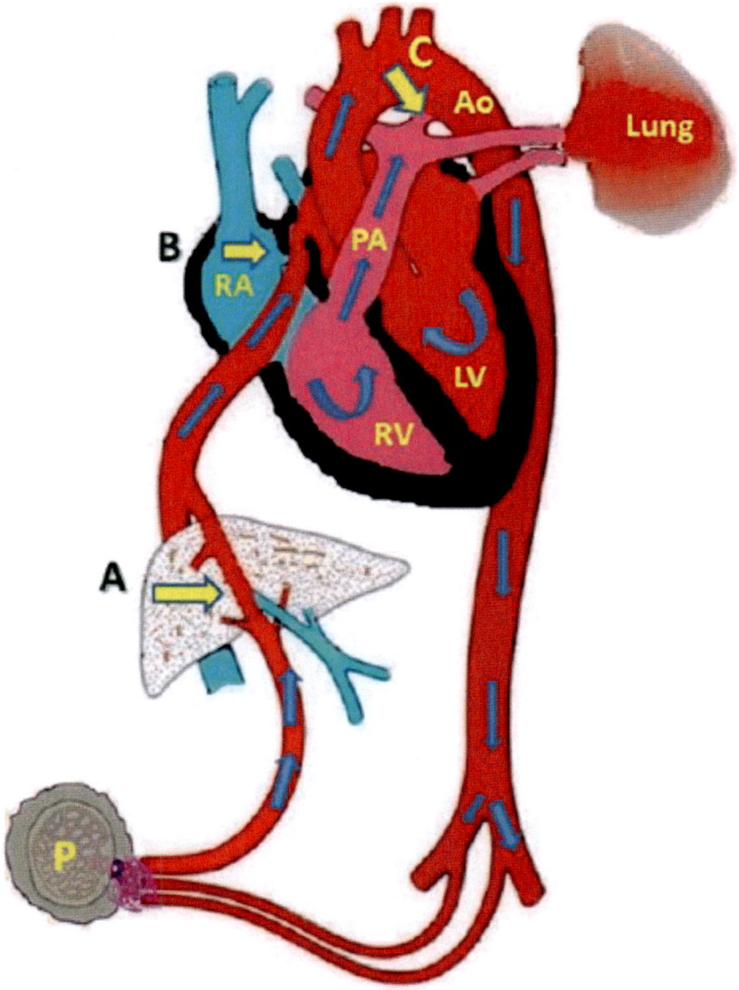

Fig. (6). It shows the fetal circulation which is a parallel arrangement of pulmonary and systemic circulations with 3 intra-cardiac and vascular passages (A,B, and C marked by yellow arrows) which allows streaming of the blood. (**A**) Ductus venosus shunts most of the left umbilical vein blood flow directly to the inferior vena cava. The blood from the placenta (P) that has been enriched with oxygen and nutrients gets *via* the umbilical vein to the liver, part flows through it and part bypasses it *via* the ductus venosus and gets *via* the v. cava inferior into the right atrium. (**B**): Foramen ovale connects between the right and left atria. Due to the higher pressure of the blood in the inferior vena cava, more blood flows from it directly into the left atrium *via* the foramen ovale which act as a valve that direct the blood stream that comes from below directly into the left atrium; hence a a small portion of the blood seeps into the right ventricle *via* the tricuspid valve. (**C**): Ductus arteriosus connects the pulmonary artery to the descending aorta and due to the high pressure in the lungs, though, a significantly larger part flows through the ductus arteriosus and goes into the aorta descendens and thus directly into the large (systemic) circulation system.

Technical settings such as acoustic focus, frequency selection, signal gain, image magnification, temporal resolution, harmonic imaging, and Doppler-related parameters should be properly tuned to get satisfactory sonographic pictures. To obtain adequate cardiac views, the fetal cardiac apex should be directed toward the anterior maternal wall. If the fetus is cephalic; the probe marker is directed to the mother's left while if the fetus is breach the probe will be in normal position and the fetal spine is posterior. Proper understanding of the fetal heart anatomy is needed to adequately interpret the obtained echocardiographic images either to diagnose or to exclude a congenital abnormality. The American Institute for Ultrasound in Medicine (AIUM) guidelines emphasized that the fetal echocardiography should include imaging of the aortic arch, ductal arch, four-chamber view, inferior vena cava, left ventricular outflow tract (LVOT), right ventricular outflow tract (RVOT), short-axis views ("low" for ventricles and "high" for outflow tracts), superior vena cava, and three-vessel and trachea views [79].

A normal fetal heart is about one-third of the thorax in size, and this proportion (cardiothoracic area, C/T area) is steady all over pregnancy with the axis of the heart lies at a 45° angle to the left of the midline [80]. There is a parallel arrangement of pulmonary and systemic circulation with presence of intra-cardiac and vascular passages that allow streaming of blood. Superior vena cava (SVC) & inferior vena cava (IVC)/ Hepatic veins are draining into the RA and foramen ovale should drain blood from RA to the LA. The atria should be of equal size and the lower atrial septum should fuse with the AV valves/ventricular septum and the flap of foramen ovale lies in the left atrial cavity. Also both ventricles are of nearly of the same size although the right side of the heart becomes larger in size as pregnancy progresses. The LV should be posterior and the RV should be anterior with intact ventricular septum. The right ventricle can be differentiated by presence of the moderator band. The examiner may be able to see pulmonary veins entering the LA; but sometime the examiner may be not able to visualize them because of fetal physiology. However, the examiner should be able to see the two atrioventricular valves (A-V valves). The two atrioventricular valves are similarly opened and differentially inserted: the septal leaflet of the tricuspid valve is inserted more apically than the mitral valve in the ventricular septum [81]. The aorta should arise from the LV and be located slightly posterior to the pulmonary artery and head rightward while pulmonary artery should arise from the RV and be anterior to the aorta and head leftward and the pulmonary artery should cross over the aorta. The pulmonary artery is about 10% larger than the aorta. The ductus arteriosus connects the pulmonary artery to the descending aorta and aortic arch is tighter curve than the ductal arch and has head vessels while ductal arch is longer, less curved-flatter, with no head vessels. The blood flow of the aorta and duct should be in the same direction. The cardiac output is expressed as combined ventricular output and is exquisitely dependant on a narrow range of heart rate which makes arrhythmias if occurs to be very poorly tolerated [82].

For complete diagnosis of a fetus with major CHDs, a systematic sequential and segmental approach should be followed. Similar to postnatal practice, the first step is to evaluate the fetal heart rate then to identify the "Situs" of the fetal heart followed by evaluation of the atrial-ventricular connections, and the ventricular-arterial alignment and lastly by evaluation of the great arteries relationship to each other. First the examiner determines position of the fetus, and then begins in an axial plane - 4 chamber view where the heart occupies about 1/3 of fetal chest. *In situs* solitus; the aorta is left and posterior to the inferior vena cava (IVC) and is posterior and to the left of the spinal cord with the liver is on the right side and the gastric air bubbles are on the left side [83]. *In situs* inversus, the aorta is located to the right of the IVC in a mirror image pattern while *in situs* ambiguous, the aorta and IVC are located on the same side of the spine in right isomerism, while the aorta is centrally located with an interrupted IVC in left isomerism [84]. After determination of the cardiac situs we should determine the cardiac position and axis. In normal conditions, the heart is located within the left chest, with the liver on the right, stomach on the left, and the apex of the heart pointed to the left (levocardia) while in dextrocardia, the heart is located within the right chest with the apex pointing to the right. In mesocardia the heart is centrally located with the apex pointing anteriorly. We should discriminate dextroposition from dextrocardia. In dextroposition, heart has normal left-sided axis but it is displaced to the right due to extracardiac reasons (for example, diaphragmatic hernia, congenital pulmonary cystic adenomatoid malformation, pleural effusion, *etc.*) [85].

The basic view of the fetal heart is the four-chamber view Figs. (**7A**) & (**7B**) which is the easiest and most important cardiac view as it can detect 43-96% of fetal congenital heart anomalies during prenatal cardiac screening. It can be easily obtained by moving the transducer cranially from the transverse abdominal view [86]. To ensure proper cutting the fetal thorax in the appropriate plane by the sonographic beam, it uses the fetal ribs as external reference points which is considered as advantage of this view. When properly done, there should be the appearance of a single rib around the fetal thorax. However, it should be noted that the fetal four-chamber is situated in a more horizontal plane than the postnatal one because of the larger liver. This view can visualize both atria, both ventricles, atrioventricular (AV) valves (mitral and tricuspid) and both the interventricular and interatrial septa [87]. To increase the detectability of CHDs by fetal echocardiography, both four-chamber view and outflow tracts should be examined meticulously. However, detecting abnormalities in the outflow tracts is more difficult and challenging than in the four-chamber view [88].

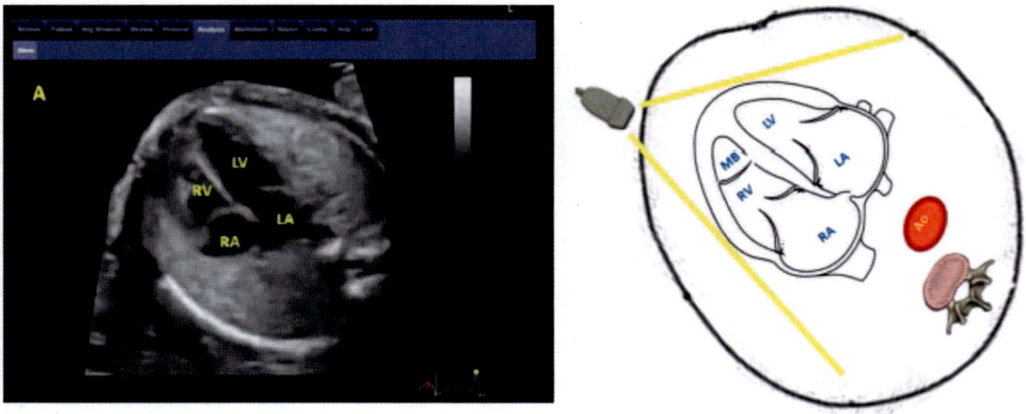

Fig. (7A). Fetal echocardiographic Apical 4-chamber view on the left panel and its cartoon demonstration on the right panel. RV can be distinguished easily by its moderator band (MB), and tricuspid valve leaflets are

more apical than that of mitral valve.

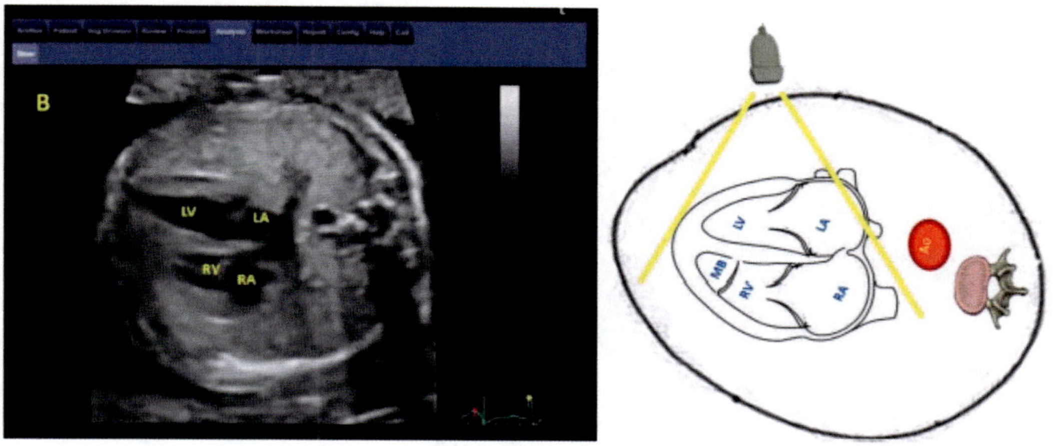

Fig. (7B). Fetal echocardiographic lateral 4-chamber view on the left panel and its cartoon demonstration on the right panel. RV can be distinguished easily by its moderator band, and tricuspid valve leaflets are more apical than that of mitral valve.

To increase the sensitivity of anomaly detection and adequate visualization of outflow tracts we can use either “Extended basic views” of left ventricular outflow tract (LVOT) and right ventricular outflow tract (RVOT) or alternatively, a comprehensive set of five short-axis projection.

The transducer is tilted 45° from the four-chamber (in a perpendicular way to the septum toward the cardiac apex) to obtain LVOT view which shows the aorta originating from the LVOT with its main great vessels of the head and neck appearing distally. It also shows the intact ventricular septum. Blood flow across the aortic valve is laminar flow with no turbulence in systole and no regurgitation in diastole (Fig. **8**).

In the same way, by further rotation of the probe in the same direction, the RVOT view Fig. (**9**) can be achieved with gentle rocking the transducer from the LVOT view toward the fetal head.

In RVOT view, visualization of pulmonary artery as it arises from the RV and divides into its main branches can be done. It also can visualize ductus arteriosus, left pulmonary artery and the ascending aorta seen centrally, wrapped by the RV and PA demonstrating crossing nature of the great arteries by moving the transducer slightly up and down [86].

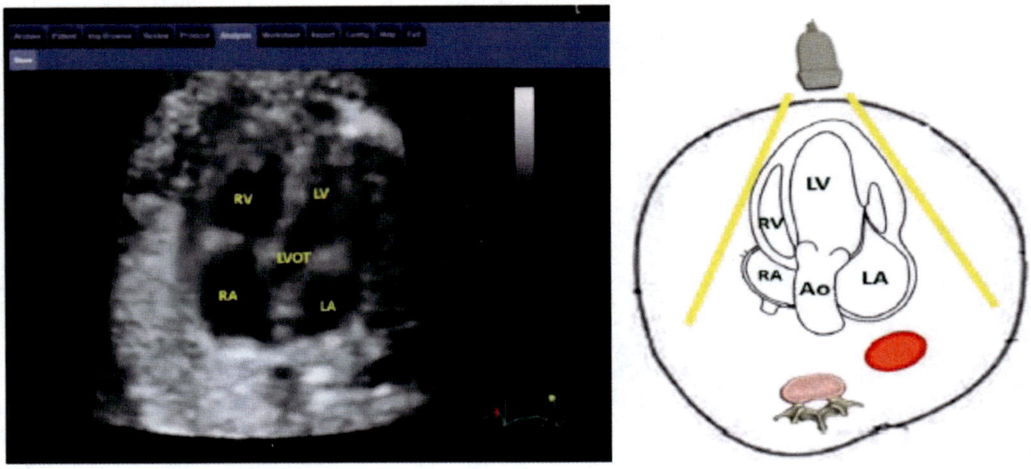

Fig. (8). Fetal echocardiographic view of LVOT on the left panel and its cartoon demonstration on the right panel. The outflow tracts are imaged by tilting the probe towards the fetal head. it showed the LVOT and ascending aorta as it arises from LV.

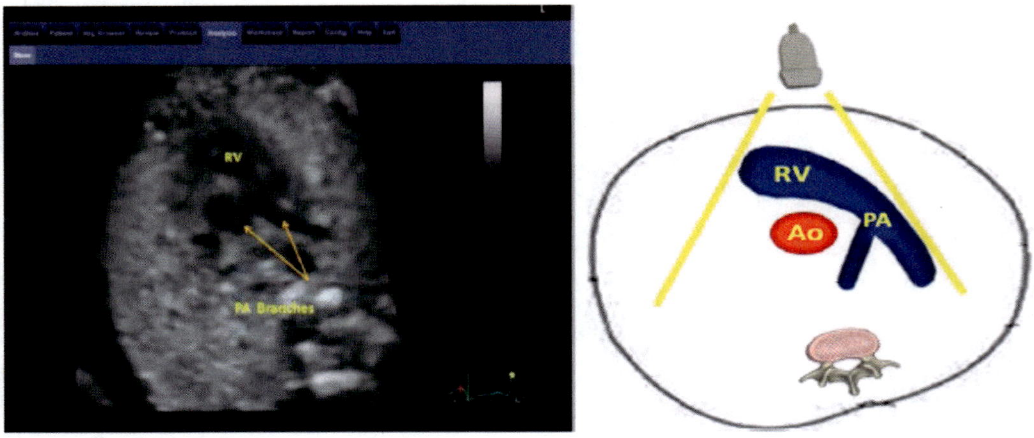

Fig. (9). Fetal echocardiographic view of RVOT on the left panel and its cartoon demonstration on the right panel. It showed the RVOT, Right ventricle gives rise to pulmonary artery (PA) and its main branches. The great vessels are be of equal size but the pulmonary artery tends to be slightly bigger (10%). They should cross at approximately 90° as they emerge from their respective ventricles (crossing perpendicular).

A comprehensive set of five short-axis projections can also be obtained by cranial or caudal tilting of the ultrasound probe from the four-chamber view with the ventricular septum parallel to the ultrasound beam and the fetal spine. In this set of views, the pulmonary artery and RVOT are seen in the most cephalad short-axis view as they course around the aorta. Also; the fetal pulmonary branches bifurcation can still be identified despite being small and the ductus arteriosus can be identified and traced into the descending aorta. More caudal and horizontal angulation from this plane, both ventricles and their respective AV valves can be identified. This set of views is adequate for the recognition of conotruncal abnormalities that could otherwise be over looked in more classic views. However, a specific diagnosis should not be made from a single plane [83].

Both fetal ventricles are almost of equal size, however, the pulmonary artery diameter is 10% larger that of aortic diameter. Two-Dimensional mode can measure the ventricular volume using the Simpson rule. M-mode combined with 2-D can evaluate RV/LV ratio, LV wall thickness, septal wall thickness, left atrial dimension, PA diameter, as well as aortic root diameter. These measures should be adjusted according to the fetal age as assessed by the biparietal diameter, fetal length or other usually used measures. Inequality of ventricular volumes can help to diagnose ventricular hypoplasia (either left or right). Also, these measures are useful to diagnose cardiomegaly due to different congenital anomalies including pericardial effusion, aneurysms, cardiomyopathies, or tumors. M-mode also can easily help to trace fetal heart motion, heart rate, wall thickness, chamber size, and motion of the valves or myocardium which can give data on wall thickness and ventricular fraction shortening as well as other functions. The fetal long axis function may give extra information about endocardial function, which is most helpful in the recognition of early ischemic changes before the development of sonographically demonstrable endocardial fibroelastosis (EFE). Color Doppler can assess vascular flow through cardiac chambers, vascular structures, and septal defects, facilitating accurate delineation of congenital defects and anomalies. It should be noted that the peak systolic velocity in the aorta increases linearly with advancing pregnancy, and it varies from around 30 cm/sec at 19 weeks to 100 cm/sec at full term. Peak systolic velocity in the aorta is more than in the pulmonary artery. At the same time, the peak systolic velocity in the pulmonary artery increases linearly with advancing pregnancy, and it achieves 100 cm/sec at full term [89 - 93].

It was observed that fetal cardiac functions in trisomy 21 were impaired irrespective of the presence or absence of CHDs. Evidence for cardiac loading (increased preload and after load) and LV systolic (in the first trimester) and later diastolic dysfunction was observed. Clur *et al.* showed significant reduction of tricuspid valve (TV) A-wave velocity and aortic valve peak velocity in trisomy 21 compared with normal fetuses. In addition, they also identified significant increases in the TV-E/A ratio and the ductus venosus-pulsatility index for veins (DV-PIV) and reduced pulmonary valve peak velocity.

There were also some evidences of left ventricular (LV) systolic dysfunction, such as decreased stroke volume (SV) and increased myocardial performance index (MPI). They also observed significant reduction of the mitral valve A-wave peak velocity and E/TVI ratio beyond 14 weeks of gestation in the trisomy 21 fetuses with normal hearts compared to the controls with increased nuchal translucency thickness [94].

Four-chamber view can visualize a complete AV canal easier than a primum ASD. Because of that; the diagnosis of primum ASD should be considered whenever a defect is noted in the part of the atrial septum near the AV valves (septum primum).

A large complete AV canal can be more obvious on the 4-chamber view during diastole when the AV valve is opened; while ASDs and VSDs can be clearly visualized above and below the closed AV valves during systole; making their diagnosis possible as early as the late first trimester.

Mixing of flow in the area of the septum primum defect, the dysplastic AV valves, and the VSD can be clearly visualized by color flow Doppler which can also show any defect in separation between the right and left ventricular inflow tracts in diastole, producing a classic "H" configuration. Color flow Doppler is also supportive in detecting and evaluating the degree of dysplastic AV insufficiency that may be severe enough to cause fetal heart failure with ascites [95].

Table **4** showed the different classification of the associated congenital anomalies associated with DS. They are classified according to detectability, severity, and according to the surgical risks [96 - 98].

Table 4. Different classification of the associated congenital anomalies associated with DS.

Classification	Grade	Criteria	Example
Detectability: by routine antenatal assessment using cardiac 4-chamber view at 18 wks' gestation	**Detectable:**	4-chamber view can detect them as they usually produce: 1- marked cardiomegaly, 2- Obvious abnormality of the AV connection. 3- Disparity between the sizes of the atria or ventricles or both.	AVSD,
	Non-Detectable:	4-chamber view fails to identify them as types of major malformations affecting the left or right heart outflows	TGA
	Possible undetectable:	could be identified or missed According to size or severity of the lesion and associated 4-chamber view changes	VSD, PS, AS, CoA,
Severity	**Complex**	If there is an atretic or hypoplastic valve or cardiac chamber	HLHS, TA, PA with VSD, DORV, DOLV
	Significant	When 4-chambers is of normal or increased size and four valves are present but require intervention	Ebstein/tricuspid valve dysplasia, significant complete AVSD, large VSD, partial AVSD, ASD, PDA, severe AS, severe PS, TGA, COA, TAPVR or TOF
	Minor	when no treatment is required	small VSD, mild AS or mild PS.
Choi Severity Classification	**normal**	No anomalies detected	
	Minor	do not require any interference	PFO, isolated peripheral PS, abnormal looking AA, simple right AA, tortuous ductus without obstruction, & mild RV dilation with or without TR (or very mild)
	Simple	simple defect or a defect completely correctable by medical treatment	VSD, ASD, and possibly CoA
	Moderate	defects that are surgically correctable with a low risk for reoperation	TOF, CoA, AVSD, and complete TGA
	Complex	defects correctable with surgery but that carry a high risk for sequelae or defects potentially suitable for a Fontan procedure	DORV, TGA with PS, critical PS, and other Fontan candidates {PA with IVS, f-SV, HLHS}

(Table 4) contd.....

Classification	Grade	Criteria	Example
Surgical risk	**High Risk**	Carries high risk of morbidity, mortality or need for reoperation	This classification has the disadvantages of having great variability between institutions and the need to change the risk stratification in accordance with future advancements in surgical treatment
	Low Risk	Carries low risk of morbidity, mortality or need for reoperation	

AA: aortic arch, AS: aortic stenosis, ASD: atrial septal defect, AVSD: artioventricular septal defect, CoA: aortic coarctation, DOLV: Double outlet left ventricle, DORV: Double outlet right ventricle, f-SV: functional single ventricle, HLHS: hypoplastic left heart syndrome, PA with VSD: Pulmonary atresia with ventricular septal defect, , PFO: Persistent Foramen Ovale, PS: pulmonary stenosis, RV: right ventricle, TA: tricuspid atresia, TAPVR: total anomalous pulmonary venous return, TGA: transposition of great arteries, TOF: Tetralogy of Fallout, TR: tricuspid regurgitation, VSD: ventricular septal defect.

2.4.2. Fetal Cardiac Magnetic Resonance Imaging (MRI)

Despite fetal echocardiography is the gold standard examination for fetal heart disease, sometimes it is inconclusive and need more advanced investigations. Fetal magnetic resonance imaging (MRI) is considered as a third-level imaging modality with a validity of diagnostic accuracy of 79% [99]. MRI provides structural and functional studies and is a secure addition that can help additional comprehensive understanding a fetus' cardiac anatomy. It can accurately determine the cardiac size, define the anatomy and size of the cardiac chambers, locate the cardiac apex and define ventricular septal thickness and angulation. It can accurately delineate the aorta, and determine the size and position of the pulmonary artery, aorta, superior vena cava and ductus arteriosus. However, pulmonary veins are sometimes difficult to be detected. It can also accurately define the ventricular geometry; relative position and kinetics [100]. Fetal MRI has many advantages over fetal echocardiography. It provides improved estimations of chamber volume and is not restricted by acoustic window. Fetal factors such as oligohydramnios and maternal factors as obesity have no effects on fetal MRI examination and MRI is less operator dependant than fetal echocardiography. It is also more able to define and evaluate fetal great vessels than fetal echocardiography [101]. However, there are some limitations for fetal MRI as it can be affected by fetal movement and there is lack of fetal MRI researches done during first trimester [102]. Mother with pacemakers or internal cardioverter defibrillators should avoid MRI. Fetal echocardiography is safer and reproducible when compared to fetal MRI. However, human fetal MRI studies did not show increased risk of morbidity of fetal MRI during three year follow-up with neither impact on intrauterine fetal growth, or change in cardiotocographic measurements [100]. Computed tomography (CT) scanning has limited applications in prenatal diagnosis.

2.5. Some Common CHDs in Children with DS

Despite that any type of congenital heart anomalies can occur in babies with DS, however, there are a number of anomalies which are well known to be common among then. As mentioned before, AVSD is the most common CHD and forms approximately 45% of all CHDs observed in DS children while VSD is the second most common CHD forms approximately 35% of all CHDs. In this section we will discuss into details some of the common CHDs in children with DS.

2.5.1. Atrioventricular Septal Defects (AVSDs)

AVSDs are congenital structural defective anomalies in the apical part or the atrial septum, basal part of the inter-ventricular septum in addition to atrio-ventricular valves. These defects arise due to faulty development of the embryonic endocardial cushions which lead to presence of a common atrioventricular junction as compared to the separate right and left atrioventricular junction in the normal heart as well as presence of defects of the muscular and membranous atrioventricular septum and an ovoid shape of the common atrioventricular junction with unwedging of LVOT from the normal position between the tricuspid and mitral valve [95]. These defects have a broad variety ranges from a primum ASD and cleft mitral valve, known as a partial atrioventricular septal defect (partial AVSD), to defects of both the primum atrial septum and inlet ventricular septum and the presence of a common atrioventricular valve, referred to as complete atrioventricular septal defect (complete AVSD) [103]. AVSDs represent about 5% of all CHDs, and are most prevalent in infants with DS. Approximately 15-20% of neonates with DS have AVSDs. Most frequently, AVSDs can be categorized into one of three groups called complete, partial (or incomplete), or transitional. Down syndrome tends to be associated with the more severe forms of AVSD which are characterized by presence of malformation involving the atrial, ventricular and atrioventricular septa and both atrioventricular valves [104]. These anomalies showed the most considerable sex and ethnic variations, with two times as many females involved and with two times as many blacks and half as many Hispanics involved compared with whites [105]. The tendency for left to right shunting across the atrioventricular septal defect is related to the bridging leaflets being attached to the atrial septum, to the ventricular septum, or floating within the AVSD. Shunting may take place at atrial and ventricular levels or exclusively at either atrial or ventricular level (Fig. **10**) [106].

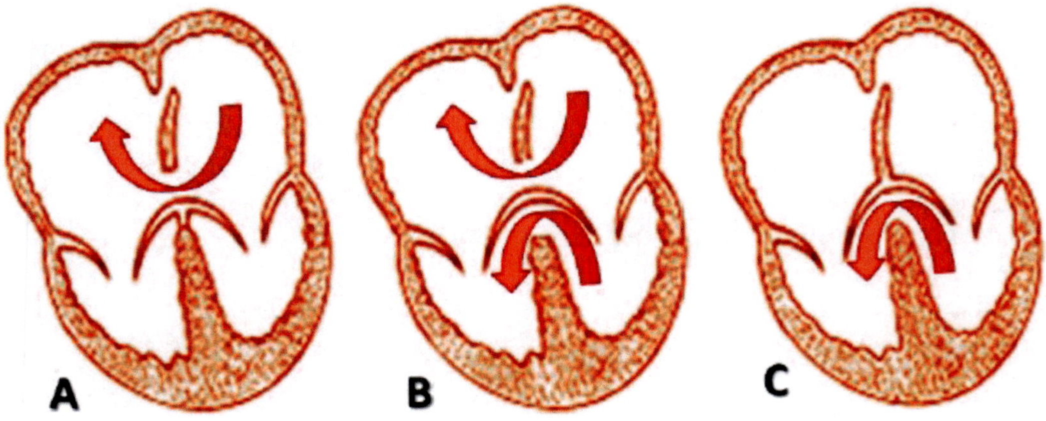

Fig. (10). Showed the level of left to right shunting across the atrioventricular septal defect. **A** : shunting is exclusively at the atrial level. **B**: shunting is at both atrial and ventricular level and **C**: shunting is exclusively at the ventricular level.

Complete AVSD may be accompanied with a number of other CHDs. ASD is also a frequent component of more complex heart problem that observed in heterotaxy syndromes. The recognition of these associated anomalies is very essential so that when counseling parents a correct hint about the outcome can be supplied. The death rate is higher in those with other associated cardiac abnormalities *e.g.* the combination of left atrial isomerism, AVSD and congenital complete heart block [106]. Nonsurgical atrioventricular (AV) conduction block is found in a considerable number of DS children with AVSD. It results from associated abnormalities in development of the AV conduction system in children with DS. The formation of the AV node and the ventricular conduction system in AVSD and DS differs from normal development, which can be a causative factor in the development of AV conduction disturbances [107]. Complete heart block is common in left atrial isomerism associated with AVSD. Subaortic stenosis is another anomaly that may be associated with AVSD. It could be due to elongation and narrowing of LVOT due to its anterior unwedged position especially notable in patients with ostium primum ASD where the superior bridging leaflet is firmly fixed to the crest of the ventricular septum. It also could occur due to fibrous subaortic shelf or fibromuscular tunnel, fibrous tissue tags or anomalous insertion of left ventricular papillary muscle [95]. In most patients with AVSD; there is a balance between the size of left and right ventricles (balanced AVSD). In few cases of AVSD, there may be dominance of one ventricle and relative hypoplasia of the other ventricle due to more commitment of common atrioventricular junction to one side (unbalanced AVSD). When there is extreme commitment of the common atrioventricular junction to the left ventricle; a condition termed as ''double inlet left ventricle with a common valve'' occurs [108]. Fallot's tetralogy is reported to occur in about 5% of all patients with AVSD. Tetralogy of Fallot associated with the atrioventricular canal defect has been usually reported in association with DS [109]. Truncus arteriosus (TA) is a rare cardiac anomaly constituting less than 1% of all congenital heart defects. It is reported is some cases with complete AVSD [110]. Other associated anomalies that can be seen in cases with AVSD are double-orifice atrioventricular valve, parachute left atrioventricular valve, and coarctation of the aorta, transposition of the great arteries and congenitally corrected transposition of the great arteries. Ebstein's anomaly, hypertrophic cardiomyopathy, cor triatrium, and absent pulmonary valve syndrome have also been reported [95].

Antenatal diagnosis is feasible by fetal echocardiography as AVSD is one of the potentially detectable lesions during the routine antenatal ultrasound anomaly scanning using the four-chamber view which is able to demonstrate the key feature of AVSD which is presence of a common atrioventricular valve with both ASD and VSD (Fig. **11**). The sensitivity of four-chamber view for antenatal detection of AVSD can be significantly improved by measuring the ratio of atrial to ventricular length (AVL). In normal fetuses; the AVL ratio did not change with gestation and the mean AVL ratio is about 0.47. This ratio is increased in AVSD with a mean of AVL ratio about 0.77 (Fig. **12**) [111]. Because of the increased frequency of associated heterotaxy syndrome with AVSD, determination of atrial situs, ventriculo-arterial connections, ventricular size and aortic arch caliber should be determined by fetal echocardiography.

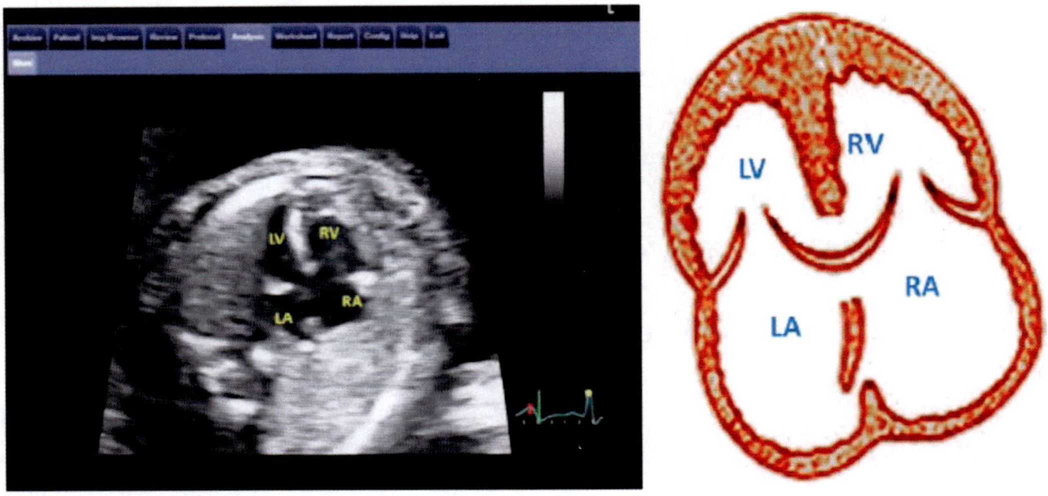

Fig. (11). Showed antenatal echocardiography with four-chamber view of the heart and its cartoonized figure. It shows the presence of a common atrioventricular valve. It is the ideal view to show the presence of a common atrioventricular valve and he defects in the atrial and ventricular septum.

After birth; the clinical picture will depend on the particular configuration of the AVSD defect and the occurrence of accompanied defects. The affected infants are usually symptomatic due to the high pulmonary blood flow coupled with presence of pulmonary hypertension, and often complicated by insufficiency of the common atrioventricular valve. In complete forms, infants usually suffer congestive heart failure, recurrent pulmonary infections, poor weight gain, disinterest in feeding, or tiring while feeding with failure to thrive within the first few months of life (usually by age 4 to 6 wk) as pulmonary vascular resistance falls. They may have a mild degree of central cyanosis due to bidirectional shunting at both the atrial and ventricular level in the presence of elevated pulmonary vascular resistance at birth. Cyanosis also may develop later in life when pulmonary artery resistances becomes higher than systemic artery resistance with reversal of the intracardiac shunt. Local chest examination may show right ventricular impulse and accentuated pulmonary component of the second heart sound. Cardiac murmur may, at this stage, be short or absent due to bidirectional shunting. The infant may have variable ejection systolic murmur, apical mid-diastolic murmur (in large left to right shunt), pansystolic murmur and gallop rhythm (with significant atrioventricular valve regurgitation). When irreversible pulmonary hypertension develops, signs of congestive heart failure improve but associated with worsening tolerance to effort [112].

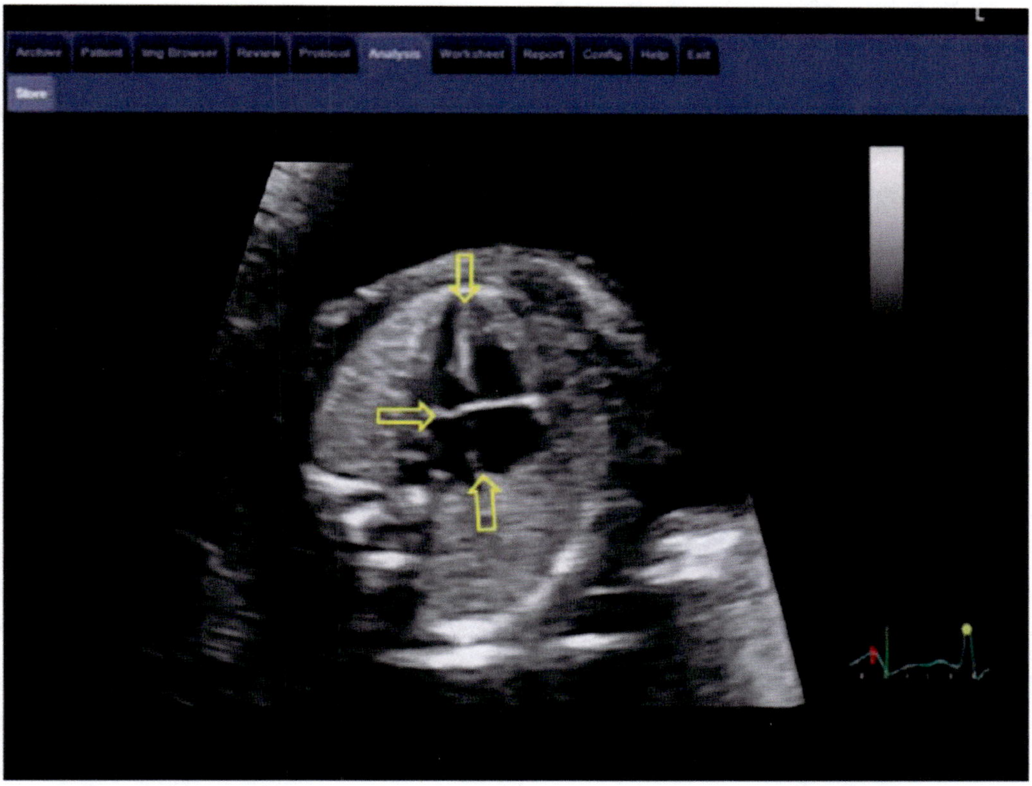

Fig. (12). Showed measurement of AVL ratio. Heart length is measured at the level of interventricular septum by placing the calipers on the epicardium at the apex of the heart and on the endocardium at the top of the atrium. Ventricular length is measured by shifting the atrial caliper to the crossing point of the ventricular septum and mitral valve. Atrial length is calculated as the difference between the heart length and ventricular length. Based on these measurements, AVL ratio is calculated.

Clinical examination alone is untrustworthy in postnatal screening for congenital heart disease in neonates with DS. Chest X-ray may show enlarged heart, signs of increased pulmonary vascular bed, prominent pulmonary conus, features of mitral valve insufficiency, left aortic arch and/or left bronchial isomerism (in associated left atrial isomerism). Electrocardiogram may reveal prolonged PR interval, superior frontal QRS axis, left axis deviation, partial right bundle branch block, bi-atrial enlargement and bi-ventricular pressure and volume overload and/or superior p wave axis (in associated left atrial isomerism). Echocardiography is the gold standard for accurate assessment and diagnosis and structural classification of this anomaly (Fig. **13**). It can show the ostium primum ASD, with the underlying common atrioventricular valve, and the defect of the ventricular septal inflow. It can show loss of normal offsetting of atrioventricular valves (absence of the atrioventricular muscular septum), abnormal configuration of the atrioventricular valves, trifoliate appearance of the left atrioventricular valve (with ''cleft''), left ventricular inlet outlet disproportion and abnormal position of the left ventricular papillary muscles [113]. AVSD should be distinguished from inlet ventricular septal defect and isolated mitral valve cleft by assessment of the left ventricular inlet/outlet ratio and percent of left atrioventricular valve guarded by the posterior leaflet [114]. Patients with "isolated" mitral cleft especially when accompanied with a VSD can have accessory chordae attached to the interventricular septum giving the impression of a common AV valve junction. A less common form of AVSD occurs when the common leaflet is fused to either the atrial septum or to the crest of the ventricular septum, creating an AVSD with no interatrial or interventricular communications correspondingly. Echocardiographic measurements of the left ventricle inlet to outlet distance ratio and the percentage of the left AV valve guarded by the mural leaflet can help in diagnosis patients with AVSD with no primum ASD [115]. Three-dimensional echocardiography can give more detailed assessment of dynamic atrioventricular valve morphology and the mechanism of valve incompetence [116]. Intra-operative monitoring of the surgical procedures can also be provided using either transesophageal or epicardial echocardiography to improve surgical outcomes and decrease the incidence of reoperation and to enable the surgeon to minimize residual defects [117].

Magnetic resonance imaging can offer images comparable to those gained by echocardiography. It allows direct visualization of defect spectrum. It is sometimes more superior to echocardiography in assessing cardiac chamber dimensions, calculating the size of the ventricular component of the defect and identifying presence/extent of ventricular hypoplasia which is a main predictor of surgical risk. It is feasible to evaluate correctly the regurgitant fraction in valve regurgitation and this may be of value not only in preoperative evaluation but in longer term follow-up [118]. An AVSD can give a typical "Goose neck" sign on a lateral left ventricular angiogram. However, angiography is no longer an element of the usual preoperative evaluation of patients with AVSD. Nowadays, the most important reason to perform cardiac catheterization in cases with AVSD is to estimate pulmonary vascular resistance especially in borderline cases before surgical correction. If the pulmonary vascular resistance is found to be elevated, reversibility with oxygen, inhaled nitric oxide and other potent pulmonary vasodilators can be assessed [119].

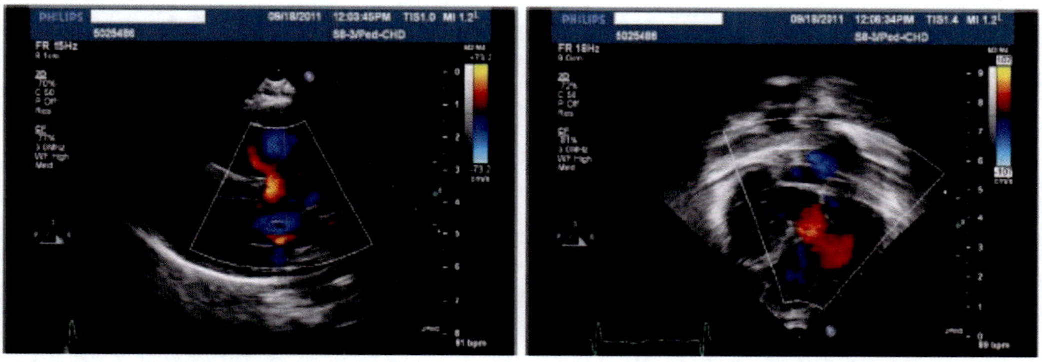

Fig. (13). The left panel showed left parasternal long axis view of 9 month old male infant with Down syndrome. It showed colored flow Doppler across a big VSD with left to right shunting. The right panel showed a subcostal view of the same infant with color flow mapping of a wide *Primum* ASD.

About 50% of infants with untreated complete AVSD expire in the first year of life mostly due to heart failure or pneumonia. In surviving children with unrepaired complete AVSD, irreversible pulmonary vascular disease (PVD) becomes increasingly common, and affects almost all children more than 2 years of age. Down syndrome is considered a risk factor for development of PVD in cases with complete AVSD.

Long-term prognosis in children with irreversible pulmonary hypertension is poor [103]. Because of the early development of PVD, primary repair should be done within the first 6 months of life usually around 2 and half months [120]. Mortality and morbidity as a result of surgical repair are low despite type of repair or presence of Trisomy 21 [121].

2.5.2. Ventricular Septal Defects (VSDs)

Ventricular septal defect (VSD) is a frequent cardiac anomaly in DS which forms about 35% of all CHDs observed in DS children. VSD might present as isolated or multiple and they are frequently accompanied with other cardiac anomalies. Different patterns of VSDs and associated anomalies exist in patients with and without DS. About one third of VSDs present in children with DS are of the muscular type, while the greater part is of the membranous and perimembranous varieties frequently of inlet type. The incidence of a cleft of the mitral valve is significantly higher in DS than non-DS children [122]. Amniocentesis is indicated for fetuses with antenatally detected VSD; due to the increased incidence of chromosomal anomalies, mostly DS [123]. The size of VSDs varies from tiny to large VSD which sometimes include more than one third of the entire ventricular septum. The defect size can be evaluated qualitatively. The defect is regarded as a large one when it is at least as large as the diameter of the aortic root. It is regarded small when it is slit-like or demonstrable only by color Doppler. Other defects are regarded as medium size [124].

Antenatal echocardiography is difficult and tricky, and VSD detection rate might be low and more operators dependent (Fig. **14**). The difficulty in antenatal detection of VSD is multifactorial. The nearly equal blood pressure in both ventricles causes no significant hemodynamic effects of VSD with non problematic blood shunting between both ventricles across the VSD. Another factor that increases the difficulty of antenatal detection of VSD is presence of artifactual areas of hypoechogenicity in the apical four-chamber view. A third factor is the complex nature and the curved appearance of interventricular septum which makes missing many of ventricular defects possible. Because of that; to diagnose VSD, it should be noticeable in at least two different planes [125]. Color Doppler echocardiography can reveal bidirectional flow across the area of defect and also allow detection of a small VSD not visible on gray-scale echocardiography. Color Doppler echocardiography may reveal the shunt location and its direction and can reveal the bidirectional flow across the defect which can help in detection of a small VSD not visible on gray-scale echocardiography. Accurate topographic diagnosis of VSD is necessary including proper definition of the affected septal segment. Small posterior defects inlet and peri-membranous subaortic defects are difficult and usually are not visible in the usual classic four-chamber view. These defects usually need modified four-chamber view and long axis view of the left ventricle, respectively for diagnosis [123]. Meticulous sonographic ruling out of other complex cardiac malformations such as tetralogy of Fallot, transposition of the great vessels, double-outlet right ventricle or other extracardiac malformations should be considered [126]. Spontaneous intrauterine closure of VSD is not rare and can occur in up to 32.5% of cases. The closure rate depends on many factors including size of defect, site of the defect, type of the defects and presence or absence of septal malalignment. Closure rate may reach 50% in small defects but large defects do not close. VSD with malalignment will never close irrespective to the size of the defect. Small perimembranous outlet defects have a relatively high intrauterine closure rate (43.8%). However, this high antenatal closure rate is unlike to occur postnatal for outlet perimembranous defects [123].

After delivery, small defects may be detected only during the routine examination because of the associated harsh systolic murmur as these defects cause little or no symptoms with normal feeding and adequate weight gain. Moderate size defects usually become symptomatic between 4 and 6 weeks of age when the pulmonary resistance begins to drop; however, the symptoms may appear earlier in premature babies. The babies may have increased respiratory rate and effort, excessive perspiration and sweating due to increased sympathetic tone, and easy fatigue with feeding. Feeding is the only exercise the baby is doing and impaired feeding is an important sign of sick baby. A thorough feeding history is essential as impaired weight gain is an important sign of heart failure in a baby. These children also may have recurrent respiratory infections due to pulmonary plethora. Large defects usually presented very early with more vigorous symptoms and signs. If cyanosis is present early, we should suspect associated Fallot's tetralogy, but if cyanosis develops later it may represent development of pulmonary hypertension and Eisenmenger's syndrome. Local examination reveals signs which are significantly correlated to the size of the defect except for the associated systolic murmur where the loudness and the intensity of the murmur are not correlated to the size of the lesion [127, 128].

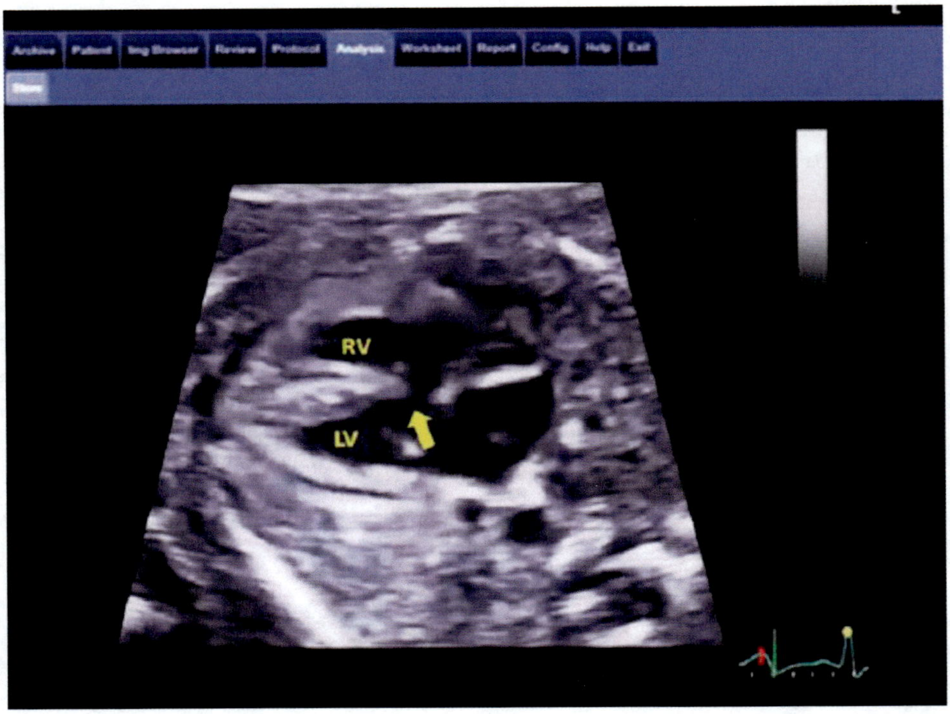

Fig. (14). Fetal echocardiographic lateral 4-chamber view. A perimembranous VSD is shown as indicated by the yellow arrow.

In small defects, there may be few signs with possible precordial impulse vigorous than usual. A harsh holosystolic murmur is maximally heard at the left sternal edge and continuous to be throughout systole but, if the defect is in the muscular portion, it becomes shorter as the defect is closing as the muscle contracts. The grade of murmur depends on the velocity of flow; the site of murmur is dependent on the site of the defect.

In moderated size defects there is vigorous apical pulsation as well as a parasternal heave and the systolic murmur, possibly with a thrill. Muscular defects can be heard along the lower left sternal border and may differ in intensity as the defect size varies with muscular contraction throughout systole. Infundibular defects shunt close to the pulmonary valve and can be auscultated best at the left upper sternal border. Perimembranous defects may have an associated systolic click of a tricuspid valve aneurysm. A prominent third sound with a short early mid-diastolic rumble is audible at the apex when pulmonary blood flow is twice the systemic flow or greater. The second heart sound is usually more narrowly split and enhanced. With large defect, central cyanosis may occur due to bidirectional shunt or sometimes right to left shunt which could be accompanied with clubbing of the fingers. A prominent right ventricular heave may be present with short or absent systolic murmur. Systolic murmur at the left lower or right lower sternal border can be heard if there is associated tricuspid regurgitation. Defects with aortic insufficiency have a diastolic decrescendo murmur along the left sternal border with the patient sitting and leaning forward. A widened pulse pressure may be present [128, 129].

Electrocardiography may be normal in small defects but can show signs of LV volume load and hypertrophy with increasing shunts. Left atrial enlargement may occur. Signs of biventricular hypertrophy and overload of the right atrium may be observed in large VSDs. If pulmonary arterial pressure is high there may be no LV hypertrophy but RV hypertrophy with right axis deviation. Large defects may include the conducting tissue and left axis deviation is observed [130]. X-ray may show no significant radiographic abnormalities in small VSD but large defects may produce signs of various degrees of chamber enlargement and cardiomegaly depending on the volume of the shunt. Signs of increased pulmonary vascular markings may also present. An enlarged left atrium may be visible in a lateral view. When pulmonary hypertension and increasing pulmonary resistance develop; decrease of pulmonary vascularity and reduction of the vasculature occur with evidence of right heart enlargement and a dilated main pulmonary artery [128].

Echocardiography is sensitive, descriptive tool of choice in diagnosing cases of VSD and can provide satisfactory information that usually needed for proper treatment plan. It has a tremendous detection ability which reaches about 88% to 95% of cases, depending on the site and size of the defect as well as technician experience. Various echocardiographic modalities including two-dimensional, Doppler, color flow imaging, three-dimensional and four-dimensional echocardiography can alleviate the need for cardiac catheterization. It can evaluate the size and site of almost all VSDs. The detection rate is high with defect sizes more than 5 mm that are situated in the membranous, inlet, or outlet portion of the septum. It is least sensitive for apical muscular defects. For better detection; a thorough echocardiographic examination with visualization of the intraventricular septum in different and multiple planes using color flow and spectral Doppler echocardiography (Fig. **15**). Two-dimensional echocardiography, along with Doppler echocardiography and color flow imaging are able to evaluate the size and site of virtually all ventricular septal defects (VSDs). Two-dimensional modes can recognize the anatomy of the defect, its size, borders and associated defects as in case aortic valve deformation and prolapse (right and non-coronary cusp) in patients with subarterial VSD. Measurement of left atrial and left ventricular diameter provides semi-quantitative data about shunt volume. Defect size is often given in terms of the size of the aortic root. Defects that are about the size of the aortic root are classified as large; those one third to two thirds of the diameter of the aorta are moderate, and those less than one third of the aortic root diameter is small [131 - 133].

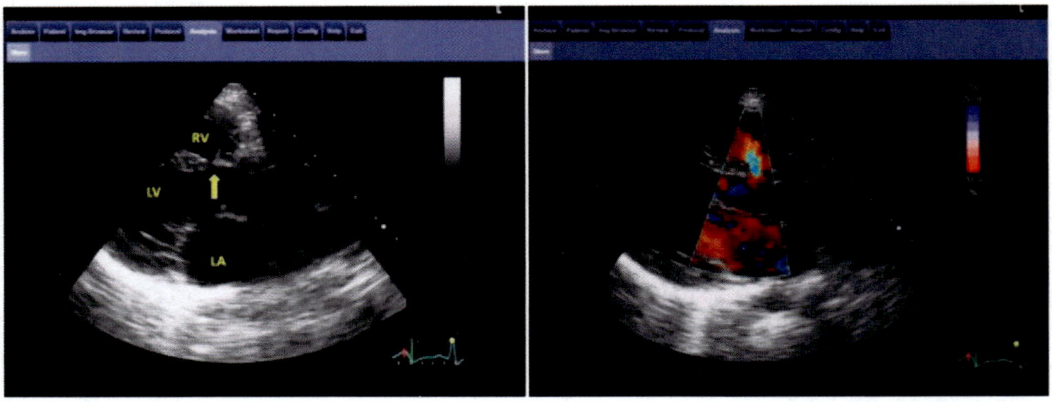

Fig. (15). Two-dimensional (Left) and Color Doppler mapping echocardiographic left parasternal views of a perimembranous VSD is shown as indicated by the yellow arrow.

Doppler echocardiography can also provide physiological data including RV pressure, pulmonary artery pressure and the pressure gradient between the ventricles. It can give a precise hemodynamic evaluation of the shunt, severity, volume overload, subpulmonic (double-chambered right ventricle) or pulmonic stenosis, pulmonary hypertension, severity of aortic regurgitation and RVOT obstruction caused by the prolapsing coronary cusp [134, 135]. When restrictions in image quality of transthoracic echocardiography hinder proper assessment of these aspects of the cardiovascular physiology, transesophageal (TEE) imaging can be done. Transesophageal echocardiography remains the diagnostic tool of choice in assessment of patients with assumed or confirmed endocarditis. It is an outstanding technique for recognition of vegetations around the borders of the defect or on adjacent valves and for the evaluation of possible complications, such as abscess formation [136]. Three-dimensional echocardiography has been proved to be sufficiently accurate in estimation of the shunt volume and can provide accurate visualization of defects that otherwise are difficult to evaluate by 2-dimensional imaging alone [137].

Angiography is infrequently indicated in evaluation of VSDs. It is indicated when other investigations are unsuccessful in clarifying the anatomy that cardiac catheterization is needed or when there are inconsistencies between echocardiographic examination and clinical judgment. It can evaluate pulmonary vascular resistance of complicated VSDs, such as those that are multiple and especially apical or those associated with pulmonary stenosis, aortic regurgitation, and pulmonary hypertension and can assess pulmonary reactivity and the reversibility of pulmonary vascular disease. Response to pulmonary vasodilators can be verified and can guide therapy. It can identify small muscular septal defects or other abnormalities that can be missed during echo exam. Shunt study, using oximetry or the indicator dilution curves, improves the diagnostic accuracy of cardiac catheterization. In cases with expected aortic regurgitation, further aortography can inspect for integrity and allows detection of aortic valve prolapse even before the appearance of its clinical feature and helps to grade the severity of aortic regurgitation [138]. Magnetic resonance imaging may be needed to define VSDs in patients with associated complex lesions.

Spontaneous closure of the defect can occur either partially or completely depend on the size, the type, the location and the associated defects. Closure of defects can occur as due to muscular growth around the defect; fibrous tissue proliferation around the growing border; or, in cases with membranous defects, an aneurysm of the tricuspid valve leaflet adheres to the edge of the defect can close it [139]. Muscular defects are more likely to close spontaneously than membranous defects. Perimembranous defects are usually larger than muscular defects, frequently require surgical intervention, and even when small have little better than a 50% chance of spontaneous closure by six years [129].

Muscular VSDs can undergo spontaneous closure as a result of muscular occlusion. Perimembranous defects can close by tricuspid valve aneurysm formation. Infundibular defects can close by prolapse of the right aortic cusp. A reduction in the size of the defect by any of these mechanisms results in changes in the hemodynamic significance of the defect [128]. Inlet and subarterial defects seldom close spontaneously because of their close proximity to the valves. However, the size of or shunt through subarterial defects can be reduced by the prolapsing of aortic valve cusps at the cost of leaflet distortion and regurgitation and occasionally can cause RVOT obstruction [139].

If the defect is not closing and left without proper management, the patients may be predisposed to have arrhythmia, endocarditis, congestive heart failure, pulmonary hypertension and even Eisenmenger syndrome. Increasing age and development of pulmonary hypertension are risk factors for arrhythmias in children with VSDs. Ventricular arrhythmias in the form of ventricular couplets, multiform ventricular ectopics, or ventricular tachycardias can occur in about one fifth of medically treated patients. The odds ratio of lethal arrhythmias increases to 1.51 for every 10-year increase in age and to 1.49 for any increase in mean pulmonary artery pressure by 10 mm Hg [140]. Infective endocarditis may develop particularly in small VSDs and patients with VSDs associated with aortic regurgitation because of the highly turbulent jet. The risk of endocarditis increases with age [141]. Congestive heart failure due to chronic volume overload of the ventricles occurs in patients with isolated medium or large VSDs. Left-sided failure can take place secondary to significant aortic regurgitation in patients with aortic valve prolapse. Right-sided heart failure can develop when the defect is associated with significant pulmonary stenosis or acquired subpulmonic stenosis (double-chambered right ventricle); it can also occur at late stages of the Eisenmenger complex [142]. Eisenmenger complex with irreversible pulmonary vascular obstructive disease can occur in 10% to 15% of patients with VSDs usually by the second or third decades of life if left untreated due to long-lasting left-to-right shunt leading to progressive pulmonary hypertension that finally end by irreversible pulmonary hypertension with reversal of the intracardiac shunt and systemic desaturation. The prognosis of patients with the Eisenmenger complex is poor, especially after onset of serious arrhythmia, hemoptysis, congestive heart failure, and significant tricuspid regurgitation [143].

Management of VSDs in infants and children depends on symptoms. A small defect does not necessitate medical management or likely need any intervention except for prophylaxis against infective endocarditis. The medium and larger defects need various degrees of medical intervention and finally surgical closure. Congestive heart failure in infants is treated with diuretics, digoxin, and after load reduction from time to time (*e.g.* angiotensin-converting enzyme) [144]. Regardless of the defect size; antibiotic prophylaxis to prevent endocarditis and serial follow-up is mandatory as infective endocarditis continues to be a possible problem until the defect is closed either surgically or spontaneously. After closure of the defect, the use of antibiotics to cover at-risk situations must be continued for a additional 6 months [145].

Surgical closure is indicated if there is uncontrolled heart failure with poor weight gain, impaired growth and failure to thrive. Even very small infants may need early surgical interference when indicated. Presence of infundibular defects indicates the needs for surgical repair regardless of the need for medical management. Surgical closure is also indicated in presence of significant shunting as indicated by presence of cardiomegaly; significant increase of Qp:Qs ratio (which reflect pulmonary circulation relative to systemic circulation) of 1.5:1 to 2:127 or other evidences of elevated pulmonary arteriolar vascular resistance during cardiac catheterization [146]. Advances in surgical and bypass skills and the ability for earlier timing of surgical repair have decreased the morbidity and mortality associated with surgical closure. Multiple "Swiss cheese" defects not controlled by medical treatment may need a palliative pulmonary artery banding. Repair using minimally invasive techniques of video-assisted cardioscopy are up to now very promising [147]. Transcatheter techniques are helpful as they avoid using cardiopulmonary bypass. However, closure of perimembranous ventricular septal defects in patients with DS, either surgically or by Amplatzer occluders, have more risk of complete heart block. The transcatheter patch might be superior in terms of cardiac conduction system protection in patients with DS after ventricular septal defect closure [148]. There some case reports about development of severe postoperative pulmonary hypertensive crisis after surgical correction of VSDs [149].

3. ACQUIRED HEART DISEASES IN DS

Despite congenital heart diseases affect a significant proportion of DS children, but the rest of those children may suffer from some postnatal cardiac problems. This is the reason for the need of ongoing cardiac surveillance and follow up for the risk of development of heart disease even for those without congenital heart defects. Neonates with DS have a higher frequency of persistent pulmonary hypertension of the neonate (PPHN), than in non-DS neonates. They are more liable to develop PPHN even in the absence of structural heart disease and should be followed until resolution of the pulmonary hypertension [150]. According to studies done by Cua *et al.* 2007 and Weijerman *et al.* 2010, the incidence of PPHN in neonates with DS is between 1.2 and 5.2% which is at least ten times higher than that in general population. This increased incidence of PPHN in neonates with DS should be considered when a neonatologist encounters such babies as their progress cannot be expected and they may need more aggressive action in identifying and treating such condition [151, 152]. The pathophysiological mechanisms underlying the development of PPHN in neonates with DS are not fully understood. One of these mechanisms is the vasoconstriction induced by the imbalance in the biosynthesis of vasoactive eicosanoids as a result of the excess thromboxane over prostacyclin in response to mild degree of hypoxia [153].

Another rare presentation in neonates with DS is the association of hypertrophic cardiomyopathy with complete atrioventricular canal defect in an infant with trisomy 21 [154]. There is also a report for development of biventricular hypertrophic cardiomyopathy and pericardial effusion as a complication of transient neonatal myeloproliferative disorder [155].

Children with DS beyond the neonatal age are also at risk of development of pulmonary hypertension (PH) even without associated congenital heart diseases. There are many predisposing factors that predispose them to PH. Obstructive sleep apnea is more common in children with DS due to the anatomy of their airway as well as the increased incidence of obesity among them which aggravate apnea. Pulmonary hypoplasia, structural lung disease and gastro-esophageal reflux (GER) are other factors increasing the incidence of PH among DS children [156].

Reflux may exaggerate upper airway obstruction, and may induce obstructive apnea or aspiration pneumonia. Examination for GER is advised for infants who have PAH, particularly those with DS who have no cardiac anomalies. This type of PH can resolved after treatment of the underlying pathology. However, persistent pulmonary hypertension may develop even in absence of structural heart disease. These children should be followed periodically by echocardiography till resolution of PH [157]. Children with DS are more liable to developed high-altitude pulmonary edema (HAPE) than non-DS children. HAPE is a fatal condition that develops after ascent in people ascending too quickly. It occurs due to change in pulmonary capillary permeability, without major activation of inflammatory mechanisms. It is characterized by presence of fine capitations, production of frothy sputum, and/or hypoxemia. Chest radiograph shows signs matching that of pulmonary edema and there is rapid clinical improvement after descent or oxygen therapy. Children with DS have many risk factor for HAPE as presence of chronic pulmonary hypertension, suffering from frequent infections, and when there is pulmonary vascular over perfusion and injury from existing or previous cardiac defects and that induce rapid development of HAPE at low altitudes. Care should be taken when traveling to even moderate altitudes with DS children [158].

Clinical and subclinical hypothyroidism is more common problem in children with DS than normal population. Pericardial effusion may be the first sign of congenital or acquired hypothyroidism. Hypothyroidism usually results in slow and gradual accumulation of fluid in the pericardium thus permitting enough time for the distensibility of the pericardium to handle it sufficiently. A number of case studies have described the presence of pericardial effusion in this group of patients. Anah *et al.* for instance, described the presence of a complex association of Down Syndrome-hypothyroidism-pericardial effusion [159]. Delay in diagnosis of hypothyroidism may favor the development of massive pericardial effusion. It present with dyspnea and cardiomegaly which sometimes becomes massive and echocardiography can easily diagnose it and electrocardiogram (ECG) shows low voltages. Features of myxedema may or may not present. Complete resolution of the effusion can occur with thyroxin therapy without the need for pericardiocentesis. The finding of pericardial effusion by echocardiography

(Fig. **16**) may indicate thyroid dysfunction. Periodic follow-up of thyroid function tests in children with DS is mandatory [160].

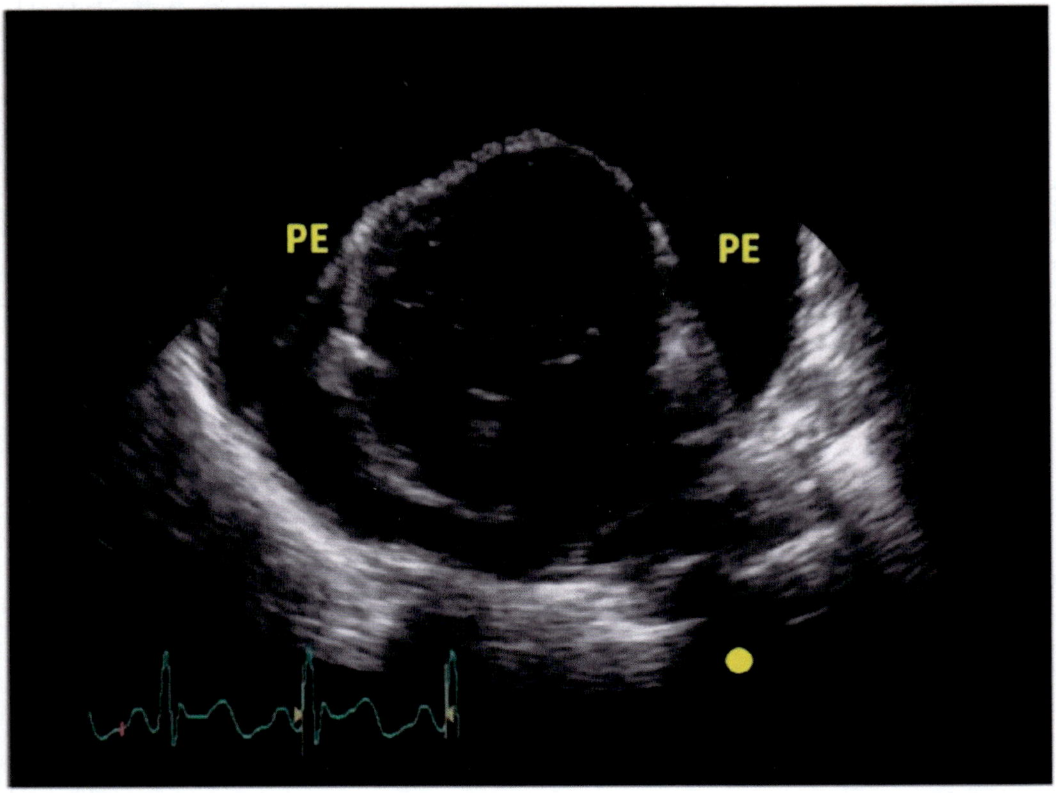

Fig. (16). Two-dimensional apical 4 chamber view showed massive pericardial effusion of 5 years old child with DS and hypothyroidism.

Children with DS may have lower systolic and diastolic blood pressure than control children. The low blood pressure observed in children with DS may be result from trisomy of type-1-angiotensin II receptor gene, causing under expression [161]. They also have higher respiratory and heart rates than the control children. The differences in respiratory and pulse rate, as well as the blood pressure, may be related to autonomic cardiac dysregulation in DS, which may be due to the autonomic dysfunction occurring at a central, brain stem, site as a result of the genetic disorder [162]. They may have also impaired systolic and diastolic cardiac functions even without structural lesions. This impaired function could be due to associated autonomic cardiac control dysregulation, abnormality in the cardiac muscle fibers with increased cardiac muscle fiber size and reduced cell number, or over expression of calcineurin. Over expression of calcineurin may lead to cardiac muscle hypertrophy [163]. Another probable mechanism that still needs confirmation is presence of significantly lower carnitine level in DS patients compared with normal children [164].

Children with DS like any other children may suffer from many acquired childhood cardiac conditions. There are some reports about development of cardiomyopathy when treated from acute myeloid leukemia which may need dose modification and reduction of anthracyclines in this patient population [165]. Mitral valve prolapse and regurgitation are quite common in adolescents with DS. Aortic insufficiency is also more common than the control. Basal septal hypertrophy with significantly protrusion into the LVOT can explain the occurrence of aortic insufficiency in some cases by ejection flow eccentrically directed to right coronary cuspid, causing a jet lesion [166]. Meticulous auscultation is most likely to be adequate to screen for valvular regurgitation, which, if found, necessitates bacterial endocarditis prophylaxis. The diagnosis can be established by echocardiography [2]. Presence of mitral valve prolapse (Fig. **17**) should attract the attention of the physician for presence of associated keratoconus which is more than 10 times more prevalent in DS than in normal population. Early identification of Keratoconus can lead to considerable decrease in corneal scarring and preventable visual loss [167].

Despite the old historical assumption that DS patients were considered protected from atherosclerotic disease and, even an "atheroma-free" example of disease, relatively recent data showed that they may really have a higher risk of death from ischemic heart disease and cerebrovascular events compared with the general population. Adelekan *et al.* demonstrated that the lipid profile of non-obese prepubertal children with DS is less favorable than that of their siblings, with higher concentrations of total cholesterol (TC), low-density lipoprotein (LDL), triglycerides (TG), and lower concentrations high-density lipoprotein (HDL) after adjustment for important confounding factors [168]. This finding is associated with a high risk for premature atherosclerosis in the general population. At the same time, high rate of obesity in children with DS is another confounding risk factor that could affect the cardiac condition among them.

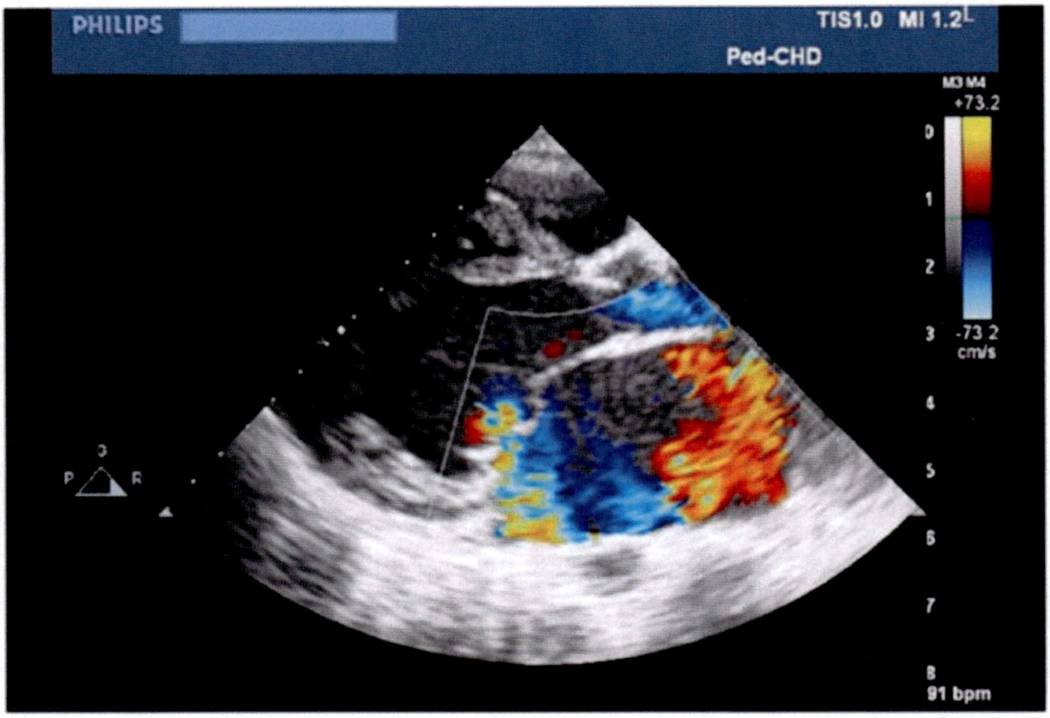

Fig. (17). Two-dimensional left parasternal long axis view showed mild mitral valve prolapse with regurgitation in 14 years old girl with DS.

4. PREVENTION OF HEART DISEASES IN DS

Primary prevention of cardiac disorders in children with DS is mainly through prevention of occurrence of DS. However, there is no way to prevent Down's syndrome despite the greet efforts by many scientists to learn more about the genetic basis of DS that could help to improve, correct or prevent many of the problems associated with the condition. Mothers with high risk to have a child with DS should consult a genetic counselor before becoming pregnant. They may get benefit from pre-implantation genetic diagnosis, which can lead to a considerably high pregnancy rate with an tremendously low risk of a DS. There some evidence that folic acid supplementation in high doses (up to 6 mg/day) together with iron supplement (150-300 mg/d of ferrous sulfate) during the first gestational month have a important protective effect against DS [169]. If pregnancy is being planned, it is generally recommended that nutritional preparations start two or three months prior to any active attempts at conception.

Foods rich in folate is to be emphasized in the diet include beans, lentils and green leafy vegetables such as spinach, kale and cabbage. There is some evidence that lack of maternal folic acid supplementation is associated with septal defects in infants with DS [16]. However, maternal folic acid supplementation does not show a protective effect on heart anomalies among infants with DS [170].

Secondary prevention of cardiac diseases in DS children is through early detection and proper treatment of both congenital and acquired heart diseases. Proper antenatal detection of CHDs as mentioned before is of paramount importance. Early surgical interference is important once applicable to prevent development of pulmonary hypertension. It is advisable to have an echocardiographic examination in the first month of life for all neonates with DS, before any cardiac surgery, as follow-up after cardiac surgery, for serial evaluation of pulmonary hypertension, before involvement in major non-cardiac surgery and before involvement in physical exercise [171]. Bacterial endocarditis prophylaxis including antibiotics prior to dental work is indicated until corrective surgery is done, if there is residual lesion remains after surgery or if there evidence of valvlar regurgitation is noted on physical examination [172]. Because of the less favorable lipid profiles in children with DS, they should be subjected to early routine screening and treatment when applicable for dyslipidemia to protect ischemic heart disease according to the guidelines of the American Academy of Pediatrics [173].

CONCLUSION

Cardiac diseases in children with DS are significant problem affecting more than half of them. Early detection and management of these disorders markedly improve life span and life style for these children. Periodic follow up by clinical examinations, laboratory investigations when needed and serial echocardiographic examination are needed for detection of any cardiac abnormalities.

CONFLICT OF INTEREST

The authors confirm that this chapter contents have no conflict of interest.

ACKNOWLEDGEMENTS

Declared None.

REFERENCES

[1] van Gameren-Oosterom HB, van Dommelen P, Schönbeck Y, Oudesluys-Murphy AM, van Wouwe JP, Buitendijk SE. Prevalence of overweight in Dutch children with Down syndrome. Pediatrics 2012; 130(6): e1520-6.
[http://dx.doi.org/10.1542/peds.2012-0886] [PMID: 23147968]

[2] Geggel RL, O'Brien JE, Feingold M. Development of valve dysfunction in adolescents and young adults with Down syndrome and no known congenital heart disease. J Pediatr 1993; 122(5 Pt 1): 821-3.
[http://dx.doi.org/10.1016/S0022-3476(06)80036-3] [PMID: 8496770]

[3] Hoffman JI, Kaplan S. The incidence of congenital heart disease. J Am Coll Cardiol 2002; 39(12): 1890-900.
[http://dx.doi.org/10.1016/S0735-1097(02)01886-7] [PMID: 12084585]

[4] Salih A. Congenital Heart Disease in Children with Down Syndrome: Experience of Kurdistan of Iraq. Duhok Med J 2011; 5(2): 24-33.

[5] Seale A, Shinebourne EA. Cardiac problems in Down syndrome. Curr Paediatr 2004; 14: 33-8.
[http://dx.doi.org/10.1016/j.cupe.2003.09.005]

[6] Freeman SB, Taft LF, Dooley KJ, *et al.* Population-based study of congenital heart defects in Down syndrome. Am J Med Genet 1998; 80(3): 213-7.
[http://dx.doi.org/10.1002/(SICI)1096-8628(19981116)80:3<213::AID-AJMG6>3.0.CO;2-8] [PMID: 9843040]

[7] Al-Jarallah AS. Down's syndrome and the pattern of congenital heart disease in a community with high parental consanguinity. Med Sci Monit 2009; 15(8): CR409-12.
[PMID: 19644417]

[8] Chéhab G, Chokor I, Fakhouri H, Hage G, Saliba Z, El-Rassi I. [Congenital heart disease, maternal age and parental consanguinity in children with Down's syndrome]. J Med Liban 2007; 55(3): 133-7.
[PMID: 17966733]

[9] Freeman SB, Bean LH, Allen EG, *et al.* Ethnicity, sex, and the incidence of congenital heart defects: a report from the National Down Syndrome Project. Genet Med 2008; 10(3): 173-80.
[http://dx.doi.org/10.1097/GIM.0b013e3181634867] [PMID: 18344706]

[10] Abbag FI. Congenital heart diseases and other major anomalies in patients with Down syndrome. Saudi Med J 2006; 27(2): 219-22.
[PMID: 16501680]

[11] Nisli K, Oner N, Candan S, *et al.* Congenital heart disease in children with Down's syndrome: Turkish experience of 13 years. Acta Cardiol 2008; 63(5): 585-9.
[http://dx.doi.org/10.2143/AC.63.5.2033225] [PMID: 19014001]

[12] Vida VL, Barnoya J, Larrazabal LA, Gaitan G, de Maria Garcia F, Castañeda AR. Congenital cardiac disease in children with Down's syndrome in Guatemala. Cardiol Young 2005; 15(3): 286-90.
[http://dx.doi.org/10.1017/S1047951105000582] [PMID: 15865831]

[13] de Rubens Figueroa J, del Pozzo Magaña B, Pablos Hach JL, Calderón Jiménez C, Castrejón Urbina R. [Heart malformations in children with Down syndrome]. Rev Esp Cardiol 2003; 56(9): 894-9.

[http://dx.doi.org/10.1016/S0300-8932(03)76978-4] [PMID: 14519277]

[14] Torfs CP, Christianson RE. Maternal risk factors and major associated defects in infants with Down syndrome. Epidemiology 1999; 10(3): 264-70.
[http://dx.doi.org/10.1097/00001648-199905000-00013] [PMID: 10230836]

[15] Khoury MJ, Erickson JD. Can maternal risk factors influence the presence of major birth defects in infants with Down syndrome? Am J Med Genet 1992; 43(6): 1016-22.
[http://dx.doi.org/10.1002/ajmg.1320430620] [PMID: 1415327]

[16] Bean LJ, Allen EG, Tinker SW, *et al.* Lack of maternal folic acid supplementation is associated with heart defects in Down syndrome: a report from the National Down Syndrome Project. Birth Defects Res A Clin Mol Teratol 2011; 91(10): 885-93.
[http://dx.doi.org/10.1002/bdra.22848] [PMID: 21987466]

[17] Moorman A, Webb S, Brown NA, Lamers W, Anderson RH. Development of the heart: (1) formation of the cardiac chambers and arterial trunks. Heart 2003; 89(7): 806-14.
[http://dx.doi.org/10.1136/heart.89.7.806] [PMID: 12807866]

[18] Aanhaanen WT, Moorman AF, Christoffels VM. Origin and development of the atrioventricular myocardial lineage: insight into the development of accessory pathways. Birth Defects Res A Clin Mol Teratol 2011; 91(6): 565-77.
[http://dx.doi.org/10.1002/bdra.20826] [PMID: 21630423]

[19] Aït Yahya-Graison E, Aubert J, Dauphinot L, *et al.* Classification of human chromosome 21 gene-expression variations in Down syndrome: impact on disease phenotypes. Am J Hum Genet 2007; 81(3): 475-91.
[http://dx.doi.org/10.1086/520000] [PMID: 17701894]

[20] Prandini P, Deutsch S, Lyle R, *et al.* Natural gene-expression variation in Down syndrome modulates the outcome of gene-dosage imbalance. Am J Hum Genet 2007; 81(2): 252-63.
[http://dx.doi.org/10.1086/519248] [PMID: 17668376]

[21] Ripoll C, Rivals I, Ait Yahya-Graison E, *et al.* Molecular signatures of cardiac defects in Down syndrome lymphoblastoid cell lines suggest altered ciliome and Hedgehog pathways. PLoS One 2012; 7(8): e41616.
[http://dx.doi.org/10.1371/journal.pone.0041616] [PMID: 22912673]

[22] Casas C, Martínez S, Pritchard MA, *et al.* Dscr1, a novel endogenous inhibitor of calcineurin signaling, is expressed in the primitive ventricle of the heart and during neurogenesis. Mech Dev 2001; 101(1-2): 289-92.
[http://dx.doi.org/10.1016/S0925-4773(00)00583-9] [PMID: 11231093]

[23] Lange AW, Molkentin JD, Yutzey KE. DSCR1 gene expression is dependent on NFATc1 during cardiac valve formation And colocalizes with anomalous organ development in trisomy 16 mice. Dev Biol 2004; 266(2): 346-60.
[http://dx.doi.org/10.1016/j.ydbio.2003.10.036] [PMID: 14738882]

[24] Fuentes JJ, Pritchard MA, Planas AM, Bosch A, Ferrer I, Estivill X. A new human gene from the Down syndrome critical region encodes a proline-rich protein highly expressed in fetal brain and heart. Hum Mol Genet 1995; 4(10): 1935-44.
[http://dx.doi.org/10.1093/hmg/4.10.1935] [PMID: 8595418]

[25] Baek KH, Zaslavsky A, Lynch RC, *et al.* Down's syndrome suppression of tumour growth and the role of the calcineurin inhibitor DSCR1. Nature 2009; 459(7250): 1126-30. [http://dx.doi.org/10.1038/nature08062] [PMID: 19458618]

[26] Li CM, Guo M, Salas M, *et al.* Cell type-specific over-expression of chromosome 21 genes in fibroblasts and fetal hearts with trisomy 21. BMC Med Genet 2006; 7: 24.

[27] Ghosh P, Bhaumik P, Ghosh S, *et al.* Polymorphic haplotypes of CRELD1 differentially predispose Down syndrome and euploids individuals to atrioventricular septal defect. Am J Med Genet A 2012; 158A(11): 2843-8. [http://dx.doi.org/10.1002/ajmg.a.35626] [PMID: 22987595]

[28] Maslen CL, Babcock D, Robinson SW, *et al.* CRELD1 mutations contribute to the occurrence of cardiac atrioventricular septal defects in Down syndrome. Am J Med Genet A 2006; 140(22): 2501-5. [http://dx.doi.org/10.1002/ajmg.a.31494]

[29] Zatyka M, Priestley M, Ladusans EJ, *et al.* Analysis of CRELD1 as a candidate 3p25 atrioventicular septal defect locus (AVSD2). Clin Genet 2005; 67(6): 526-8. [http://dx.doi.org/10.1111/j.1399-0004.2005.00435.x] [PMID: 15857420]

[30] Ackerman C, Locke AE, Feingold E, *et al.* An excess of deleterious variants in VEGF-A pathway genes in Down-syndrome-associated atrioventricular septal defects. Am J Hum Genet 2012; 91(4): 646-59. [http://dx.doi.org/10.1016/j.ajhg.2012.08.017] [PMID: 23040494]

[31] Horsley V, Pavlath GK. NFAT: ubiquitous regulator of cell differentiation and adaptation. J Cell Biol 2002; 156(5): 771-4. [PMID: 11877454]

[32] Abu-Harb M, Wyllie J, Hey E, Richmond S, Wren C. Antenatal diagnosis of congenital heart disease and Down's syndrome: the potential effect on the practice of paediatric cardiology. Br Heart J 1995; 74(2): 192-8. [http://dx.doi.org/10.1136/hrt.74.2.192] [PMID: 7547001]

[33] Caserta L, Ruggeri Z, D'Emidio L, *et al.* Two-dimensional fetal echocardiography: where we are. J Prenat Med 2008; 2(3): 31-5. [PMID: 22439025]

[34] Sharland G. Fetal cardiac screening and variation in prenatal detection rates of congenital heart disease: why bother with screening at all? Future Cardiol 2012; 8(2): 189-202. [http://dx.doi.org/10.2217/fca.12.15] [PMID: 22413979]

[35] Nicolaides KH, Snijders RJ, Gosden CM, Berry C, Campbell S. Ultrasonographically detectable markers of fetal aneuploidy. Lancet 1992; 340: 704-7.

[36] Persutte WH, Hobbins J. Single umbilical artery: a clinical enigma in modern prenatal diagnosis. Ultrasound Obstet Gynecol 1995; 6(3): 216-29. [http://dx.doi.org/10.1046/j.1469-0705.1995.06030216.x] [PMID: 8521073]

[37] Prefumo F, Güven MA, Carvalho JS. Single umbilical artery and congenital heart disease in selected and unselected populations. Ultrasound Obstet Gynecol 2010; 35(5): 552-5. [http://dx.doi.org/10.1002/uog.7642] [PMID: 20443197]

[38] Gossett DR, Lantz ME, Chisholm CA. Antenatal diagnosis of single umbilical artery: is fetal echocardiography warranted? Obstet Gynecol 2002; 100(5 Pt 1): 903-8. [http://dx.doi.org/10.1016/S0029-7844(02)02148-8] [PMID: 12423851]

[39] Bornstein E, Sheiner E, Barnhard Y, *et al.* The association of maternal BMI with fetal echogenic intracardiac foci and echogenic bowel. J Matern Fetal Neonatal Med 2010; 23(8): 781-4. [http://dx.doi.org/10.3109/14767050903314176] [PMID: 19921962]

[40] Bronshtein M, Jakobi P, Ofir C. Multiple fetal intracardiac echogenic foci: not always a benign sonographic finding. Prenat Diagn 1996; 16(2): 131-5. [http://dx.doi.org/10.1002/(SICI)1097-0223(199602)16:2<131::AID-PD823>3.0.CO;2-Q] [PMID: 8650123]

[41] Rodriguez R, Herrero B, Bartha JL. The continuing enigma of the fetal echogenic intracardiac focus in prenatal ultrasound. Curr Opin Obstet Gynecol 2013; 25(2): 145-51. [http://dx.doi.org/10.1097/GCO.0b013e32835e14eb] [PMID: 23340246]

[42] Petrikovsky BM, Challenger M, Wyse LJ. Natural history of echogenic foci within ventricles of the fetal heart. Ultrasound Obstet Gynecol 1995; 5(2): 92-4. [http://dx.doi.org/10.1046/j.1469-0705.1995.05020092.x] [PMID: 7719874]

[43] Nyberg DA, Souter VL, El-Bastawissi A, Young S, Luthhardt F, Luthy DA. Isolated sonographic markers for detection of fetal Down syndrome in the second trimester of pregnancy. J Ultrasound Med 2001; 20(10): 1053-63. [PMID: 11587012]

[44] Wax JR, Cartin A, Pinette MG, *et al.* Sonographic grading of fetal intracardiac echogenic foci in a population at low risk of aneuploidy. J Clin Ultrasound 2003; 31(1): 31-8. [http://dx.doi.org/10.1002/jcu.10127] [PMID: 12478650]

[45] Wax JR, Mather J, Steinfeld JD, Ingardia CJ. Fetal intracardiac echogenic foci: current understanding and clinical significance. Obstet Gynecol Surv 2000; 55(5): 303-11. [http://dx.doi.org/10.1097/00006254-200005000-00024] [PMID: 10804537]

[46] Wax JR, Royer D, Mather J, *et al.* A preliminary study of sonographic grading of fetal intracardiac echogenic foci: feasibility, reliability and association with aneuploidy. Ultrasound Obstet Gynecol 2000; 16(2): 123-7. [http://dx.doi.org/10.1046/j.1469-0705.2000.00206.x] [PMID: 11117080]

[47] Shipp TD, Bromley B, Lieberman E, Benacerraf BR. The frequency of the detection of fetal echogenic intracardiac foci with respect to maternal race. Ultrasound Obstet Gynecol 2000; 15(6): 460-2. [http://dx.doi.org/10.1046/j.1469-0705.2000.00138.x] [PMID: 11005111]

[48] Shanks AL, Odibo AO, Gray DL. Echogenic intracardiac foci: associated with increased risk for fetal trisomy 21 or not? J Ultrasound Med 2009; 28(12): 1639-43. [PMID: 19933476]

[49] Zhao BW, Yang Y, Pan M, Li P, Wang B, Tang FG. Color Doppler twinkling artifact in fetuses with echogenic intracardiac foci: echocardiographic observation and clinical significance. Ultrasound Obstet Gynecol 2010; 35(5): 548-51. [http://dx.doi.org/10.1002/uog.7641] [PMID: 20336698]

[50] Roberts DJ, Genest D. Cardiac histologic pathology characteristic of trisomies 13 and 21. Hum Pathol 1992; 23(10): 1130-40.
[http://dx.doi.org/10.1016/0046-8177(92)90031-W] [PMID: 1398642]

[51] Renna MD, Pisani P, Conversano F, *et al.* Sonographic markers for early diagnosis of fetal malformations. World J Radiol 2013; 5(10): 356-71.
[http://dx.doi.org/10.4329/wjr.v5.i10.356] [PMID: 24179631]

[52] Nicolaides KH, Brizot ML, Snijders RJ. Fetal nuchal translucency: ultrasound screening for fetal trisomy in the first trimester of pregnancy. Br J Obstet Gynaecol 1994; 101(9): 782-6.
[http://dx.doi.org/10.1111/j.1471-0528.1994.tb11946.x] [PMID: 7947527]

[53] Park J, Sofka M, Lee S, Kim D, Zhou SK. Automatic nuchal translucency measurement from ultrasonography. Med Image Comput Comput Assist Interv 2013; 16(Pt 3): 243-50.
[http://dx.doi.org/10.1007/978-3-642-40760-4_31] [PMID: 24505767]

[54] Nicolaides KH, Heath V, Cicero S. Increased fetal nuchal translucency at 11-14 weeks. Prenat Diagn 2002; 22(4): 308-15.
[http://dx.doi.org/10.1002/pd.308]

[55] von Kaisenberg CS, Prols F, Nicolaides KH, Maass N, Meinhold-Heerlein I, Brand-Saberi B. Glycosaminoglycans and proteoglycans in the skin of aneuploid fetuses with increased nuchal translucency. Hum Reprod 2003; 18(12): 2544-61.
[http://dx.doi.org/10.1093/humrep/deg499] [PMID: 14645170]

[56] Berger A. What is fetal nuchal translucency? BMJ 1999; 318(7176): 85.
[http://dx.doi.org/10.1136/bmj.318.7176.81a] [PMID: 9880279]

[57] Hackshaw AK, Wald NJ. Assessment of the value of reporting partial screening results in prenatal screening for Down syndrome. Prenat Diagn 2001; 21(9): 737-40.
[http://dx.doi.org/10.1002/pd.132] [PMID: 11559909]

[58] Souka AP, Krampl E, Bakalis S, Heath V, Nicolaides KH. Outcome of pregnancy in chromosomally normal fetuses with increased nuchal translucency in the first trimester. Ultrasound Obstet Gynecol 2001; 18(1): 9-17.
[http://dx.doi.org/10.1046/j.1469-0705.2001.00454.x] [PMID: 11489218]

[59] Bilardo CM, Müller MA, Pajkrt E, Clur SA, van Zalen MM, Bijlsma EK. Increased nuchal translucency thickness and normal karyotype: time for parental reassurance. Ultrasound Obstet Gynecol 2007; 30(1): 11-8.
[http://dx.doi.org/10.1002/uog.4044] [PMID: 17559183]

[60] Hyett J, Perdu M, Sharland G, Snijders R, Nicolaides KH. Using fetal nuchal translucency to screen for major congenital cardiac defects at 10-14 weeks of gestation: population based cohort study. BMJ 1999; 318(7176): 81-5.
[PMID: 17559183]

[61] Ghi T, Huggon IC, Zosmer N, Nicolaides KH. Incidence of major structural cardiac defects associated with increased nuchal translucency but normal karyotype. Ultrasound Obstet Gynecol 2001; 18(6): 610-4.
[http://dx.doi.org/10.1046/j.0960-7692.2001.00584.x] [PMID: 11844199]

[62] Schwärzler P, Carvalho JS, Senat MV, Masroor T, Campbell S, Ville Y. Screening for fetal aneuploidies and fetal cardiac abnormalities by nuchal translucency thickness measurement at 10-14 weeks of gestation as part of routine antenatal care in an unselected population. Br J Obstet Gynaecol 1999; 106(10): 1029-34.
[http://dx.doi.org/10.1111/j.1471-0528.1999.tb08109.x] [PMID: 10519427]

[63] Mavrides E, Cobian-Sanchez F, Tekay A, *et al.* Limitations of using first-trimester nuchal translucency measurement in routine screening for major congenital heart defects. Ultrasound Obstet Gynecol 2001; 17(2): 106-10.
[http://dx.doi.org/10.1046/j.1469-0705.2001.00342.x] [PMID: 11251916]

[64] Wald NJ, Morris JK, Walker K, Simpson JM. Prenatal screening for serious congenital heart defects using nuchal translucency: a meta-analysis. Prenat Diagn 2008; 28(12): 1094-104.
[http://dx.doi.org/10.1002/pd.2124] [PMID: 19009556]

[65] Clur SA, Ottenkamp J, Bilardo CM. The nuchal translucency and the fetal heart: a literature review. Prenat Diagn 2009; 29(8): 739-48.
[http://dx.doi.org/10.1002/pd.2281] [PMID: 19399754]

[66] Kagan KO, Valencia C, Livanos P, Wright D, Nicolaides KH. Tricuspid regurgitation in screening for trisomies 21, 18 and 13 and Turner syndrome at 11+0 to 13+6 weeks of gestation. Ultrasound Obstet Gynecol 2009; 33(1): 18-22.
[http://dx.doi.org/10.1002/uog.6264] [PMID: 19031473]

[67] DeVore GR. Trisomy 21: 91% detection rate using second-trimester ultrasound markers. Ultrasound Obstet Gynecol 2000; 16(2): 133-41.
[http://dx.doi.org/10.1046/j.1469-0705.2000.00203.x] [PMID: 11117082]

[68] Geipel A, Gembruch U. [Screening performance of first trimester nuchal translucency, ductus venosus blood flow and tricuspid regurgitation for cardiac defects]. Z Geburtshilfe Neonatol 2012; 216(4): 157-61.
[http://dx.doi.org/10.1055/s-0032-1316345] [PMID: 22926815]

[69] Pavlícek J, Gruszka T, Matura D, Petros M, Jabůrek L. [Fetal tricuspid regurgitation]. Ceska Gynekol 2011; 76(4): 306-15.
[PMID: 22026072]

[70] Zalel Y, Achiron R, Yagel S, Kivilevitch Z. Fetal aberrant right subclavian artery in normal and Down syndrome fetuses. Ultrasound Obstet Gynecol 2008; 31(1): 25-9.
[http://dx.doi.org/10.1002/uog.5230] [PMID: 18098348]

[71] Willruth AM, Dwinger N, Ritgen J, *et al.* Fetal aberrant right subclavian artery (ARSA) - a potential new soft marker in the genetic scan? Ultraschall Med 2012; 33(7): E114-8.
[PMID: 21614745]

[72] Paladini D, Sglavo G, Pastore G, Masucci A, D'Armiento MR, Nappi C. Aberrant right subclavian artery: incidence and correlation with other markers of Down syndrome in second-trimester fetuses. Ultrasound Obstet Gynecol 2012; 39(2): 191-5.
[http://dx.doi.org/10.1002/uog.10053] [PMID: 21793087]

[73] Güçer S, Ince T, Kale G, *et al.* Noncardiac malformations in congenital heart disease: a retrospective

analysis of 305 pediatric autopsies. Turk J Pediatr 2005; 47(2): 159-66.
[PMID: 16052857]

[74] Paladini D, Tartaglione A, Agangi A, *et al.* The association between congenital heart disease and Down syndrome in prenatal life. Ultrasound Obstet Gynecol 2000; 15(2): 104-8.
[http://dx.doi.org/10.1046/j.1469-0705.2000.00027.x] [PMID: 10775990]

[75] Johnson B, Simpson LL. Screening for congenital heart disease: a move toward earlier echocardiography. Am J Perinatol 2007; 24(8): 449-56.
[http://dx.doi.org/10.1055/s-2007-986681] [PMID: 17992711]

[76] Patterson AJ, Zhang L. Hypoxia and fetal heart development. Curr Mol Med 2010; 10(7): 653-66.
[http://dx.doi.org/10.2174/156652410792630643] [PMID: 20712587]

[77] Parker MJ, Joubert GI, Levin SD. Portal vein thrombosis causing neonatal cerebral infarction. Arch Dis Child Fetal Neonatal Ed 2002; 87(2): F125-7.
[http://dx.doi.org/10.1136/fn.87.2.F125] [PMID: 12193520]

[78] Crossley KJ, Allison BJ, Polglase GR, Morley CJ, Davis PG, Hooper SB. Dynamic changes in the direction of blood flow through the ductus arteriosus at birth. J Physiol 2009; 587(Pt 19): 4695-704.
[PMID: 19675069]

[79] American Institute for Ultrasound in Medicine (AIUM). AIUM practice guideline for the performance of fetal echocardiography. Laurel, MD: AIUM; 2010. Available at: https://www.smfm.org/attachedfiles/fetalEchoaiumsmfm.pdf. 2010.

[80] Paladini D, Chita SK, Allan LD. Prenatal measurement of cardiothoracic ratio in evaluation of heart disease. Arch Dis Child 1990; 65(1 Spec No): 20-3.
[http://dx.doi.org/10.1136/adc.65.1_Spec_No.20] [PMID: 2407198]

[81] Allan L. Technique of fetal echocardiography. Pediatr Cardiol 2004; 25(3): 223-33.
[http://dx.doi.org/10.1007/s00246-003-0588-y] [PMID: 15360115]

[82] Lee MY, Won HS. Technique of fetal echocardiography. Obstet Gynecol Sci 2013; 56(4): 217-26.
[http://dx.doi.org/10.5468/ogs.2013.56.4.217] [PMID: 24328006]

[83] Simpson JM. Impact of fetal echocardiography. Ann Pediatr Cardiol 2009; 2(1): 41-50.
[http://dx.doi.org/10.4103/0974-2069.52806] [PMID: 20300268]

[84] Carvalho JS, Ho SY, Shinebourne EA. Sequential segmental analysis in complex fetal cardiac abnormalities: a logical approach to diagnosis. Ultrasound Obstet Gynecol 2005; 26(2): 105-11.
[http://dx.doi.org/10.1002/uog.1970] [PMID: 16041685]

[85] Caserta L, Ruggeri Z, D'Emidio L, *et al.* Two-dimensional fetal echocardiography: where we are. J Prenat Med 2008; 2(3): 31-5.
[PMID: 22439025]

[86] Allan LD. A practical approach to fetal heart scanning. Semin Perinatol 2000; 24(5): 324-30.
[http://dx.doi.org/10.1053/sper.2000.16551] [PMID: 11071373]

[87] Silverman NH, Golbus MS. Echocardiographic techniques for assessing normal and abnormal fetal cardiac anatomy. J Am Coll Cardiol 1985; 5(1) (Suppl.): 20S-9S.
[http://dx.doi.org/10.1016/S0735-1097(85)80140-6] [PMID: 3880776]

[88] Lee W, Allan L, Carvalho JS, *et al.* ISUOG Fetal Echocardiography Task Force. ISUOG consensus statement: what constitutes a fetal echocardiogram? Ultrasound Obstet Gynecol 2008; 32(2): 239-42. [http://dx.doi.org/10.1002/uog.6115] [PMID: 18663769]

[89] Allan L. Technique of fetal echocardiography. Pediatr Cardiol 2004; 25(3): 223-33. [http://dx.doi.org/10.1007/s00246-003-0588-y] [PMID: 15360115]

[90] Naderi S, McGahan JP. A primer for fetal cardiac imaging: a stepwise approach for 2-dimensional imaging. Ultrasound Q 2008; 24(3): 195-206. [http://dx.doi.org/10.1097/RUQ.0b013e3181862b84] [PMID: 18776813]

[91] Allan LD, Joseph MC, Boyd EG, Campbell S, Tynan M. M-mode echocardiography in the developing human fetus. Br Heart J 1982; 47(6): 573-83. [PMID: 7082505]

[92] Stamm ER, Drose JA. The fetal heart. In: Rumack CA, Wilson SR, Charboneau WJ, Eds. Diagnostic ultrasound. (2nd ed.) St. Louis, MO: Mosby 1998; pp. 1123-59.

[93] Gardiner HM. Fetal echocardiography: 20 years of progress. Heart 2001; 86 (Suppl II ii12± ii22). [http://dx.doi.org/10.1136/heart.86] [PMID: 11709530]

[94] Clur SA, Oude Rengerink K, Ottenkamp J, Bilardo CM. Cardiac function in trisomy 21 fetuses. Ultrasound Obstet Gynecol 2011; 37(2): 163-71. [http://dx.doi.org/10.1002/uog.8819] [PMID: 20814928]

[95] Craig B. Atrioventricular septal defect: from fetus to adult. Heart 2006; 92(12): 1879-85. [http://dx.doi.org/10.1136/hrt.2006.093344] [PMID: 17105897]

[96] Abu-Harb M, Hey E, Wren C. Death in infancy from unrecognised congenital heart disease. Arch Dis Child 1994; 71(1): 3-7. [http://dx.doi.org/10.1136/adc.71.1.3] [PMID: 8067789]

[97] Choi EY, Lee CH, Yoon MJ, *et al.* Impact of fetal diagnosis of congenital heart disease on parents. Korean J Pediatr 2006; 49: 1073-8. [http://dx.doi.org/10.3345/kjp.2006.49.10.1073]

[98] Cha S, Kim GB, Kwon BS, *et al.* Recent trends in indications of fetal echocardiography and postnatal outcomes in fetuses diagnosed as congenital heart disease. Korean Circ J 2012; 42(12): 839-44. [http://dx.doi.org/10.4070/kcj.2012.42.12.839] [PMID: 23323122]

[99] Manganaro L, Vinci V, Bernardo S, *et al.* Magnetic resonance imaging of fetal heart: anatomical and pathological findings. J Matern Fetal Neonatal Med 2014; 27(12): 1213-9. [http://dx.doi.org/10.3109/14767058.2013.852174] [PMID: 24102352]

[100] Loomba RS, Chandrasekar S, Shah PH, Sanan P. The developing role of fetal magnetic resonance imaging in the diagnosis of congenital cardiac anomalies: A systematic review. Ann Pediatr Cardiol 2011; 4(2): 172-6. [http://dx.doi.org/10.4103/0974-2069.84665] [PMID: 21976881]

[101] Yamamura J, Schnackenburg B, Kooijmann H, *et al.* Magnetic resonance angiography of fetal vessels: feasibility study in the sheep fetus. Jpn J Radiol 2010; 28(10): 720-6. [http://dx.doi.org/10.1007/s11604-010-0498-x] [PMID: 21191736]

[102] Roy CW, Seed M, van Amerom JF, *et al.* Dynamic imaging of the fetal heart using metric optimized gating. Magn Reson Med 2013; 70(6): 1598-607.
[http://dx.doi.org/10.1002/mrm.24614] [PMID: 23382068]

[103] Calabrò R, Limongelli G. Complete atrioventricular canal. Orphanet J Rare Dis 2006; 5: 1-8.
[http://dx.doi.org/10.1186/1750-1172-1-8] [PMID: 16722604]

[104] Freeman SB, Bean LH, Allen EG, *et al.* Ethnicity, sex, and the incidence of congenital heart defects: a report from the National Down Syndrome Project. Genet Med 2008; 10(3): 173-80.
[http://dx.doi.org/10.1097/GIM.0b013e3181634867] [PMID: 18344706]

[105] Blom NA, Ottenkamp J, Deruiter MC, Wenink AC, Gittenberger-de Groot AC. Development of the cardiac conduction system in atrioventricular septal defect in human trisomy 21. Pediatr Res 2005; 58(3): 516-20.
[http://dx.doi.org/10.1203/01.PDR.0000179388.10921.44] [PMID: 16148066]

[106] Anderson RH, Wessels A, Vettukattil JJ. Morphology and morphogenesis of atrioventricular septal defect with common atrioventricular junction. World J Pediatr Congenit Heart Surg 2010; 1(1): 59-67.
[http://dx.doi.org/10.1177/2150135109360813] [PMID: 23804724]

[107] Huggon IC, Cook AC, Smeeton NC, Magee AG, Sharland GK. Atrioventricular septal defects diagnosed in fetal life: associated cardiac and extra-cardiac abnormalities and outcome. J Am Coll Cardiol 2000; 36(2): 593-601.
[http://dx.doi.org/10.1016/S0735-1097(00)00757-9] [PMID: 10933376]

[108] Unolt M, Putotto C, Marino D. Double-orifice left atrioventricular valve in patients with atrioventricular septal defect with and without down syndrome. Ann Thorac Surg 2013; 95(5): 1843-4.
[http://dx.doi.org/10.1016/j.athoracsur.2012.11.048] [PMID: 23608283]

[109] Vergara P, Digilio MC, De Zorzi A, *et al.* Genetic heterogeneity and phenotypic anomalies in children with atrioventricular canal defect and tetralogy of Fallot. Clin Dysmorphol 2006; 15(2): 65-70.
[http://dx.doi.org/10.1097/01.mcd.0000198925.94082.ea] [PMID: 16531730]

[110] Chintala K, Gurczynski J, Aggarwal S. Prenatal diagnosis of complete atrioventricular septal defect with truncus arteriosus. Prenat Diagn 2007; 27(6): 560-2.
[http://dx.doi.org/10.1002/pd.1716] [PMID: 17380467]

[111] Machlitt A, Heling KS, Chaoui R. Increased cardiac atrial-to-ventricular length ratio in the fetal four-chamber view: a new marker for atrioventricular septal defects. Ultrasound Obstet Gynecol 2004; 24(6): 618-22.
[http://dx.doi.org/10.1002/uog.1750] [PMID: 15517546]

[112] Kumar S, Donofrio M, Frank L, He D, Jonas R. Complete atrioventricular canal with guarded primum septal defect. Pediatr Cardiol 2011; 32(4): 503-5.
[http://dx.doi.org/10.1007/s00246-010-9869-4] [PMID: 21188369]

[113] Smallhorn JF, Tommasini G, Anderson RH, Macartney FJ. Assessment of atrioventricular septal defects by two dimensional echocardiography. Br Heart J 1982; 47(2): 109-21.
[http://dx.doi.org/10.1136/hrt.47.2.109] [PMID: 7059391]

[114] Sulafa AK, Tamimi O, Najm HK, Godman MJ. Echocardiographic differentiation of atrioventricular septal defects from inlet ventricular septal defects and mitral valve clefts. Am J Cardiol 2005; 95(5):

607-10.
[http://dx.doi.org/doi:10.1016/j.amjcard.2004.11.007] [PMID: 15721100]

[115] Lange A, Mankad P, Walayat M, Palka P, Burns JE, Godman MJ. Transthoracic three-dimensional echocardiography in the preoperative assessment of atrioventricular septal defect morphology. Am J Cardiol 2000; 85(5): 630-5.
[http://dx.doi.org/10.1016/S0002-9149(99)00823-1] [PMID: 11078279]

[116] Kim HK, Kim WH, Hwang SW, *et al.* Predictive value of intraoperative transesophageal echocardiography in complete atrioventricular septal defect. Ann Thorac Surg 2005; 80(1): 56-9. [http://dx.doi.org/10.1016/j.athoracsur.2005.01.060] [PMID: 15975339]

[117] Ali S. Echocardiographic diagnosis of atrioventricular septal defect without primum atrial septal defect: a relatively "common" congenital heart defect in Down's syndrome. Anadolu Kardiyol Derg 2011; 11(2): 183-5.
[http://dx.doi.org/10.5152/akd.2011.044] [PMID: 21362598]

[118] Parsons JM, Baker EJ, Anderson RH, *et al.* Morphological evaluation of atrioventricular septal defects by magnetic resonance imaging. Br Heart J 1990; 64(2): 138-45.
[http://dx.doi.org/10.1136/hrt.64.2.138] [PMID: 2393612]

[119] Wu CS, Chiu IS, Wu SJ, *et al.* Correlation between pulmonary vascular change and hemodynamics in patients with complete atrioventricular septal defect. J Formos Med Assoc 2005; 104(2): 82-8.
[PMID: 15765161]

[120] Lange R, Guenther T, Busch R, Hess J, Schreiber C. The presence of Down syndrome is not a risk factor in complete atrioventricular septal defect repair. J Thorac Cardiovasc Surg 2007; 134(2): 304-10.
[http://dx.doi.org/10.1016/j.jtcvs.2007.01.026] [PMID: 17662766]

[121] Atz AM, Hawkins JA, Lu M, *et al.* Pediatric Heart Network Investigators. Surgical management of complete atrioventricular septal defect: associations with surgical technique, age, and trisomy 21. J Thorac Cardiovasc Surg 2011; 141(6): 1371-9.
[http://dx.doi.org/10.1016/j.jtcvs.2010.08.093] [PMID: 21163497]

[122] Marino B, Papa M, Guccione P, Corno A, Marasini M, Calabrò R. Ventricular septal defect in Down syndrome. Anatomic types and associated malformations. Am J Dis Child 1990; 144(5): 544-5.
[http://dx.doi.org/10.1001/archpedi.1990.02150290038021] [PMID: 2139542]

[123] Paladini D, Palmieri S, Lamberti A, Teodoro A, Martinelli P, Nappi C. Characterization and natural history of ventricular septal defects in the fetus. Ultrasound Obstet Gynecol 2000; 16(2): 118-22.
[http://dx.doi.org/10.1046/j.1469-0705.2000.00202.x] [PMID: 11117079]

[124] Shen O, Lieberman S, Farber B, Terner D, Lahad A, Levy-Lahad EA. prenatal Isolated Ventricular Septal Defect May Not Be Associated with Trisomy 21. J Clin Med 2014; 3: 432-9.
[http://dx.doi.org/10.3390/jcm3020432]

[125] Axt-Fliedner R, Schwarze A, Smrcek J, Germer U, Krapp M, Gembruch U. Isolated ventricular septal defects detected by color Doppler imaging: evolution during fetal and first year of postnatal life. Ultrasound Obstet Gynecol 2006; 27(3): 266-73.
[http://dx.doi.org/10.1002/uog.2716] [PMID: 16485323]

[126] Chaoui R, Bollmann R. [Fetal color Doppler echocardiography. Part 2: Abnormalities of the heart and great vessels]. Ultraschall Med 1994; 15(3): 105-11.
[http://dx.doi.org/10.1055/s-2007-1003942] [PMID: 8091194]

[127] Hussain M, Hussain S, Krishin J, Abbasi S. Presentation of congestive cardiac failure in children with ventricular septal defect. J Ayub Med Coll Abbottabad 2010; 22(4): 135-8.
[PMID: 22455281]

[128] Minette MS, Sahn DJ. Ventricular septal defects. Circulation 2006; 114(20): 2190-7.
[http://dx.doi.org/10.1161/CIRCULATIONAHA.106.618124] [PMID: 17101870]

[129] Turner SW, Hunter S, Wyllie JP. The natural history of ventricular septal defects. Arch Dis Child 1999; 81(5): 413-6.
[http://dx.doi.org/10.1136/adc.81.5.413] [PMID: 10519715]

[130] Ellis JH IV, Moodie DS, Sterba R, Gill CC. Ventricular septal defect in the adult: natural and unnatural history. Am Heart J 1987; 114(1 Pt 1): 115-20.
[http://dx.doi.org/10.1016/0002-8703(87)90315-2] [PMID: 3604855]

[131] Pieroni DR, Nishimura RA, Bierman FZ, *et al.* Second natural history study of congenital heart defects. Ventricular septal defect: echocardiography. Circulation 1993; 87(2) (Suppl.): I80-8. [PMID: 8425326].
[PMID: 8425326]

[132] Sutherland GR, Godman MJ, Smallhorn JF, Guiterras P, Anderson RH, Hunter S. Ventricular septal defects. Two dimensional echocardiographic and morphological correlations. Br Heart J 1982; 47(4): 316-28. [PMID: 0007066116].
[http://dx.doi.org/10.1136/hrt.47.4.316] [PMID: 7066116]

[133] Andrade JL. The role of Doppler echocardiography in the diagnosis, follow-up, and management of ventricular septal defects. Echocardiography 1991; 8(4): 501-16. [PMID: 0010149268].
[http://dx.doi.org/10.1111/j.1540-8175.1991.tb01010.x] [PMID: 10149268]

[134] Ludomirsky A, Huhta JC, Vick GW III, Murphy DJ Jr, Danford DA, Morrow WR. Color Doppler detection of multiple ventricular septal defects. Circulation 1986; 74(6): 1317-22. [PMID: 0003779917].
[http://dx.doi.org/10.1161/01.CIR.74.6.1317] [PMID: 3779917]

[135] Garg A, Shrivastava S, Radhakrishnan S, Dev V, Saxena A. Doppler assessment of interventricular pressure gradient across isolated ventricular septal defect. Clin Cardiol 1990; 13(10): 717-21. [PMID: 0002257713].
[http://dx.doi.org/10.1002/clc.4960131009] [PMID: 2257713]

[136] Bayer AS, Bolger AF, Taubert KA, *et al.* Diagnosis and management of infective endocarditis and its complications. Circulation 1998; 98(25): 2936-48. [PMID: 0009860802].
[http://dx.doi.org/10.1161/01.CIR.98.25.2936] [PMID: 9860802]

[137] Ishii M, Hashino K, Eto G, *et al.* Quantitative assessment of severity of ventricular septal defect by three-dimensional reconstruction of color Doppler-imaged vena contracta and flow convergence region. Circulation 2001; 103(5): 664-9.
[http://dx.doi.org/10.1161/01.CIR.103.5.664] [PMID: 11156877]

[138] Santamaria H, Soto B, Ceballos R, Bargeron LM Jr, Coghlan HC, Kirklin JW. Angiographic differentiation of types of ventricular septal defects. AJR Am J Roentgenol 1983; 141(2): 273-81. [PMID: 0006603117].
[http://dx.doi.org/10.2214/ajr.141.2.273] [PMID: 6603117]

[139] Ammash NM, Warnes CA. Ventricular septal defects in adults Ann Intern Med 2001; 135(9): 812-24.
[http://dx.doi.org/10.7326/0003-4819-135-9-200111060-00011] [PMID: 11694106]

[140] Wolfe RR, Driscoll DJ, Gersony WM, *et al.* Arrhythmias in patients with valvar aortic stenosis, valvar pulmonary stenosis, and ventricular septal defect. Results of 24-hour ECG monitoring. Circulation 1993; 87(2) (Suppl.): I89-I101. [PMID: 0008425327].
[PMID: 8425327]

[141] Gersony WM, Hayes CJ, Driscoll DJ, *et al.* Bacterial endocarditis in patients with aortic stenosis, pulmonary stenosis, or ventricular septal defect. Circulation 1993; 87(2) (Suppl.): I121-6. [PMID: 0008425318].
[PMID: 8425318]

[142] Kidd L, Driscoll DJ, Gersony WM, *et al.* Second natural history study of congenital heart defects. Results of treatment of patients with ventricular septal defects. Circulation 1993; 87(2) (Suppl.): I38-51. [PMID: 0008425321].
[PMID: 8425321]

[143] Neutze JM, Ishikawa T, Clarkson PM, Calder AL, Barratt-Boyes BG, Kerr AR. Assessment and follow-up of patients with ventricular septal defect and elevated pulmonary vascular resistance. Am J Cardiol 1989; 63(5): 327-31. [PMID: 0002913735].
[http://dx.doi.org/10.1016/0002-9149(89)90340-8] [PMID: 2913735]

[144] Montigny M, Davignon A, Fouron JC, Biron P, Fournier A, Elie R. Captopril in infants for congestive heart failure secondary to a large ventricular left-to-right shunt. Am J Cardiol 1989; 63(9): 631-3.
[http://dx.doi.org/10.1016/0002-9149(89)90915-6] [PMID: 2645762]

[145] Penny DJ, Vick GW 3rd. Ventricular septal defect. Lancet 2011; 377(9771): 1103-2.
[http://dx.doi.org/10.1016/S0140-6736(10)61339-6] [PMID: 21349577]

[146] Lun K, Li H, Leung MP, *et al.* Analysis of indications for surgical closure of subarterial ventricular septal defect without associated aortic cusp prolapse and aortic regurgitation. Am J Cardiol 2001; 87(11): 1266-70.
[http://dx.doi.org/10.1016/S0002-9149(01)01517-X] [PMID: 11377352]

[147] Sanfelippo PM, Hector DA. Considerations in the surgical management of ventricular septal defect and aortic insufficiency--a case report. Angiology 1998; 49(4): 321-5.
[http://dx.doi.org/10.1177/000331979804900411] [PMID: 9555936]

[148] Zeinaloo A, Macuil B, Zanjani KS, Sideris E. Transcatheter patch occlusion of ventricular septal defect in Down syndrome. Am J Cardiol 2011; 107(12): 1838-40.
[http://dx.doi.org/10.1016/j.amjcard.2011.02.316] [PMID: 21481831]

[149] Soneda J, Ban T, Okamoto Y, Matsuda K, Sakamoto K, Yamada T. [Severe postoperative pulmonary hypertensive crisis in a case of ventricular septal defect with Down's syndrome]. Nippon Kyobu Geka Gakkai Zasshi 1989; 37(6): 1247-50.

[PMID: 2530290]

[150] Shah PS, Hellmann J, Adatia I. Clinical characteristics and follow up of Down syndrome infants without congenital heart disease who presented with persistent pulmonary hypertension of newborn. J Perinat Med 2004; 32(2): 168-70. [http://dx.doi.org/10.1515/JPM.2004.030] [PMID: 15085894]

[151] Cua CL, Blankenship A, North AL, Hayes J, Nelin LD. Increased incidence of idiopathic persistent pulmonary hypertension in Down syndrome neonates. Pediatr Cardiol 2007; 28(4): 250-4. [http://dx.doi.org/10.1007/s00246-006-0011-6] [PMID: 17486396]

[152] Weijerman ME, van Furth AM, van der Mooren MD, *et al.* Prevalence of congenital heart defects and persistent pulmonary hypertension of the neonate with Down syndrome. Eur J Pediatr 2010; 169(10): 1195-9. [http://dx.doi.org/10.1007/s00431-010-1200-0] [PMID: 20411274]

[153] Fukushima H, Kosaki K, Sato R, *et al.* Mechanisms underlying early development of pulmonary vascular obstructive disease in Down syndrome: An imbalance in biosynthesis of thromboxane A2 and prostacyclin. Am J Med Genet A 2010; 152A(8): 1919-24. [http://dx.doi.org/10.1002/ajmg.a.33555] [PMID: 20583254]

[154] Benjamin W. Eidem, Carolyn Jones, Frank Cetta. Unusual Association of Hypertrophic Cardiomyopathy with Complete Atrioventricular Canal Defect and Down Syndrome. Tex Heart Inst J 2000; 27(3): 289-91. [PMID: 11093415]

[155] Wacker A, Scheel-Walter HG, Neunhoeffer F. [Biventricular hypertrophic non-obstructive cardiomyopathy as a symptom of transient myeloproliferative disorder in a newborn with Down syndrome]. Z Geburtshilfe Neonatol 2009; 213(2): 64-6. [http://dx.doi.org/10.1055/s-0029-1214406] [PMID: 19319796]

[156] King P, Tulloh R. Management of pulmonary hypertension and Down syndrome. Int J Clin Pract Suppl 2011; (174): 8-13. [http://dx.doi.org/10.1111/j.1742-1241.2011.02823.x] [PMID: 22171818]

[157] Seki M, Kato T, Masutani S, Matsunaga T, Senzaki H. Pulmonary arterial hypertension associated with gastroesophageal reflux in a 2-month-old boy with Down syndrome. Circ J 2009; 73(12): 2352-4. [http://dx.doi.org/10.1253/circj.CJ-08-0993] [PMID: 19491506]

[158] Durmowicz AG. Pulmonary edema in 6 children with Down syndrome during travel to moderate altitudes. Pediatrics 2001; 108(2): 443-7. [http://dx.doi.org/10.1542/peds.108.2.443] [PMID: 11483813]

[159] Anah MU, Ansa VO, Etiuma AU, Udoh EE, Ineji EO, Asindi AA. Recurrent pericardial effusion associated with hypothyroidism in Down Syndrome: a case report. West Afr J Med 2011; 30(3): 210-3. [PMID: 22120489]

[160] Dinleyici EC, Ucar B, Kilic Z, Dogruel N, Yarar C. Pericardial effusion due to hypothyroidism in Down syndrome: report of four cases. Neuroendocrinol Lett 2007; 28(2): 141-4. [PMID: 17435671]

[161] Wiseman FK, Alford KA, Tybulewicz VL, Fisher EM. Down syndrome--recent progress and future prospects. Hum Mol Genet 2009; 18(R1): R75-83.
[http://dx.doi.org/10.1093/hmg/ddp010] [PMID: 19297404]

[162] Iellamo F, Galante A, Legramante JM, *et al.* Altered autonomic cardiac regulation in individuals with Down syndrome. Am J Physiol Heart Circ Physiol 2005; 289(6): H2387-91.
[http://dx.doi.org/10.1152/ajpheart.00560.2005] [PMID: 16024564]

[163] Al-Biltagi M, Serag AR, Hefidah MM, Mabrouk MM. Evaluation of cardiac functions with Doppler echocardiography in children with Down syndrome and anatomically normal heart. Cardiol Young 2013; 23(2): 174-80.
[http://dx.doi.org/10.1017/S1047951112000613] [PMID: 22717046]

[164] Seven M, Cengiz M, Tüzgen S, Iscan MY. Plasma carnitine levels in children with Down syndrome. Am J Hum Biol 2001; 13(6): 721-5.
[http://dx.doi.org/10.1002/ajhb.1117] [PMID: 11748810]

[165] O'Brien MM, Taub JW, Chang MN, *et al.* Cardiomyopathy in children with Down syndrome treated for acute myeloid leukemia: a report from the Children's Oncology Group Study POG 9421. J Clin Oncol 2008; 26(3): 414-20.
[http://dx.doi.org/10.1200/JCO.2007.13.2209] [PMID: 18202418]

[166] Saraiva LR, Brindeiro Filho D, Carneiro RW, De França NA. [Aortic insufficiency and septal hypertrophy in a boy with Down's syndrome]. Arq Bras Cardiol 1991; 57(2): 133-6.
[PMID: 1840434]

[167] Howells G. Mitral valve prolapse, keratoconus and Down's syndrome. J R Soc Med 1992; 85(12): 773.
[PMID: 1494176]

[168] Adelekan T, Magge S, Shults J, Stallings V, Stettler N. Lipid profiles of children with Down syndrome compared with their siblings. Pediatrics 2012; 129(6): e1382-7.
[http://dx.doi.org/10.1542/peds.2011-1262] [PMID: 22585768]

[169] Czeizel AE, Puhó E. Maternal use of nutritional supplements during the first month of pregnancy and decreased risk of Down's syndrome: case-control study. Nutrition 2005; 21(6): 698-704.
[http://dx.doi.org/10.1016/j.nut.2004.10.017] [PMID: 15925294]

[170] Meijer WM, Werler MM, Louik C, Hernandez-Diaz S, de Jong-van den Berg LT, Mitchell AA. Can folic acid protect against congenital heart defects in Down syndrome? Birth Defects Res A Clin Mol Teratol 2006; 76(10): 714-7.
[http://dx.doi.org/10.1002/bdra.20312] [PMID: 17051586]

[171] Al-Biltagi M. Echocardiography in children with Down syndrome. World J Clin Pediatr 2013; 2(4): 36-45.
[http://dx.doi.org/10.5409/wjcp.v2.i4.36] [PMID: 25254173]

[172] Nishimura RA, Carabello BA, Faxon DP, *et al.* ACC/AHA 2008 Guideline Update on Valvular Heart Disease: Focused Update on Infective Endocarditis. A Report of the American College of Cardiology/American Heart Association Task Force on Practice Guidelines. Circulation 2008; 118(8): 887-96.

[http://dx.doi.org/10.1161/CIRCULATIONAHA.108.190377] [PMID: 18663090]

[173] Bamba V. Update on screening, etiology, and treatment of dyslipidemia in children. J Clin Endocrinol Metab 2014; 99(9): 3093-102.
[http://dx.doi.org/10.1210/jc.2013-3860] [PMID: 24848708]

CHAPTER 5

Respiratory Problems in Children with Down Syndrome

Mohammed Al-Biltagi*

Pediatric Department, Faculty of Medicine, Tanta University, Egypt

Abstract: Children with Down syndrome (DS) are more prone to have respiratory disorders which can be categorized into congenital structural disorders of the airways and lungs, acquired disorders, and sleep-related disorders and obstructive sleep apnea. Children with DS have a high incidence of airway anomalies; both upper and lower compared to non-DS children. The most important findings are hypoplasia of midface with dysfunction of malformed Eustachian tube, a short palate, hypoplastic nasal bones, choanal stenosis, macroglossia, enlarged adenoids and tonsils, lingual tonsils, and narrow oropharynx, and nasopharynx, abnormal oropharyngeal structures, laryngomalacia, tracheomalacia, congenital subglottic stenosis, tracheo-oesophageal fistula, bronchomalacia and branching and lung anomalies. Among the acquired respiratory disorders encountered in children with DS are respiratory infections including acute bronchiolitis due to infection with respiratory syncytial virus, pneumonia, infection with H1n1 stains of flu virus, high incidence of acute lung injury, occurrence of pulmonary hemosiderosis, increase incidence of pulmonary hypertension, GERD, and the possibility of having asthma. Sleep disorders are common and important problems, frequently under-recognized in children with DS and can be a significant distressing factor to their families. The prevalence of these disorders in children with DS is very high, particularly in boys. Vaccinations help to prevent a considerable number of infectious diseases. The immune dysfunctions of DS are not a contraindication for the currently available vaccines: their immunogenicity and safety are not significantly different from those observed in the general population.

Keywords: Adenotonsillar hypertrophy, Abronchomalacia, Children, Down syndrome, Esophageal atresia, Glue ear, Immune stimulation, Hypotonia, Laryngomalacia, Lung hypoplasia, Hypothyroidism, Macroglossia, Pulmonary

* **Corresponding Author Dr. Mohammed Al-Biltagi:** Pediatric Department, Faculty of Medicine, Tanta University, Egypt; Tel: (+973)39545472; Fax: (+973) 1759 0495; Email: mbelrem@hotmail.com

hypertension, Reflux, Respiratory problem, Subglottic stenosis, Tracheal atresia, Tracheal bronchus, Tracheoesophageal fistula, Tracheomalacia.

1. INTRODUCTION

Children with Down syndrome (DS) suffer a major health load and troubles, especially the young children who frequently encounter cardiac and respiratory problems. DS can affect the respiratory tract (both upper and lower) in different ways and can impact upon and lower respiratory functions, giving rise to a wide variety of respiratory manifestations. Respiratory problems are common reasons for increased morbidity and mortality in children with DS. These respiratory problems include structural anomalies of the airways and lungs, glue ears, frequent lower respiratory tract infections and increased incidence of obstructive sleep apnoea. Additionally, other organ systems or extrinsic factors may play a role *e.g.* congenital heart diseases (CHD), gastrointestinal malformations, autoimmune conditions, thyroid dysfunction, hematological disorders, and associated immunodeficiency [1 - 3]. They are also at a higher risk of pulmonary arterial hypertension (PAH) than healthy children, partly due to upper airway obstruction and CHD [4]. They are also more liable to have obstructive sleep apnea and sleep-related breathing disorders which are associated with a wide range of symptoms, including developmental delay, behavioral difficulties, impaired growth, easy tiredness and pulmonary hypertension [5]. In this chapter we will discuss the common respiratory disorders in children with DS, their etiology, prevalence, diagnosis and the possible management.

2. ETIOLOGY OF RESPIRATORY DISORDERS IN DOWN SYNDROME CHILDREN

Down syndrome is the most common chromosomal abnormalities and is related to many health medical issues. The presence of an extra copy of HSA21 chromosome in persons with DS causes over expression of about 30-50% of HSA21 genes. This up-regulation can, in turn, activate a deregulation of the expression of non-HSA21 genes. Moreover, the overdose of HSA21 microRNAs (miRNAs) may initiate down-regulation of its target genes [6]. Gene over expression has been recognized as a major influential factor for the unique DS phenotypes. Previous genetic study had discovered a range of gene expressions accountable for many of the characteristic traits observed in DS patients including cardiovascular, brain, and gastrointestinal anomalies. However, the molecular/genetic basis underlying the pulmonary anomalies are not yet clarified enough, even though respiratory complications are the primary reason of morbidity and mortality in DS patients [7].

Dosage imbalance of genes on chromosome 21 (Hsa21) disturbs the complex gene-regulatory interactions and modifies the development to result in a wide range of phenotypes, together with the unique facial dysmorphology. Craniofacial changes may lead to wide spectrum of complications including breathing, eating, and communication problems. Proponents of the "amplified developmental instability" hypothesis argue that trisomy 21 results in a generalized genetic imbalance that disturbs evolutionarily preserved developmental pathways by diminishing developmental homeostasis and accuracy all over development. Recognition of facial prominences in the DS sample exhibiting increased changeable asymmetry during facial morphogenesis which affords an evidence for increased developmental instability in DS faces [8]. Trisomy change the expression of non-trisomic genes implicated in development leading to craniofacial structural changes associated with DS [9].The phenotypic expression of trisomy 21 generates changeable, though unique, facial morphology. Though certain facial appearance has been standardized quantitatively and qualitatively as distinctive features of DS (*e.g.* epicanthic folds, macroglossia, and hypertelorism), all of these features may present in other craniofacial disorders with a fundamental genetic etiology. Facial characters are affected in a differential way in DS, as evidenced by statistically significant variation in combination both within and between facial regions [10]. Laryngomalacia with obstruction of the upper airway is the result of increased dosage of some genes due to partial Trisomy 11q syndrome. Some genes in 11q14q25 may be responsible for laryngomalacia. A comparable effect could be observed in trisomy 21 cases that have an increased rate of laryngomalacia compared with non-syndromic children, however; studies confirmed an etiological base [11].

Human congenital pulmonary anomalies that are due to defective Sonic hedgehog (SHH) signaling comprise lung hypoplasia, tracheoesophageal fistula, tracheal atresia, and esophageal atresia. SHH controls branching morphogenesis and affects differentiation of the peripheral lung mesenchyme needed for formation of bronchial and vascular smooth muscle. SHH expression is initially discovered in the tracheal diverticulum during the embryonic stage. Down syndrome critical region gene 1-like 1 (Dscr1l1 AB061524) is one along with numerous genes which are affected by up-regulation in lungs, which may explain the reason for increased incidence of different bronchial and lung pathologies occurred in DS including lung hypoplasia, tracheoesophageal fistula, tracheal atresia, and esophageal atresia [12].

The incidence of pulmonary hypertension is high in DS newborn which reaches as high as 6% of all DS births over a 4-year period [13]. One of the potential mechanisms is an unusual production of nitric oxide (NO) and impaired pulmonary vasodilatation in response to NO in DS patients *versus* controls [14]. Mutation of bone morphogenetic protein receptor (BMPR) gene was found to raise NO production and showed an increased incidence of pulmonary arterial hypertension in a subset of DS patients. Persistent Pulmonary Hypertension of the Newborn observed in neonates with DS was also accompanied with high incidence of congenital diaphragmatic hernia, alveolar capillary hypoplasia, and renal agenesis [15].

Individuals with DS have an increased incidence of immunological deviation with high vulnerability to bacterial and viral infections especially of the respiratory tract. Activation of immune system is revealed by changes in gene expression profiles of immune competent blood cells. There is significant down regulation of 13 genes concerned with immune system function (BCL2, CCL3, CCR7, CD19, CD28, CD40, CD40LG, CD80, EDN1, IKBKB, IL6, NOS2 and SKI) and significant up-regulation of other immune system-related 4 genes in children with DS which could explain the molecular mechanism underlying DS pathology and reinforce the secondary effects of the presence of a third copy of HSA21 [16].

In addition to the presence of these congenital and structural respiratory tract disorders, the presence of other systemic factors such as by hypotonia, congenital heart diseases and obesity add more loads to children with DS. The incidence of overweight and obesity is elevated in children with DS more than that observed in the general population, and appear to be more liable to be overweight at a younger age [17, 18]. Cardiomegaly and enlargement of the pulmonary arteries (*e.g.* that result from lesions associated with a left to right shunt, such as ventricular septal defect, atrial septal defect or patent ductus arteriosus) may cause compression of the airways and result in malacia of the airways. Those children also are more liable to develop pulmonary hypertension more rapid than non-syndromic children with CHD due to increase pulmonary vascular fragility. Surgical correction of the cardiac defects can results in various respiratory complications such as development of chylothorax, injury to the recurrent laryngeal nerve, diaphragmatic paralysis, and subglottic stenosis which further impair the respiratory functions [19, 20]. Recurrent aspiration due to associated gastroesophageal reflux disease (GERD) can cause both clinically evident acute lower respiratory infections and chronic inflammation and damage of the lower airways which may go unobserved for some time, but eventually may cause both bronchiectasis and lung parenchymal damage. Once bronchiectasis has developed, this additionally weakens the clearance of airway secretions and predisposes to lower airway infections [21].

3. RESPIRATORY DISORDERS IN CHILDREN WITH DOWN SYNDROME

Children with DS are at a higher risk for respiratory problems. The respiratory problems can be categorized into 3 main categories; congenital structural disorders of the airways and lungs, acquired disorders, and sleep-related disorders and obstructive sleep apnea.

3.1. Congenital Disorders

Down syndrome is the most frequent chromosomal disorders in humans. Numerous congenital anomalies associated with DS have been illustrated. Children with DS and respiratory manifestations have an elevated prevalence of airway anomalies compared with non-DS children. The most important findings are laryngomalacia, tracheomalacia, tracheal bronchus, and bronchomalacia [22]. These anomalies include also other upper and lower airway abnormalities. Upper airway abnormalities include narrowing of the nasopharyngeal passages, macroglossia, adenotonsillar hypertrophy and laryngomalacia, which is worsened by reflux. Lower airway abnormalities include subglottic stenosis (may be more likely following intubation, as tracheal diameter is smaller), tracheo-oesophageal fistula, tracheobronchomalacia, tracheal stenosis, branching anomalies, pulmonary hypoplasia and subpleural cyst.

3.1.1. Upper Airway Diseases

Infants with DS are more prone to upper airway obstruction which is frequently a complex and occurs at multi-levels. This is due to hypoplasia of midface with malformation and dysfunction of the Eustachian tube, a short palate, hypoplastic nasal bones, choanal stenosis, macroglossia, enlarged adenoids and tonsils, lingual tonsils, narrow oropharynx and nasopharynx, abnormal oropharyngeal structures and generalized muscular hypotonia. The tonsils are displaced medially and cause more obstruction in the back of the throat, and adenoids sitting in a contracted nasopharynx and thus causing more obstruction. Other obstructive elements may contribute such as presence of excessive secretions, and glossoptosis [23].

These morphological variants affect children with DS in different ways including high incidence of recurrent otitis media, sinusitis and sleep apnea syndrome. Infants with DS and severe chronic upper airway obstruction may develop cor-pulmonale and heart failure. Features of the sleep apnea syndrome are obvious; specifically, noisy breathing with retraction, cyanosis, frequent apnea during sleep, and daytime lethargy and somnolence. The clinical picture may be confused with cyanotic congenital heart disease. Arterial blood gas analyses showed alveolar hypoventilation, especially during sleep. The nature of the obstructive element is variable [24]. Abnormalities in the paranasal sinuses as a result of the mid-facial hypoplasia, the tardy maturation of the immunological system, or the existence of ciliary dyskinesia provoke common infections in the upper respiratory tracts and chronic sinusitis [25].

Children with DS have midface hypoplasia and mandibular hypoplasia causing the upper airway size to be smaller than in other children. In addition, children with DS have a relative enlargement of the tongue, medially displaced tonsils that cause more obstruction in the back of the throat, adenoids sitting in a contracted nasopharynx and thus causing more obstruction, as well as hypotonia of the upper airway with resultant collapse at multiple levels of the airway during sleep. Increased upper airway infections, nasal secretions, obesity and hypotonia further contribute to both oropharyngeal and hypopharyngeal collapse and obstruction during sleep [26]. Narrowing of the oropharynx and nasopharynx can lead to increased incidence of postextubation stridor post-operatively as they are more likely to require multiple intubations. This has important clinical significance as many children with DS require major corrective cardiac or otolaryngeal surgeries [27]. A complete and individualized approach is imperative in managing upper airway obstruction in children with DS. Children with DS and upper airway obstruction may need surgical interventions including tonsillectomy, adenoidectomy, tonsillar pillar plication, uvulopalatopharyngoplasty, anterior tongue reduction, tongue-hyoid suspension, laryngotracheoplasty, and tracheotomy [28].

3.1.2. Lower Airway Diseases

Congenital anomalies of the lower airways form about 7.5 to 20% of all congenital anomalies of the respiratory tract and are extensively more frequent in children with DS, mostly if there are associated cardiac anomalies. They are divided into 3 main groups; stenotic or malacic (airway collapse) anomalies, tracheo-oesophageal fistula and branching and lung anomalies. However, the lower airways cannot be managed in isolation; a large number of what are considered as lower airway symptoms relate to upper airway problems. Tracheobronchial anomalies arise between the third and sixteenth week of gestation, and they mainly affect the main bronchi. Most of the tracheobronchial anomalies are restricted to the right upper lobe bronchus (47%) and are distinguished by an abnormality at its origin, either agenesis or a supernumerary bronchus. Tracheal bronchus, congenital tracheal stenosis and laryngomalacia are among the recorded anomalies in children with DS [29].

3.1.2.1. Stenotic and Malacic (Airway Collapse) Anomalies

The airways and lungs in children with DS are found to be smaller than normal. This is of particular importance during intubation as there is increased risk of difficult intubation as well as the risk of subluxation. Those children usually need a smaller endotracheal tube than predicted; even when adjusted for age and height. A noteworthy reduction in both the coronal and sagittal diameter of the trachea in adults with DS has also been described.

Tracheobronchomalacia

Tracheomalacia is one of the common respiratory tract dysplasia in children characterized by excessive collapsibility of the trachea, typically during expiration. Congenital forms are associated with severe symptoms. Milder forms often present after the neonatal period. Tracheobronchomalacia is frequently under-diagnosed because of the nonspecific symptoms, variable and atypical features and the unreliable routine methods in the assessment of tracheobronchomalacia in children. In addition, many physicians are confused about its clinical characteristics. One study showed that the incidence of bronchomalacia in left lung was 11%, while that of right lung was 53.3%. Meanwhile, bronchomalacia of both lungs are noticed in 35.6%. It is more common in boys under the age of 2 years. It can present with recurrent chest infections, expiratory stridor with or without cough, and/or wheezing. The wheezing is classically monophonic in the contrary to the polyphonic wheezing observed in asthma or bronchiolitis. Tracheobronchomalacia is also a cause of failure to extubation either following anesthesia or from mechanical ventilatory support. Children with tracheomalacia are at a high risk of sudden death syndrome due to occurrence of sudden collapse of the floppy and easily collapsible airway. When the child starts to be panic, the intra-thoracic pressure increases exerting more pressure on the easily collapsible airway, increasing the obstruction and squeeze the trachea more and more, eventually leading to collapse. At the same time, if the child is diagnosed as corticosteroid/β2-agonist-resistant asthma, presence of tracheobronchomalacia should be considered. Patients with severe airway malacia are more liable to develop severe pneumonia compared with those with slight or moderate malacia. Improvements or even elimination of malacia is noticed with the aging of the children and the proper anti-infection therapy [30, 31].

Diagnosis of Tracheobronchomalacia can be done by both bronchoscopy and bronchography; however functional bronchoscopy is still not standardized. Opposite to the old bronchograph system where a big quantity of a hyperosmolar contrast medium was inserted into the lungs; a extremely tiny quantity (about 0.5 ml) of iohexol is inserted. This defines the airways and may demonstrate remarkable narrowing during expiration. Dynamic airway CT is a promising tool for noninvasive diagnosis. Multidetector CT has enhanced the ability to noninvasively diagnose tracheobronchomalacia with the potential to decrease the morbidity and mortality associated with this disorder [32, 33].

Medical approaches aim to reduce the associated symptoms of tracheomalacia. Treatment may be conservative in mild-to-moderate cases with just observation as many of the children outgrow with aging and supplementation with oxygen when needed. Antibiotics as well as chest physiotherapy are obviously required in less severe disease. Continuous positive airway pressure (CPAP) and bi-level positive airway pressure (BiPAP) *via* a nasopharyngeal or tracheostomy tube may be needed in moderate to severe cases until correction is done by surgery. Relatively high pressures (20 cm H_2O) may be essential to open the airway and maintain it open. Bronchoscopy and stent insertion lead to significant improvement, but with a high complication rate. Surgical approaches aim to improve the caliber of the airway (airway stenting, aortopexy, tracheopexy). Surgical lateropexia, tracheal resection, and surgical external stabilization are options. The most commonly performed surgery in children is aortopexy [34, 35].

Congenital Tracheal Stenosis

Generally, kids with DS have narrower airways than other kids. This is due to the generalized reduction in the diameter of the tracheal lumens with considerable reduction in both the coronal and sagittal diameter compared with normal controls. The first intubation of a child with DS should be done with an endotracheal tube as a minimum two sizes lesser than would be used in a child of the similar age without DS, to prevent potential trauma to the airway [36]. Congenital tracheal stenosis (CTS) is uncommon in the general population but is found a bit more often in patients with DS. The most common type of CTS in patients with DS appears to be segmental 'hourglass' stenosis. CTS may be the consequence of an intrinsic anomaly of the trachea itself or might be the consequence of outside forces squeezing the airway, such as cardiovascular malformations. However, the regular feature in all cases of CTS is an intrinsic narrowing of the trachea creating airway obstruction. In the greater part of cases, it made of a funnel-shaped part of the trachea distinguished by complete circular cartilaginous tracheal rings (Fig. **1**). CTS may include only a short segment of the trachea, or it may include greater than 50% of the trachea, involving the main bronchi. The second type of stenosis is referred to as long-segment tracheal stenosis (LSTS) and is the most severe and difficult variety of CTS. Except for some cases of mild CTS, all forms of CTS are usually serious, critical, and life threatening [37]. It is a true challenging and life-threatening obstructive airway disease.

The incidence of congenital tracheal stenosis in children with congenital heart disease, which is seen in about 40-50% of children with DS, has been noted to be 1.2%. Patients with DS also are predisposed to have other pathologies with upper airway obstruction such as nasopharyngeal, oropharyngeal, and subglottic compromise [38]. Congenital tracheal stenosis is frequently accompanied with other congenital anomalies of the respiratory, cardiovascular, and gastrointestinal systems. Vascular rings are among the most frequent associated anomalies in children with CTS. An associated pulmonary artery sling is a frequent trait that is found in about 30% to 50% of children with CTS. This association was nominated as the ring-sling complex by Berdon [39]. These things, coupled with the raised incidence of cardiac disease, place these children at high risk for acute and chronic cardiopulmonary vulnerability and compromise [40].

It usually manifests in early infancy and can present with a broad range of symptoms and varying levels of severity. Signs may consist of biphasic stridor, tachypnea, retractions, nasal flaring, apnea, cyanosis, wheezing, noisy breathing, recurrent upper respiratory "cold symptoms," persistent croup, and pneumonia. Dysphagia has also been described which may be associated with apnea or cyanotic spells when an infant or a child with CTS tries to swallow a solid food.

Failure to thrive may be a result of increased work of breathing, leading to increased energy expenditure and poor feeding. Patients may have hyperextend heads in a try to "stent" the trachea to open and improve breathing. Life-threatening crisis may be triggered by an acute respiratory disease and disastrous near-death episode necessitating cardiopulmonary resuscitation [41].

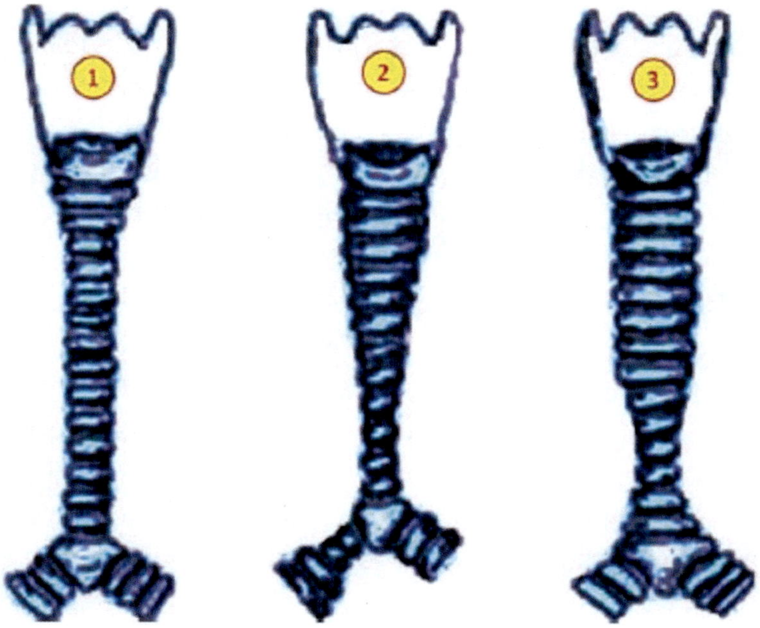

Fig. (1). Showed types of tracheal stenosis; 1: generalized tracheal hypoplasia; 2: funnel type stenosis with one normal end and the other one stenotic, 3: segmental stenosis with two or three cartilage rings involved.

The identification of an airway problem somewhat often takes place when those children are going for cardiac surgery, subjected to diagnostic radiography with sedation, or they are going through induction and intubation for anesthesia. Plain x-ray may illustrate abnormal air distribution, shifting of the heart and mediastinum, evidence of tracheal compression, and changed tracheo-bronchial angles, frequently the consequence of abnormal vasculature (*i.e.* pulmonary artery sling) impinging on the normal course of the main bronchi [42]. Other diagnostic tests may include barium esophagography, tracheobronchography, bronchoscopy, echocardiography, and cardiac catheterization. Computed tomography (CT) can visualize vascular abnormalities of the aortic arch and great arteries. Spiral sequencing or 3-dimensional reformatting of the CT scans and virtual bronchoscopy can be done to rebuild the trachea and proximal bronchi. Magnetic resonance imaging may be the most excellent procedure for identification of the vascular anatomy of the mediastinum without added risk of radiation exposure. Bronchoscopy together with bronchography is a simple tool, cheaper than CT, and has outstanding topographic and temporal resolution [43].

There is no standardized technique for CTS repair. An individualized approach selected for each patient and airway lesion is necessary to optimize patient management. However; there is an agreement that the segmental resection and anastomosis is the ideal and the best for the short segment stenosis while slide tracheoplasty is most successful technique for the long-segment ones. Conservative management can be applied for selected group of patients with careful and close follow up. Slide tracheoplasty with concomitant repair of cardiac lesions is presently the favorite management for long-segment stenosis. Management of such patients remains a real challenge for both the clinicians and the patients' families, and needs a multidisciplinary approach. Survival following surgical management has improved over the years, but mortality continued to be high, predominantly in a particular subset of patients presenting at an age less than 1 month with associated cardiac anomalies [44, 45].

Subglottic Stenosis

The subglottic stenosis is well recognized possible condition in children with DS. However, this anomaly and its effect on laryngeal and respiratory function are often missed. Congenital subglottic stenosis is less frequent than the acquired one. Acquired subglottic stenosis may occur as a sequel of neonatal endotracheal intubation (Fig. **2**). The child usually attends with stridor and increasing inspiratory effort with use of accessory muscles which raise the negative intrathoracic pressure producing tracheal tug, intercostal, subcostal, and sternal recession. Easy fatigability with shortness of energy for playing or talking occurs with major stenosis. Increased respiratory and pulse rates are common in these circumstances but cyanosis and bradycardia are warning signs of decompensation. Stridor in subglottic stenosis is inspiratory at the beginning but may become biphasic with increasing severity of the obstruction [46].

Flexible nasopharyngeal laryngoscopy with local anaesthesia can be used to evaluate the pathology in the nose, nasopharynx, oropharynx, hypopharynx, larynx, arytenoids, epiglottis and vocal cords. However; rigid bronchoscopy is the best in evaluation of the pathology in the glottis and subglottis regions. The severity of the clinical presentation is well correlated with the degree of obstruction to the lumen of the airway. The severity of the obstruction can be graded I – IV. Grade I has an obstruction of 0 – 50% of the lumen while grade II has an obstruction of 51 – 70% of the lumen. Grade III has an obstruction of 71 – 99% of the lumen while grade IV has 100% obstruction or no detectable lumen [47].

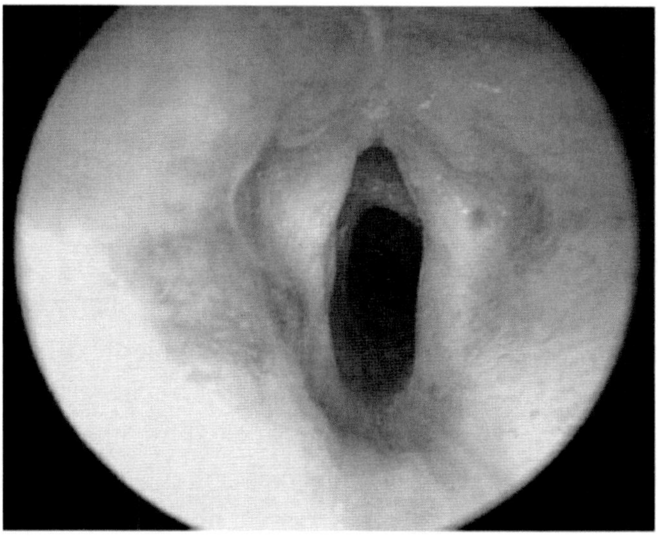

Fig. (2). Showed acquired subglottic stenosis after mechanical ventilation.

When subglottic stenosis occurs in a child with DS, the ordinary intubation procedure may need adjustment. In these children, an endotracheal tube of a size appropriate to the patient's age may be too rigid in the subglottic area. By irritating a previously asymptomatic subglottic stenosis, long-term endotracheal intubation in this type of patient may be more possible to induce a clinically significant subglottic stenosis. The approach of treatment will depend on the severity of clinical manifestations and the response to therapy. Subglottic stenosis in children with DS is more complex to repair and is associated with lower success rates of decannulation. Surgical repair of subglottic stenosis intends to offer a sufficiently widened lumen while conserving the vocal quality with airway protection. Furthermore, it is imperative during management of these children not to induce an even more severe subglottic stenosis. Treatment success depends on a thorough and adequate preoperative assessment and adjusting the repair to address the severity and position of the individual lesion. Understanding the complex pathophysiology of subglottic stenosis along with the wide variety of available surgical options will aid the surgeon in achieving a successful outcome [48, 49].

3.1.2.2. Esophageal Atresia/Tracheo-Esophageal Fistula

DS is one among many well-known chromosomal aberrations observed in patients with tracheo-esophageal fistula. Tracheo-esophageal fistula is present in about 0.4% of children with DS and is observed more often in infants of younger mothers and Hispanics. It also represents only 4% of congenital anomalies of the esophagus.

Development of EA/TEF is under the control of many genes and genetic pathways; but only a few genes have been shown to be involved in humans. About 50% of the cases with EA/TEF are coupled with other congenital anomalies such as vertebral, anal, cardiovascular, tracheoesophageal, renal, and limb abnormalities [50]. Many patients are affected by other malformations, such as microcephaly, micrognathia, pyloric stenosis, duodenal atresia, single umbilical artery, and anomalies of the genitourinary, respiratory and gastrointestinal systems. There are five main subtypes of tracheo-esophageal fistula and atresia, according to the presence of atresia, its location and the type of connection between trachea and esophagus [51].

Presence of Esophageal atresia in the fetus should be suspected if there is maternal polyhydramnios. Newborns with esophageal atresia usually have profuse, fine white frothy bubbles of mucus filling both mouth and nose. Secretions come again in spite of continuous suctioning. The newborn could present with episodic cyanotic and coughing spells with associated respiratory distress during oral feeds as in H type fistula. Symptoms become worse during feeding in the presence of a TEF. Repeated and unexplained pulmonary infections which dominantly involve lower lobes are encountered since birth with choking and cyanosis at feeding time due to frequent aspiration of food or gastrointestinal secretions. The symptoms triggered by malignant TEFs include cough, aspiration, and fever. Abdominal distention may increase due to accumulation of air in the stomach. The average duration of symptoms from onset to diagnosis is about 12 days. Early diagnosis of H-type tracheoesophageal fistula is usually hard to be done due to its nonspecific symptoms that can be attributed to more frequent conditions such as gastroesophageal reflux and swallowing disorders or other anomalies such as laryngeal cleft [52].

Antenatal diagnosis of congenital TEFs can be attained. Antenatal ultrasound may show polyhydramnios, absence of fluid-filled stomach, small abdomen, small for gestational age, lower-than-expected fetal weight, and a distended esophageal pouch. Absence of stomach gas on prenatal ultrasound is a sign of esophageal atresia. Plain chest x-ray may show tracheal compression and deviation. Absence of a gastric bubble indicates either esophageal atresia without a TEF or esophageal atresia with a proximal TEF. Insertion of a nasogastric tube may show coiling in the mediastinum of patients who have associated esophageal atresia which is a diagnostic sign of TEFs associated with esophageal atresia. Chest X-ray can make the diagnosis of TEF in most cases of congenital TEF, and other diagnostic tools are rarely needed. It also can show presence of complications such as pneumonia. Aspiration pneumonia in the posterior segments of the upper lobes may occur due to aspiration of the gastric contents from the esophageal pouch or stomach. Recurrent or massive aspiration may cause acute lung injury in some patients [53, 54].

Contrast studies are rarely needed to confirm the diagnosis because of the risk of aspiration pneumonitis and pulmonary injury, and the little information obtained and added to the diagnostic workup. If the contrast study should be done; only 1-2 mL of barium is infused through an 8 F catheter inserted into the esophagus. Chest X-rays are taken in the lateral decubitus position as well as the anteroposterior position to detect any leak of the contrast into the trachea [55]. Preoperative esophageal endoscopy can verify the fistula with insertion of a gastric tube which stops at the fistula. Multidetector-row CT scans with 3-dimensional (3D) visualizes many organs and structures and is able to properly diagnose and confirm presence of TEF with high quality images and offer crucial data helping in planning for surgery, and, without contrast medium, it is a less invasive examination [56]. Magnetic resonance imaging may be utilized to diagnose and localize H-type TEF safely and accurately in a sick preterm infant. The display of the fistula on MRI together with the clinical picture are adequate for the diagnosis if the initial investigation is negative or could not be done [57]. Once the diagnosis is established, clinician should search other disorders including those belong to the respiratory system, which are quite common [58].

Treatment is always surgical and must be performed early for more favorable prognosis. Neonate born with esophageal atresia and tracheoesophageal fistula often requires intubation and mechanical ventilation. Too much gas enters into gastrointestinal tract would cause gastric dilatation, which often leads to neonatal death. Rapid control of the fistula is imperative to improve ventilation efficiency and relieve gastric dilatation, which is essential for complete surgical repair [59]. Surgical therapy of the TEF is evolving, with open thoracic ligation being the gold standard; however thoracoscopic ligation is increasingly being performed. Repair of the EA depends on the distance between the proximal and distal pouch. For short gap EA, primary repair is the preferred approach with reconnection of the two ends of the baby's esophagus to each other. For long-gap esophageal atresia; the Foker technique with axial traction or the Kimura advancement with extrathoracic spit fistula are surgical options. Postoperative gastroesophageal reflux is common after repair of the fistula [60].

3.1.2.3. Branching and Lung Anomalies

Tracheal bronchus is an unusual congenital anomaly seen in DS consisting of an aberrant or accessory bronchus originating from the trachea in which the right upper lobe has its origin in the trachea rather than distal to the carina (Fig. **3**). It may occur either as an isolated anomaly or as a part of multiple airway anomalies especially tracheoesophageal fistula, and fused or hypoplastic first and second ribs [22]. While this may be an incidental finding, it may also be associated with respiratory disease, particularly recurrent right upper lobe pneumonia. An aberrant right upper lobe bronchus originating from the trachea (tracheal bronchus) should be considered in all cases presented with recurrent pneumonia. It can be diagnosed with bronchoscopy done because of persistent or recurrent respiratory symptoms. It may show that the bifurcation of the carina is higher than usual.

Computed tomography can reveal associated tracheal stenosis and tracheal bronchus. Complications like bronchiectasis or bronchial stenosis can also be discovered by bronchography. The clinician should have a high index of doubt for presence of airway anomalies in DS patients who have chronic respiratory symptoms. The presence of a clinically important tracheal bronchus should be thought about in every child with repeated right upper lobe pneumonia, particularly in children with DS syndrome or rib abnormalities. If bronchiectasis or bronchial stenosis is found, surgical resection should be done [61]. The majority of patients with tracheal bronchus can be managed conservatively. Correction of the primary anomalies is of supreme importance for the relief of respiratory symptoms [62].

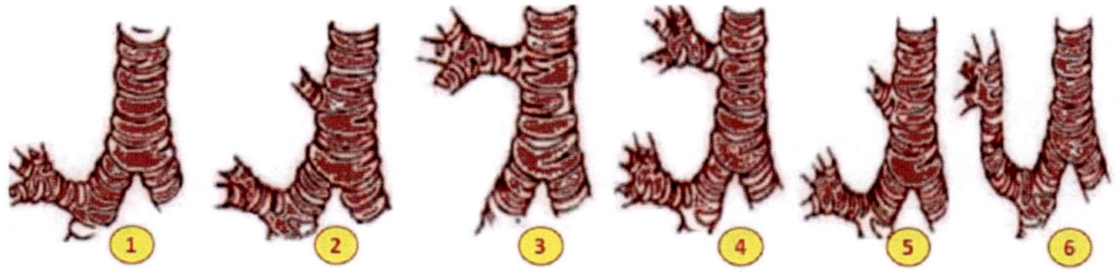

Fig. (3). Showed tracheal branching anomalies and tracheal bronchus. 1: Normal; 2: Displaced apical bronchus; 3: Displaced lobar bronchus; 4: Super numerical lobar bronchus; 5: Super numerical apical bronchus; 6: Aberrant apical bronchus.

Children with DS have a high incidence of inherited developmental lung anomalies than the non-syndromic children. This risk increased among those who have heart disease. In a postmortem study of DS children who died due to cardiac problem, six out of seven of those children had hypoplastic lungs with diminished lung volume and characteristic alveolar hypoplasia, decreased number of terminal lung units, decreased number of the acini contained alveoli, distension of the alveolar ducts and decreased number of large alveoli. This alveolar hypoplasia is due to deficiency of elastic fibers -in the entrance- rings of alveoli and the number of alveoli contained in a lobule is smaller than normal. A double capillary network is also commonly found in DS patients. The effect of these abnormalities on lung function has not been clearly established [2]. The hypoplastic lung tissue in patients with DS is more susceptible to the mechanical stress and injury during mechanical ventilation and this is most likely to be reason for postoperative respiratory failure. Cardiac and respiratory system involvement is the most frequent reason of morbidity and mortality in children with DS [63].

Displaced lobar bronchus; 4: Super numerical lobar bronchus; 5: Super numerical apical bronchus; 6: Aberrant apical bronchus.

Down syndrome patients typically have inflated subpleural cystic airspaces on computed tomography (CT) imaging and on lung biopsy, occasionally concomitant with endogenous lipoid pneumonia (cholesterol clefts, foamy macrophages, and lymphocytic inflammation). Subpleural cysts are almost specific to DS, where they have been well recognized, and may be linked to the high risk of pulmonary hypoplasia. They may result from decreased postnatal production of peripheral small air passages and alveoli, which consecutively may be a sign of slow rate of cell proliferation that looks to be a general feature of DS [64]. A relationship with prematurity was observed. The subpleural cysts can be diagnosed by computed tomography but not by standard radiography. Down syndrome is typically associated with distended airspaces and widened alveolar ducts, which seem to be changes occurs due to impaired postnatal alveolarization rather than primary lung hypoplasia. However, decline in airway branching in the lungs of patients with DS implies interference with development took place before birth [65, 66].

In some infants and children with DS, there may in addition be both radiographic and pathologic evidence of subpleural cysts within the periphery of the lung. Lung biopsies from DS patients are considered as one of the most complicated conditions for a pathologist to analyze as there are frequently due to numerous superimposed forms of injury. For example, a DS patient with atrioventricular canal and aspiration may have impaired lung function and anatomy due partially to the underlying chromosomal syndrome as well as hemodynamic effects of the underlying congenital heart disease and chemical injury from repeated aspiration and/or infection. The mechanisms of impaired alveolar development concomitant with other forms of congenital heart disease are not well clarified though it is possible that the intrauterine hemodynamics within the pulmonary vasculature affects the degree of alveolarization [67].

3.2. Acquired Disorders

Respiratory problems are an important reason of morbidity and mortality in children with DS. Respiratory illnesses (aspiration, pneumonia and influenza) were the second most common cause of death for children with DS aged up to 19 years, and the most common cause across all age groups. Respiratory illnesses also are the most common primary reason for admission for children under the age of 3 years [3, 68]. It has been documented that up to 88% of children with DS will need hospitalization at some age before their 16th birthday, and about 16% of them will have more than four hospitalizations [69, 70]. Among the acquired respiratory disorders encountered in children with DS are respiratory infections including acute bronchiolitis due to infection with respiratory syncytial virus (RSV), pneumonia, infection with H1N1 stains of flu virus, high incidence of acute lung injury, occurrence of pulmonary hemosiderosis, increase incidence of pulmonary hypertension, GERD, and the possibility of having asthma in children with DS.

3.2.1. Increased Rate of Respiratory Infections

There is an increased rate of respiratory infections in children with DS due to decreased levels of IgG2 and reduced numbers of lymphocytes, CD4+ T cells, CD4+ iNKT cells and Tregs, relative to their corresponding healthy siblings. This could result in high rate of repeated lower respiratory infections (RTI) and related hospitalization. Another important cause of RTI in children with DS is the presence of CHD in about 440-50% of them. Children with DS and CHD are more liable for hospitalization for RTI and needed more frequent ventilatory support than children with DS who do not have CHD [71].

3.2.1.1. Otitis Media and Glue Ear

Children with DS have a higher rate of Eustachian tube dysfunction which precipitates those children to have chronic otitis media with effusion. The principal site of pathology in otitis media in children with DS is the Eustachian tube; and the pathogenesis is related to abnormal functions of this tube. Eustachian tube connects the tympanic cavity with the nasopharynx. It is the primary defense mechanism of the middle ear as it allows equilibration of middle ear pressure with atmospheric pressure. It protects the middle ear from reflux of nasopharyngeal secretions; and drain secretions from the middle ear into the nasopharynx. Unlike adults, child's Eustachian tube is more horizontally aligned. This allows for easier spread of infection from the nasopharynx to the middle ear. Otitis media passes through the following stages: tubal occlusion, pre-suppuration, suppuration, and resolution or complication [72]. Acute otitis media presents with ear pain, fever, impaired hearing and sometimes a purulent discharge (otorrhea) through a perforation of the tympanic membrane (or tympanotomy tube). In infants, the age group most liable to otitis media; symptoms are frequently non-specific and may include irritability, restlessness, bouts of screaming, anorexia, vomiting, fever and occasionally, convulsions. Pulling and rubbing of the ears with restlessness may be an indirect evidence of acute otitis media. The clinical picture of acute otitis media in older children may also be non-specific. It is recommended therefore, to exclude acute otitis media before any child with fever is labeled as having pyrexia of unknown origin [73].

Otitis media with effusion (OME or glue ear) is an accumulation of fluid in the middle ear and is the most frequent cause of impaired hearing in children of > 6 months of age. Children with DS are more liable than children without DS to have glue ear, which is an accumulation of non-infected sticky liquid in their ear on the far side of the ear drum. OME is almost universal in all children with DS, begins at a younger age and persists to older ages than in children without DS with a peak of ≥60 % around 1 and 6-7 years. The rate of otitis media shows a declining trend in older children. Mild to moderate hearing loss can develop in children with bilateral OME [74]. This leads to hearing difficulties, which can lead to language and communication problems. Grommet insertion can be difficult or impossible in children with DS, as the morphological features include narrow ear canals. Amplification devices can be used to alleviate the hearing losses consequent upon the glue ear but conventional behind-the-ear hearing aids are often not tolerated [75].

3.2.1.2. Acute and Chronic Rhinosinusitis

Chronic sinusitis is a common problem in patients with DS. About 17.6% of children with DS were reported to have continuous runny nose. There are different factors that working together to increase the incidence of sinusitis in DS children including altered craniofacial dimensions with narrow nasal passages, low skull bases, and poorly developed sinuses; possible allergic factors; depressed immune function; and abnormal cilia ultra-structures. These abnormal cilia ultra-structures may include partial lack of the A subunits walls of some peripheral doublets which are associated with abnormal mucociliary transport. The Narrow nasopharynx can lead to airway obstruction by the normally growing adenoid tissues predisposing those patients to frequent nasal congestion and consequently infections [76].

The diagnosis of rhinosinusitis is primarily a clinical diagnosis based on the duration of illness and complex of signs and symptoms. Imaging of the paranasal sinuses is indicated for suspected or confirmed complications of sinusitis or when a surgical intervention is being considered for chronic rhinosinusitis. Plain X-ray is the preferred initial examination to start with. It can be used as a screening tool before enrollment of other tomographic techniques. Conventional pluridirectional tomography is now replaced by CT scanning, which has the benefit of offering both good bone detail and soft tissue imaging. Children with questionable orbital or CNS complications should have CT scanning of the paranasal sinuses [77].

It is critical to maintain nasal hygiene in these children using nasal saline sprays which can be used 5 times or more per day and with even a higher frequency if the child is developing an upper respiratory infection. Aggressive medical and surgical interventions have led to a good control of the chronic rhinitis. Treatment of the nasal drainage can be done in the same way as in the general population, with nasal irrigation, nasal steroids, antihistamines, decongestants and even antibiotics when needed. High-dose amoxicillin together with saline nasal irrigation can relieve the symptoms of acute sinusitis more rapidly and more frequent than using saline nasal irrigation alone. However, antibiotic treatment for acute sinusitis grants only a little therapeutic advantage over nasal irrigation. Surgical therapy for chronic rhinosinusitis should be implemented using a stepwise approach after medical therapy fails [78, 79].

3.2.1.3. Acute Bronchiolitis

Children with DS usually suffer more frequently and more severely from repeated respiratory tract infections. Respiratory syncytial virus (RSV) is one of the pathogens most frequently identified as a cause of lower respiratory tract infections in infants and children with increasing severity in high-risk groups. Down syndrome is a well known independent significant risk factor for severe RSV lower respiratory tract infections in children. This severity is due to presence of different factors including impaired both innate and adoptive immune systems, abnormal respiratory functions in terms of anatomical abnormalities in the lungs and airways, and abnormal histological and physiological factors. All of these factors influence the course of RSV infection in such high risk groups in a complex manner [80].

Pulmonary hypertension is a common complication accompanying congenital heart disease in about half of DS patients. Presence of pulmonary hypertension is an important criterion in increasing the severity of acute bronchiolitis, and is considered as a prognostic factor and an item for management guidance [81]. On the other hand, DS itself without congenital heart disease is a significant risk factor for severe RSV infections. Bronchomalacia and tracheomalacia is frequently seen in persons with DS as well as lung hypoplasia and emphysematous changes. There are also reported cases of aspiration pneumonia and obliterating bronchiolitis associated with RSV infections. DS patients are in addition known to have small thymi with low amount of T-cell receptor excision circles (TRECs), low peripheral blood naïve CD4+ T cell count. Moreover, the overall T-cell count, and the B-cell count; all are decreased, which may also be related to susceptibility to severe respiratory viral infections. Thus, in DS, these anatomical, functional and histological abnormalities, as well as quantitative and qualitative abnormalities in immunological parameters, should be taken into consideration when assessing the risk of severe RSV infections [82 - 84].

RSV bronchiolitis is an important health problem in children with DS. Children with DS have a 6-fold more risk of hospitalization due to RSV lower respiratory tract infections in the first 2 years of life than those without DS with increased severity of disease when hospitalized. The incidence of hospitalization due to infection with RSV in children with DS was found to be 9.9%–17.6% in large cohorts, which is much higher than the hospitalization rate observed in the normal population (about 1%) [85]. Children with DS have a significantly longer hospitalization stay; and they usually require mechanical ventilatory support more frequently with higher mortality rate than non-DS children. Unlike the normal children, the increased risk for hospitalization in children with DS continues beyond 24 months of age. The risk is further increased in presence of other comorbidities *e.g.* CHD or pulmonary hypertension. There is a higher risk of recurrent wheezing, though the role of RSV in recurrent wheezing in DS is not yet well-known [86]. Infection by RSV has a wide range of clinical manifestations and severity from mild symptoms in the upper respiratory tract to bronchiolitis and even pneumonia, and may progress to severe form, requiring admission to ICU, intubation, mechanical ventilation, and even at times can lead to death [87].

RSV can only be prevented but not cured. Adequate hand washing and proper health education are the main approaches in primary prevention. Efforts to decrease the morbidity from RSV lower RTI have focused on identification of medical and environmental risk factors, and control of environmental factors. In the absence of a vaccine, palivizumab prophylaxis for groups of children at high risk for RSV hospitalization is at present the most excellent method to decrease the severity of the disease and its related hospitalization and mortality [88]. The treatment of acute viral bronchiolitis caused by RSV is supportive. There are different concepts of treatment. Hydration is of utmost importance. A Mega dose of vitamin A is found not useful in the treatment of children with RSV infection. Bronchodilators are occasionally helpful and may be tried on a personal basis to find out whether there is benefit. Inhaled and systemic corticosteroids are not helpful and not recommended, and the use of ribavirin, leukotrienes, DNase, antibiotics and chest physiotherapy do not improve outcomes. Inhaled hypertonic saline showed no benefit in combination with epinephrine. More recently, a combination of epinephrine and dexamethasone is found to be beneficial in children with bronchiolitis [89, 90]. Palivizumab treatment is the mainstay of treatment in infant and young children with high risk. It decreases the duration of wheezing in otherwise healthy-late preterm infants. This might be important for children with DS, as they have an increased risk of recurrent wheezing, although the role of RSV in recurrent wheezing in DS is not yet established [91].

3.2.1.4. Pneumonia

Children with DS have high susceptibility to lower respiratory tract infection, such as *Streptococcus pneumoniae, Haemophilus influenzae, Staphylococcus aureus, mycoplasma pneumoniae*, Chlamydophila pneumoniae, Moraxella catarrhalis, Gram-negative aerobic bacteria, as well as anaerobic organisms, Gram-negative bacilli (*Mycobacterium tuberculosis*), aerosolized pathogens (*Legionella*), and pathogens disseminated haematogenically (*S. aureus* from endocarditis) or by contiguity with other organs. Viruses such as *influenza virus, adenovirus, respiratory syncytial virus* and other uncommon microbes are potential causative agents. Viral or atypical organisms may lead to a more severe type of pneumonia. Patients with DS are very liable to respiratory tract infections, predominantly during the first two years of age though they can also have such infections at older ages. The occurrence of repeated respiratory infections in DS is due to both structural and functional anomalies of the respiratory system, the presence of congenital heart malformations as well as IgG deficits [92, 93].

Pneumococcal disease can be caused by *Streptococcus pneumoniae* bacteria which is an important cause of vaccine-preventable illness and death. Pneumococcal pneumonia is a common problem in DS patients; a frequent reason for hospitalization and one of the main causes of death in DS patients. Persons with DS have impaired immune system functions which predispose them to a high risk of invasive Pneumococcal disease. Children with DS may have a fulminant course of pneumococcal pneumonia, because of their tendency to have an increased anti-inflammatory response. They show a significant increase in IL-10 production upon stimulation with *S. pneumoniae* compared to their healthy siblings [94].

Treatment of pneumococcal infections in children with DS using penicillin and other antibiotics is usually more successful and effective. However; some strains of these bacteria became resistant to these drugs. Because of that, prevention of the disease, through adequate and effective vaccination program, becomes even more important. Pneumococcal polysaccharide vaccine (PPSV) gives immune response against 23 types of pneumococcal bacteria, including stains known to cause severe disease. However; elderly people, children under 2 years of age, and people with some long-term illnesses might have insufficient or no immune response at all. Another kind of pneumococcal vaccine (pneumococcal conjugate vaccine, or PCV) is a part of routine vaccination recommended for children below 5 years of age. Persons with DS develop satisfactory serotype-specific antibody response to all conjugated and nearly all unconjugated serotypes used [95].

Children with DS have several risk factors for having severe influenza diseases such as congenital heart disease (in about 50% of patients), childhood obesity or excess weight (in the majority), and a higher prevalence of type 1 diabetes than in age-matched control children. In addition, specific impairment in immune response are frequently found, such as leukopenia, chemotactic defects, reduced immunoglobulin G4 levels, as well as T- and B-cell abnormalities with decrease number of B lymphocytes [96]. All these factors expose children with DS to a serious type of influenza pneumonia with increased need for hospitalization as well as increased risk of death especially when coupled with reduced access to healthcare [97]. Although it is not easy to differentiate clinically between bacterial and viral types of pneumonia; inflammatory markers may be useful. Inflammatory marker, procalcitonin, has a comparable sensitivity to C-reactive protein (sensitivity 86%) but it has more specificity for bacterial pneumonia in children (specificity 88%) [98].

Mycoplasma pneumonia (MP) is usually accompanied with cold agglutinin syndrome, and sometimes both cold IgM and warm IgG autoantibodies are identified. This type of pneumonia may further be complicated with either non-immune or autoimmune hemolytic anemia which adds more hazards to the general condition of the already compromised patient. When young children with DS develop pneumonia, physicians should consider *Mycoplasma pneumoniae* as a possible etiologic agent [99].

Legionella pneumophila is a Gram-negative intracellular microbe that frequently causes severe and life-threatening pneumonia. Legionnaires' disease is a well recognized common cause of pneumonia in adults but is considered to be uncommon in children. Infection with *Legionella pneumophila* primarily occurs in immunosuppressed patients such as kidney transplantation and DS. The clinical picture and natural course of Legionnaires' disease in children is not obvious. The legionnaire pneumonia cannot be differentiated from pneumonias caused by other infectious agents. Clinical picture, radiological and biological findings are indistinguishable from other nosocomially acquired pneumonias. The overall mortality rate in children can reach 33% of cases and reaches even higher rate in immunosuppressed children. So; Legionellosis should be included in the differential diagnosis of the respiratory illness in the immune compromised children including DS [100, 101]. Newer macroazalides are among the first-line therapies and can be used in severe infections, mainly those occurring in immune compromised patients. Azithromycin is the drug of choice in children. Delay in starting adequate therapy is a principal factor associated with a poor prognosis. Thus, all cases of pneumonia complicated with respiratory failure, or shock or if associated with underlying disease causing severe immune deficiency should initially receive an agent active against *Legionella spp.,* at least when the causative agent remains unknown. Supportive measures may improve the prognosis in critically ill patients. In intubated patients with delayed recovery, superinfection by *Pseudomonas aeruginosa* or co-infection by other microbes should be excluded [102].

Recurrent pneumonia or persistent pulmonary infiltrate on chest X-rays should be distinguished from other reasons of respiratory disorders that are quite common in DS. Picard *et al.* described two cases of Morgagni hernia that were previously diagnosed as recurrent pneumonia. They concluded that when a child with DS has a persistent lower lobe infiltrate on chest radiograph, the possibility of a diaphragmatic defect should be entertained [103]. Pneumonia may also be a manifestation of allergy to foods or other allergens. Children with DS reported respiratory symptoms relating to food allergy more frequently than non-syndromic children who have a food allergy [104].

3.2.2. Increased Incidence of Acute Lung Injury

The increased severity and the high rates of morbidity and mortality associated with having acute respiratory infections in DS children are related to the occurrence of a higher incidence of acute lung injury (ALI). Bruijn *et al.* reported significantly higher rate of ALI and Adult Respiratory Distress Syndrome (ARDS) in mechanically ventilated children with DS (58% & 46% respectively) than that noted in the general pediatric population who require mechanical ventilatory support (13% and 7% respectively) [105].

Long-term effects of ALI on the health of children with DS are unknown and need to be clarified by assessment of the lung functions. The mechanism leading to the elevated rate of ALI in children with DS is still doubtful. Initial ventilator settings have recently been shown to be a risk factor for the development of ARDS [106]. Apoptosis or programmed cell death has a fundamental role in the pathogenesis of injurious states of the pulmonary system such as of ALI/ARDS; so that the increased rate of ALI/ARDS may be due to a high rate of apoptosis in children with DS. An increased rate of apoptosis in DS has been shown in several cells including neurons, thymocytes, and granulocytes. It has been proposed that increased apoptosis in DS cells is due to the incapacity to handle the excess oxidative stress, causing accumulation of free reactive oxygen radicals and cell injury [107, 108].

3.2.3. Increased Incidence of Pulmonary Hypertension

Pulmonary hypertension (PH) is distinguished by a continuous elevation of the pulmonary vascular resistance that increasingly causes remodeling of the pulmonary vessels and eventually right ventricular failure. It is defined as a mean PA pressure of more than 25 mmHg at rest or 30 mmHg with exercise [109]. Patients with DS have an increased tendency to develop pulmonary hypertension compared with age-matched controls (1.2% compared to 0.1%). The pathology is now well defined and major progress has been achieved in understanding the pathobiological mechanisms. Many factors may contribute to PH associated with DS, such as upper airway obstruction, lung hypoplasia, alveolar simplification (which may be worse in the presence of CHD), CHD, changes in the production and secretion of pulmonary surfactant, elevated plasma levels of asymmetric dimethyl arginine (ADMA), hypothyroidism, obstructive airway disease, sleep apnea, reflux, and aspiration [110]. High plasma levels of ADMA may be involved in development of vascular dysfunction in adults with idiopathic pulmonary hypertension. ADMA reduces NO production in DS patients with PH.

ADMA levels could be used a promising biomarker for PH in DS patients [13].

Most of the symptoms of pediatric PH are non-specific and usually go as subtle till end stage. Because of the nonspecific symptoms and the subtle physical findings, the diagnosis of the disease is frequently delayed till later stages. At birth, affected newborns frequently suffer cyanosis. Clinical examination may show hepatomegaly, an active right ventricle on palpation with a loud pulmonary second sound on auscultation. Persistent pulmonary hypertension of the newborn (PPHN) may be hard to treat but the condition may improve with time and therapy to allow home discharge. If left untreated, the idiopathic PH most commonly present with breathlessness, and children frequently present have poor appetite, faltering growth, lethargy, tachypnea, tachycardia, and irritability. Symptomatic severity has been connected to prognosis, emphasizing the importance of early diagnosis and management. The natural course of pulmonary arterial hypertension is usually progressive and fatal [111, 112].

There are various diagnostic tests and procedures that exclude other diseases and ensure an accurate diagnosis of PAH. These diagnostic procedures include thorough clinical history and physical examination, ECG, chest X-ray, transthoracic Doppler echocardiography, pulmonary function tests, arterial blood gas analysis, ventilation and perfusion lung scan, high-resolution computed tomography of the lungs, contrast-enhanced spiral computed tomography of the lungs and pulmonary angiography, blood tests and immunology, abdominal ultrasound scan, exercise capacity assessment, and hemodynamic evaluation. Invasive and non-invasive markers of disease severity, either biomarkers or physiological parameters and tests that can be widely applied, have been proposed to reliably monitor the clinical course. Recent treatment strategies in children have improved their prognosis over the past decade since the introduction of new therapeutic agents [4].

3.2.4. Increased Incidence of Gastro-Esophageal Reflux Disease (GERD)

Gastroesophageal reflux is a retrograde movement of gastric contents (solids or liquids) into the esophagus. Mild cases present commonly in children as spitting up while present with even forcefully vomiting in severe cases. Though some spitting up in infants is common and may be treated as normal; it considered abnormal when it results in either distress in the child or complications to the child's health such as pneumonia, esophagitis or slow growth. Down syndrome is frequently associated with gastrointestinal disorders, especially in early infancy and often necessitating therapy. Gastroesophageal reflux disease (GERD) is the most frequent motility disorder. It is often misdiagnosed because of its atypical manifestations. In addition, the involvement of the enteric nervous system in the pathophysiology of GERD in DS is not yet fully understood but looks supported by many evidences [113].

The diagnosis of gastroesophageal reflux disease (GERD) may be challenging with a lot of controversies due to the wide variation in symptoms. The most evident signs of reflux are repeated spitting up and/or vomiting. While normal infants may spit up occasionally, the infant with reflux will spit up or vomit after nearly every feeding. Another difference between spitting up and vomiting is the force. Vomiting is more powerful and forceful, usually due to spasms of the pylorus muscle. 85% of all infants with GER become symptomatic by the age of 7 days, with another 10% showing signs by the 6th week of life. Early diagnosis of esophageal functional disorders is necessary to prevent development of respiratory problems, growth retardation in children, weight loss in adults, and to set up the proper type of surgery when needed. Diagnosis of GERD has to be inferred by doing tests demonstrating presence of excessive rate or duration of reflux events, esophagitis, or a clear association of symptoms and signs with reflux events in the absence of alternative diagnoses. These tests involve barium meal for anatomy, endoscopy for esophagitis, and pH monitoring to confirm a time relation between (acid) GER and symptoms. Multiple intraluminal impedance adds more information than pH monitoring, but is more expensive and has limited therapeutic impact as long as drugs are mainly "anti-acid [114].

A proper differential diagnosis between GER, GERD and other possible conditions mimicking reflux is vital in order to direct the treatment, avoiding the overuse of acid suppressive medications which currently represents a main source of debate. In fact DS is frequently accompanied with motor disorders and this proof must be considered in the choice of therapy: in particular all options available to improve motility seem to be useful in such patients. The effectiveness of therapy is firmly correlated with the degree of mental impairment, so that modulating therapy is essential, especially in view of the severity of the neurological status [115]. Lifestyle modifications are stressed on as a first-line therapy in both GER and GERD, whereas medications are clearly indicated only for patients with GERD. Surgical treatments are reserved for children with intractable symptoms or who are at risk for life-threatening complications of GERD. Caution should be done when using promoters of gastric emptying and motility. Improper use of proton pump inhibitors in the pediatric population should be avoided [116].

3.2.5. Increased Incidence of Pulmonary Hemosiderosis

Idiopathic pulmonary hemosiderosis (IPH) is a clinical condition and a rare reason of diffuse alveolar hemorrhage distinguished by unusual deposition of hemosiderin iron in the macrophages of pulmonary alveoli. It is a serious and potentially lethal condition which occurs mainly in infants and children below 10 years of age. Although an inflammatory pulmonary capillaritis is present in most patients with DS, IPH is a distinct entity in which pulmonary inflammatory changes are lacking. Most cases occur in children [117]. It is characterized by a triad of hemoptysis, opacities in X-ray, and anemia, in which the etiology is still unknown. Therefore, the diagnosis depends only on exclusion of other disorders in which diffuse alveolar hemorrhage is a fundamental sign. Acute episodes may occur frequently, eventually ending with pulmonary fibrosis in the chronic stage [118]. The association between DS and IPH is rare, having been reported only thrice [119 - 121], and no underlying mechanism has been proposed for this association. However, it has been shown that patients with DS have a high rate of respiratory problems.

IPH was diagnosed on the basis of: 1) an open lung biopsy showing focal alveolar edema and hemorrhage without parenchymal inflammatory alterations, 2) a bronchoalveolar lavage showing hemosiderin-laden macrophages, and 3) exclusion of infectious or immunologic causes of hemoptysis [122]. Bronchoalveolar lavage fluid is yellow in color due to Haemosiderin-laden macrophages. Microscopic examination of the lung tissue specimens obtained by transbronchial lung biopsy (TBLB) reveals hemorrhage and numerous hemosiderin-laden macrophages in the alveoli but no vasculitis or capillaritis. CT scan chest may show patchy areas of ground glass appearance in lung lobes occasionally pleural nodules [123]. Usually, the treatment consists of high doses of corticosteroids, which can be used together with immunosuppressive agents. First-line conventional treatment of IPH is traditionally based on systemic corticosteroids; however, many steroid-sparing agents are being increasingly used as add on to the corticosteroids in children with recurrent or refractory bleeding. The use of these drugs is especially promising for maintenance treatment, because it tends to avoid the side effects of long-term corticosteroids [119].

3.2.6. Asthma in Down Syndrome

Recurrent wheezing occurs in about 33% of children with DS and many cases were incorrectly diagnosed and treated as asthma. Poor responses to anti-asthmatic medication may imply existence of other causes of wheezing in DS children other than asthma [124 - 126]. Diagnosis of asthma is rarely established in children with DS as the diagnosis is hindered by the difficulty in doing pulmonary function testing in such children. Wheezes in children with DS are more likely to have a different pathophysiology from that of asthma. Exclusion of underlying structural lesions of wheezes such as tracheobronchomalacia, muscle hypotonia, compression of the intrathoracic airways by congenital heart defects and upper airway obstruction should be performed [124, 127]. Recurrent wheezing is very prevalent in children with DS. However, infection with Respiratory syncytial virus did not notably share in increasing the risk of developing recurrent wheezing in such children [126]. At the same time, those children have low prevalence of allergic rhinitis, unlikely to have positive skin prick test (SPT) reactions to common aeroallergens and less frequency of atopic sensitization [128].

The prevalence of asthma in children with DS is less frequent when compared with their siblings or controls. However; there are no differences in eczema and hay fever prevalence between children with DS and their siblings. Autoimmune diseases like coeliac disease, hypothyroidism and diabetes mellitus are much more frequent in DS patients that may imply presence of imbalance T-helper cell 1/2 ratio and disordered regulatory T-cell dysfunction in DS. Increased incidence of wheezing in DS children is multifactorial. Increased incidence of congenital lung anomalies reduce the elastic recoil of lung parenchyma and could reduce intrathoracic airway patency in DS. The airway itself is more liable to be soft and collapsible which causes increased frequency and severity of respiratory infections in young children with DS and hence the associated wheezing. Muscle hypotonia and upper airway collapse may also contribute to wheeze prevalence and severity in those children [127].

3.3. Sleep-Related Disorders

Sleep disorders are common and important problems, frequently under-recognized in children with DS and can be significant distressing factor to their families. The prevalence of these disorders in children with DS is very high, particularly in boys [129]. Their sleeping patterns and architecture differ from that of children without DS beginning in infancy and these patterns continue throughout childhood, adolescence, and early adulthood. Children with DS may have considerable abnormalities in the REM sleep phase, including a decreased percentage of time spent in REM, a decrease in REM activity, and an increase in time to initiation of REM sleep. They have frequent sleep fragmentation, night waking, and undifferentiated sleep, as well as lower sleep efficiency (% of time in bed spent asleep) than typically developing children [130].

The amounts of both REM and non-REM sleep may have significant effects on learning, memory, and behavior, which have more important implications on this population who already have a baseline neurocognitive impairment [131]. Sleep problems appear to be correlated with prevalent comorbidities such as enlarged adenoids or tonsils, a diagnosis of asthma or reactive airway disease and autism. Consideration of sleep disturbances other than obstructive sleep apnea may improve the clinical care of children with DS. Broader screening for both respiratory and non-respiratory sleep disturbances could be clinically useful in decreasing the impact of sleep disturbances on this population. Close follow-up for children identified with sleep concerns appears to be an important component of clinical care for children with DS, as some treatments (such as adenotonsillectomy for obstructive sleep apnea) may not be curative [132].

Children with DS are affected by many other craniofacial abnormalities including mid-face hypoplasia and glossomegaly as well as adenotonsillar hypertrophy and truncal obesity, all of which increase the propensity for sleep related upper airway obstruction and therefore may affect sleep. Generalized pharyngeal collapse dominates in DS children who present with sleep-disordered breathing and is independent of age, gender, and BMI. Additionally, because of global hypotonia, children with DS may be at increased risk of sleep related airway closure, yet not generate sufficient airflow rates to result in palatal vibration necessary to produce the sound of snoring [133].

Obstructive sleep apnea syndrome in children is a one of the manifestations of sleep-disordered breathing and is accompanied with a number of complications. Anatomical narrowing of the upper airway conjoined with impaired compensation for reduction of the neuromuscular tone is an important factor in the pathogenesis. Adenotonsillar hypertrophy is the most important predisposing factor. However, many other causes of craniofacial defects may coexist [134]. Children with DS are at great risk for obstructive sleep apnea (OSA) especially at high altitude. Significant relationships are found between OSA and dysphagia, CHD, prematurity, GERD, and other functional and anatomic gastrointestinal (GI) conditions. These disorders may help to identify infants who are at greater risk of OSA and may warrant evaluation [135]. Escalating elevation and high altitude aggravate the underlying respiratory problems and deteriorate the sleep quality in non-DS persons. Higher altitude can modulate the severity of OSA in DS which increases with increasing altitude. At elevations >1500 m, children with DS and OSA have an unreasonably greater risk of hospitalizations than non-syndromic children with OSA [136].

In one study the prevalence of OSA in children with DS may reach 59% of cases. Amusingly, nearly 40% of children with DS and OSA did not have regular snoring [137]. Early detection of OSA in children with DS is recommended because of its potentially adverse effects on development. Children with DS have nearly the same symptoms with slightly poorer gas exchange compared with the non-syndromic children. They usually have more severe OSA than the typically developing children, suggesting a relative reluctance by parents or doctors to investigate symptoms of OSA in children with DS. These findings highlight the need for formal screening tools for OSA to improve detection of this condition in this high-risk group [138]. Children with DS and OSA have a higher NREM apnea-hypopnea index (AHI), which becomes worse in the recumbent position, perhaps indicating a positional effect compounded by underlying hypotonia inherent to DS [139]. Evident apnea during sleep is an independent positive predictive factor for development of OSA in children. A child with observable apnea during sleep must be referred to a specialized sleep laboratory for polysomnography (PSG) [140]. Diagnosis of OSA is mainly based on an overnight PSG. This investigation is expensive, time consuming and not widely available. Upper airway imaging could be a useful tool for investigating OSA and in establishing the site(s) of obstruction. Several radiological techniques (lateral neck radiography, cephalometry, computerized tomography, magnetic resonance imaging and post-processing of these images using computational fluid dynamics) have been used to study the role of structural alterations in the aetio-pathogenesis. Dynamic cine MRI studies can identify the level of obstruction so that the treatment made more focused. Preoperative echocardiography may be needed to verify presence of right-sided heart failure, which when present is an indication for cardiac catheterization to determine pulmonary venous and arterial pressures [134].

Although from the clinical point of view; many children with DS respond differently well to the continuous positive airway pressure (CPAP) therapy. However; the efficacy of CPAP therapy in such patient group is still in need for more studies. There are a wide range of treatment options for these children, which can give other choices replacing continuous positive airway pressure or tracheostomy [141]. A considerable figure of infants with DS may recover from OSA within several months. This is especially important during treatment choice, particularly between CPAP and tracheostomy, because it may only be needed for a short time [142]. The surgical treatment of sleep-related breathing disorders in children depends on the cause of the upper airway obstruction, which can be located in the nasal fossae, pharynx (the most frequent is adenotonsillar hyperplasia), or larynx (laryngomalacia, cysts...). Adenotonsillectomy is the most frequently performed and effective (70-80%) procedure. The aim of this technique is to normalize nocturnal respiratory parameters and daytime symptoms, as well as to revert, or at least to halt, cardiovascular complications, neurocognitive disturbances, growth delay and enuresis, which can develop if treatment is not provided or is delayed. However, despite its effectiveness, adenotonsillectomy more frequently leads to complications in children with sleep apnea-hypopnea syndrome (SAHS) than in those undergoing this procedure for other reasons. Other obstructive disorders of the upper airway must also be treated, although less frequently due to their lower incidence. These disorders include choanal atresia or stenosis, laryngomalacia, and hypoplasia of the midface or mandible. Tracheotomy will sometimes be required [143]. More aggressive surgeries to treat OSA in children with DS may be needed as a combination of tongue reduction, tongue hyoid advancement, uvulopalatopharyngoplasty, and maxillary or midface advancement. The patient may improve clinically, and the symptoms as snoring, and noisy breathing and alleviated and the patient will need less oxygen requirements. However, some symptoms of residual airway obstruction are frequent after surgery [144].

4. RESPIRATORY PROPHYLAXIS

Vaccinations help to prevent a considerable number of infectious diseases. The immune dysfunctions of DS are not a contraindication for the currently available vaccines: their immunogenicity and safety are not significantly different from those observed in the general population. Some of these vaccines induce somewhat lower humoral responses to the usual ones (mumps, measles, acellular pertussis), but obtaining levels considered protective. These determining factors require that this group must strictly adhere to the systematic vaccine guidelines established in each Community, and their inclusion among the risk groups that must have the benefit of receiving vaccines which have selective indications [145].

4.1. Respiratory Syncytial Virus Prophylaxis

Respiratory syncytial virus (RSV) is a seasonal contagious disease and is one of the most important viral pathogens causing acute respiratory infections in children. It is responsible for about 3.4 million hospitalizations every year in children under the age of five. Because of the more significant risk for RSV infection and related hospitalization in children with DS; prevention of the disease is the ideal strategy. Palivizumab is an anti-RSV monoclonal antibody, intended to offer passive immunity against serious lower respiratory tract infection caused by RSV and thereby prevent or decrease the severity of RSV infection in children at high risk including DS [91]. It is given intramuscularly at a dose of 15 mg/kg on monthly basis. The efficacy and safety of palivizumab has been documented and a large number of economic studies have tested its cost-effectiveness. It is efficient in minimizing the frequency of RSV infection-related hospitalizations *i.e.* in decreasing the rate of severe lower respiratory tract RSV infections in children with chronic lung disease, congenital heart disease or preterm babies [146]. Palivizumab use resulted in a 3.6-fold reduction in the incidence rate ratio for RSV-related hospitalization in children with DS during the first 2 years of life [147]. The incremental cost-effectiveness ratios (ICER) values differ significantly from study to another, from highly cost-effective to not cost-effective. The availability of low-cost palivizumab would reduce its unbalanced distribution across the countries, so that RSV prophylaxis would be available to the poorest countries where children are at greatest risk [146].

4.2. Pneumococcal Prophylaxis

Streptococcus pneumoniae is the most important bacterial reason of respiratory illness. Invasive pneumococcal diseases include pneumonia, meningitis and septicemia. DS children had reduced expansion of T and B cell lymphocytes pool in the first years of life. Though T lymphocytes ultimately reach a level near the expected normal levels, B lymphocytes continued to be reduced. Children with DS have unusual percentage of peripheral blood lymphoid subsets, cellular dysfunction, and thymic and T cell aberrations. DS has been shown to be a risk condition for the development of invasive pneumococcal disease. DS children frequently suffer from acute otitis media, sinusitis and pneumonias and their lethality for sepsis is particularly high: a principal aetiological agent of these processes is *pneumococcus*. There are 2 main types of pneumococcal vaccines. One used for children below the age of 2 years (*e.g.* Prevanar which contains extracts from thirteen of the most common types of *Streptococcus pneumoniae* bacteria) and one used for older children and adults (*e.g.* Pneumovax which contains 23 serotypes contained in the vaccine as 1, 2, 3, 4, 5, 6B, 7F, 8, 9N, 9V,

10A, 11A, 12F, 14, 15B, 17F, 18C, 19F, 19A, 20, 22F, 23F, and 33F) [148].

Despite the normal IgG antibody response to pneumococcal vaccine is still not yet defined, a 2- to 4-fold increase in post-immunization antibody levels generally denotes a satisfactory response. Children with DS produce sufficient serotype-specific antibody response to all conjugated and nearly all unconjugated pneumococcal serotypes used. They have also intact and normal opsonophagocytosis activity against pneumococcal serotypes 9N, 19F and 23F in individuals with age between 6-24 years. However, some children with DS may have low response to some types of pneumococcal vaccine [95]. Meanwhile, the protective level may varies with the age of the person and may fluctuate with various pneumococcal serotypes. There is a delay in maturation of the acquisition of the polysaccharide antigen response, which shows very poor immunogenic response in infants. A specific antibody response to polysaccharide antigens is complete in children after the age of 2 years [149, 150].

4.3. Flu Prophylaxis

Many risk factors for catching influenza found in children with DS including congenital heart disease, altered immunity and anatomical abnormalities. Despite persons with DS are at high risk for flu related respiratory complications, they are not clearly listed in groups that should have priority vaccination or for early treatment of influenza. The immune response to the inactivated influenza vaccine in children with DS is mildly impaired than the immune response in the control cases [151, 152]. However, because of the increased risk for flu-related hospitalization and death for patients with DS and influenza-like illness; patients with DS should receive the vaccine against the seasonal influenza viruses. Early treatment of DS patients for influenza-like illness should be encouraged by health systems and DS organizations [153].

4.4. Haemophilus Influenzae Prophylaxis

The *Haemophilus influenzae* serotype b (Hib) conjugate vaccine stimulates both the antibody production and immunological memory and is very effective in preventing invasive Hib disease. The incidence of invasive Hib disease reduced significantly within 2 years across all age groups, possibly through a mixture of direct and indirect protection (herd immunity) within 1 year after initiation of this vaccine. In general, more than 50% of e children reported with Hib vaccine failure have antibody levels below the levels known to confer long-term protection, which implies that these children could be at additional risk of invasive Hib disease and would benefit from another dose of Hib vaccine [154].

4.5. Immunomodulation With Pidotimod

Different kinds of biologically active immunostimulants substances; of natural and artificial origins and with diverse modes of action have been launched in some countries for the prevention of acute respiratory tract infections (ARTIs) in children. These substances act generally by enhancing the immune response or stimulating the child's innate defense mechanisms. Pidotimod (3-L-pyroglutam-l-L-thiaziolidine-4carboxylic acid) is an artificial dipeptide molecule with immunomodulatory properties and is constitutionally similar to Piracetam. Pidotimod use is associated with up regulation of a number of genes concerned with the stimulation of innate immune responses and in antimicrobial activity. Interestingly the ratio of Flu-specific IgG1/IgG3 is distorted in pidotimod-treated individuals, suggesting a privileged activation of complement-dependent effector mechanisms. Pidotimod has an immunostimulatory and immunoregulatory activity on T lymphocytes and strengthens and stimulates immunological mechanisms involved in both the humoral and cellular immunity mediated by T lymphocytes. At the same time, it stimulates and increases macrophage migration, which is an essential and central to the cellular immune response which serves the purpose of obtaining an adequate phagocytosis and elimination of the infectious agent. Pidotimod can potentiate the beneficial effect of immunization, possibly resulting in a stronger activity of both innate and adaptive immune responses [155, 156].

Pidotimod treatment is able to significantly reduce the number of children with upper and lower airways symptoms, and medications use, increase school attendance, and reduce the pediatric visits for recurrent respiratory infections [157]. Because of its efficacy and safety, pidotimod may be rated as an excellent drug in the recurrent respiratory infections management in children. It has a prophylactic action and effective and efficient protection against infections by

Gram-positive and gram-negative bacteria. For treatment of acute respiratory infection, 400 mg of Pidotimod are taken twice daily for 15 days (2 hours before or 2 hours after food), while for prevention of recurrent infection it can be used as 400 mg twice daily for 60 days [158].

CONCLUSION

Children with DS are more liable to have congenital and acquired respiratory problems. Every effort should be done to prevent respiratory diseases in this vulnerable group of population.

CONFLICT OF INTEREST

The authors confirm that this chapter contents have no conflict of interest.

ACKNOWLEDGEMENTS

Declared none.

REFERENCES

[1] Pandit C, Fitzgerald DA. Respiratory problems in children with Down syndrome. J Paediatr Child Health 2012; 48(3): E147-52. [http://dx.doi.org/10.1111/j.1440-1754.2011.02077.x] [PMID: 21535288]

[2] Watts R, Vyas H. An overview of respiratory problems in children with Down's syndrome. Arch Dis Child 2013; 98(10): 812-7. [http://dx.doi.org/10.1136/archdischild-2013-304611] [PMID: 23814080]

[3] Yang Q, Rasmussen SA, Friedman JM. Mortality associated with Down's syndrome in the USA from 1983 to 1997: a population-based study. Lancet 2002 Mar 23; 359(9311): 1019-25.

[4] Hawkins A, Langton-Hewer S, Henderson J, Tulloh RM. Management of pulmonary hypertension in Down syndrome. Eur J Pediatr 2011; 170(7): 915-21. [http://dx.doi.org/10.1007/s00431-010-1378-1] [PMID: 21203772]

[5] Shires CB, Anold SL, Schoumacher RA, Dehoff GW, Donepudi SK, Stocks RM. Body mass index as an indicator of obstructive sleep apnea in pediatric Down syndrome. Int J Pediatr Otorhinolaryngol 2010; 74(7): 768-72. [http://dx.doi.org/10.1016/j.ijporl.2010.03.050] [PMID: 20452066]

[6] Fillat C, Altafaj X. Gene therapy for Down syndrome. Prog Brain Res 2012; 197: 237-47. [http://dx.doi.org/10.1016/B978-0-444-54299-1.00012-1] [PMID: 22541296]

[7] Salinas M, Elawabdeh N, Lin J, Naguib MM, Hodge MG, Shehata BM. The spectrum of pulmonary malformation in trisomy-21 patient. A review with emphasis on the molecular-genetic basis. Fetal

Pediatr Pathol 2013; 31(1): 38-42.
[http://dx.doi.org/10.3109/15513815.2012.659415] [PMID: 22497682]

[8] Starbuck JM, Cole TM III, Reeves RH, Richtsmeier JT. Trisomy 21 and facial developmental instability. Am J Phys Anthropol 2013; 151(1): 49-57.
[http://dx.doi.org/10.1002/ajpa.22255] [PMID: 23505010]

[9] Billingsley CN, Allen JR, Baumann DD, *et al.* Non-trisomic homeobox gene expression during craniofacial development in the Ts65Dn mouse model of Down syndrome. Am J Med Genet A 2013; 161A(8): 1866-74.
[http://dx.doi.org/10.1002/ajmg.a.36006] [PMID: 23843306]

[10] Starbuck J, Reeves RH, Richtsmeier J. Morphological integration of soft-tissue facial morphology in Down Syndrome and siblings. Am J Phys Anthropol 2011; 146(4): 560-8.
[http://dx.doi.org/10.1002/ajpa.21583] [PMID: 21996933]

[11] Lall M, Thakur S, Puri R, Verma I, Mukerji M, Jha PA. A 54 Mb 11qter duplication and 0.9 Mb 1q44 deletion in a child with laryngomalacia and agenesis of corpus callosum. Mol Cytogenet 2011; 21(4)
[http://dx.doi.org/10.1186/1755-8166-4-19] [PMID: 21936942]

[12] Miller LA, Wert SE, Clark JC, Xu Y, Perl AK, Whitsett JA. Role of Sonic hedgehog in patterning of tracheal-bronchial cartilage and the peripheral lung. Dev Dyn 2004; 231(1): 57-71.
[http://dx.doi.org/10.1002/dvdy.20105] [PMID: 15305287]

[13] Cua CL, Blankenship A, North AL, Hayes J, Nelin LD. Increased incidence of idiopathic persistent pulmonary hypertension in Down syndrome neonates. Pediatr Cardiol 2007; 28(4): 250-4.
[http://dx.doi.org/10.1007/s00246-006-0011-6] [PMID: 17486396]

[14] Cannon BC, Feltes TF, Fraley JK, Grifka RG, Riddle EM, Kovalchin JP. Nitric oxide in the evaluation of congenital heart disease with pulmonary hypertension: factors related to nitric oxide response. Pediatr Cardiol 2005; 26(5): 565-9.
[http://dx.doi.org/10.1007/s00246-004-0767-5] [PMID: 16132310]

[15] Roberts KE, McElroy JJ, Wong WP, *et al.* BMPR2 mutations in pulmonary arterial hypertension with congenital heart disease. Eur Respir J 2004; 24(3): 371-4.
[http://dx.doi.org/10.1183/09031936.04.00018604] [PMID: 15358693]

[16] Zampieri BL, Biselli-Périco JM, de Souza JE, *et al.* Altered expression of immune-related genes in children with Down syndrome PLoS One 2014; 15(9): e107218-337.
[http://dx.doi.org/10.1371/journal.pone.0107218] [PMID: 25222269]

[17] Charleton PM, Dennis J, Marder E. Medical management of children with Down syndrome. Paediatr Child Health 2010; 20: 331-7.
[http://dx.doi.org/10.1016/j.paed.2010.06.006]

[18] Rubin SS, Rimmer JH, Chicoine B, Braddock D, McGuire DE. Overweight prevalence in persons with Down syndrome. Ment Retard 1998; 36(3): 175-81.
[PMID: 9638037]

[19] Irving CA, Chaudhari MP. Cardiovascular abnormalities in Down's syndrome: spectrum, management and survival over 22 years. Arch Dis Child 2012; 97(4): 326-30.
[http://dx.doi.org/10.1136/adc.2010.210534] [PMID: 21835834]

[20] Weijerman ME, van Furth AM, van der Mooren MD, *et al.* Prevalence of congenital heart defects and persistent pulmonary hypertension of the neonate with Down syndrome. Eur J Pediatr 2010; 169(10): 1195-9.
[http://dx.doi.org/10.1007/s00431-010-1200-0] [PMID: 20411274]

[21] Arvedson J, Rogers B, Buck G, Smart P, Msall M. Silent aspiration prominent in children with dysphagia. Int J Pediatr Otorhinolaryngol 1994; 28(2-3): 173-81.
[http://dx.doi.org/10.1016/0165-5876(94)90009-4] [PMID: 8157416]

[22] Bertrand P, Navarro H, Caussade S, Holmgren N, Sánchez I. Airway anomalies in children with Down syndrome: endoscopic findings. Pediatr Pulmonol 2003; 36(2): 137-41.
[http://dx.doi.org/10.1002/ppul.10332] [PMID: 12833493]

[23] Morales-Angulo C, Gallo-Terán J, Azuara N, Rama Quintela J. [Otorhinolaryngo logical manifestations in patients with Down syndrome]. Acta Otorrinolaringol Esp 2006; 57(6): 262-5. [http://dx.doi.org/10.1016/S0001-6519(06)78705-2] [PMID: 16872101]

[24] Levine OR, Simpser M. Alveolar hypoventilation and cor pulmonale associated with chronic airway obstruction in infants with Down syndrome. Clin Pediatr (Phila) 1982; 21(1): 25-9.
[http://dx.doi.org/10.1177/000992288202100104] [PMID: 6459903]

[25] Kovesi T, Sinclair B, MacCormick J, Matzinger MA, Carpenter B. Primary ciliary dyskinesia associated with a novel microtubule defect in a child with Down's syndrome. Chest 2000; 117(4): 1207-9.
[http://dx.doi.org/10.1378/chest.117.4.1207] [PMID: 10767266]

[26] Barr E, Dungworth J, Hunter K, McFarlane M, Kubba H. The prevalence of ear, nose and throat disorders in preschool children with Down's syndrome in Glasgow. Scott Med J 2011; 56(2): 98-103.
[http://dx.doi.org/10.1258/smj.2011.011036] [PMID: 21670137]

[27] de Jong AL, Sulek M, Nihill M, Duncan NO, Friedman EM. Tenuous airway in children with trisomy 21. Laryngoscope 1997; 107(3): 345-50.
[http://dx.doi.org/10.1097/00005537-199703000-00013] [PMID: 9121311]

[28] Jacobs IN, Gray RF, Todd NW. Upper airway obstruction in children with Down syndrome. Arch Otolaryngol Head Neck Surg 1996; 122(9): 945-50.
[http://dx.doi.org/10.1001/archotol.1996.01890210025007] [PMID: 8797558]

[29] Sánchez I, Navarro H, Méndez M, Holmgren N, Caussade S. Clinical characteristics of children with tracheobronchial anomalies. Pediatr Pulmonol 2003; 35(4): 288-91.
[http://dx.doi.org/10.1002/ppul.10256] [PMID: 12629626]

[30] Pan W, Peng D, Luo J, *et al.* Clinical features of airway malacia in children: a retrospective analysis of 459 patients Int J Clin Exp Med 2014; 15(7(9)): 3005-12.
[PMID: 25356175]

[31] Kugler C, Stanzel F. Tracheomalacia. Thorac Surg Clin 2014; 24(1): 51-8.
[http://dx.doi.org/10.1016/j.thorsurg.2013.09.003] [PMID: 24295659]

[32] Xia Y, Huang Y, Li QB, *et al.* Analysis of 53 cases with bronchoscopically confirmed pediatric tracheobronchomalacia. Zhonghua Er Ke Za Zhi 2007; 45(2): 96-.
[PMID: 17456335]

[33] Lee EY, Boiselle PM. Tracheobronchomalacia in infants and children: multidetector CT evaluation. Radiology 2009; 252(1): 7-22.
[http://dx.doi.org/10.1148/radiol.2513081280] [PMID: 19561247]

[34] Goyal V, Masters IB, Chang AB. Interventions for primary (intrinsic) tracheomalacia in children. Cochrane Database Syst Rev 2012; 17(10): CD005304.
[http://dx.doi.org/10.1002/14651858.CD005304.pub3] [PMID: 23076914]

[35] Bohadana SC. Interventions for primary (intrinsic) tracheomalacia in children. Sao Paulo Med J 2013; 131(1): 66.
[http://dx.doi.org/10.1590/S1516-31802013000100013] [PMID: 23538600]

[36] Shott SR. Down syndrome: analysis of airway size and a guide for appropriate intubation. Laryngoscope 2000; 110(4): 585-92.
[http://dx.doi.org/10.1097/00005537-200004000-00010] [PMID: 10764002]

[37] Phipps LM, Raymond JA, Angeletti TM. Congenital tracheal stenosis. Crit Care Nurse 2006; 26(3): 60-9.
[PMID: 16717388]

[38] Shapiro NL, Huang RY, Sangwan S, Willner A, Laks H. Tracheal stenosis and congenital heart disease in patients with Down syndrome: diagnostic approach and surgical options. Int J Pediatr Otorhinolaryngol 2000; 31(54): 137-42.
[http://dx.doi.org/10.1016/S0165-5876(00)00361-XPMID] [http://dx.doi.org/10967384]

[39] Berdon WE. Rings, slings, and other things: vascular compression of the infant trachea updated from the midcentury to the millennium--the legacy of Robert E. Gross, MD, and Edward B. D. Neuhauser, MD. Radiology 2000; 216(3): 624-32.
[http://dx.doi.org/10.1148/radiology.216.3.r00se40624] [PMID: 10966687]

[40] Russell HM, Backer CL. Pediatric thoracic problems: patent ductus arteriosus, vascular rings, congenital tracheal stenosis, and pectus deformities. Surg Clin North Am 2010; 90(5): 1091-113.
[http://dx.doi.org/10.1016/j.suc.2010.06.009] [PMID: 20955885]

[41] Acosta AC, Albanese CT, Farmer DL, Sydorak R, Danzer E, Harrison MR. Tracheal stenosis: the long and the short of it. J Pediatr Surg 2000; 35(11): 1612-6.
[http://dx.doi.org/10.1053/jpsu.2000.18330] [PMID: 11083434]

[42] Elliott M, Roebuck D, Noctor C, *et al.* The management of congenital tracheal stenosis. Int J Pediatr Otorhinolaryngol 2003; 67 (Suppl. 1): S183-92.
[http://dx.doi.org/10.1016/j.ijporl.2003.08.023] [PMID: 14662192]

[43] Dodge-Khatami A, Tsang V, Roebuck D, Elliott M. Management of congenital tracheal stenosis: a multidisciplinary approach. Images Paediatr Cardiol 2000; 2(1): 29-39.
[PMID: 22368577]

[44] Wijeweera O, Ng SB. Retrospective review of tracheoplasty for congenital tracheal stenosis. Singapore Med J 2011; 52(10): 726-9.
[PMID: 22009391]

[45] Herrera P, Caldarone C, Forte V, *et al.* The current state of congenital tracheal stenosis. Pediatr Surg Int 2007; 23(11): 1033-44.

[http://dx.doi.org/10.1007/s00383-007-1945-3] [PMID: 17712567]

[46] Morrissey MS, Bailey CM. Diagnosis and management of subglottic stenosis after neonatal ventilation. Arch Dis Child 1990; 65(10): 1103-4.
[http://dx.doi.org/10.1136/adc.65.10.1103] [PMID: 2248497]

[47] Loi HD, Parhr AS, Subramaniam SK, Choo KE, Ng HP. Neonatal post-intubation subglottic stenosis. Med J Malaysia 2004; 59(1): 126-8.
[PMID: 15535351]

[48] Miller R, Gray SD, Cotton RT, Myer CM III, Netterville J. Subglottic stenosis and Down syndrome. Am J Otolaryngol 1990; 11(4): 274-7.
[http://dx.doi.org/10.1016/0196-0709(90)90089-E] [PMID: 2146897]

[49] Brodner DC, Guarisco JL. Subglottic stenosis: evaluation and management. J La State Med Soc 1999; 151(4): 159-64.
[PMID: 10234887]

[50] Freeman SB, Torfs CP, Romitti PA, *et al.* Congenital gastrointestinal defects in Down syndrome: a report from the Atlanta and National Down Syndrome Projects. Clin Genet 2009; 75(2): 180-4.
[http://dx.doi.org/10.1111/j.1399-0004.2008.01110.x] [PMID: 19021635]

[51] Brosens E, Ploeg M, van Bever Y, *et al.* Clinical and etiological heterogeneity in patients with tracheo-esophageal malformations and associated anomalies. Eur J Med Genet 2014; 57(8): 440-52.
[http://dx.doi.org/10.1016/j.ejmg.2014.05.009] [PMID: 24931924]

[52] Perry M, Eick J, Jakob K, Adolph V, Uwaifo O. Clinical images - a quarterly column: early presentation of h-type tracheoesophageal fistula. Ochsner J 2013; 13(4): 483-5.
[PMID: 24357993]

[53] Khorshid EA, Dokhan AL, Turkistani AF, Shadi SM, Hassab MH. Five year experience in prenatal ultrasound diagnosis of esophageal atresia in Saudi Arabia. Ann Saudi Med 2003; 23(3-4): 132-4.
[PMID: 16985300]

[54] Spitz L. Oesophageal atresia. Orphanet J Rare Dis 2007.
[http://dx.doi.org/10.1186/1750-1172-2-24]

[55] Parolini F, Morandi A, Macchini F, *et al.* Esophageal atresia with proximal tracheoesophageal fistula: a missed diagnosis. J Pediatr Surg 2013; 48(6): E13-7.
[http://dx.doi.org/10.1016/j.jpedsurg.2013.04.018] [PMID: 23845651]

[56] Davari HR, Latifi S. Successful airway management in a patient with tracheal stenosis and tracheoesophageal fistula: a case report. Acta Med Iran 2014; 52(7): 565-8.
[PMID: 25135268]

[57] Gunlemez A, Anik Y, Elemen L, Tugay M, Gökalp AS. H-type tracheoesophageal fistula in an extremely low birth weight premature neonate: appearance on magnetic resonance imaging. J Perinatol 2009; 29(5): 393-5.
[http://dx.doi.org/10.1038/jp.2008.198] [PMID: 19399000]

[58] El Biache I, Lechqar M, Rami M, Bouabdallah Y. Isolated congenital tracheoesophageal fistula: report of 2 cases. Pan Afr Med J 2014; 22(17): 304.
[http://dx.doi.org/10.11604/pamj.2014.17.304.3958] [PMID: 25328600]

[59] Ni Y, Yao Y, Liang P. Simple strategy of anesthesia for the neonate with tracheoesophageal fistula: a case report. Int J Clin Exp Med 2014; 15(327): 8.
[PMID: 24482727]

[60] Nabzdyk CS, Chiu B, Jackson CC, Chwals WJ. Management of patients with combined tracheoesophageal fistula, esophageal atresia, and duodenal atresia. Int J Surg Case Rep 2014; 5(12): 1288-91.
[http://dx.doi.org/10.1016/j.ijscr.2013.09.016] [PMID: 25460495]

[61] McLaughlin FJ, Strieder DJ, Harris GB, Vawter GP, Eraklis AJ. Tracheal bronchus: association with respiratory morbidity in childhood. J Pediatr 1985; 106(5): 751-5.
[http://dx.doi.org/10.1016/S0022-3476(85)80348-6] [PMID: 3998915]

[62] Wong KS, Lien R, Lin TY. Clinical and computed tomographic features of tracheal bronchus in children. J Formos Med Assoc 1999; 98(9): 646-8.
[PMID: 10560243]

[63] Yamaki S, Horiuchi T, Takahashi T. Pulmonary changes in congenital heart disease with Down's syndrome: their significance as a cause of postoperative respiratory failure. Thorax 1985; 40(5): 380-6.
[http://dx.doi.org/10.1136/thx.40.5.380] [PMID: 3161204]

[64] Gonzalez OR, Gomez IG, Recalde AL, Landing BH. Postnatal development of the cystic lung lesion of Down syndrome: suggestion that the cause is reduced formation of peripheral air spaces. Pediatr Pathol 1991; 11(4): 623-33.
[http://dx.doi.org/10.3109/15513819109064794] [PMID: 1835001]

[65] Biko DM, Schwartz M, Anupindi SA, Altes TA. Subpleural lung cysts in Down syndrome: prevalence and association with coexisting diagnoses. Pediatr Radiol 2008; 38(3): 280-4.
[http://dx.doi.org/10.1007/s00247-007-0699-3] [PMID: 18097658]

[66] Schloo BL, Vawter GF, Reid LM. Down syndrome: patterns of disturbed lung growth. Hum Pathol 1991; 22(9): 919-23.
[http://dx.doi.org/10.1016/0046-8177(91)90183-P] [PMID: 1833304]

[67] Dishop MK. Diagnostic Pathology of Diffuse Lung Disease in Children. Pediatr Allergy Immunol Pulmonol 2010; 23(1): 69-85. r
[http://dx.doi.org/10.1089/ped.2010.0007] [PMID: 22332032]

[68] So SA, Urbano RC, Hodapp RM. Hospitalizations of infants and young children with Down syndrome: evidence from inpatient person-records from a statewide administrative database. J Intellect Disabil Res 2007; 51(Pt 12): 1030-8.
[http://dx.doi.org/10.1111/j.1365-2788.2007.01013.x] [PMID: 17991010]

[69] Selikowitz M. Health problems and health checks in school-aged children with Down syndrome. J Paediatr Child Health 1992; 28(5): 383-6.
[http://dx.doi.org/10.1111/j.1440-1754.1992.tb02697.x] [PMID: 1389451]

[70] Turner S, Sloper P, Cunningham C, Knussen C. Health problems in children with Down's syndrome. Child Care Health Dev 1990; 16(2): 83-97.
[http://dx.doi.org/10.1111/j.1365-2214.1990.tb00641.x] [PMID: 2139819]

[71] Broers CJ, Gemke RJ, Weijerman ME, Kuik DJ, van Hoogstraten IM, van Furth AM. Frequency of

lower respiratory tract infections in relation to adaptive immunity in children with Down syndrome compared to their healthy siblings. Acta Paediatr 2012; 101(8): 862-7. [http://dx.doi.org/10.1111/j.1651-2227.2012.02696.x] [PMID: 22548641]

[72] Oni AA, Bakare RA, Nwaorgu OG, Ogunkunle MO, Toki RA. Bacterial agents of discharging ears and antimicrobial sensitivity patterns in children in Ibadan, Nigeria. West Afr J Med 2001; 20(2): 131-5. [PMID: 11768012]

[73] Roddey OF Jr, Hoover HA, Earle R Jr. Physical examination for otitis media. Pediatr Infect Dis J 2003; 22(7): 673. [http://dx.doi.org/10.1097/01.inf.0000076543.05393.5a] [PMID: 12867848]

[74] Maris M, Wojciechowski M, Van de Heyning P, Boudewyns A. A cross-sectional analysis of otitis media with effusion in children with Down syndrome. Eur J Pediatr 2014; 173(10): 1319-25. [http://dx.doi.org/10.1007/s00431-014-2323-5] [PMID: 24816633]

[75] Fortnum H, Leighton P, Smith MD, *et al.* . Assessment of the feasibility and clinical value of further research to evaluate the management options for children with Down syndrome and otitis media with effusion: a feasibility study Health Technol Assess 2014; 18(60): 1-47. [http://dx.doi.org/10.3310/hta18600] [PMID: 25270051]

[76] McLean L, MacCormick J, Robb I, Carpenter B, Pothos M. Cilia ultrastructure in children with Down syndrome. J Otolaryngol 2003; 32(6): 379-83. [http://dx.doi.org/10.2310/7070.2003.13923] [PMID: 14967083]

[77] Lloyd GA. Diagnostic imaging of the nose and paranasal sinuses. J Laryngol Otol 1989; 103(5): 453-60. [http://dx.doi.org/10.1017/S0022215100156622] [PMID: 2754313]

[78] Khoshdel A, Panahande GR, Noorbakhsh MK, Malek Ahmadi MR, Lotfizadeh M, Parvin N. A comparison of the efficacy of amoxicillin and nasal irrigation in treatment of acute sinusitis in children. Korean J Pediatr 2014; 57(11): 479-83. [http://dx.doi.org/10.3345/kjp.2014.57.11.479] [PMID: 25550702]

[79] Magit A. Pediatric rhinosinusitis. Otolaryngol Clin North Am 2014; 47(5): 733-46. [http://dx.doi.org/10.1016/j.otc.2014.06.003] [PMID: 25213280]

[80] Mori M, Morio T, Ito S, *et al.* Risks and prevention of severe RS virus infection among children with immunodeficiency and Down's syndrome. J Infect Chemother 2014; 20(8): 455-9. [http://dx.doi.org/10.1016/j.jiac.2014.05.001] [PMID: 24929631]

[81] Bardi-Peti L, Ciofu EP. [Bronchiolitis and pulmonary hypertension]. Pneumologia 2010; 59(2): 95-100. [PMID: 20695366]

[82] Thorburn K. Pre-existing disease is associated with a significantly higher risk of death in severe respiratory syncytial virus infection. Arch Dis Child 2009; 94(2): 99-103. [http://dx.doi.org/10.1136/adc.2008.139188] [PMID: 18653625]

[83] Bloemers BL, van Furth AM, Weijerman ME, *et al.* Down syndrome: a novel risk factor for respiratory syncytial virus bronchiolitis--a prospective birth-cohort study. Pediatrics 2007; 120(4):

e1076-81.
[http://dx.doi.org/10.1542/peds.2007-0788] [PMID: 17908728]

[84] Bull MJ. Pulmonary complications and chronic conditions of Down syndrome during childhood: an agenda for clinical care and research. J Pediatr 2011; 158(2): 178-9.
[http://dx.doi.org/10.1016/j.jpeds.2010.11.006] [PMID: 21168154]

[85] van Beek D, Paes B, Bont L. Increased Risk of RSV Infection in Children with Down's Syndrome: Clinical Implementation of Prophylaxis in the European Union Clin Dev Immunol 2013. 2013: 801581 Epub Jun 25
[http://dx.doi.org/10.1155/2013/801581] [PMID: 23878586]

[86] Megged O, Schlesinger Y. Down syndrome and respiratory syncytial virus infection. Pediatr Infect Dis J 2010; 29(7): 672-3.
[http://dx.doi.org/10.1097/INF.0b013e3181d7ffa5] [PMID: 20228692]

[87] Alvarez AE, Marson FA, Bertuzzo CS, Arns CW, Ribeiro JD. Epidemiological and genetic characteristics associated with the severity of acute viral bronchiolitis by respiratory syncytial virus. J Pediatr (Rio J) 2013; 89(6): 531-43.
[http://dx.doi.org/10.1016/j.jped.2013.02.022] [PMID: 24035870]

[88] Paes BA, Mitchell I, Banerji A, Lanctôt KL, Langley JM. A decade of respiratory syncytial virus epidemiology and prophylaxis: translating evidence into everyday clinical practice. Can Respir J 2011; 18(2): e10-9.
[PMID: 21499597]

[89] Mitchell I. Treatment of RSV bronchiolitis: drugs, antibiotics. Paediatr Respir Rev 2009; 10 (Suppl. 1): 14-5.
[http://dx.doi.org/10.1016/S1526-0542(09)70007-7] [PMID: 19651393]

[90] Plint AC, Johnson DW, Patel H, *et al.* Epinephrine and dexamethasone in children with bronchiolitis. N Engl J Med 2009; 14(360(20)): 89-15.
[http://dx.doi.org/10.1056/NEJMoa0900544] [PMID: 19439742]

[91] Wang D, Bayliss S, Meads C. Palivizumab for immunoprophylaxis of respiratory syncytial virus (RSV) bronchiolitis in high-risk infants and young children: a systematic review and additional economic modelling of subgroup analyses. Health Technol Assess 2011; 15(5): iii-iv, 1-124.
[http://dx.doi.org/10.3310/hta15050] [PMID: 21281564]

[92] Hermida Pérez JA, Hernandez Guerra JS. Community-acquired pneumonia in adults with Down syndrome. Three clinical cases and a review of the literature. Rev Med Int Sindr Down 2010; 14(2): 25-30.
[http://dx.doi.org/10.1016/S2171-9748(10)70008-8]

[93] Chetty K, Thomson AH. Pneumonia due to viral and atypical organisms and their sequelae Childhood respiratory infections. Paediatr Drugs 2007; 9(6): 401-11.
[http://dx.doi.org/10.2165/00148581-200709060-00007] [PMID: 18052410]

[94] Broers CJ, Gemke RJ, Morré SA, Weijerman ME, van Furth AM. Increased production of interleukin-10 in children with Down syndrome upon *ex vivo* stimulation with Streptococcus pneumoniae. Pediatr Res 2014; 75(1-1): 109-3.
[http://dx.doi.org/10.1038/pr.2013.173] [PMID: 24126819]

[95] Kusters MA, Manders NC, de Jong BA, van Hout RW, Rijkers GT, de Vries E. Functionality of the pneumococcal antibody response in Down syndrome subjects. Vaccine 2013 Dec 16; 31(52): 6261-5. [http://dx.doi.org/10.1016/j.vaccine.2013.09.070] [PMID: 24200977]

[96] Pérez-Padilla R, Fernández R, García-Sancho C, *et al.* Pandemic (H1N1) 2009 virus and Down syndrome patients. Emerg Infect Dis 2010; 16(8): 1312-4. [http://dx.doi.org/10.3201/eid1608.091931] [PMID: 20678334]

[97] Medrano López C, García-Guereta Silva L, Lirio Casero J, García Pérez J. Grupo CIVIC, Grupo de Trabajo de Infecciones de la Sociedad Española de Cardiología Pediátrica y Cardiopatías Congénitas. [Respiratory infections, Down's syndrome and congenital heart disease: the CIVIC 21 study]. An Pediatr (Barc) 2009; 71(1): 38-46. [http://dx.doi.org/10.1016/j.anpedi.2008.11.007] [PMID: 19423411]

[98] Moulin F, Raymond J, Lorrot M, *et al.* Procalcitonin in children admitted to hospital with community acquired pneumonia. Arch Dis Child 2001; 84(4): 332-6. [http://dx.doi.org/10.1136/adc.84.4.332] [PMID: 11259234]

[99] Cassimos D, Bezirgiannidou Z, Pantelidou D, Christoforidis A, Chatzimichael A, Maritinis G. Warm autoimmune hemolytic anemia following recurrent *mycoplasma pneumonia* infections in a child with Down syndrome. Pediatr Hematol Oncol 2008; 25(7): 693-8. [http://dx.doi.org/10.1080/08880010802237492] [PMID: 18850483]

[100] Noda R, Takaya J, Hasui M, Araki A, Kaneko K. Severe concurrent lung infection caused by legionella and mycoplasma in a 3-year-old patient with Down syndrome and tuberous sclerosis. Pediatr Int 2009; 51(3): 413-4. [http://dx.doi.org/10.1111/j.1442-200X.2009.02825.x] [PMID: 19500283]

[101] Rodríguez JC, Masiá M, Gutiérrez F, Royo G. Legionella pneumophila in community acquired pneumonia: interpretation of microbiological techniques. Med Clin (Barc) 2004; 28(122(7)): 277-8. [http://dx.doi.org/10.1093/jac/dkg191] [PMID: 15012882]

[102] Roig J, Rello J. Legionnaires' disease: a rational approach to therapy. J Antimicrob Chemother 2003; 51(5): 1119-29. [http://dx.doi.org/10.1093/jac/dkg191] [PMID: 12668578]

[103] Picard E, Ben Nun A, Fisher D, Schwartz S, Goldberg M, Goldberg S. Morgagni hernia mimicking pneumonia in Down syndrome. J Pediatr Surg 2007; 42(9): 1608-11. [http://dx.doi.org/10.1016/j.jpedsurg.2007.04.039] [PMID: 17848258]

[104] Bade MA, Rammeloo EM, Hermans J, de Vries Locher AL, de Graaf EA, Mearin ML. Symptoms of disease and food allergy in children with Down syndrome. Ned Tijdschr Geneeskd 1995; 19;139(33):-4 PMID: 1995; 19(139(33)): 1680-4. [PMID: 7566230]

[105] Bruijn M, van der Aa LB, van Rijn RR, Bos AP, van Woensel JB. High incidence of acute lung injury in children with Down syndrome. Intensive Care Med 2007; 33(12): 2179-82. [http://dx.doi.org/10.1007/s00134-007-0803-z] [PMID: 17673975]

[106] Gajic O, Frutos-Vivar F, Esteban A, Hubmayr RD, Anzueto A. Ventilator settings as a risk factor for acute respiratory distress syndrome in mechanically ventilated patients. Intensive Care Med 2005;

31(7): 922-6.
[http://dx.doi.org/10.1007/s00134-005-2625-1] [PMID: 15856172]

[107] Martin TR, Nakamura M, Matute-Bello G. The role of apoptosis in acute lung injury. Crit Care Med 2003; 31(4) (Suppl.): S184-8.
[http://dx.doi.org/10.1097/01.CCM.0000057841.33876.B1] [PMID: 12682438]

[108] Busciglio J, Yankner BA. Apoptosis and increased generation of reactive oxygen species in Down's syndrome neurons *in vitro*. Nature 1995; 21(28)(378(6559)): 776-9.1995;
[http://dx.doi.org/10.1038/378776a0] [PMID: 8524410]

[109] Machado C, Brito I, Souza D, Correia LC. Etiological frequency of pulmonary hypertension in a reference outpatient clinic in Bahia, Brazil. Arq Bras Cardiol 2009; 93(6): 629-636, 679-686.
[PMID: 20379644]

[110] Ivy DD, Abman SH, Barst RJ, *et al.* Pediatric pulmonary hypertension. J Am Coll Cardiol 2013; 24(62) (25): D117-26.
[http://dx.doi.org/10.1016/j.jacc.2013.10.028.Review] [PMID: 24355636]

[111] Widlitz A, Barst RJ. Pulmonary arterial hypertension in children. Eur Respir J 2003; 21(1): 155-76.
[http://dx.doi.org/10.1183/09031936.03.00088302] [PMID: 12570125]

[112] Manes A, Campana C. Pulmonary hypertension: classification and diagnostic algorithm. Ital Heart J 2005; 6(10): 834-9.
[PMID: 16270476]

[113] Macchini F, Leva E, Torricelli M, Valadè A. Treating acid reflux disease in patients with Down syndrome: pharmacological and physiological approaches. Clin Exp Gastroenterol 2011; 4: 19-22.
[http://dx.doi.org/10.2147/CEG.S15872] [PMID: 21694868]

[114] Vandenplas Y. Challenges in the diagnosis of gastroesophageal reflux disease in infants and children. Expert Opin Med Diagn 2013; 7(3): 289-98.
[http://dx.doi.org/10.1517/17530059.2013.789857] [PMID: 23581607]

[115] Quitadamo P, Ummarino D, Staiano A. GER and GERD in children: to treat or not to treat? Minerva Pediatr 2015; 67(2): 187-97.
[PMID: 25645256]

[116] Lightdale JR, Gremse DA. Section on Gastroenterology, Hepatology, and Nutrition. Gastroesophageal reflux: management guidance for the pediatrician Pediatrics 2013; 131(5): e1684-95.
[http://dx.doi.org/10.1542/peds.2013-0421] [PMID: 23629618]

[117] Maalej S, Drira I, Fennira H, *et al.* Idiopathic pulmonary hemosiderosis in adults. Rev Pneumol Clin 2005; 61(2): 109-1.
[http://dx.doi.org/RPC-03-2005-61-2-0761-8417-101019-200513950] [PMID: 16012364]

[118] Willms H, Gutjahr K, Juergens UR, *et al.* Diagnostics and therapy of idiopathic pulmonary hemosiderosis. Med Klin (Munich) 2007; 15(102(6)): 445-50.
[PMID: 17571219]

[119] Aceti A, Sciutti R, Bracci PR, Bertelli L, Melchionda F, Cazzato S. Idiopathic pulmonary haemosiderosis in a child with Down's syndrome: case report and review of the literature. Sarcoidosis Vasc Diffuse Lung Dis 2012; 29(1): 58-61.

[PMID: 23311126]

[120] Niimi A, Amitani R, Kurasawa T, *et al.* [Two cases of idiopathic pulmonary hemosiderosis: analysis of chest CT findings]. Nihon Kyobu Shikkan Gakkai Zasshi 1992; 30(9): 1749-55.
[PMID: 1447853]

[121] Galant S, Nussbaum E, Wittner R, DeWeck AL, Heiner DC. Increased IgD milk antibody responses in a patient with Down's syndrome, pulmonary hemosiderosis and cor pulmonale. Ann Allergy 1983; 51(4): 446-9.
[PMID: 6226218]

[122] Airaghi L, Ciceri L, Giannini S, Ferrero S, Meroni PL, Tedeschi A. Idiopathic pulmonary hemosiderosis in an adult. Favourable response to azathioprine. Monaldi Arch Chest Dis 2001; 56(3): 211-3.
[PMID: 11665500]

[123] Mu XD, Su L, Nie LG, Na J, Wang RG, Li HC. Idiopathic pulmonary hemosiderosis in adults: report of two cases and literature review. Monaldi Arch Chest Dis 2001; 56(3): 211-3.
[PMID: 23311126]

[124] McDowell KM, Craven DI. Pulmonary complications of Down syndrome during childhood. J Pediatr 2011; 158(2): 319-25.
[http://dx.doi.org/10.1016/j.jpeds.2010.07.023] [PMID: 20846671]

[125] Schieve LA, Boulet SL, Boyle C, Rasmussen SA, Schendel D. Health of children 3 to 17 years of age with Down syndrome in the 1997-2005 national health interview survey. Pediatrics 2009; 123(2): e253-60.
[http://dx.doi.org/10.1542/peds.2008-1440] [PMID: 19171577]

[126] Bloemers BL, van Furth AM, Weijerman ME, *et al.* High incidence of recurrent wheeze in children with down syndrome with and without previous respiratory syncytial virus lower respiratory tract infection. Pediatr Infect Dis J 2010; 29(1): 39-42.
[http://dx.doi.org/10.1097/INF.0b013e3181b34e52] [PMID: 19907362]

[127] Weijerman ME, de Winter JP. Clinical practice. The care of children with Down syndrome. Eur J Pediatr 2010; 169(12): 1445-52.
[http://dx.doi.org/10.1007/s00431-010-1253-0] [PMID: 20632187]

[128] Mannan SE, Yousef E, Hossain J. Prevalence of positive skin prick test results in children with Down syndrome: a case-control study. Ann Allergy Asthma Immunol 2009; 102(3): 205-9.
[http://dx.doi.org/10.1016/S1081-1206(10)60082-8] [PMID: 19354066]

[129] de Miguel-Díez J, Villa-Asensi JR, Alvarez-Sala JL. Prevalence of sleep-disordered breathing in children with Down syndrome: polygraphic findings in 108 children. Sleep 2003; 15(26(8)): 1006-9.
[PMID: 14746382]

[130] Levanon A, Tarasiuk A, Tal A. Sleep characteristics in children with Down syndrome. J Pediatr 1999; 134(6): 755-60.
[http://dx.doi.org/10.1016/S0022-3476(99)70293-3] [PMID: 10356146]

[131] Nisbet LC, Phillips NN, Hoban TF, O'Brien LM. Characterization of a sleep architectural phenotype in children with Down syndrome. Sleep Breath 2014; 12.

[PMID: 25500979]

[132] Hoffmire CA, Magyar CI, Connolly HV, Fernandez ID, van Wijngaarden E. High prevalence of sleep disorders and associated comorbidities in a community sample of children with Down syndrome. J Clin Sleep Med 2014; 15(10(4)): 411-9.
[PMID: 24733987] [http://dx.doi.org/10.5664/jcsm.3618]

[133] Fung E, Witmans M, Ghosh M, Cave D, El-Hakim H. Upper airway findings in children with Down syndrome on sleep nasopharyngoscopy: case-control study. J Otolaryngol Head Neck Surg 2012; 41(2): 138-44.
[PMID: 22569015]

[134] Slaats MA, Van Hoorenbeeck K, Van Eyck A, *et al.* Upper airway imaging in pediatric obstructive sleep apnea syndrome. Sleep Med Rev 2014; 21(pii: S1087-0792 (14)): 00082-3.
[http://dx.doi.org/10.1016/j.smrv.2014.08.001] [PMID: 25438733]

[135] Goffinski A, Stanley MA, Shepherd N, *et al.* Obstructive sleep apnea in young infants with Down syndrome evaluated in a Down syndrome specialty clinic. Am J Med Genet A 2015; 167A(2): 324-30.
[http://dx.doi.org/10.1002/ajmg.a.36903] [PMID: 25604659]

[136] Jensen KM, Sevick CJ, Seewald L, *et al.* Greater Risk of Hospitalization in Children with Down Syndrome and Obstructive Sleep Apnea at Higher Elevation. Chest 2015; 5
[http://dx.doi.org/10.1378/chest.14-1883]

[137] Ng DK, Hui HN, Chan CH, *et al.* Obstructive sleep apnoea in children with Down syndrome. Singapore Med J 2006; 47(9): 774-9.
[PMID: 16924359]

[138] Lin SC, Davey MJ, Horne RS, Nixon GM. Screening for obstructive sleep apnea in children with Down syndrome. J Pediatr 2014; 165(1): 117-22.
[http://dx.doi.org/10.1016/j.jpeds.2014.02.032] [PMID: 24679609]

[139] Nisbet LC, Phillips NN, Hoban TF, O'Brien LM. Effect of body position and sleep state on obstructive sleep apnea severity in children with Down syndrome. J Clin Sleep Med 2014; 15(10(1)): 81-.2014;
[http://dx.doi.org/10.5664/jcsm.3368] [PMID: 24426825]

[140] Chang L, Wu J, Cao L. Combination of symptoms and oxygen desaturation index in predicting childhood obstructive sleep apnea. Int J Pediatr Otorhinolaryngol 2013; 77(3): 365-71.
[http://dx.doi.org/10.1016/j.ijporl.2012.11.028] [PMID: 23246417]

[141] Rosen D. Management of obstructive sleep apnea associated with Down syndrome and other craniofacial dysmorphologies. Curr Opin Pulm Med 2011 Nov ; 17(6): 431-6.
[http://dx.doi.org/10.1097/MCP.0b013e32834ba9c0] [PMID: 21918449]

[142] Rosen D. Some infants with Down syndrome spontaneously outgrow their obstructive sleep apnea. Clin Pediatr (Phila) 2010; 49(11): 1068-71.
[http://dx.doi.org/10.1177/0009922810378037] [PMID: 20724331]

[143] Fernández Julián E. [Surgical treatment of sleep-related breathing disorders in children]. Acta Otorrinolaringol Esp 2010; 61 (Suppl. 1): 53-9.
[http://dx.doi.org/10.1016/S0001-6519(10)71247-4] [PMID: 21354495]

[144] Lefaivre JF, Cohen SR, Burstein FD, *et al.* Down syndrome: identification and surgical management

of obstructive sleep apnea. Plast Reconstr Surg 1997; 99(3): 629-37.
[http://dx.doi.org/10.1097/00006534-199703000-00004] [PMID: 9047180]

[145] International medical review on down'S syndrome. Vaccination schedule for people with Down's syndrome, 2012. Rev Med Int Sindr Down 2011; 15(3): 45-7.
[http://dx.doi.org/10.1016/S2171-9748(11)70015-0]

[146] Andabaka T, Nickerson JW, Rojas-Reyes MX, Rueda JD, Bacic Vrca V, Barsic B. Monoclonal antibody for reducing the risk of respiratory syncytial virus infection in children. Cochrane Database Syst Rev 2013 Apr; 30(4): CD006602.
[http://dx.doi.org/10.1002/14651858.CD006602.pub4]

[147] Yi H, Lanctôt KL, Bont L, *et al.* CARESS investigators. Respiratory syncytial virus prophylaxis in Down syndrome: a prospective cohort study. Pediatrics 2014; 133(6): 1031-7.
[http://dx.doi.org/10.1542/peds.2013-3916] [PMID: 24799541]

[148] Yildirim I, Shea KM, Little BA, *et al.* Vaccination, Underlying Comorbidities, and Risk of Invasive Pneumococcal Disease. Pediatrics 2015; 2(pii: peds.2014-2426)
[http://dx.doi.org/10.1542/peds.2014-2426] [PMID: 25647674]

[149] Costa-Carvalho BT, Martinez RM, Dias AT, *et al.* Antibody response to pneumococcal capsular polysaccharide vaccine in Down syndrome patients. Braz J Med Biol Res 2006; 39(12): 1587-92.
[http://dx.doi.org/10.1590/S0100-879X2006001200010] [PMID: 17160268]

[150] Balmer P, North J, Baxter D, *et al.* Measurement and interpretation of pneumococcal IgG levels for clinical management. Clin Exp Immunol 2003; 133(3): 364-9.
[http://dx.doi.org/10.1046/j.1365-2249.2003.02232.x] [PMID: 12930362]

[151] Joshi AY, Abraham RS, Snyder MR, Boyce TG. Immune evaluation and vaccine responses in Down syndrome: evidence of immunodeficiency? Vaccine 2011 Jul 12; 29(31): 5040-6.
[http://dx.doi.org/10.1016/j.vaccine.2011.04.060] [PMID: 21596078]

[152] Kusters MA, Bok VL, Bolz WE, Huijskens EG, Peeters MF, de Vries E. Influenza A/H1N1 vaccination response is inadequate in down syndrome children when the latest cut-off values are used. Pediatr Infect Dis J 2012; 31(12): 1284-5.
[http://dx.doi.org/10.1097/INF.0b013e3182737410] [PMID: 22986705]

[153] Pérez-Padilla R, Fernández R, García-Sancho C, *et al.* Pandemic (H1N1) 2009 virus and Down syndrome patients. Emerg Infect Dis 2010; 16(8): 1312-4.
[http://dx.doi.org/10.3201/eid1608.091931] [PMID: 20678334]

[154] Ladhani S, Heath PT, Ramsay ME, *et al.* Long-term immunological follow-up of children with haemophilus influenzae serotype b vaccine failure in the United Kingdom Clin Infect Dis 2009; 1(49(3)): 372-80.
[http://dx.doi.org/10.1086/600292] [PMID: 19580418]

[155] Zuccotti GV, Mameli C. Pidotimod: the past and the present. Ital J Pediatr 2013; 6(39:75): 372-80.
[http://dx.doi.org/10.1186/1824-7288-39-75] [PMID: 24314100]

[156] Zuccotti GV, Mameli C, Trabattoni D, *et al.* Immunomodulating activity of Pidotimod in children with Down syndrome. J Biol Regul Homeost Agents 2013; 27(1): 253-8.
[PMID: 23489705]

[157] Licari A, De Amici M, Nigrisoli S, *et al.* Pidotimod may prevent recurrent respiratory infections in children. Minerva Pediatr 2014; 66(5): 363-7.
[PMID: 25253184]

[158] Careddu P. Role of immunoactivation with pidotimod in recurrent respiratory infections in childhood. Arzneimittelforschung 1994; 44(12A): 1506-11.
[PMID: 7857353]

CHAPTER 6

Are Gastrointestinal Disorders of Real Concern in Children with Down Syndrome?

Mohammed Al-Biltagi*

Pediatric Department, Faculty of Medicine, Tanta University, Egypt

Abstract: Down syndrome (DS) is a systemic disorder affecting the whole body including the gastrointestinal (GI) tract; from the oral cavity and ending with the anal canal that are involved in the food digestion absorption and excretion. These disorders could be anatomical or functional. About 10% of children born with DS have one or more forms of the structural abnormalities which may include tracheoesophageal fistula, congenital diaphragmatic hernia, small bowel obstruction, annular pancreas, and anal anomalies. Functional gastrointestinal disturbances include oral, esophageal, gastric and/or intestinal motility dysfunctions leading to feeding difficulties, prolonged feeding duration, dysphagia, gastro-oesophageal reflux disease, increased risk of aspiration, delayed gastric emptying, constipation, Hirschprung's disease and malnutrition with its effects on general health and physical compromise. These functional disturbances may be difficult to treat and may, in sequence, affect the prognosis of corrective surgeries, and hence need more cautions.

Keywords: Anal anomalies, Annular pancreas, Aspiration, Atresia, Congenital diaphragmatic hernia, Constipation, Delayed gastric emptying, Down syndrome, Duodenal stenosis, Dysphagia, Feeding difficulties, Gastroesophageal reflux disease, Gastrointestinal, Hirschprung's disease, Imperforate annus, Malnutrition, Motility dysfunctions, Small bowel obstruction, Tracheoesophageal fistula, Trisomy.

1. INTRODUCTION

Down syndrome is a systemic disorder affecting the whole body including the gastrointestinal (GI) tract which includes wide parts of the body; starting from the oral cavity and ending with the anal canal that are involved in the food

* **Corresponding Author Dr. Mohammed Al-Biltagi:** Pediatric Department, Faculty of Medicine, Tanta University, Egypt; Tel: (+973)39545472; Fax: (+973) 1759 0495; Email: mbelrem@hotmail.com

digestion absorption and excretion. The link between gastrointestinal diseases and DS is well recognized. About 77% of neonates with DS have or will suffer gastrointestinal disorders at one time. It can cause both structural and functional abnormalities of GI tract. Children with DS are more prone to develop these disorders more than in the general population. These abnormalities can appear very early even in the early neonatal period or appear later in life in adulthood. It also can appear as serious and life threatening condition, causing immediate problems in a newborn or appear more slowly and insidious that can be missed by the parents and even the doctors. Children with DS may also develop any of the usual disorders that can be encountered by other children. Even in absence of structural and functional abnormalities of GI tract; children and adults with DS may display gastrointestinal symptoms from time to time such as vomiting, diarrhea, constipation, abdominal pain and discomfort that improve with few or no intervention much as in others. In this chapter we will shed some light on these disorders in children with DS [1].

2. STRUCTURAL ABNORMALITIES

Down syndrome is well known to be associated with gastrointestinal abnormalities and is considered as a probable predisposing state for gut anomalies and congenital heart disease as part of the VATER syndrome. About 10% of children born with DS have one or more form of the structural abnormalities which may include tracheoesophageal fistula, congenital diaphragmatic hernia, small bowel obstruction, annular pancreas, Hirschprung's disease, and anal anomalies. Esophageal atresia is noted more frequently in offspring of younger mothers and Hispanics. Hirschsprung disease is more common in boys and in infants of younger mothers and blacks, while anal stenosis/atresia is present more frequently amongst females and Asians [2]. Because of the complexity of embryonic development of the gastrointestinal (GI) tract, there is an increased risk of developmental abnormality especially in presence of chromosomal and genetic disorders including DS. These abnormalities may be structural or functional and may be complex and multiple with more than one part of the gut affected or other systems involved.

2.1. Tracheoesophageal Fistula and Atresia

Esophageal atresia and tracheoesophageal fistula (EA/TEF) are serious congenital anomalies affecting 1:3500 live births. There are five subtypes of EA/TEF have been described, based on the site of the atresia and the type of anastomosis between trachea and esophagus (Fig. **1**). Fifty percent of the patients have other associated anomalies like cardiovascular, tracheoesophageal, anal, renal, vertebral, and limb abnormalities (occurring together in the VACTERL association). DS is one of the very well studied chromosomal abnormalities that are noted in EA/TEF patients. Surgery is the best treatment; aimed to reconnect the two ends of the baby's esophagus to each other. However, in some children, a big part of the esophagus is missing so that the two ends can't be easily connected. This is known as long-gap esophageal atresia [3].

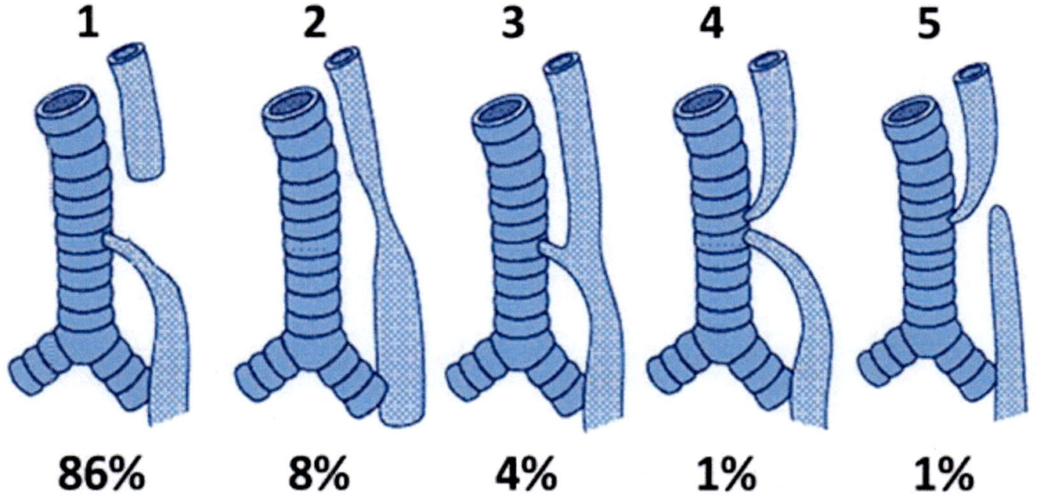

Fig. (1). Shows Different Types of Tracheoesophageal Fistula And Atresia; **1:** Atresia With Distal Fistula Which is The Most Common Type (86%), **2:** Isolated Esophageal Atresia which is The Second Most Common Type (8%), **3:** Isolated Tracheoesophageal Fistula (H type) Which is The Third Most Common Type (4%), **4:** Atresia With Double Fistula Which is a Rare Type (1%) , And **5:** Atresia With Proximal Fistula Which is a Rare Type (1%).

2.2. Congenital Diaphragmatic Hernia

Congenital diaphragmatic hernia (CDH) is an abnormality characterizes by presence of defective part in the diaphragm due to failure of complete closure of the diaphragmatic muscles during the fetal development in utero. Failure of diaphragm to completely separate the chest cavity from the abdominal cavity permits some of the abdominal organs (like stomach, intestines, and even the liver) to move up into the chest cavity through the opening present in the diaphragm. Presence of abdominal organs inside the thoracic cavity diminishes full development of the lungs causing variable degrees of pulmonary hypoplasia and prevents further normal development of the heart. There are two main categories of diaphragmatic hernia; posterolateral Bochdalek hernia and anterior Morgagni hernia (Fig. **2**). Bochdalek hernia is the most common type (85% of cases) and involves an opening on the back of right or left side of the diaphragm where the stomach, intestines and liver or spleen usually raise up into the chest cavity. Bilateral hernias are uncommon and pose very difficult problems. Morgagni hernia is rarer than Bochdalek type (3%), tends to be small and includes a defect in the front of the diaphragm (foramen of Morgagni), just behind the sternum where the liver or intestines may ascend up into the chest cavity. Hiatus hernia is a third type but it is considered as functional rather than a structural in origin and needs repair only if symptoms are severe [4].

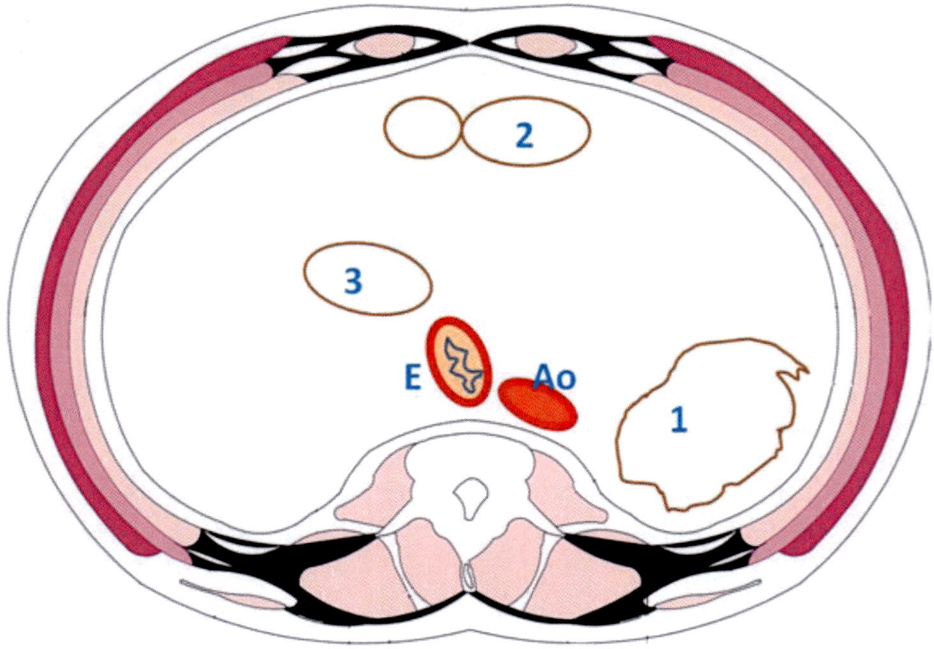

Fig. (2). Showed The 3 Main Types of Congenital Diaphragmatic Hernia; **1:** is The Posterior Bochdalek Hernia (85%), **2:** The Anterior Morgagni Hernia (3%), **3:** Central Type, Ao: Aorta, E; Esophagus.

About one tenth of all cases with CDH have chromosome anomalies. The most frequent associated anomalies are trisomy 18 and isochromosome 12p. Though infants with DS may have either Bochdalek or Morgagni hernia, generally the frequency of CDH in DS appears to be low. Morgagni hernias are more frequently described than Bochdalek hernias, signifying that it is the most frequent type of CDH among individuals with DS [5]. Morgagni hernias frequently manifests with recurrent chest infection and has a high rate of associated anomalies, commonly congenital heart diseases [6].The age of presentation differs from neonatal age till the age of 12 years. The way of presentation varied from being asymptomatic and discovered accidentally during routine examination to presentation with respiratory distress. Isolated case report of retroperitoneal teratoma in a person with DS and Morgagni hernia had also been described. Fascinatingly, identical twins of DS with the same congenital heart disease and Morgagni hernia have been described [7].

Despite those children with DS constitute only few numbers of patients with Morgagni hernia; a genetic component to Morgagni hernia may be suggested. This significant relationship between the hernia of Morgagni and trisomy 21 may be a sign of imperfect dorsoventral migration of rhabdomyoblasts from the paraxial myotomes, due to the increased cellular adhesiveness in DS [8]. Prenatal anticipation of Morgagni hernias can be done when the by antenatal ultrasound detect presence of polyhydramnios, and presence of abdominal organs in the thoracic cavity. Increased thickness of nuchal translucency (NT) in presence of CDH is associated with a bad prognosis and is linked to an early intrathoracic compression [9]. The diagnosis of Morgagni hernias may be strikingly delayed when associated with DS or other severe congenital anomalies. It should be strongly considered in patients with DS who presented with repeated chest infections. In general; children with DS who presented with respiratory distress or chest deformity, diaphragmatic hernia should be considered as a potential reason of respiratory distress and chest deformity besides congenital heart disease and pulmonary reasons. Chest x-rays in 2 planes may help in its diagnosis. Previously normal chest x-ray should not preclude the diagnosis of Morgagni's hernia even when bilateral. The diagnosis is more difficult in cases of bilateral Morgagni hernias especially if one of the hernial sacs is empty. CT scan is of great help in diagnosis of bilateral hernias. Both open and laparoscopic methods have proven satisfactory as operative treatment of Morgagni hernias. Trans-abdominal approach is preferred in bilateral cases because it allows simple reduction, proper inspection of contents, easy access and repair of bilateral hernias, and adequate correction of accompanied malrotation if present. Recurrences were seen in patients with DS, which may be corrected by laparotomy or laparoscopically [10, 11].

2.3. Small Bowel Obstruction

Small bowel obstruction is a common disorder in newborns, infants and children with DS; congenital duodenal obstruction is the most common form. Internal duodenal obstruction is coupled with other major congenital gastrointestinal anomalies in about 38-55% of patients such as intestinal malrotation and preduodenal portal vein, esophageal atresia, and different types of imperforate anus. Renal anomalies and other combinations of anomalies such as VATER/ VACTERALS may also present. Despite superior mesenteric artery syndrome is a very uncommon disorder in childhood; but it most frequently results in duodenal obstruction in the adulthood. Chromosomal anomalies, mainly DS, is found in about 15-27% of affected patients [12, 13].

Intestinal obstruction can be either complete or partial. In complete obstruction, part of the bowel has failed to develop completely (duodenal or jejunal atresia) while in partial obstruction, the bowel has developed partially where is narrower than it should be (duodenal stenosis) or there is a membrane (web-like) compromising the lumen (Fig. **3**). The most common site of intestinal obstruction due to duodenal web is the second part of duodenum (85% - 90%); followed by the third part (20%) and lastly by the fourth part (10%). The duodenum is also the most common site for small intestine stenosis and atresia; while the ileum is the least affected. However, these birth defects can affect multiple sites of the intestine. The pancreas can also obstruct the intestine if it encircles the duodenum causing narrowing or blockage (as in case of annular pancreas) [14].

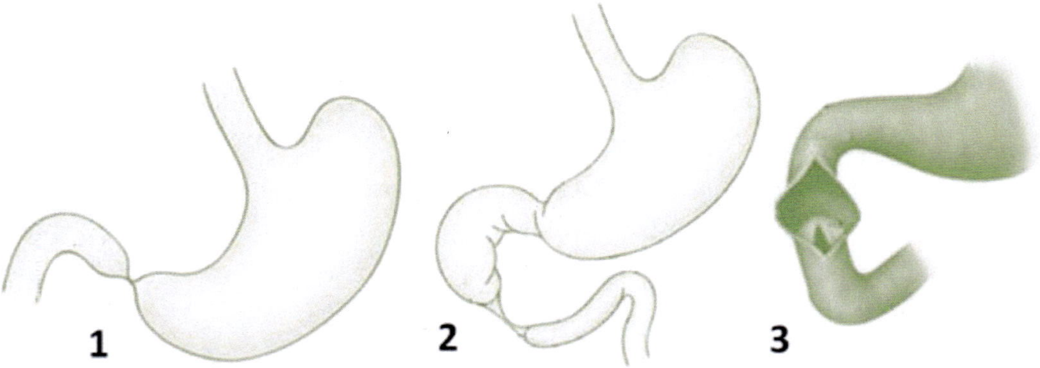

Fig. (3). Shows Different Types of Gastrointestinal Obstruction; **1:** Pyloric Stenosis, **2:** Duodenal Atresia, **3:** Duodenal web.

Obstructive symptoms of duodenal stenosis or atresia usually appear early in infancy and the primary diagnosis is usually done in the neonatal period. There is a frequent history of polyhydramnios, feeding difficulties, and emesis which could be bilious in severe obstruction. Antenatal expectation of the disease can be there; if there is polyhydramnios, dilated bowel, ascites, or a combination. Antenatal ultrasound can diagnose the condition. In less severe degrees of obstruction, the diagnosis can be made by late childhood. The children may have intermittent, repeated bilious vomiting, with distension of the upper abdomen. Sometimes they have also postprandial right upper quadrant abdominal pain. However, presence of the associated mental retardation observed in children with DS may delay the perception of such symptoms which could be overlooked because of the associated mental and physical retardation [15]. Plain X-ray of the abdomen shows dilatation of the duodenum while contrast studies show impaired transit of contrast media with a filling defect in the second part of the duodenum in an infant or child with repeated prolonged vomiting. Flexible endoscopy can discover over distension of the duodenum, projection of the duodenal web and, if any, the mucosal diaphragm in the stenotic lumen of the duodenum [13].

Treatment is generally surgical. This involves removing the obstructed part of the bowel and then connecting it up again. It is a major surgical operation, but it is essential for surviving of most the affected babies. In a few number of milder cases; the obstruction can he managed without surgery *via* dietary modification.

Duodeno-duodenostomy is the treatment of choice for cases with either duodenal stenosis or atresia while exploratory laparotomy is needed for a second web at the time of the surgery. Associated anomalies in children with DS (such as cardiac defects, anorectal defects or tracheoesophageal defects) may need multiple staged operations and carry greater intraoperative and postoperative morbidity and mortality risks. Children with DS who have intestinal stenosis have a higher long-term mortality rate than the non-syndromic children [12, 13].

2.4. Annular Pancreas

Annular pancreas is rare condition but it occurs comparatively more frequent in children with DS than non-syndromic children. About one fourth of annular pancreas cases occur in DS patients. In annular pancreas, there is a thin band of normal pancreatic tissue surrounded the second part of the duodenum either completely or partially due to abnormal rotation of the ventral primordium. There are two types; complete and partial or incomplete. In complete annular pancreas, the pancreatic tissue or annular duct is surrounding the 2nd part of duodenum completely (Fig. **4**); while in incomplete type; the annulus does not surround the duodenum completely, giving a 'crocodile jaw' appearance. It is commonly associated with other anomalies in more than two thirds of cases including gut malrotation, intrinsic duodenal obstruction, and duodenal bands. It is more common in girls and women and the presentation can be in the first postnatal life or delayed till the fourth decade of life [16].

Recently, antenatal diagnosis and advances in imaging have led to increased experience with this condition. The antenatal 2-D ultrasound examination in the 2nd trimester is a good method for screening and accurate diagnosis of annular pancreas. Annular pancreas can be suspected if there is double bubble sign. Other signs include hyperechogenic bands around the duodenum [17]. Vomiting is the most common presenting symptom of annular pancreas. Delayed presentation may occur in adult with recurrent postprandial right upper abdominal pain, sometimes associated with abdominal vomiting, pancreatitis, or abnormal liver tests. Computerized tomography can show the pancreatic tissue surrounding the 2nd part of duodenum either completely or incompletely. It also can show the accompanied duodenal narrowing and dilatation of proximal duodenum.

MRI/MRCP (Magnetic Resonance Cholangiopancreatography) can assess pancreatic ductal anatomy better [15]. Children are more likely to require surgery because of the increased frequency of associated anomalies. They can be managed with duodenal bypass. Close long-term follow-up is essential for infants treated for annular pancreas because many of them can be expected to develop complications, even if the initial postoperative period is uncomplicated and survival is excellent [18].

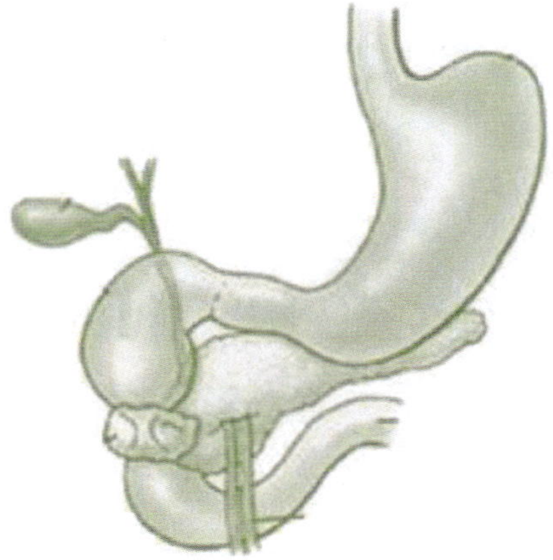

Fig. (4). Showed complete form of annular pancreas where pancreatic parenchyma completely surround the 2nd part of duodenum.

2.5. Imperforate Annus

Patients with DS have a higher incidence of anorectal malformation than non-syndromic patients. Anorectal anomalies include broad spectrum of anatomical abnormalities, affect both sexes, involve the distal anus and rectum as well as the urinary and genital tracts and are frequently hard to assess. The incidence of these anomalies is approximately 1/5000 live births. The anomaly may be very minor and easily to be treated with outstanding functional outcome, or may be complex, hard to handle, frequently associated with other anomalies, and have a poor functional outcome [19]. These anomalies can also be classified according to the level of termination of the rectum in relation to the pubococcygeal and ischiatic lines into high, intermediate, and low types. The low anorectal malformation with or without a fistula is generally the type encountered in DS children (Fig. **5**).

However, the mechanism of inheritance of these malformations and its genetic relation with DS is still unknown, despite the association (Anorectal malformation-Down's syndrome) appears not to be by chance. So; this specific benign type of defects can be expected to occur in most patients with DS [20].

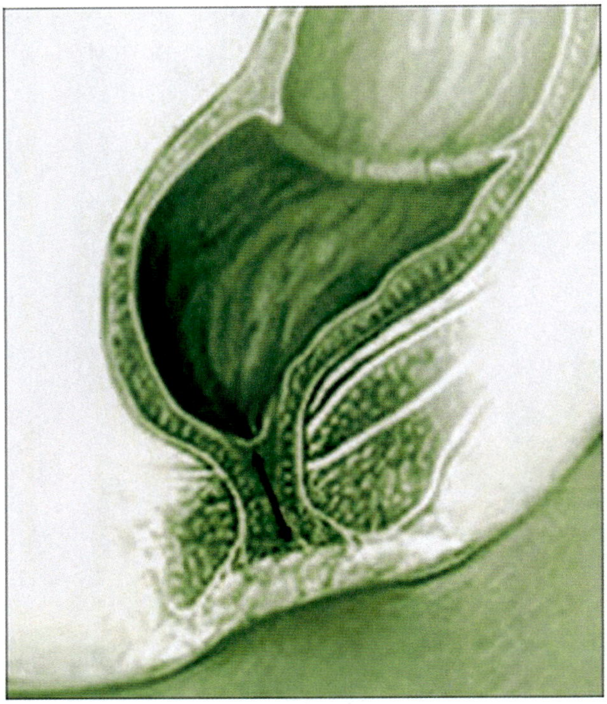

Fig. (5). Shows imperforate anus: there are 3 types; high, intermediate, and low types.

Imperforate anus without fistula is a rare anorectal malformation and is accompanied by DS in 50% of cases. This anomaly is described as absence of annus, with a blind rectal pouch, located about 2 cm above perineal skin, has a common wall with the urethra or vagina and is accompanied with a higher rate of other congenital disorders. A colostrogram done before the ultimate surgical repair is imperative; together with consideration of the intraopetative findings (height and diameter of rectal pouch). The incidence of post-operative anal prolapse is very high and may be precipitated by presence of hypotonia characteristic to children with DS. Association of DS in cases of anorectal malformations should not be considered as a contraindication to for surgical repairing of the imperforate anus and to closing the colostomy. Strict postoperative follow up is needed with early and adequate controlling of post-operative constipation which is usually very severe [21, 22].

3. FUNCTIONAL DISORDERS

Children with DS are associated with different types of functional gastrointestinal disturbances including oral, esophageal, gastric and intestinal motility problems causing feeding difficulties, increase risk of aspiration, prolonged feeding duration, constipation and malnutrition with its physical sequelae. Dysfunction of the foregut motility results in several problems such as dysphagia from oesophageal dysmotility, gastro-oesophageal reflux disease, and prolonged gastric emptying time. Also, there is high rate of developing constipation and Hirschsprung disease. These functional disturbances may be difficult to treat and may, in sequence, affect the prognosis of corrective surgeries, and hence need more cautions [23].

These functional impairment is related to occurrence of both micro-anatomy and functional impairment of the enteric nervous system. The abnormal brain development, function and the consequential intellectual impairment associated with DS may result from the genetic imbalance induced by the trisomy of chromosome 21. Functional esophageal and colonic motility disorders are not rare. It could be either congenital or acquired. The most famous of these disorders are esophageal dysmotility syndromes (*e.g.* achalasia, gastroesophageal reflux, dysphagia) and chronic constipation. Hirschsprung's disease occurs in about 2-15% of cases with DS as chromosome 21 itself; is considered as a site of a gene modifier for Hirschsprung's disease. Lately; well recognized candidate genetic mechanisms supply distinctive insight into the genetic bases of the neurological and cognitive problems associated with DS. Although the role of the triplicated chromosome 21 and genetic dosage imbalance stay important, the extra functions of other chromosome 21 genes in the pathogenesis of the enteric nervous system developmental anomalies remains uncertain and needs further studies [24].

3.1. Feeding Difficulties

Children with DS are suffering from different degrees of feeding difficulties. These difficulties could be a real challenge and a source of stress for children and parents alike. Children with genetic disorders like DS commonly have feeding disorders and swallowing dysfunction as a result of complex interplays between structural, medical, functional, physiological, and behavioral factors. Feeding problems accompanying these genetic disorders may also result in feeding to be distasteful, negative, or even painful and hard experience for both the child and his family because of repeated choking, coughing, gagging, fatigue, or emesis, enforcing the child to withhold eating and to develop undesired behaviors that make it more difficult, if not impossible. This is coupled with the limited experiences about dealing with problems of oral intake associated with the medical or physical conditions, frequently associated with DS such as prematurity, which often impair the normal development of the child's oral motor skills. Neuromotor coordination impairments associated with DS (*e.g.* hypotonia, poor tongue control, and open mouth posture) often hinder gaining of efficient and adequate oral-motor skills and results in feeding difficulties [25].

Besides lagging of development of oral-motor function in children with DS behind intellectual development, it also tracks a deviant path. In particular, specific aspects of There are impairments of tongue and jaw functions together with problems beginning and maintaining a smooth series of feeding actions due to the impact of functional and anatomical characteristics of DS on oral health and feeding abilities. Orofacial dysfunction is also caused by the reduced neuromotor control, muscle weakness, dental abnormalities, dysmorphology and associated systemic illness. This orofacial dysfunction impairs feeding and swallowing in particular [26].

At the same time, the parent-child interactions tend to be more controlling as well as the parents of DS children do not spontaneously report the extent of their child's feeding problems except when specific question arises, especially if accompanied by observation of feeding [27]. Meanwhile, children with DS are more liable for increased frequency of respiratory problems which can seriously affect the feeding and swallowing capabilities and sequentially the feeding and swallowing skills can affect respiration [28]. Poor airway protection during swallowing has serious impacts on the infant's respiratory status as result of chronic aspiration during feeding and may provoke recurrent respiratory illness, pneumonia, and lung damage [29].

Management of these feeding disorders depends on an incorporated approach to ensure safety of a practical feeding program which maintains the optimal growth of the child. One of these approaches is behavioral therapy of the feeding disorders. It includes manipulations in the presentation of foods and drink and consequences for food refusal and acceptance (*e.g.* praise, extinction, contingent access to preferred foods). Multidisciplinary team is usually needed because the child feeding inability is multifactorial. This interdisciplinary team usually consists of a behavioral psychologist, pediatric gastroenterologist, speech pathologist, nutrition, and sometimes other specialties [25].

3.2. Gastro-Esophageal Reflux Disease

GERD is one of the commonest esophageal motility disorders observed in DS and is frequently undervalued and overlooked. About 45% of the GERD-related complications occur in patients with DS specially those related to oropharyngeal aspiration that can cause pneumonia and aspiration syndromes which are frequently occur in patients with neurological dysphagia, such as DS [24, 30].

GERD is a status that occurs when reflux of stomach contents causes bothering symptoms and/or complications. Symptoms differ by age and are bothersome when they have side effect(s) on the health of children (Fig. **6**). Asymptomatic reflux or bilious vomiting should not be mistaken with GERD. However, the classic manifestations of GERD are hard to be assessed in neurologically inadequate children who lack adequate cognitive ability that enable them to report symptoms. GERD may manifest also with complications like esophagitis, hemorrhage, stricture, Barrett's esophagus and even adenocarcinoma [31, 32].

Children with neurodevelopmental disabilities such as DS have increased incidence of GERD compared with neurologically intact children. They often fail to respond to medical treatment and may necessitate surgical treatment [23]. They frequently have uncommon symptoms of this condition. However, a high index of doubt is required to discover hidden GERD and early discover it early complications [33]. Patients with DS may have primary and secondary esophageal motility disorders, for unknown causes. They may have repeated esophageal symptoms and/or atypical manifestations such as food rejection, repeated vomiting, coughing, and failure to thrive and they should be evaluated for esophageal function. Early diagnosis and management of esophageal functional disorders is essential to prevent respiratory problems, growth retardation in children, weight loss in adults, and to set up the correct type of surgery if needed [34].

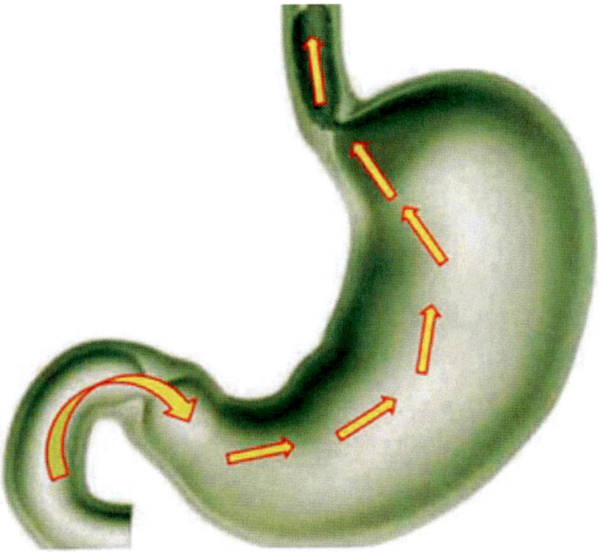

Fig. (6). Show passage of the food and acid back up into the esophagus from the stomach in GERD.

Confirmation of presence of GERD can be done by different diagnostic techniques. However; 24-hour pH-metry remain the gold standard to diagnose GERD. Radiography and pulmonary scintiscan can help to identify presence of aspiration which is a frequent association with GERD. Barium contrast study of upper gastrointestinal tract is also helpful to identify presence of hiatus hernia, strictures, swallowing disturbances, the motility of esophagus and stomach and to rule out anatomical anomalies. Gastroscopy is useful in identifying reflux esophagitis and biopsies can be obtained to assess its severity. Esophageal manometry is helpful to detect motor esophageal disorders (especially in neurologically impaired patients) and the competence of the lower esophageal sphincter [35]. Lifestyle changes are highlighted as first-line therapy in both GER and GERD, whereas medications are clearly indicated only for patients with GERD. Surgical therapies are reserved for children with intractable symptoms or who are at risk for life-threatening complications of GERD [36].

3.3. Achalasia

Achalasia is a rare primary oesophageal motility disorder that presents as a functional obstruction at the oesophago-gastric junction with an estimated prevalence of eight per 100,000 people. The prevalence of achalasia in DS is much higher (3.4%), which implies a unique association between these two uncommon conditions. Although the exact etiology of achalasia is unknown, studies have proposed that its pathogenesis is related to autoimmune, infectious or genetic factors, leading to the intrinsic loss of inhibitory myenteric neurons in both the oesophagus and lower oesophageal sphincter (Fig. 7).

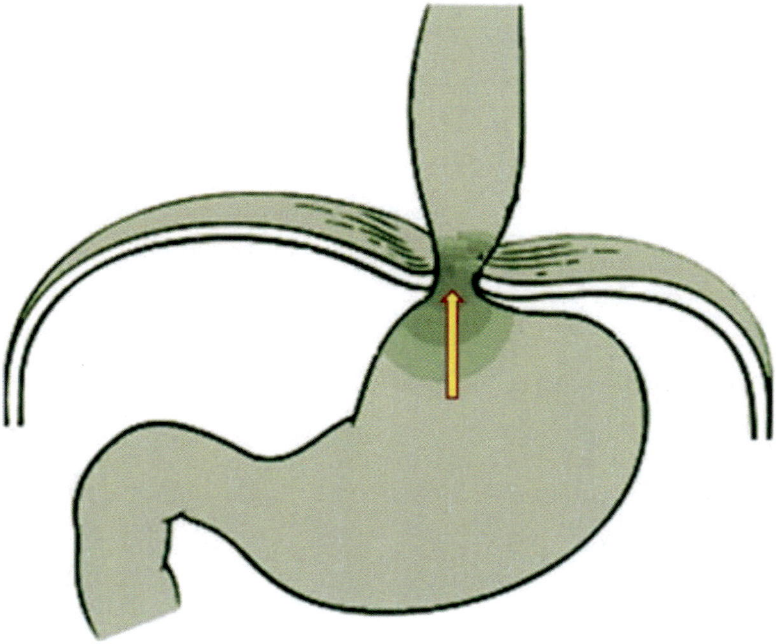

Fig. (7). Shows failure of the lower esophagus to relax with swallowing.

The mechanism of achalasia in DS is related to the genetic imbalance present in DS that result in abnormal development of the nervous system, including that of the gut (enteric), which may be due to decreased neuronal migration or abnormal dendritic development. Autoimmunity is another possible mechanism. The aberrant immune response in DS, which is responsible for increased risk of infection, may also be a causal factor in the pathogenesis of achalasia, as certain viruses such as varicella-zoster and measles viruses have previously been implicated in the etiology of achalasia [24, 34, 37].

3.4. Dysphagia

Difficult swallowing (dysphagia) has similar presentations in both children and adults. Infants and children with particular developmental and/or medical circumstances are at more risk to have dysphagia than normally developed infants and children. The structural and physiological characteristics of DS have direct effects on oral health causing orofacial dysfunctions together with impaired feeding and swallowing. These abnormalities that increase the risk of dysphagia in DS include presence of macroglossia, hypotonia, small oral mechanism, and tongue protrusion. Pharyngeal dysphagia is common and more persistent in children with DS and should be routinely explored especially in patients with a tracheotomy or significant neurologic delays who are more likely to have worsening or prolonged pharyngeal dysphagia [38]. If left untreated, it can result in aspiration pneumonias, gastroesophageal reflux, and/or the incapability to set up and sustain appropriate nutrition and hydration in infants and children with failure to thrive. Aspiration can be expected by presence of coughing with swallowing, postprandial wheezing, laryngeal gurgling and recurrent pneumonia. Early recognition of dysphagia in those children is essential to avoid or reduce complications [39].

The main purposes of managing DS dysphagic child are to improve and preserve satisfactory nutrition for good health and growth and to avoid further complications related to food aspiration into the lungs. Because most of these aims can be done at home, it is essential to encourage a family-centered approach as a part of the treatment strategies. The family should be educated about the different approaches for oral feeding, how to prepare various and nutritious meals, how to position the child whilst feeding, how to determine progression of the child's swallowing skills, the positive interactive behaviors and the accessibility of adaptive equipment. Various technical approaches are planned to prevent the development of orofacial dysfunction in DS. One of these approaches is early myofunctional therapy coupled with appliance wear. These approaches showed promising successful over the long term when multidisciplinary management is possible [40].

3.5. Constipation

Constipation is passage of hard or thick hard or pellet-like, pasty stools with discomfort and frequency less than 3 times per week. It is mainly due to decrease water content of the stool or due to stasis of the stool in the rectum which allow absorption of water from the stool by the colonic mucosa. Low muscle tone and decreased motor activity are two important factors exist in children with DS predisposing them to have constipation. The two factors do not allow adequate pressure to develop inside the abdominal cavity when the child tries to pass a motion. This causes stagnation of the stool in the colon for longer time leading to loss of water from the stool. Other clinical conditions commonly present in children with DS predisposing them to have constipation; include are food allergy, Hirschsprung disease, Celiac Disease, and hypothyroidism [41, 42].

Constipation is in addition one of the cardinal features of hypothyroidism which is a frequent comorbid condition in DS. Because the manifestations of hypothyroidism can be overlooked in children with DS, a regular thyroid function testing is advised every 1-2 years, even if the child is asymptomatic and growing well. If Hirschsprung disease, Celiac Disease, and hypothyroidism are excluded; the caregivers and physicians should work together to explore safe laxative medications. Chronic constipation can induce incontinence of the bladder, nausea, vomiting, lack of appetite and abdominal distension. Untreated constipation can lead to rectal fissures, fecal impaction; and stretching of the rectum causing loss of the urge sensation to evacuate the bowel. Chronic constipation is also linked to a poor immune system. High fiber diet has an important role to prevent constipation. It is advisable to substitute refined grains and grain products, such as white flour, white rice, and white pasta with whole-grain equivalents, and promote the child to eat more fruit and vegetables. In some situations; the cause of constipation is related to behavioral concerns. Developmental-behavioral specialist can provide help to overcome these situations [43].

3.6. Hirschsprung's Disease "Aganglionic Megacolon"

DS is the most common chromosomal anomaly associated with Hirschsprung's disease (HD). The association of HD with DS is well-recognized with an incidence of 2-10%. It is an anomaly of the lower part of the large intestine due to abnormal innervations of the bowel wall with missing nerve cells which impairs the normal work of pushing stools along to the anus, producing constipation (Fig. **8**). Occasionally, there is abnormal innervation of a long segment of bowel wall which usually gives early manifestations during the neonatal period and the newborn does not pass any stools. The children with affected long segments may present with chronic constipation, distended abdomen, vomiting, and ultimately poor weight gain. However, cases with short segmented are less symptomatic and could be overlooked as a case of simple constipation; so that it is imperative to think about the possibility of short segment Hirschprung's disease in any child with persistent constipation despite dietary measures and simple laxatives [44]. The diagnosis once suspected could be confirmed by plain abdominal radiograph, contrast enema radiographs of the colon, anal manometry, and biopsy of the bowel. The plain x-ray can show a dilated small intestines or proximal colon while contrast enema can show dilatation of proximal portion of the colon with non-dilated diseased segment with a "transition zone" (the point where the normal bowel becomes aganglionic) may be visible. However, certain precaution should be in mind with the contrast enema. It could be normal in the first 3 months of life, till the colon start to dilate. Also, it should be avoided if enterocolitis is suspected because of the increased risk of inducing perforation. Anal manometry (balloon distention of the rectum) reveals absence of the internal anal sphincter relaxation upon rectal distention. Contrast enema and anal manometry are nearly equal in sensitivity and specificity. Rectal suction biopsy may reveal absence of ganglion cells and the presence of hypertrophic nerve trunks [45].

Treatment usually includes surgical removal of the affected abnormal part of the bowel. Occasionally it is essential to let the remaining lower part of the bowel 'rest' by using a colostomy. Association of DS with Hirschprung's disease results in poorer prognosis and outcomes regarding the postoperative complications, continence and mortality. Compared to Non-DS children, children with DS have significantly increased incidence of postoperative complications and a longer hospitalization. A large number of patients with DS continue to have persistent bowel dysfunction after surgical treatment of HD. During the post-operative period; long-term follow-up of those patients with DS have suffering from severe constipation. They also have increased incidence of postoperative enterocolitis. Coexistence of HD and DS is associated with increased rates of pre-/postoperative enterocolitis, poorer functional outcomes and increased mortality [46].

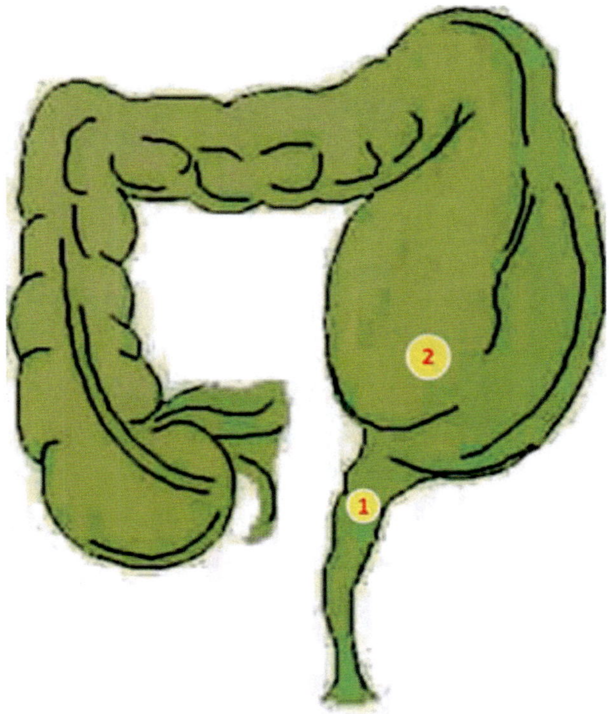

Fig. (8). Shows hirschsprung's disease, where certain nerve cells (Ganglion Cells) in a portion of the colon are missing. The figure shows shrunken rectum which lacks ganglion nerve cells (1), causing swelling in the area above it (2).

3.7. Malabsorption Syndrome

Many children with DS suffer from malabsorption, celiac disease and lactose intolerance; which contribute to increased health risks from other associated diseases as cardiovascular and respiratory problems. Other causes of malabsorption may be due to pancreatic deficiency, reduced intestinal absorptive ability, hypochlorhydria, food allergies or other causes. Insufficient digestive action in the stomach is observed in some cases with DS. The malabsorption-induced chronic malnutrition could result in the neuropathologic signs of Alzheimer's disease which usually start to appear at or slightly earlier than the fourth decade in all patients with DS [47].

3.7.1. Celiac Disease (CD)

Celiac disease (CD) is a chronic autoimmune induced permanent intolerance to gluten that occurs in genetically predisposed persons when gluten, a major protein found in wheat, barley, and rye is given in the diet. It is characterized by polygenic predisposition with the human leukocyte antigen (HLA) locus as the leading genetic element. It has an autoimmune nature. It is predominantly asymptomatic or has atypical clinical course. It has also a tendency of high frequency in patients with DS and some other diseases. It is an inflammatory enteropathy causing atrophy of the small bowel mucosa and villi, resulting in nutrients malabsorption, muscle wasting, and chronic diarrhea which are the classical or typical symptoms of CD. It affects up to 1% of the population with high prevalence in DS patients being reported in several countries. The risk of having CD in individuals with DS is about six-fold than that of non-DS persons [48, 49]. This association between CD and DS is not fully unknown, and the variability of CD frequency in different populations of DS patients, is not fully understood. The prevalence of celiac disease in DS, ranging from 4 to 5% which is much higher than the prevalence of the disease in the general population and thus a connection can thus be suggested between the presence of DS and the occurrence of CD in an individual [50, 51].

Classically, CD is characterized by manifestations of malabsorption syndrome like chronic diarrhea, passage of large massive stools, steatorrhea, excess flatus, bloating, weight loss, short stature, failure to thrive, fatigue, and personality changes. Diarrhea occurs because of anti-gliadin antibody damage sustained by the intestines. However, most cases are asymptomatic or present with mild and non-specific, which makes the diagnosis difficult especially in children with DS and other co-morbid conditions. Also; the subtle symptoms of the disease can overlap with the natural history of DS [52].

Physical examination may reveal presence of emaciation, pallor, hypotension, edema, dermatitis herpetiformis, easy bruising, changes related bone, skin and/or mucous membrane due to the associated vitamin deficiencies, abdominal protrusion or distension due to intestinal motility dysfunction, and loss of different sensations in extremities including vibration, position and light touch due to associated vitamin deficiencies. Signs of severe vitamin/mineral deficiencies may include deep tendon hyporeflexia, muscle spasms (due to magnesium and/or calcium deficiency), bone tenderness and bone pain (due to osteomalacia) and/or gluten ataxia [53].

Early diagnosis and detection of CD is required to prevent various complications, and even malignancy which may develop in long-term persistence of untreated CD. Small bowel biopsy is the gold standard for the diagnosis of CD [54]. There is no consistency in standardization of the current serological tests. *Celiac Blood Panel or Cascade* is a group of serological tests which aid the physician in diagnosis. The tests may consist of, but not restricted to: Immunoglobulin A anti-endomysium antibodies (EMA), IgA anti-gliadin antibodies (AGA), IgG anti-gliadin antibodies (AGA), Deamidated gliadin peptide antibody (DGP), and IgA anti-tissue transglutaminase (tTGA). Deamidated gliadin peptide (DGP) antibodies tests in combination with Tissue transglutaminase (TTG) antibodies have enhanced diagnostic accuracy than the usual gliadin antibodies. Multiplex immunoassay (MIA) is a diagnostic test able to measure multiple antibodies at the same time. It provides accurate diagnosis with reduced turnaround time and cost. Combination testing helps to identify patients who need intestinal biopsy. Test panels include AGA to decide if a person's body makes adequate IgA antibodies for the EMA and TTG results to be trustworthy. IgA deficiency is, in itself not harmful. These diagnostic tests must be done before restricting gluten, to make sure the most correct diagnosis [55]. In asymptomatic cases of CD, a high rate of positive antiendomysial antibodies may propose presence of hidden CD that is evident with immunologic markers but not yet with clinical symptoms. Screening of CD can be expected by presence of high levels of Anti-Tissue Transglutaminase Antibodies in DS Population [56].

Presence of low hemoglobin is an important risk factor, so all children with DS, particularly those with anemia should be screened for celiac disease [57]. CD should be considered in all cases of sideropenic anaemia not responding to iron oral therapy in children with DS. In this situation; the treatment of sideropenic anaemia and its complications, alongside iron preparations, also needs compliance with a gluten-free diet [58].

The treatment is mainly based on total lifelong avoidance of gluten intake and the foods that contain gluten as wheat, rye, and barley. The symptoms usually resolve within a few weeks from starting gluten-free diet with normalization of nutritional status, enhancement of growth rate in both weight and height (with resultant normal stature), and correction of hematological and biochemical parameters [59].

3.7.2. Lactose Intolerance

Lactose malabsorption (LM) is characterized by inability to break down lactose into glucose and galactose, due to deficiency of mucosal lactase in the small intestine. As a result, lactose accumulates in the colon. The colonic bacteria break lactose down to short-chain fatty acids, CO_2, and H_2 which cause bloating, cramps, osmotic diarrhea, and other symptoms of irritable bowel syndrome. These can be seen in about 50% of lactose malabsorbers. Ethnic and geographic variations of LM are known. LM is common in regions that traditionally consume low amounts of milk, such as Asia, South America and Africa [60]. Many studies showed increased frequency of lactose intolerance among children with DS [61]. Diagnosis of lactose intolerance depends mainly on the clinical grounds and the response to dietary lactose restriction. Assessment of lactose malabsorption can be done using lactose breath hydrogen test and by direct assessment of lactase enzyme activity performed on small intestinal tissue biopsy samples [62].

Lactose malabsorption may play a pivotal role in worsening of the mental functions. This is especially important in DS children who already have some degree of mental impairment. In lactose malabsorption; high intestinal lactose contents may impair L-tryptophan metabolism and hence affect 5-hydroxytryptamine (serotonin) availability. Lactose malabsorption should be thought-out in patients with signs of mental impairment [63]. Lactose intolerance can be treated with various therapeutic approaches including lactose-reduced diet and enzyme replacement. The response to multiple enzyme replacement may help to guide the rational dietary management; however, the clinical efficacy of this approach needs more studies [64].

3.7.3. Toddler Diarrhea

Toddler diarrhea occurs when a young child passes several loose stools/day while he has otherwise good health status with excellent growth and normal examination. Toddler diarrhea may occur in children with DS during treatment of constipation due to excessive intake of fruit juice and undigested vegetable matter in an attempt to overcome constipation. It is important to exclude any underlying medical problem, and then assure the parents and involve dieticians in management of these children. If reducing the amount of taken fruit juice did not succeed to stop diarrhea; decreasing dietary fibers may be helpful. On the other hand; Calogen which is along chain triglyceride dietary supplement showed significant ability to reduce the bulk of stooling in a significant portion of affected children [65].

3.8. Autoimmune Gastrointestinal Disorders

DS has been associated with several gastrointestinal and hepatobiliary autoimmune diseases, as celiac disease, inflammatory bowel diseases, autoimmune chronic hepatitis and sclerosing cholangitis. Several observational epidemiological studies have observed higher incidence and prevalence of autoimmune diseases among DS individuals than in the rest of the population [66].

3.8.1. Autoimmune Hepatitis

Despite Hepatitis B is the more usual cause of chronic hepatitis in DS, but also may be of autoimmune in nature. Although autoimmune hepatitis is a rare condition but it probably occurs relatively more frequently in children with DS than non syndromic children. It may manifest with generalized fatigue, malaise and vague pains or occasionally with more definite arthropathy. It may also present with jaundice. So, it should be differentiated from other causes of jaundice in DS children as hypothyroidism and gall stones. A high index of suspicion is required [67]. Autoimmune hepatitis may be one of the presentations of antiphospholipid syndrome with increased antiphospholipids and in particular an increased frequency of anticardiolipin antibodies. Screening children with DS for certain clinical findings including autoimmune hepatitis may prove useful [68].

Liver enzymes may not be severely raised even in the presence of relatively active hepatitis. However; the serum aminotransferase levels may be elevated from 1.5 to 50 times the reference ranges with increasing of the serum immunoglobulin levels, mainly immunoglobulin G (IgG) and mildly to moderately raised serum bilirubin and alkaline phosphatase. Other autoimmune antibodies may be seropositive such as antinuclear antibodies (ANAs), smooth-muscle antibodies (SMAs), liver-kidney microsomal type 1 (LKM-1) or anti-liver cytosol 1 (anti-LC1) antibodies. Hypoalbuminemia and prolongation of prothrombin time may be observed with severe hepatic synthetic dysfunction, such as active disease or decompensated cirrhosis [69]. It is important to recognize this condition early so that better management can be achieved. Steroid therapy in proper dosing showed satisfactory response with normalization of the liver functions and restoration of normal liver histological appearances [70].

3.8.2. Inflammatory Bowel Disease (IBD)

Inflammatory bowel disease (IBD) is a chronic relapsing inflammation of the intestine, characteristically begins in early adulthood. IBD is generally classified into two subtypes, according to the clinical and histological features: Crohn disease and ulcerative colitis (UC). IBD, especially ulcerative colitis, are quite infrequent in DS patients with a prevalence of about 0.1-0.2 " which could be explain "by chance" without any pathophysiology binding mechanism between both entities [65]. The data about the association between DS and IBD are controversial. Some authors concluded that genetic factors (like trisomy 21) could be important determinants of susceptibility in IBD and other authors claimed "by chance" association [71, 72]. Pathophysiologic relationship between DS and IBD is unclear and the data came from series of cases and affirmation of DS as a predisposing factor to develop IBD cannot be made.

3.9. Toilet Training

Toileting can be one of the most sensitive and stressful periods in parenting. There is a wide difference in the age at which the child with DS can reach independent toileting and a comparable range in the length of time, effort and power that has to be given by the parents to accomplish it. Readiness for toileting depends on many factors including; the age of the child, the bladder control with the child ability to completely empty the bladder, presence of predictable stooling patterns, the degree of development of the child motor skills and the ability to walk to and from the bathroom independently, the ability of the child to respond to simple directions and the child ability to express his needs and desire to go to the bathroom. The majority of DS children reach day and night dryness by the age of 4-5 years, which is about 1 year delayed than the normal children. However, only about one third of DS children (35%) are toilet trained at age 4. At 11 years; one third remains enuretic. Children with mental impairment usually take a longer time to achieve toileting abilities. These children typically have difficulties in awareness; initiation; sequencing, memory; and manual dexterity in handling their clothes. Physiological readiness for toileting is desirable prior to starting toilet training programs [73, 74].

Children with DS usually follow the classic developmental succession and sex-differentiated pattern, but on a tardy schedule. There is an association between the capability to differentiate between the desire for urination and the urge for defecation and their cognitive ability to talk about one's own feelings and thoughts. This observation may imply the complexity of this function, and the possible significance of body awareness and sensory integration for skill acquisition. More studies are required to understand the reason of delay of bladder and bowel control in children with DS, and to be able to provide support and guide to parents as regard to this matter [75].

3.10. Gall Bladder Stone

Gall stones are rare, but increasing, finding in DS children and usually discovered by chance during radiological examination. The reason for association between DS and gall bladder stone is not known but patients with DS have lower gall-bladder contraction index which suggests gallbladder hypomotility. This hypomotility may be a feature related to the high prevalence of gallstones in DS [76]. Gall bladder motility disorder was also identified in children with severe constipation which is quite common in children with DS [77].

4. INCREASED INCIDENCE OF GASTROINTESTINAL AND HEPATOBILIARY INFECTIONS

Helicobacter pylori (H. pylori) are main bacterial cause of gastrointestinal disorders. Infection with H. pylori usually starts since early life. Children with neurological impairment have significantly higher risk of H. pylori infection than the control and the risk is significantly correlated with the severity of the chronic disease. Children with DS have multiple immunologic defects and more risk factors that expose them to different infections as being living in institutions and overcrowding. Different studies showed high seropositivity for H. pylori in DS which could be attributed to overcrowding, sanitary conditions, and dietary regimen that affect the rout of H. pylori transmission and infection [78]. However, the rate of seropositivity was found to be low in non- institutionalized DS children [79].

There is an increase in the incidence of hepatotrophic virus (A, B and C) in institutionalized patients with DS. Poor sanitary circumstances and impaired immunological conditions might predispose DS children to infection with these hepatotrophic viruses. Sanitary conditions directly influence HAV transmission cycle.

Poor socioeconomic levels, poor hygienic conditions, including children with DS and the length of attendance in the day-care settings are important risk factors for the high prevalence of HAV infection. Such findings suggest that if hepatitis A vaccination should become available as a routine policy, and the target group should be infants less than two years. Moreover, those children should receive the vaccine before they start to attend the day-care centers [80].

Markers of hepatitis B virus (HBV) are found with high frequency in immuno-compromised individuals. Children with DS acquire HBV infection easily and this occurs when they attend the school independently that the school is a closed or an open institution. They also become more frequently HBV chronic carriers and they maintain HBV replication; so, they must be vaccinated before they begin to attend school and they must be treated with antiviral agents as soon as possible [81]. Due to the increased risk hepatitis B infection in both open and closed institutions for mentally retarded patients, recombinant hepatitis B vaccine is strongly recommended to such population with high immunogenicity. Children with DS are capable of responding adequately to hepatitis B vaccine with seroconversion with one month after vaccination [82, 83]. Hepatitis C was found in some studies to be less common in children with DS when compared to the prevalence of Hepatitis B [84]. However, IFN therapy for HCV infection in patients with DS may be unfavorable as compared with non-DS children [85].

CONCLUSION

Gastrointestinal disorders are quite common in children with DS. Meticulous attention should be paid to these issues for early detections and proper management.

CONFLICT OF INTEREST

The authors confirm that this chapter contents have no conflict of interest.

ACKNOWLEDGEMENTS

Declared none.

REFERENCES

[1] Spahis JK, Wilson GN. Down syndrome: perinatal complications and counseling experiences in 216 patients. Am J Med Genet 1999; 89(2): 96-9.
[PMID: 10559764]

[2] Freeman SB, Torfs CP, Romitti PA, *et al.* Congenital gastrointestinal defects in Down syndrome: a report from the Atlanta and National Down Syndrome Projects. Clin Genet 2009; 75(2): 180-4.
[http://dx.doi.org/10.1111/j.1399-0004.2008.01110.x] [PMID: 19021635]

[3] de Jong EM, Felix JF, de Klein A, Tibboel D. Etiology of esophageal atresia and tracheoesophageal fistula: "omind the gap"?. Curr Gastroenterol Rep 2010; 12(3): 215-22.
[http://dx.doi.org/10.1007/s11894-010-0108-1] [PMID: 20425471]

[4] McGivern MR, Best KE, Rankin J, Wellesley D, *et al.* Epidemiology of congenital diaphragmatic hernia in Europe: a register-based study. Arch Dis Child Fetal Neonatal Ed 2014; 100(2): 137-44.
[http://dx.doi.org/10.1136/archdischild-2014-306174] [PMID: 20425471]

[5] Pober BR. Overview of epidemiology, genetics, birth defects, and chromosome abnormalities associated with CDH. Am J Med Genet C Semin Med Genet 2007; 145C(2): 158-71.
[http://dx.doi.org/10.1002/ajmg.c.30126]

[6] Al-Salem AH, Zamakhshary M, Al Mohaidly M, Al-Qahtani A, Abdulla MR, Naga MI. Congenital

Morgagni's hernia: a national multicenter study. J Pediatr Surg 2014; 49(4): 503-7. [http://dx.doi.org/10.1016/j.jpedsurg.2013.08.029] [PMID: 24726101]

[7] Parmar RC, Tullu MS, Bavdekar SB, Borwankar SS. Morgagni hernia with Down syndrome: a rare association -- case report and review of literature. J Postgrad Med 2001; 47(3): 188-90. [PMID: 11832621]

[8] Honoré LH, Torfs CP, Curry CJ. Possible association between the hernia of Morgagni and trisomy 21. Am J Med Genet 1993; 47(2): 255-6. [PMID: 8213915]

[9] Spaggiari E, Stirnemann J, Ville Y. Outcome in fetuses with isolated congenital diaphragmatic hernia with increased nuchal translucency thickness in first trimester. Prenat Diagn 2012; 32(3): 268-71. [http://dx.doi.org/10.1002/pd.3819] [PMID: 22430726]

[10] Jetley NK, Al-Assiri AH, Al-Helal AS, Al-Bin Ali AM. Down's syndrome as a factor in the diagnosis, management, and outcome in patients of Morgagni hernia. J Pediatr Surg 2011; 46(4): 636-9. [http://dx.doi.org/10.1016/j.jpedsurg.2010.10.001] [PMID: 21496530]

[11] Al-Salem AH. Bilateral congenital Morgagni-Larrey's hernia. World J Pediatr 2010; 6(1): 76-80. [http://dx.doi.org/10.1007/s12519-010-0011-8] [PMID: 20143216]

[12] Escobar MA, Ladd AP, Grosfeld JL, *et al.* Duodenal atresia and stenosis: long-term follow-up over 30 years. J Pediatr Surg 2004; 39(6): 867-71. [http://dx.doi.org/10.1016/j.jpedsurg.2004.02.025] [PMID: 15185215]

[13] Lee SS, Hwang ST, Jang NG, *et al.* A case of congenital duodenal web causing duodenal stenosis in a down syndrome child: endoscopic resection with an insulated-tip knife. Gut Liver 2011; 5(1): 105-9. [http://dx.doi.org/10.5009/gnl.2011.5.1.105] [PMID: 21461083]

[14] Mustafawi AR, Hassan ME. Congenital duodenal obstruction in children: a decade's experience. Eur J Pediatr Surg 2008; 18(2): 93-7. [http://dx.doi.org/10.1055/s-2008-1038478] [PMID: 18437652]

[15] Savino A, Rollo V, Chiarelli F. Congenital duodenal stenosis and annular pancreas: a delayed diagnosis in an adolescent patient with Down syndrome. Eur J Pediatr 2007; 166(4): 379-80. [http://dx.doi.org/10.1007/s00431-006-0241-x] [PMID: 17043846]

[16] Zyromski NJ, Sandoval JA, Pitt HA, *et al.* Annular pancreas: dramatic differences between children and adults. J Am Coll Surg 2008; 206(5): 1019-25. [http://dx.doi.org/10.1016/j.jamcollsurg.2007.12.009] [PMID: 18471747]

[17] Dankovcik R, Jirasek JE, Kucera E, Feyereisl J, Radonak J, Dudas M. Prenatal diagnosis of annular pancreas: reliability of the double bubble sign with periduodenal hyperechogenic band. Fetal Diagn Ther 2008; 24(4): 483-90. [http://dx.doi.org/10.1159/000178759]

[18] Lin YT, Chang MH, Hsu HY, Lai HS, Chen CC. A follow-up study of annular pancreas in infants and children. Zhonghua Min Guo Xiao Er Ke Yi Xue Hui Za Zhi 1998; 39(2): 89-93. [PMID: 9599896]

[19] Levitt MA, Peña A. Anorectal malformations. Orphanet J Rare Dis 2007 Jul 26; 2 [http://dx.doi.org/10.1186/1750-1172-2-33] [PMID: 17651510]

[20] de Buys Roessingh AS, Mueller C, Wiesenauer C, Bensoussan AL, Beaunoyer M. Anorectal malformation and Down's syndrome in monozygotic twins. J Pediatr Surg 2009; 44(2): e13-6. [http://dx.doi.org/10.1016/j.jpedsurg.2008.10.116] [PMID: 19231514]

[21] Fanjul M, Molina E, Cerdá J, *et al.* [Characteristics of the anorectal atresia without fistula. Based on 12 cases]. Cir Pediatr 2009; 22(1): 45-8. [PMID: 19323083]

[22] Torres R, Levitt MA, Tovilla JM, Rodriguez G, Peña A. Anorectal malformations and Down's syndrome. J Pediatr Surg 1998; 33(2): 194-7. [http://dx.doi.org/10.1016/S0022-3468(98)90430-4] [PMID: 9498385]

[23] Sullivan PB. Gastrointestinal disorders in children with neurodevelopmental disabilities. Dev Disabil Res Rev 2008; 14(2): 128-36. [http://dx.doi.org/10.1002/ddrr.18] [PMID: 18646021]

[24] Moore SW. Down syndrome and the enteric nervous system. Pediatr Surg Int 2008; 24(8): 873-83. [http://dx.doi.org/10.1007/s00383-008-2188-7] [PMID: 18633623]

[25] Cooper-Brown L, Copeland S, Dailey S, *et al.* Feeding and swallowing dysfunction in genetic syndromes. Dev Disabil Res Rev 2008; 14(2): 147-57. [http://dx.doi.org/10.1002/ddrr.19] [PMID: 18646013]

[26] Faulks D, Collado V, Mazille MN, Veyrune JL, Hennequin M. Masticatory dysfunction in persons with Down's syndrome. Part 1: aetiology and incidence. J Oral Rehabil 2008; 35(11): 854-62. [http://dx.doi.org/10.1111/j.1365-2842.2008.01877.x] [PMID: 18702629]

[27] Spender Q, Stein A, Dennis J, Reilly S, Percy E, Cave D. An exploration of feeding difficulties in children with Down syndrome. Dev Med Child Neurol 1996; 38(8): 681-94. [http://dx.doi.org/10.1111/j.1469-8749.1996.tb12138.x] [PMID: 8761164]

[28] Roth DE, Caulfield LE, Ezzati M, Black RE. Acute lower respiratory infections in childhood: opportunities for reducing the global burden through nutritional interventions. Bull World Health Organ 2008; 86(5): 356-64. [http://dx.doi.org/10.2471/BLT.07.049114] [PMID: 18545738]

[29] Miller CK. Feeding issues and interventions in infants and children with clefts and craniofacial syndromes. Semin Speech Lang 2011; 32(2): 115-26. [http://dx.doi.org/10.1055/s-0031-1277714] [PMID: 21948638]

[30] Hillemeier C, Buchin PJ, Gryboski J. Esophageal dysfunction in Down's syndrome. J Pediatr Gastroenterol Nutr 1982; 1(1): 101-4. [http://dx.doi.org/10.1097/00005176-198201010-00017] [PMID: 6224922]

[31] Pace F, Bazzoli F, Fiocca R, *et al.* The Italian validation of the Montreal Global definition and classification of gastroesophageal reflux disease. Eur J Gastroenterol Hepatol 2009; 21(4): 394-408. [http://dx.doi.org/10.1097/MEG.0b013e32830a70e2] [PMID: 19262401]

[32] Sherman PM, Hassall E, Fagundes-Neto U, *et al.* [A global, evidence-based consensus on the definition of gastroesophageal reflux disease in the pediatric population]. Arch Pediatr 2010; 17(11): 1586-93. [http://dx.doi.org/10.1016/j.arcped.2010.08.030] [PMID: 20943357]

[33] de Veer AJ, Bos JT, Niezen-de Boer RC, BÖhmer CJ, Francke AL. Symptoms of gastroesophageal reflux disease in severely mentally retarded people: a systematic review. BMC Gastroenterol 2008 Jun 11; 8(23)
[http://dx.doi.org/10.1186/1471-230X-8-23]

[34] Zárate N, Mearin F, Gil-Vernet JM, Camarasa F, Malagelada JR. Achalasia and Down's syndrome: coincidental association or something else? Am J Gastroenterol 1999; 94(6): 1674-7.
[http://dx.doi.org/10.1111/j.1572-0241.1999.01161.x] [PMID: 10364043]

[35] Lightdale JR, Gremse DA. Section on Gastroenterology, Hepatology, and Nutrition. Gastroesophageal reflux: management guidance for the pediatrician. Pediatrics 2013; 131(5): e1684-1695.
[http://dx.doi.org/10.1542/peds.2013-0421] [PMID: 23629618]

[36] Gremse DA. GERD in the pediatric patient: management considerations. MedGenMed 2004 may 5; 6(2): 13.
[PMID: 15266239]

[37] Viegelmann G, Low Y, Sriram B, Chu HP. Achalasia and Down syndrome: a unique association not to be missed. Singapore Med J 2014; 55(7): e107-8.
[http://dx.doi.org/10.11622/smedj.2013260] [PMID: 24379117]

[38] O'Neill AC, Richter GT. Pharyngeal dysphagia in children with Down syndrome. Otolaryngol Head Neck Surg 2013; 149(1): 146-50.
[http://dx.doi.org/10.1177/0194599813483445] [PMID: 23525851]

[39] Prasse JE, Kikano GE. An overview of pediatric dysphagia. Clin Pediatr (Phila) 2009; 48(3): 247-51.
[http://dx.doi.org/10.1177/0009922808327323] [PMID: 19023104]

[40] Faulks D, Mazille MN, Collado V, Veyrune JL, Hennequin M. Masticatory dysfunction in persons with Down's syndrome. Part 2: management. J Oral Rehabil 2008; 35(11): 863-9.
[http://dx.doi.org/10.1111/j.1365-2842.2008.01878.x] [PMID: 18793251]

[41] Yin H, Boyd T, Pacheco MC, Schonfeld D, Bove KE. Rectal biopsy in children with Down syndrome and chronic constipation: Hirschsprung disease *vs* non-hirschsprung disease. Pediatr Dev Pathol 2012; 15(2): 87-95.
[http://dx.doi.org/10.2350/11-01-0957-OA.1] [PMID: 21991983]

[42] Gale L, Wimalaratna H, Brotodiharjo A, Duggan JM. Down's syndrome is strongly associated with coeliac disease. Gut 1997; 40(4): 492-6.
[http://dx.doi.org/10.1136/gut.40.4.492] [PMID: 9176077]

[43] Nurko S, Zimmerman LA. Evaluation and treatment of constipation in children and adolescents. Am Fam Physician 2014 Jul 15; 90(2): 13-496.
[PMID: 25077577]

[44] Kessmann J. Hirschsprung's disease: diagnosis and management. Am Fam Physician 2006; 74(8): 1319-22.
[PMID: 17087425]

[45] De Lorijn F, Reitsma JB, Voskuijl WP, *et al.* Diagnosis of Hirschsprung's disease: a prospective, comparative accuracy study of common tests. J Pediatr 2005; 146(6): 787-92.
[http://dx.doi.org/10.1016/j.jpeds.2005.01.044] [PMID: 15973319]

[46] Friedmacher F, Puri P. Hirschsprung's disease associated with Down syndrome: a meta-analysis of incidence, functional outcomes and mortality. Pediatr Surg Int 2013; 29(9): 937-46. [http://dx.doi.org/10.1007/s00383-013-3361-1] [PMID: 23943251]

[47] Abalan F, Jouan A, Weerts MT, Solles C, Brus J, Sauneron MF. A study of digestive absorption in four cases of Down's syndrome. Down's syndrome, malnutrition, malabsorption, and Alzheimer's disease. Med Hypotheses 1990; 31(1): 35-8. [http://dx.doi.org/10.1016/0306-9877(90)90051-F] [PMID: 2138242]

[48] Cerqueira RM, Rocha CM, Fernandes CD, Correia MR. Celiac disease in Portuguese children and adults with Down syndrome. Eur J Gastroenterol Hepatol 2010; 22(7): 868-71. [http://dx.doi.org/10.1097/MEG.0b013e3283328341] [PMID: 20545028]

[49] Mårild K, Stephansson O, Grahnquist L, Cnattingius S, Söderman G, Ludvigsson JF. Down syndrome is associated with elevated risk of celiac disease: a nationwide case-control study. J Pediatr 2013; 163(1): 237-42. [http://dx.doi.org/10.1016/j.jpeds.2012.12.087] [PMID: 23399451]

[50] Størdal K, Bakken IJ, Surén P, Stene LC. Epidemiology of coeliac disease and comorbidity in Norwegian children. J Pediatr Gastroenterol Nutr 2013; 57(4): 467-71. [http://dx.doi.org/10.1097/MPG.0b013e3182a455dd] [PMID: 23863325]

[51] Boudraa G, Hachelaf W, Benbouabdellah M, Belkadi M, Benmansour FZ, Touhami M. Prevalence of coeliac disease in diabetic children and their first- degree relatives in west Algeria: screening with serological markers. Acta Paediatr Suppl 1996; 412: 58-60. [http://dx.doi.org/10.1111/j.1651-2227.1996.tb14254.x] [PMID: 8783762]

[52] Mackey J, Treem WR, Worley G, Boney A, Hart P, Kishnani PS. Frequency of celiac disease in individuals with Down syndrome in the United States. Clin Pediatr (Phila) 2001; 40(5): 249-52. [http://dx.doi.org/10.1177/000992280104000502] [PMID: 11388673]

[53] Husby S, Murray JA. New aspects of the diagnosis of celiac disease in children, adolescents, and adults. Mayo Clin Proc 2013; 88(6): 540-3. [http://dx.doi.org/10.1016/j.mayocp.2013.03.018] [PMID: 23660481]

[54] Uibo O, Teesalu K, Metskula K. Screening for celiac disease in Down's syndrome patients revealed cases of subtotal villous atrophy without typical for celiac disease HLA-DQ and tissue transglutaminase antibodies. World J Gastroenterol 2006 Mar 7; World J Gastroenterol 2006 Mar 7; 12(9): 1430-4. [PMID: 16552815]

[55] Hill ID, Dirks MH, Liptak GS, *et al.* Guideline for the diagnosis and treatment of celiac disease in children: recommendations of the North American Society for Pediatric Gastroenterology, Hepatology and Nutrition. J Pediatr Gastroenterol Nutr 2005; 40(1): 1-19. [http://dx.doi.org/10.1097/00005176-200501000-00001] [PMID: 15625418]

[56] Webb C, Norström F, Myléus A, *et al.* Celiac disease can be predicted by high levels of anti-tissue transglutaminase antibodies in population-based screening. J Pediatr Gastroenterol Nutr 2015; 60(6): 787-91. [http://dx.doi.org/10.1097/MPG.0000000000000688] [PMID: 25564816]

[57] Bhat AS, Chaturvedi MK, Saini S, *et al.* Prevalence of celiac disease in Indian children with Down syndrome and its clinical and laboratory predictors. Indian J Pediatr 2013; 80(2): 114-7. [http://dx.doi.org/10.1007/s12098-012-0838-1] [PMID: 22791400]

[58] Pavlović M, Radlović N, Leković Z, Berenji K, Stojsić Z, Radlović V. Coeliac disease as the cause of resistant sideropenic anaemia in children with Down's syndrome: case report. Srp Arh Celok Lek 2010; 138(1-2): 91-4. [http://dx.doi.org/10.2298/SARH1002091P] [PMID: 20422917]

[59] Akobeng AK, Thomas AG. Systematic review: tolerable amount of gluten for people with coeliac disease. Aliment Pharmacol Ther 2008; 27(11): 1044-52. [http://dx.doi.org/10.1111/j.1365-2036.2008.03669.x]

[60] Babu J, Kumar S, Babu P, Prasad JH, Ghoshal UC. Frequency of lactose malabsorption among healthy southern and northern Indian populations by genetic analysis and lactose hydrogen breath and tolerance tests. Am J Clin Nutr 2010; 91(1): 140-6. [http://dx.doi.org/10.3945/ajcn.2009.27946]

[61] Pueschel SM. Gastrointestinal concerns and nutritional issues in persons with Down's syndrome. Down Syndrome Quarterly 1999; 4(4): 1-11.

[62] Sibley E. Genetic variation and lactose intolerance: detection methods and clinical implications. Am J Pharmacogenomics 2004; 4(4): 239-45. [http://dx.doi.org/10.2165/00129785-200404040-00003]

[63] Ledochowski M, Sperner-Unterweger B, Fuchs D. Lactose malabsorption is associated with early signs of mental depression in females: a preliminary report. Dig Dis Sci 1998; 43(11): 2513-7. [http://dx.doi.org/10.1023/A:1026654820461] [PMID: 9824144]

[64] Misselwitz B, Pohl D, Frühauf H, Fried M, Vavricka SR, Fox M. Lactose malabsorption and intolerance: pathogenesis, diagnosis and treatment. United European Gastroenterol J 2013; 1(3): 151-9. [http://dx.doi.org/10.1177/2050640613484463] [PMID: 24917953]

[65] Powell CV, Jenkins HR. Toddler diarrhoea: is it a useful diagnostic label? Arch Dis Child 2012; 97(1): 84-6. [http://dx.doi.org/10.1136/adc.2010.191825] [PMID: 21831872]

[66] Souto-Rodríguez R, Barreiro-de-Acosta M, Domínguez-Muñoz JE. Down's syndrome and inflammatory bowel disease: is there a real link? Rev Esp Enferm Dig 2014; 106(3): 220-2. [PMID: 25007021]

[67] Kaushik SP, Kaye G, Clarke AC. Autoimmune hepatobiliary disease in trisomy 21. J Clin Gastroenterol 2000; 30(3): 330-2. [http://dx.doi.org/10.1097/00004836-200004000-00029] [PMID: 10777202]

[68] RequeníSilla Y, Rosenfield CG, Miller LC. Antiphospholipid antibodies and Down syndrome: a case series. J Pediatr Hematol Oncol 2002; 24(7): 575-8. [http://dx.doi.org/10.1097/00043426-200210000-00018] [PMID: 12368700]

[69] Czaja AJ. Autoimmune hepatitis--approach to diagnosis. MedGenMed 2006 may 23; 8(2): 55.

[70] O'Mahony D, Whelton MJ, Hogan J. Down syndrome and autoimmune chronic active hepatitis: satisfactory outcome with therapy. Ir J Med Sci 1990; 159(1): 21-2. [http://dx.doi.org/10.1007/BF02937210] [PMID: 2138593]

[71] Yamamoto M, Abo W, Hori T, *et al.* Crohn's disease in a child with Down syndrome. Pediatr Int 2002; 44(5): 537-9. [http://dx.doi.org/10.1046/j.1442-200X.2002.01598.x] [PMID: 12225558]

[72] Hampe J, Schreiber S, Shaw SH, *et al.* A genomewide analysis provides evidence for novel linkages in inflammatory bowel disease in a large European cohort. Am J Hum Genet 1999; 64(3): 808-16. [http://dx.doi.org/10.1086/302294] [PMID: 10053016]

[73] Mancini MC, Carvalho e Silva P, Gonçalves SC, Martins SdeM. [Comparison of functional performance among children with Down syndrome and children with age-appropriate development at 2 and 5 years of age]. Arq Neuropsiquiatr 2003; 61(2B): 409-15. [http://dx.doi.org/10.1590/S0004-282X2003000300016] [PMID: 12894276]

[74] Dolva AS, Coster W, Lilja M. Functional performance in children with Down syndrome. Am J Occup Ther 2004; 58(6): 621-9. [http://dx.doi.org/10.5014/ajot.58.6.621] [PMID: 15568546]

[75] Frank K, Esbensen AJ. Fine motor and self-care milestones for individuals with Down syndrome using a Retrospective Chart Review. J Intellect Disabil Res 2014; 23 [http://dx.doi.org/10.1111/jir.12176] [PMID: 25533735]

[76] TaşYdemir HA, Cetinkaya MC, Polat C, Belet U, Kalayci AG, AkbaşY S. Gallbladder motility in children with Down syndrome. J Pediatr Gastroenterol Nutr 2004; 39(2): 187-91. [http://dx.doi.org/10.1097/00005176-200408000-00012] [PMID: 15269626]

[77] Veras Neto MC, Yamada RM, da Costa Pinto EA. Gallbladder motility in children with chronic constipation. J Pediatr Gastroenterol Nutr 2008; 46(4): 414-8. [http://dx.doi.org/10.1097/MPG.0b013e31813347c4] [PMID: 18367954]

[78] Douraghi M, Goudarzi H, Rostami MN, Mirsamadi ES. Helicobacter pylori seropositivity in institutionalized children with Down syndrome. Pediatr Infect Dis J 2011; 30(12): 1123-4. [http://dx.doi.org/10.1097/INF.0b013e318227879f] [PMID: 22105426]

[79] Jaber SM. Helicobacter pylori seropositivity in children with chronic disease in Jeddah, Saudi Arabia. Saudi J Gastroenterol 2006; 12(1): 21-6. [http://dx.doi.org/10.4103/1319-3767.27740] [PMID: 19858580]

[80] Queiroz DA, Cardoso DD, Martelli CM, *et al.* Risk factors and prevalence of antibodies against hepatitis A virus (HAV) in children from day-care centers, in Goiania, Brazil. Rev Inst Med Trop Sao Paulo 1995; 37(5): 427-33. [http://dx.doi.org/10.1590/S0036-46651995000500008] [PMID: 8729753]

[81] Findor JA, Sordá JA, Rey J, Fernández J, Kohan A, Díaz Lestrem M. [Hepatitis B (HBV) and C (HBC) virus infections in Down's syndrome and in neuropsychiatric patients without Down's syndrome]. Gen 1992; 46(3): 208-12. [PMID: 1340826]

[82] Van Damme P, Vranckx R, Meheus A. Immunogenicity of a recombinant DNA hepatitis B vaccine in

institutionalized patients with Down's syndrome. Vaccine 1990; 8 (Suppl:S53-5). [http://dx.doi.org/10.1016/0264-410X(90)90236-F] [PMID: 2139285]

[83] García O, Bruguera M, Mayor A, Sánchez-Tapias JM, Vall O, Rodés J. [Hepatitis B at an open institution for the mentally retarded. Immunogenic effect of a recombinant anti-hepatitis-B vaccine]. Enferm Infecc Microbiol Clin 1990; 8(3): 148-52. [PMID: 2151250]

[84] Lunding S, Hansen KS, Krogsgaard K, Rosdahl N, Smith E, Wantzin PS. Occurrence of hepatitis B and C among mentally retarded. Ugeskr Laeger 1999; 161(31): 4393-6. [PMID: 10487103]

[85] Miyoshi Y, Tajiri H, Okaniwa M, *et al.* Hepatitis C virus infection and interferon therapy in patients with Down syndrome. Pediatr Int 2008; 50(1): 7-11. [http://dx.doi.org/10.1111/j.1442-200X.2007.02515.x] [PMID: 18279197]

CHAPTER 7

Infection in Children with Down Syndrome

Nermin K. Saeed*

Pathology Department, Salmaniya Medical Complex, Kingdom of Bahrain

Abstract: Infections are an important reason of increased morbidity and mortality in children with DS. Infection in children with DS characterized by increased severity of infection due to accentuated inflammatory response; increased the need for intensive care; prolonged duration of illness and need for extra or augmented treatment to cure the same infections compared with the normal population. In this chapter we will discuss the causes of increased infections in children with DS, the relation of infection to the pathogenesis of DS, the common infection in DS and immune modulation of children with DS. Every effort should be done to minimize the risk of infection and to improve their immunity.

Keywords: Air way anomalies, Antioxidants, Bacterial pneumonia, Breast feeding, Children, Congenital ear anomalies, Congenital Heart Diseases, Down syndrome, Gastro-oesophageal reflux, Hygiene, Immune aging, Immune modulation, Immunodeficiency, Infections, Nutritional deficiencies, Otitis media, Palivizumab, Pidotimod, Respiratory syncytial virus, Vaccination.

1. INTRODUCTION

Down syndrome (DS) is the most frequent chromosomal anomaly in the human being which results from incomplete or complete trisomy of the human chromosome 21. It causes various complex phenotypes which affect the whole body including the immune system. Infections are a significant reason of increased rate of sickness and death in children with DS. Infection in children with DS is characterized by increasing severity due to accentuated inflammatory response; increased the need for intensive care; prolonged duration of illness and

* **Corresponding Author Nermin K Saeed:** Pathology Department, Salmaniya Medical Complex, Kingdom of Bahrain; Mobile: (+973)39910076; Fax: (+973) 1759 0495; Email: nkamalh@hotmail.com

the need for extra or augmented treatment to cure the same infections compared with the normal population. In this chapter we will discuss the causes of increasing infections in children with DS, the relation of infection to the pathogenesis of DS, the common infection of DS and immune modulation of children with DS [1].

2. CAUSES OF RAISED RATE AND SEVERITY OF INFECTIONS IN DS CHILDREN

The raised rate of infection in DS children is due to different factors. Immune deficiency increases both frequency of infection and the severity of associated inflammation. Anatomical co-morbidities are important factors that could precipitate infections or exaggerate its severity.

There are different airways anatomical abnormalities, congenital ear abnormalities, increased prevalence of gastroesophageal reflux disease (GERD), muscular hypotonia, and increased incidence of congenital heart disease.

Nutritional deficiencies may be another factor in areas where adequate care is not available to this cohort of patients. Children with DS may have also a poor vaccination response.

2.1. Immunodeficiency in Children with Down Syndrome

The immune system plays an essential but complex role to protect against infections with different microbes. It also controls the degree of inflammation that results from these infections.

Without adequate immune status, recurrent or life threatening infections are inevitable and severe inflammatory response with undesirable tissue damage may be triggered in response to infections. Relative immunodeficiency is commonly underestimated in children with DS that could place those patients at great risk (Fig. **1**).

2.1.1. Genetic Basis of Immunodeficiency in Down Syndrome

Partial or complete triplication of chromosome 21 may be associated with gene over expression which could be responsible for many disturbances in the immune system of patients with DS.

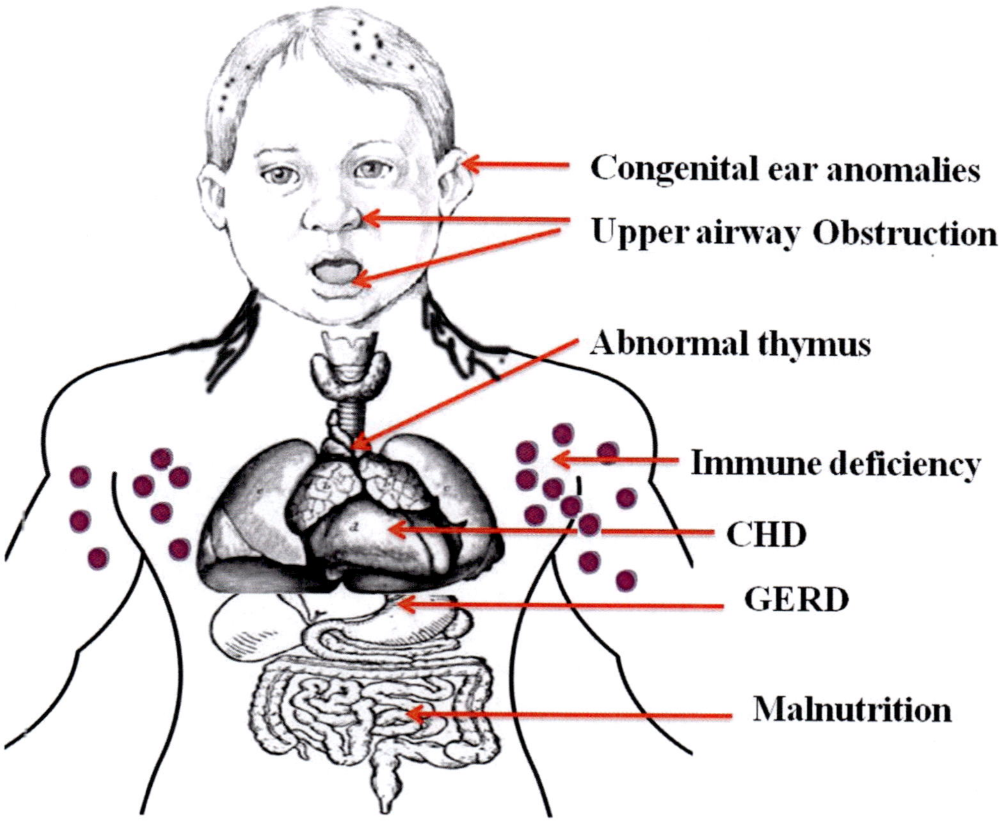

Fig. (1). Showed causes of immune deficiency in children with down syndrome.

Chromosome 21 has a 21q22 gene-rich R bands which called the "Down syndrome region and contains about 225 genes. Among these genes; many genes encode for many proteins responsible for the proper functioning of the immune system. Among these are the genes that encode for CuZn-superoxide dismutase (SOD-1), the regulator of calcineurin 1 (RCAN1), CD18-beta chain of LFA-1, interferon receptor, APP-amyloid precursor protein, and protein S-100 beta. RCAN1 is a transcription factor that depresses the signal transduction provoked by the nuclear factor of activated T cells (NFAT), and has been found to decrease the inflammatory responses in mice by maintaining an inhibitor of nuclear factorkappa B cells (NF-kB). Over expression of these molecules may play a role in thymic derangement which causes abnormal maturation leading to functionally impaired T cells, changes in cell-mediated immunity, phagocytosis, antibodies-mediated immunity and increased prevalence of autoantibodies in DS children. For example, there is 150% over expression of a gene on chromosome 21 that encodes for superoxide disimutase-1 (SOD1). The over activity of this enzyme causes increased rate of switch of superoxides to peroxides in individuals' blood resulting in elevated levels of peroxides that may harm DNA and lipids structures, and in low levels of the superoxides which unfavorably influence the functions of phagocytes that are vital for killing microbes such as *Staphylococcus aureus* and *Candida albicans*. Another example is over-expression of the gene that encodes for lymphocyte function associated antigen-1(LFA-1), which can cause an unusual interaction between cells from the thymus, inducing aberrant T-cell maturation and selection. Over expression of the gene for CD18, one of the subunits of family of leucocyte integrin adhesion molecules vital in immunity and in inflammation might influence leucocyte behavior in DS. This CD18 molecule regulates the interaction of all leucocytes with other leucocytes, endothelium, and other tissues and with microorganisms and its over expression may cause striking immunodeficiency. Over-expression of the interferon receptor and numerous novel adhesion molecules genes also present on chromosome 21 is frequent in DS and can play a role in immune deficiency as well [2 - 4].

Over expression of genes present on Chromosome 21 may be associated with down regulation of other genes located in chromosomes other than 21 that can affect negatively the activity of the immune system. VAV2 is a gene located within the critical region for the tuberous sclerosis gene, TSC1, on human chromosome 9q34. There is down-regulation of VAV2 expression in DS neonates. The gene is an activator of Cdc42, Rac1 and RhoA which control actin dynamics and gene expression. Down-regulation of VAV2 could impair leukocyte migration, for knockdown of VAV2 hinders Rac activation in some cells. Leukocyte trans-endothelial migration is imperative for immune surveillance and inflammation [5].

2.1.2. Impairment of T Cells in Down Syndrome

Thymus is a triangular bi-lobed gland that is considered as a primary immune organ formed of reticular connective tissue with cuboidal epithelial cells and is responsible for generating functional T cells. Histologically; it is differentiated into mesenchymal capsule and two main sub-compartments; the cortex, and the medulla with a reticular connective tissue like any lymphoid tissues that act as a support to blood cells inside the gland. Inside the gland, maturation of immature lymphocytes into T-lymphocytes occurs under the effect of a group of hormones known collectively as thymosins which help migration and development of these immature thymocytes from the medulla to the cortex [6].

T cells play an essential task in cell-mediated immunity. These cells are called T cells because they originated from thymocytes present in thymus gland. Normally; only 2% of thymocytes developed to T-cells. There are 6 basic types of T cell; T - Helper (CD4+ T cells), cytotoxic T cells (CD8+ T cells), memory T cells (either CD4+ or CD8+), regulatory T cells (Known as Treg cells or suppressor T cells), natural killer T cells and mucosal associated invariant T cells. T cells can be distinguished from other lymphocytes by the presence of a T-cell receptor (TCR) on the cell surface which is responsible for T cell activation by simultaneous engagement with co-stimulatory molecule (like CD28, or ICOS) on the T cell by the major histocompatibility complex (MHCII) peptide and co-stimulatory molecules on the antigen-presenting (APC) which is needed for construction of an adequate immune response. In DS, there is an altered distribution and function of T cell populations mostly due to abnormal thymic function. There is reduction of T cell population below the 10th percentile in almost 90% of DS children with a smaller thymus size and decreased T cell expansion in infancy and decreased T-cell receptors. There are variable histological changes in thymus gland which could reach up to fibrotic involution of the thymus gland. There is moderate to severe cortical thymocyte reduction with decreased thickness of the cortex and poor demarcation to a complete loss of the corticomedullary junction. There is also decrease or absence of interdigitating reticulum cells approximately correlated with the severity of morphologic changes of DS with enlarged Hassal's corpuscles in DS and cystic changes in most cases and fibrosis in 46 to 77% of them. The complex structural and cellular thymic changes, affecting both cortical and medullary microenvironment, could be correlated with the imbalances of immunity in DS patients [7]. There is an average increase of 3.9-fold higher in cells constitutive levels of TNF-alpha mRNA in the trabeculae, corticomedullary junctions, and medulla of DS thymuses than in age-matched control thymuses. DS thymuses also contained an average of 3 fold higher numbers of cells with mast cell morphology. There are 2.4-fold in discrete cells expressing IFN-gamma mRNA distinctly localized to the cortical region of DS thymuses. These two cytokines (TNF-alpha and IFN-gamma) regulate thymocyte proliferation. The over-expression of both of these cytokines in DS thymuses suggests abnormal regulation in cytokine production in DS and may supply a clarification for the abnormal thymic structure and thymocyte development and maturation associated with DS [8]. There is also significantly lower number of signal-joint T cell receptor (sj-TREC+) lymphocytes, the levels of which were strongly correlated with age.

Children with DS show slightly reduced proliferative responses of thymocytes to IL-4 *in vitro* and as a result, T-cell differentiation and maturation might be deteriorated in DS. Down syndrome thymocytes have a markedly reduced percentage of cells expressing high levels of the alpha, beta T cell receptor (TCR alpha, beta) and the associated CD3+ molecule. There are also significant decrease of CD1+, CD4+ and CD8+ naive (RA+CCR7+) lymphocytes, significant increase of CD4+ and CD8+ central memory (RA-CCR7+), and terminally differentiated (TD) (RA+CCR7-) lymphocytes [9]. There are also significant changes of T cell differentiation, with increased proliferative T cell response to IL-15 in DS children, along with increased amount of Tregs and of cells expressing markers of apoptosis [10]. This may indicate precocious thymic involution occurring in DS as reflected by an increased production of IL-7 and IL-15, which is vital for cell survival and proliferation. This complex changes present in the peripheral blood is probably the consequence of a compensatory mechanism. This overproduction of homeostatic cytokines could be a response to the decreased intrathymic production of T lymphocytes and/or to the expansion of Treg in the periphery, and could be necessary to permit the survival of T cells [11]. This disparity in the percents of T cell subpopulations observed in DS peripheral blood lymphocytes may be responsible to the increased vulnerability to infection associated with DS and may signify a reduced effectiveness in the production of newly differentiated T cells by the DS thymus [12]. There is clear proof that serum levels of thymic hormones are low with increased thymic factors inhibitory activity. It is suggested that the immunodeficiency of DS results from a defect restricted mainly to the epithelial cells of the thymus which fail to synthesize or secrete one or more hormones essential for the differentiation of T-lymphocytes [13].

The absolute numbers of T-cells including absolute counts of CD4 and CD8 T-cell subsets are significantly lower in children with DS at all ages particularly in the first two years of life. With increasing age differences become smaller. The CD4/CD8 ratio is constant with age, but lesser in DS than in healthy controls [14]. It is also observed that the number of "avid" T cells, is considerably elevated in the DS than in the control group. However, the blastogenic response of the T cells to mitogen is considerably reduced specially after the age of 10 years. T lymphocytes in the peripheral blood from DS patients showed a major lack of membrane mitochondrial potential (MMP) and altered T cell intracellular signalling [15]. This could explain the lowered T cell function including the response to specific antigens and some mitogens. Proliferation upon stimulation with anti-CD3 is depressed in children with DS. They have a deviant pattern of the signaling pathway after CD3 cross-linking, distinguished by the lack of tyrosine phosphorylation of a part of the proteins implicated in the cascade. On the contrary, the gamma chain of the IL-2-receptor is normally expressed and properly phosphorylated during cell activation in DS [16].

There is also a reduction in T cell proliferation in children with DS in response to the particular viral antigens of Influenza A and B, and also to tetanus toxoid which is mostly due to a diminished response of CD4 T-cells. This effect is partly overcome in the presence of monocytes and B-cells [17]. T-lymphocytes of children with DS are significantly more sensitive to inhibition of proliferation by interferon. However, there is a reciprocal relationship between stimulation with tetanus toxoid and the effect of interferon on this stimulation. Low levels of toxoid-stimulated proliferation causes increased stimulation by interferon in DS; while in controls at high levels, interferon has a more inhibitory effect on proliferation [18]. Other T lymphocyte functions also could be deteriorated in children with DS. Antibody-dependent cellular cytotoxic (ADCC) activities of T lymphocytes are vital because of their possible role in protection against tumors and viral infections and in controlling various lymphocyte reactions. Different studies showed that ADCC is reduced in children with DS in comparison to healthy controls [19].

In children with DS, there is an over-expression of the gene located on chromosome 21 that encodes for lymphocyte functional antigen-1 (LFA-1). This antigen expressed on the cell surface of lymphocytes has a function in intercellular adhesion and consequently the cellular-mediated immune response. Over-expression of LFA-1 may lead to enhanced aggregation of cells and therefore causes cellular immune dysfunction [20]. Children with DS have a number of proinflammatory CD14(dim)CD16(+) monocytes that perform an important task in the onset and maintenance of chronic inflammatory diseases in DS. This inflammatory response augments the harmful effects of the associated infections [21]. There is also amplified early apoptotic cells (especially T cells) and premature immunologic aging in DS children probably due to accelerated thymic involution which may confirm the fact that the function of cells- and not their number- is key mechanism responsible for the deterioration of the immune system in DS children and may as well add to the known fact that cellular immunity is more severely affected than humoral immunity in these children [22].

2.1.3. Impairment of B Cells in Down Syndrome

B cell is a type of lymphocyte with characteristic B-cell receptor and formed in the bone marrow. It plays the major role in the humoral immunity of the adaptive immune system as it is responsible for antibodies formation; performs the role of antigen-presenting cells (APCs); and evolves into memory B cells as a result of antigenic activation. It is recently proved to have a suppressive function as well [23]. Both number and function of B lymphocyte were impaired in children with DS. Most of researches showed severe reduction of the B lymphocyte population throughout childhood.

Children with DS lack the primary increase and expansion of B-lymphocytes that usually occurs in healthy children in the first years of age. Lack of this expansion may result from reduced maturation of B-lymphocytes due to intrinsic abnormality of the adaptive immune system in DS [17]. There were contradictory researches about the function of B lymphocytes and serum levels of immunoglobulin M, A, and G and/or Ig G subclasses in children with DS. Some studies showed normal serum levels of IgA and IgG [24] while other studies showed elevated levels of these antibodies in children with DS relative to the healthy children [25, 26]. This elevation of serum levels of IgG and IgA could be a result rather than a reason. It could be explained by excess stimulation of the immune system and increased production of antibodies as a result of failure to clear the infectious agents in children with DS as well as increased frequency of these infections. Elevation of Ig G is not uniform to all IgG subclasses. There is elevation of both IgG1 and IgG3 levels (which are important to fight infections with encapsulated bacteria) while there is decrease in IgG2 and IgG4 levels. There are also diminished levels of IgM in children with DS [17]. The combined association of B lymphocytopenia and hypergammaglobulinemia in children with DS supports the presence of disorder in T-lymphocyte help, with the likelihood that immunoglobulins are oligoclonal in DS, and specific T-cell– dependent antibody responses are inadequate [27].

2.1.4. Impairment of Neutrophils and Monocytes

Neutrophils of children with DS have numerous abnormalities and showed impaired chemotaxis, phagocytosis and the oxidative burst which predispose to diminished resistance to infection. It has also impaired intracellular calcium which serves as a second messenger and controls different functions in numerous cell types, including neutrophils. Significant higher intracellular calcium with prolonged response of intracellular calcium to N-formyl-methionyl-leu-yl-phenylalanine was observed in neutrophils from subjects with DS which indicates presence of intrinsic cellular defects in DS [28]. Oxidative burst occurs in neutrophils in response to certain stimuli with generation of a series of reactive oxygen metabolites which is a key event in the function of these cells during infection and inflammation. Neutrophils from DS children have a low level of superoxide and a decreased activity of H_2O_2-myeloperoxidase-halide system than that observed in normal children. These alterations in the enzymatic activities of the Cu/Zn-Superoxide dismutase and myeloperoxidase induce imbalance in the release of reactive oxygen species in activated neutrophils which increase the oxidative injury observed in children with DS [29].Children with trisomy 21 demonstrated, a cellular defect of chemotaxis and a decreased cellular capacity of the killing of *Staphylococcus aureus* and of *Escherichia coli.* However, phagocytosis of these bacteria kept normal [30]. Like neutrophils, monocytes showed significantly impaired chemotaxis; even though chemokinesis was significantly increased [31].

The defect in chemotactic migration of neutrophils and reduced mononuclear phagocytes observed in DS could be due to either an intrinsic defect of the leukocytes of DS (*e.g.* a shorter half-life), or enzymatic defects, or shifts in the migrating subpopulations of leukocytes. However, the random mobility (without chemotactic gradient) for both types of cells is not impaired [32]. Despite the low total number of monocytes in children with DS, but they had plenty of proinflammatory CD14(dim)CD16(+) monocytes. This raised level of CD14(dim)CD16(+) monocytes may perform a significant task in initiating and maintaining chronic inflammatory disease in DS [21]. PMN phagocytosis in DS children may be normal or impaired when compared to the control. Rosner and Kozinn showed reduced *in vitro* phagocytic capacity of peripheral blood neutrophils to ingest live *Candida albicans* and reduced neutrophil adhesiveness in DS compared with controls [33]. The vitro killing of *Candida albicans* by neutrophils was also significantly lower in DS children than control [34]. Granulocytes also showed inadequate response to the effect of granulocyte macrophage colony-stimulating factor (GM-CSF) and IL-5, which are well known cytokines that help to maintain the survival, endurance, and activation of granulocytes, with less protective effect on apoptosis in DS than in controls [35].

2.1.5. Impairment of Natural Killer (NK) Cells

There are high numbers of some types of NK cells like CD16_CD57 NK cells in DS patients during both childhood and adulthood which could be explained by precocious ageing of immune system. However, there are lesser numbers of CD16 CD56 natural killer (NK) cells in children with DS [17, 36]. As regard to NK cell functions, there are conflicting results. Some studies showed to some extent more increase in NK activity in adult patients with DS, both in peripheral blood mononuclear cells (PBMCs) and monocyte depleted PBMCs. However, other studies showed reduced NK cytotoxic activity in children and adults with DS compared to controls [37, 38].

2.1.6. Impaired Portal of Immunity

The route of entry and exit of the microorganisms of the human body is called portal of entry and exit, mostly the upper respiratory tract and mouth or damaged skin. Nasal cilia are microscopic filaments that coat the mucous membranes in the nose and immersed in nasal mucus that help to humidify the air, filters dust (and other allergens and particles), chemicals, bacteria and viruses that enter the nose with breathing. Some researchers showed that the nature of the mucociliary defect in DS cannot be attributed to primary cilia ultrastructure abnormalities or due to a primitive defect of cilia but mostly due to changes in mucus properties as in rheological parameters [39]. The mucociliary dysfunction could be due to abnormal mucociliary transport [40]. Presence of normal cilia is suggestive that the impaired nasal ciliary function is a result rather than a cause of repeated respiratory infections.

A lower rate of immunoglobulin secretions by parotid was also noted in individuals with DS which reflects presence of immunodeficiency of the humoral mucosal immune response. Study of young and older adults with DS showed severe decrease in both total IgA levels and specific IgA to common oral microbes in saliva relative to the control [41]. It could be a possible factor involved in increasing their susceptibility to recurrent respiratory infections and gingivitis compared to controls [41 - 43]. Children with DS have high concentrations of circulating IgG or IgA specific for gliadin with very few numbers of CD4 circulating cells, and their plasma IL-6 concentrations correlated with those of antigliadin IgG. An overload of dietary antigens and deteriorated nutrient absorption secondary to distorted functioning of the gastrointestinal mucosa might hinder the normal immune responses by inducing programmed cell death in CD4 T-cells [44].

2.1.7. Poor Response to Vaccination

One of the possible causes of immunodeficiency in children with DS is their poor response to vaccination. The particular antibody responses of DS children to different vaccinations were found to be inadequate, although most of them develop protective IgG titers. The specific IgG titers to the neoantigen bacteriophage phi174 in DS children were lesser than the average range [45]. Joshi *et al.*; suggested presence of subtle changes in both humoral and cellular arms of the immune response in children with DS as compared with the normal children in response to two vaccines [T-independent (type 2 – pneumococcal polysaccharide vaccine) and T-dependent Ab responses (with inactivated seasonal influenza vaccine)]. They showed decreased class-switched memory B cells and an increase in the activated CD21 and low B cell population. In addition, children with DS had decreased CD4 T cells and lower thymic output and function as compared with controls [46]. Also; the response to type I oral Poliovirus was considerably less in children with DS [47]. The response to the tetanus and influenza antigenic stimulation was also impaired including interleukin 2 (IL 2) productions [48]. However, specific antibody responses are induced in DS children, though with titers lower than in non-DS control individuals, which is constant with frequent infections.

2.1.8. Premature Aging of The Immune System

Apoptosis and functional deterioration of granulocytes may add to the increased risk of infections in children with DS. Enhanced apoptosis of granulocytes may also be a factor to avoid chronic airway inflammation and bronchial asthma in DS individuals [35]. Thymus in children with DS is small, abnormal and naive Tc and naive Th cells lack the expansion that is usually observed in the first years of life. These alterations in T lymphocyte subset observed in DS children are the result of (partial) failure of T lymphocyte generation, an intrinsic T lymphocyte defect, an increased apoptosis, or a combination of these factors as well as precocious aging of the immune system due to the relative lower number of CD4_CD45RA_ naive T lymphocytes and lower T cell-receptor excision circle counts in DS children [49].

It was observed that dysgammaglobulinaemia is rising with age in association with hyperglobulinaemia of the IgG, IgA and IgD types, sparing immunoglobulins IgM and Ig E. In addition the transformation capacity of peripheral blood lymphocytes decreased with age. This could be explained as the result of premature aging of the thymus-dependent immune system [50]. Presence of autoantibodies (*e.g.* rheumatoid factor, anti-mitochondrial (AMA), smooth-muscle (SMA), liver-kidney microsomal (LKM), nuclear (ANA), gastric parietal cell (GPC) and neutrophil cytoplasmic (ANCA) antibodies) in children and adolescents with DS might be related to the aging of the immune system or could be an earlier indicator of autoimmune diseases in these patients [51].

2.2. Anatomical Co-morbidities

There is an increased rate of associated co morbidities in DS children that posed them to increased incidence of infections. Among these co morbidities are congenital airway anomalies, congenital heart diseases, gastrointestinal tract anomalies, associated autoimmune diseases including hypothyroidism and celiac disease, hypotonia, relative obesity and occurrence of hematological disorders such as acute lymphoblastic leukemia and transient myeloproliferative disease. All these co morbidities increase the incidence of various infections as a complication of the disease itself or as a complication of treatment.

2.2.1. Air Way Anomalies

Upper and lower, small and large airways could be affected in children with DS and present in about 75% of DS children who had recurrent respiratory symptoms and underwent fiberoptic bronchoscopy. These anatomical anomalies of the airways may hinder the clearance of secretions and ease infections [1]. Anomalies of the upper airway include mid-face hypoplasia, relatively large adenoids, tonsils and tongue, relative glossoptosis and small upper airway volume which is about 2/3 normal volume. The distinctive mid-face hypoplasia, macroglossia and mandibular hypoplasia predispose them to obstructive sleep apnea. These together with relatively large tonsils and adenoids, add to airway obstruction and increases vulnerability to infections [52]. Laryngomalacia is present in 50% of children with DS who have recurrent respiratory infections. Laryngomalacia is due to different factors including hypotonia and is worsened by presence of gastroesophageal reflux [53].

Congenital anomalies of the lower airways are frequent and strongly associated with cardiovascular anomalies. Vascular compression of the large airways can occur due to cardiomegaly or due to aberrant or distended vessels like vascular slings or rings and aberrant pulmonary or innominate arteries. Tracheobronchomalacia, bronchomalacia and tracheal bronchus are probably under diagnosed disorders in DS children who have frequent respiratory infections and should be in mind [54]. The upper and the lower airways as well as both lugs are small in children with DS relative to their peers. Children with DS have lung hypoplasia more often than observed in non-DS children. These children have reduced number of terminal lung units, the acini contain reduced number of alveoli, the alveolar ducts are spacious and distended and there are reduced numbers of the large alveoli [55]. Aspiration from impaired oropharyngeal coordination or gastroesophageal reflux is another major cause of respiratory problems in children with DS. Hypotonia has important implication. Any hypotonic child has a high risk of respiratory disorders due to incompetent respiratory muscles and inefficient cough to clear secretions as well as malacia of the airways (Laryngomalacia, tracheomalacia, bronchomalacia, airway malacia). Neurological developmental delay in children with DS can affect coordination of swallowing as well as the immune system development [56].

2.2.2. Congenital Ear Anomalies

Stenosis of external ear canal is observed in 40-50% of infants with DS. Small and narrow Eustachian tube and tube dysfunction caused by the enlarged adenoid contribute to development of middle ear effusion and otitis media which may end with chronic otitis media, glue ear and impaired hearing. These changes can clarify the reasons for the elevated prevalence of hearing loss and the delayed language development observed in DS. Chronic Eustachian tube dysfunction lasts longer in children with DS than in the general population, which predispose them to higher incidence of chronic ear infections. However, ear canals grow with age, and may no longer be of concern after age of three [57].

2.2.3. Congenital Heart Diseases

There is an increased rate of congenital heart diseases (CHD) in children with DS which could reach 40%-60% and children with DS comprise approximately 10%

of all children with CHD. The most common CHDs associated with DS are (Atrioventricular Canal, Ventricular Septal Defect, Atrial Septal Defects, Patent Ductus Arteriosus, and Tetralogy of Fallot) [58]. Faria *et al.*; showed the association of CHD with severe infections in children with DS including pneumonia and sepsis due to increased frequency of respiratory problems caused by cardiac failure as well as the cardiac effects on the large airways [59].

2.2.4. Gastro-oesophageal Reflux Disease (GERD)

Gastroesophageal reflux is the most common motility disorders observed in children with DS due to hypotonia and decreased the pharyngeal and esophageal muscle tone. It occurs mainly in early infancy and often be misdiagnosed because of its atypical manifestations. Serious complications can occur in about 43% of GERD when presents in children with DS. Gastric contents aspiration into airway can cause pulmonary inflammation, aspiration syndromes, chemical pneumonitis, and induces reflex spasm of lower oesophagus and bronchospasm. Silent GERD could cause recurrent subclinical aspiration of thin fluids and increase the incidence of lower respiratory tract infections. It may be responsible for up to 42% of chronic respiratory symptoms in DS children. So, a high index of suspicion is needed to detect GERD and its complications [38, 60].

2.2.5. Associated Nutritional Deficiencies

Nutritional status of children with DS strongly affects the immune system. A well-nourished DS child living in appropriate environment and physically free from associated co-morbidities will not suffer from infections that are commonly associated in children with primary immunodeficiency. Zinc is one of extensively studied micronutrient in children with DS and is needed for various immunologic mechanisms including SOD activity. Changes in zinc plasma levels can affect the immune status in children with DS and is linked to the raised risk of infectious diseases, which represents the major reason of death in affected individuals. Soto-Quintana *et al.* showed significantly diminished zinc plasma levels in children with DS [61]. Cocchi *et al.* also demonstrated presence of zinc deficiency which might be only transient, and found that plasma levels of zinc were normal at birth and decrease over time after 5 years of age [24]. Zinc deficiency could be due to malnutrition or due to mal absorption. However, normalization of cellular zinc levels in patients with DS does not always correct the immune defect [62].

3. COMMON INFECTIONS IN CHILDREN WITH DOWN SYNDROME

Children with DS are more liable to frequent infections with a tendency for slower resolutions and more complications as they behave with infections in a different way from that with normal children. Both upper and lower respiratory tract infections and hepatitis B infections are among the most frequent infections encountered in children with DS which could trigger autoimmune-mediated endocrine disorders as well as other autoimmune disorders due to immune dysregulation. At the same times; children with DS have a significantly higher mortality risk and rate from infection than children without DS [63]. Table **1** shows some common infections in children with DS

Table 1. Common infections in children with DS.

Respiratory infections
- Otitis media with/without effusion
- Cholesteatoma
- Bacterial pharyngitis, tonsillitis.
- Bacterial tracheitis (pseudomembranous croup)
- Respiratory syncytial virus (RSV): bronchiolitis and/or pneumonia
- Other viral, bacterial pneumonia, *Mycoplasma pneumonia*
Digestive system infections:
- Oral Candidiasis.
- Juvenile periodontitis & gingivitis
- Helicobacter Pylori gastritis
- Viral hepatitis (A, B, C)
Cardiovascular system infections
- Infective endocarditis
- Pacemaker-associated infections
Nervous system infections:
- Mycotic aneurysm
- Meningoencephalitis
- Tuberculous meningitis and Tuberculous radiculomyelitis

(Table 1) contd.....

Malignancy-associated infections:
- Fulminant sepsis, bacteremia, pneumonia, systemic candidiasis
- Cutaneous infections, mucositis, and cellulitis.
Other Infections:
- Cytomegalovirus (CMV) infection
- Polyomaviruses infections

3.1. Respiratory Infections in Children with DS

Respiratory infections are the most frequent infections in DS children which could be viral, bacterial, fungal or mixed infections. The percentage of major lower respiratory infections in DS children may reach up to 8% and are the most frequent cause for acute hospital admission [64, 65]. The highest percentage of admissions in those children is between 1 and 5-year-old children, followed by infants younger than 1 year of age and then by children with age between 5-17 years. These infections are associated with marked low IgG2 levels; dramatically reduced numbers of total lymphocytes, CD4(+) T lymphocytes, CD4(+) invariant natural killer (iNKT) cells and regulatory T cells in the DS group which are important reasons to catch these infections [66]. Presence of congenital heart disease is an important predisposing factor for severe and prolonged lower respiratory tract infections and more likely to require admission to an ICU and ventilatory support. Aspiration from improper oropharyngeal coordination or gastroesophageal reflux is a major reason of respiratory problems in the DS population. Evaluation of feeding abilities and gastroesophageal reflux is vital in the assessment of respiratory problems in DS population [56]. Other local factors like diminutive facial bone structures; shallow or absent cavities of the paranasal sinuses; small narrow ear canals with a shallow drainage angle; and a narrow airways with a shallow high-arched palate may also take part in increasing severity and incidence of respiratory tract infections. Repeated respiratory infections have a long term effects on children with DS. These repeated infections further impair the mental and motor development; and induce more behavioral problems and poor quality of life with impaired school achievements [67].

There are high risk and increased prevalence of otitis media with effusion (OME) in DS children, with a peak of ≥60 % around 1 and 6-7 years. A declining trend is seen in older children (≥8 years). Mild to moderate hearing loss was present in children with bilateral OME [68]. The recovery rate for otitis media with effusion is lesser in DS children than in the control children. Consequences of otitis media with effusion (atelectatic eardrum, permanent perforation of the eardrum, middle ear cholesteatoma and hearing loss) considerably occur more frequently in DS children than the non-syndromic children [69]. The increased rate of complications is related to different factors; including the depressed immunity; residual mesenchyme, fixation and superstructure deformity of the stapes, hypoplasia or sclerosis of mastoid bones and large facial canal dehiscence; including dehiscence of the fallopian canal [70]. Cholesteatoma is also a real difficult problem in DS children. It should be suspected in each DS child presenting with alarming symptoms such as otorrhea and hearing loss. If there is any suspicion on inspection, additional imaging studies (high-resolution computed tomography) are indicated [71]. The efficacy of grommet ear tube insertion (tympanostomy tube) in DS children is markedly reduced than that observed in control children. They have more frequent periods of otorrhea from the ear tubes than the control children and emerging of antibiotic-resistant-bacteria are more frequent. The majority of them may require two or more sets of tubes insertion during their childhood. Conservative treatment is the treatment of first choice. Insertion of tympanostomy tubes should be reserved only when middle ear effusion causes severe degree of hearing loss or when there are impending pathological changes of the eardrum, such as adhesion and deep retraction pocket formation [69]. It should be noted that the efficacy of adenoidectomy in children with DS is significantly less than that in controls and should influence surgical decision making in these children [72].

Children with DS have large tonsils & adenoids. Group A *Streptococcus* (*Streptococcus pyogenes*; or GAS) is the most common cause of bacterial pharyngitis, but other *streptococci* such as group C and G β-hemolytic *streptococci* may also cause acute pharyngitis. More specifically, *Streptococcus pyogenes* is generally associated with upper respiratory tract infections such as tonsillitis and pharyngitis, and also causes bronchitis. Children with DS are more frequently affected by episodes of pharyngitis and tonsillitis as a result of immune system anomalies and possibly clinical complications arising from the syndrome.

They are also more susceptible to infection or colonization by non-GAS when compared to controls [73].

Bacterial tracheitis (pseudomembranous croup) is characterized by inflammatory upper airways obstruction with fever. Bronchoscopy showed presence of purulent tracheal secretions and a normal epiglottis. Most cases are due to *Staphylococcus aureus,* but *Haemophilus influenzae* (before using *Haemophilus influenzae* vaccine) and various *streptococci* had also been implicated. CANT *et al.*; reported four children with DS seen over three years with severe airways obstruction due to tracheitis with *Haemophilus influenzae* (Hib) as the causative organism. Bacterial tracheitis should be considered when a child with DS presents with upper airways obstruction [74]. Tracheitis may require urgent bronchoscopy and intubation. The patients should be cared for in a unit with adequate facilities for managing this life-threatening condition. However, the routine use of the Hib vaccine all over the world, markedly reduced the rate of invasive Hib disease.

Infection with respiratory syncytial virus (RSV) is the most significant and severe cause of lower respiratory tract infections in all DS children especially premature infants. Being a child with DS is an independent risk factor for severe RSV infection and hospitalization [75]. Children with DS have a drastically higher risk than did children without DS for being hospitalized (raised from 0.5% to 2% in general pediatric population to 9% among children with DS) with RSV-related lower respiratory tract infections (as bronchiolitis and pneumonia), even in the absence of other underlying conditions or coexisting risk factors. However, DS children with congenital heart disease (CHD) or low immunoprophylaxis against RSV carry higher risks than DS children without CHD [76]. Pulmonary hypertension (which frequently occurs in children with DS more than in non-syndromic children) is an additional possible risk factor for serious RSV infection. Frequent occurrence of apnea in children with DS (due to abnormal upper airway physiology) may trigger respiratory viral infections especially with RSV. This augmented with decreased lung function and impaired immune system could predispose children with DS to serious condition if they become infected with RSV [77]. These children have the potential to be infected with RVS till an older age than healthy controls. They present more often with fever, consolidation and more often have radiographic consolidation detected on chest radiography. They usually need longer hospitalization, necessitate more frequent ventilatory support and have an elevated mortality rate probably indicating the association with cardiac disease. However, hospitalization for RSV-provoked lower respiratory tract infection in DS children does not raise notably the risk for recurrent wheezing or long-term airway morbidity [75].

Other respiratory viral infections have severe outcome in children with DS. The H1N1 pandemic occurred in 2009 showed that patients with DS had unfavorable results in cases with influenza-like illness (ILI) and serious acute respiratory illness (SARI) during the first months of the outbreak of influenza A pandemic (H1N1) 2009 virus. Increased pro-inflammatory cytokines production results in unnecessary inflammation and a more severe clinical course, which may explain the increased severity and morbidity of influenza A infection in DS children [78]. Those patients had greater risk for hospitalization, endotracheal intubation, mechanical ventilation, and even death. Patients with DS are more probably liable to develop pneumonia, severe influenza and high risk of death during hospitalization [66]. Herpes simplex pneumonia was also described in a child with DS. He presented with interstitial pneumonitis with nonspecific physical, X-ray, and laboratory findings, and unfortunately he died. Diagnosis of herpes simplex pneumonia was confirmed by isolation of herpes simplex virus from autopsy lung cultures and by displaying the antigen in the tissue using immunoperoxidase procedure. However, herpes simplex pneumonia is probably a treatable condition. Early virologic studies are advised in immunocompromised patients including children when presenting with progressive pneumonitis of undetermined cause [79].

Bacterial pneumonia when present may be severe and may need aggressive treatment in children with DS. Pneumonias are usually encountered in children less than 5 years of age. Recurrent pneumonia due to aspiration is frequent in DS children due to the associated GERD. *Mycoplasma pneumoniae* is a common organism for atypical pneumonia in children with DS. It could present with fever, cough, wheezing, irritability, and tachypnea. Children may have bilateral consolidations on their chest X-ray and may progress to respiratory distress, which may necessitate hospitalization. They may experience serious mycoplasma infections early in life because of the associated immune abnormalities in DS

[80]. *Mycoplasma pneumonia* is mostly coupled with cold agglutinin syndrome, whereas both cold IgM and warm IgG autoantibodies can be induced. These warm IgG autoantibodies, following mycoplasma infection can cause warm autoimmune hemolytic anemia [81]. *Mycoplasma pneumoniae* should be suspected as a potential reason for pneumonia in young children with DS. When having a severe infection; extracorporeal membrane oxygenation might have a valuable role in the management [82].

3.2. Digestive System Infections in Children with DS

The mouth is one of the most diversified sources of microorganisms specially *Candida*. Childhood is one of the most favorable conditions for increasing frequency of infection by *Candida*. In addition; DS children are more prone to colonization and infections with *Candida albicans*. There are different anatomic and physiologic factors that may contribute to the increased oral carriage of *C. albicans*. These factors include large tongue, oral muscles incompetence, repeated respiratory infections, motor difficulty and immune deficiency particularly of cellular immunity and decrease salivary IgA. Colonization with *C. albicans* can be accompanied by simultaneous erythematous or white pseudomembranous lesions of the oral mucosa and is positively correlated to age [83]. The morphology and typing of *Candida albicans* isolates obtained from children with DS tend to form fringes regardless of size and highly proteolytic more than that observed in the controls [84].

Persons with DS have a high prevalence of juvenile periodontitis compared with normal age-matched control people and also when compared with other mentally retarded persons of matching age. They have inflamed gingiva together with an increased amount of plaque that is related to age and reduced oral hygiene. They have immune-inflammatory over response of the tissues, reduced oral hygiene, decreased attendance to dental care and weakened cell-mediated and humoral immunity with deficient phagocytic system [85]. Mouth breathing with the associated mouth dryness and tongue and lip fissuring are additional factors predisposing to periodontitis. Decrease muscle tone of head and oral cavity including lips and cheeks contributes to inefficient mastication and natural cleansing mechanism of the teeth with more food may be impacted between the teeth after eating. There is a strong relationship between defective neutrophil chemotaxis and the progression of periodontal disease in DS [86]. Children with DS show higher susceptibility to *Helicobacter pylori* infection which could be due to immunodeficiency and poor hygienic conditions. Seropositivity for *Helicobacter pylori* was found in about 50% of mentally retarded children including children with DS [87, 88].

Despite that hepatitis A virus (HAV) infection is still one of the most frequent causes of acute liver disease and more prevalent in children, yet studies showed no increased risk among children with DS [89]. Children with DS can acquire easily Hepatitis B Virus (HBV) infection than normal children especially when they start to attend school independently whether the school is a closed or an open institution. However, the prevalence of Hepatitis B in children with DS is similar to that other institutionalized mentally retarded patients. Children with DS are also more liable to be chronic HBV carriers and they maintain HBV replication due to their immature immune response. So, they must be vaccinated before they begin to attend school and they must be treated with antiviral agents once they are diagnosed [90]. It was observed that children with DS frequently carry hepatitis B surface antigen (HBsAg) even in population with low infection rate which could suggest inadequate immunological handling of the hepatitis B virus (HBV) in DS patients due to an abnormal immune response [89]. They have also low seroconversion rate in response to hepatitis B vaccine. So with, all patients with DS should be vaccinated against hepatitis B virus and should be followed and monitored by clinicians [91]. It also should be noted that DS children with hepatitis C viral infection showed less favorable response to treatment with interferon (IFN) as compared with non-DS children [92].

Despite that acute appendicitis is the most frequent surgical emergency in childhood, but its incidence is strikingly lesser in DS patients than in the non-syndromic children. Although the biological reasons and mechanisms for this low incidence still unknown, this observation should be considered during assessment of acute abdomen in DS patients [93].

However, it should be kept in mind. There is one case report describing occurrence of intra-thoracic appendicitis within a Morgagni hernia in a child with

DS. The diagnosis was a challenge due to the unusual anatomical position [94].

3.3. Cardiovascular System Infections in DS Children

DS children are at a high risk for CHD. This predisposes them to pathophysiological conditions, medications and procedures associated with immunodeficiency which may increase the chance of cardiovascular complications including infections. In one study in Dublin, children with DS form about 10% of cases with infective endocarditis [95]. Another case study described occurrence of very rare endocarditis caused by lactobacilli in DS adolescent female who did have surgical repair of atrioventricular septal defect because of early development of Eisenmenger's syndrome [96]. Pacemakers are occasionally needed in children with DS if there is atrioventricular conduction disorder either due to congenital heart disease or following its correction. Down syndrome is a significant risk factor in development of infection after pacemaker implantation [97].

3.4. Infections of The Nervous System in DS Children

There are very few studies about infections of the nervous system in DS children; most of them are single case reports that illustrate unusual etiologies, which most likely do not correspond to the main infections common to DS children. There was a description of DS child who had infective endocarditis and presented with mycotic aneurysm of the middle cerebral artery that occurred as a complication. The child was successfully managed medically without the need for surgical intervention [98]. There is another case report described a 2 years DS child who was complicated with Moyamoya syndrome following central nervous invasion by the measles virus. Moyamoya like cerebrovascular lesions occur more often and is more aggressive in DS children than in non-syndromic children and their clinical presentation is always of the infarction type [99]. Another case described occurrence of severe meningoencephalitis following *Mycoplasma pneumoniae* infection who recovered completely within few weeks. Infection with *Mycoplasma pneumoniae* should be suspected in all cases presented with acute encephalopathy [100]. Tuberculous radiculomyelitis (TBRM) is an uncommon complication of TB meningitis. It was described in a 10-year-old Asian girl with

DS who presented with acute urinary retention and fever then she had acute neurological deterioration and found to have evidence of TB meningitis [101]. Aseptic meningitis was reported in 1-year-old male infant with DS. He was treated using many antimicrobials including cefotaxime and ceftriaxone for bacterial meningitis caused by *Haemophilus influenzae type b*. Despite of using many antibiotics, he continued to have high fever for more than a month. After, discontinuation of the antibiotics, the fever subsided and cerebrospinal fluid findings normalized, confirming the cause as drug induced aseptic meningitis. This case emphasizes about the importance of proper recognition and diagnosis of this rare occurrence of drug-induced aseptic meningitis. It is simply treated by withdrawal of the offending medications, and its recurrence can be easily prevented [102].

3.5. Infections in Children with DS with Malignancy

DS children are at a higher risk of malignancy and treatment complications especially acute leukemia than the remaining pediatric population. Malignancy itself adds further burden of the already exhausted immune system in DS children. This burden could be linked to the tumor itself through invasion and depression of the bone marrow and immune system like pancytopenia that results from invasion of bone marrow by leukemic cells in acute lymphoblastic leukemia (ALL) or related to the hematologic toxicity due to chemotherapy. Complications related to chemotherapy are a major reason of increased morbidity and mortality in DS children leading to numerous modifications in treatment protocols. There is a high incidence of infections like pneumonia and bacteremia in children with ALL which sometimes need interruption of treatment or dose reduction. Fulminant sepsis due to *Candida* infection and other organisms may be a cause of death in those children [103]. Children with DS and ALL had deeper, more prolonged neutrophil and monocyte count nadirs; more risk of toxicity; more prolonged hospitalizations; and more frequent microbiologically documented infections, mucositis, and cellulitis. The high risk of severe neutropenia, monocytopenia, and increase risk of cellulitis in DS-ALL increases the need to stress on the skin hygiene, caution, attention and aggressive treatment of cutaneous infections [104]. Viral etiology of infection should also be considered if the routine diagnostic tools do not show the etiologic agent. A case of human coronavirus OC43 pneumonia was described in a pediatric leukemia patient with DS and febrile neutropenia. It is important and relevant to consider viral etiology and to routinely utilize polymerase chain reaction-based diagnostic utilities to reveal the etiology of a significant group of "pneumonias of unidentified cause" in immunocompromised pediatric patients [105]. It should be noted that the susceptibility to the malignancy associated infection differs according to the type of malignancy. For example; children with DS and acute myeloid leukemia (AML) have significantly less infectious toxicity and complications during treatment and have a more favorable infection profile then children with DS and ALL [106].

3.6. Other Infections in Children with DS

Cytomegalovirus (CMV) infection is highly prevalent among children attending day-care centers including children with DS. CMV infection is very common in children with DS attending this special day-care center and prevalence of the CMV IgG antibody may reach up to 76%. This high rate of CMV infection in children with DS is due to the associated mental retardation, poor understanding of the basic principles of hygiene, and because they produce excess saliva due to protrusion of the tongue with high prevalence of CMV shedding in the urine or saliva by these children [107]. Children with DS are significantly more sensitive to random chromosomal breakage after Varicella virus infection than control subjects. However, the chromosomal breaks reverted back to the preinfection range within one month [108]. Polyomaviruses infections are extremely frequent childhood and young adult infections. Most of these infections are asymptomatic or cause mild problems but usually symptomatic in immunosuppressed patients, old age or post-transplantation and can cause Merkel cell carcinoma, progressive multifocal leukoencephalopathy (PML) and BK virus nephropathy. Children with DS showed higher prevalence rate (greater-than-double prevalence rates) of urinary polyomavirus infection and in viral titers. This may be due to several factors including diminish humoral and especially cell-mediated immunological surveillance in DS [109].

4. COULD INFECTIONS PREDISPOSE TO HAVING A CHILD WITH DOWN SYNDROME?!

The genetic basis of DS is well known. However, environmental factors are probably participating in its pathogenesis. These factors may include higher socio-economic status, use of oral contraception, maternal smoking, exposure to ionizing radiation, certain paternal occupations and housing near risky waste sites. Study done by McNally *et al.* showed that space-time clustering amongst cases of DS suggests that relevant etiological agents may cluster in space-time. The types of etiological cause involved are likely to be infectious [110]. A study done by Annerén *et al.* showed overrepresentation of Herpes Simplex Virus type-2 antibody positivity among DS mothers. However, there was no enough number of studies to confirm the role of HSV-2 as a major cause of DS. Other studies failed to find a relation between maternal Hepatitis A and Hepatitis B infections during pregnancy [111, 112].

5. PREVENTION OF INFECTIONS IN DS CHILDREN

Because of the increased risk of infection and the infection-related complications, improving the immunity and preventing the infection are of utmost importance to children with DS. These aims can be achieved by various ways like proper hygiene, adequate diet, vitamins supplement, immunomodulations and proper vaccinations.

5.1. Breast Feeding

Breast feeding has many advantages to typical newborns. These advantages are more needed to children with DS. However, breast feeding is complex and a real challenge to mothers of DS children due to the associated cardiac anomaly, low muscle tone and poor sucking ability. Maternal depression and frustration as result of having a child with DS and the frequent admission of the new DS baby to the hospital either for a diagnostic work-up or to treat a health problems are other factors for poor breast feeding in DS children. However, children with DS can be breast fed successfully, with proper support, encouragement of their mothers, sound information, and assisted to set realistic expectations. Lactation consultant and other members of the health care team should support the mother to do what she can and wants to do for her infant. Breast feeding gives an extra protection against infections which are more common in children with DS. It also improves mouth and tongue coordination and provides additional stimulation for the baby who is usually sleepy as well as enhancing mother-infant bonding [113, 114].

5.2. Proper Hygiene

Proper hygiene is important to prevent infections and its complications. Care of skin is mandatory as it is one of the portals of entry for the immune system which protect the body. Dryness of the skin is very common in children with DS that can occur up to 90% of DS children. Dry skin can induce itching, skin cracking (particularly of the hands, feet, wrists and elbows) and skin infection which could be a focus for a systemic infection. Proper moisturizing the skin and daily application of hypoallergenic barrier cream can help to keep the skin healthy and intact. Over exposure to sunlight should be minimized and use of sun screen is judicious [115]. Periodontal disease is a significant oral health problem seen in children with DS, which may be related to immune deficiency factors, poor oral hygiene, teeth grinding and/or crowding. Proper teeth brushing should be done at least twice-daily. Teeth should be evaluated at age of 2 years for early detection of dental decay and periodontitis by a pediatric dentist; then follow up every 6 months for early detection of delay, alterations in the sequence of tooth eruption or gingivitis and periodontal disease which can occur early and progresses rapidly. If the child has congenital heart disease or with residual lesion after correction, he should have prophylaxis against bacterial endocarditis [116].

5.3. Prophylaxis Against Respiratory Infections

Children with DS are at significant risk for respiratory syncytial virus (RSV) infection and related hospitalization specially if there are other co morbidities like cardiac diseases. Palivizumab is a monoclonal antibody used to prevent RSV infections in high-risk infant as with prematurity or other medical problems such as DS or congenital heart disease. Palivizumab used in intramuscular monthly dose of 15 mg/kg of body weight is associated with reduction of the incidence rate for RSV-related hospitalization by about 3.6-fold in children with DS during the first 2 years of life [117]. Pidotimod (Polimod) is an artificial immunomodulator dipeptide compound with biological and immunological activity on both the adaptive and the innate immune responses. Pidotimod can decrease the frequency of recurrent infections of the upper respiratory and urinary tracts in children. The use of Pidotimod is accompanied with the up regulation of a number of genes included in the activation of innate immune responses and in antimicrobial activity. Amusingly, these effects are more evident in the setting of immune defects such as DS [118, 119]. Pidotimod in a daily dose of 400 mg is markedly able to decrease in the number of days of fever, degree of severity of the signs and symptoms of the acute episodes and use of antibiotics and antipyretic drugs in children with DS. Pidotimod is well tolerated and no significant clinical, hematological or biochemical side-effects are noted [120]. The use of Levamisole as an immune modulating agent in children with DS showed an adequate immune modulation in some children with DS but it failed in others [121].

5.4. Antioxidants Supplement in DS Children

DS children have a greater incidence of infections, largely due to the poorly functioning immune system which is partially due to oxidative stress (excess of oxidative free radicals) and low levels of antioxidants. Individuals with DS have high levels of oxidative stress throughout their life. Genes that are over expressed on chromosome 21 are accompanied with oxidative stress and neuronal apoptosis. There are many trials to use antioxidants to combat oxidative stress in children with DS [122]. Children with DS have below normal plasma levels of selenium. Selenium supplementation was found to augment Ig G2 and Ig G4 level through stimulation of immunoglobulin production with parallel decrease in incidence of infection rate and improvement in resistance to infection [123]. Zinc supplements seemed to benefit children with DS. Zinc affects the metabolism of thyroid hormones in children with DS. Zinc supplements can normalize the thyroid stimulating hormone and thyroxine levels. Oral zinc supplementation can significantly affect the immune system. It can normalize thymulin and zinc plasma levels and normalize lymphocyte proliferation and polymorphonuclear activity after zinc supplementation. Zinc supplementation has a helpful clinical effect in these children, since a decreased rate of infections was found [124]. Ascorbic acid deficiency in the blood was found in many children with DS. There is a strong evidence of the link between ascorbic acid deficiency and increase incidence of infections. Vitamin C supplement is recommended to prevent and to treat recurring infections. It has valuable antioxidant properties that can be exploited in combating cell deterioration [125]. Dietary supplementation with alpha-lipoic acid and L-cysteine significantly decreases septic oxidative stress and increases total antioxidant status of the serum in children with DS which could help them to overcome sepsis associated oxidative stress and enhances their ability to fight infections [126]. Many children with DS showed manifestations of vitamins deficiencies which could be another factor for their poor immunity. Multivitamin supplementation *e.g.* vitamins A, C and E, all can help to improve their resistance to infection with fewer infections and fewer days off school.

5.5. Vaccination of Children with Down Syndrome

Despite many studies showed fewer efficacies of many vaccines given to children with DS [91, 127, 128], but other studies proved its efficacy [129]. Immunodeficiency associated with DS is not a contraindication for vaccination. Vaccinations can prevent a good number of infectious diseases that children with DS could be exposed to. Immunogenicity and safety of most of the vaccines are not significantly different from those observed in the normal children. Despite some vaccines produce lower humoral responses to the usual ones (mumps, measles, acellular pertussis, hepatitis, pneumococcal and meningococcal), but still able to produce an accepted protective effects which necessitate strict adherence to vaccination schedules [130]. Early intake of hepatitis B is recommended as the efficacy of the vaccine may decrease with age due to the associated co morbidities of the syndrome. Early BCG vaccine is also recommended in countries with high incidence of tuberculosis.

Pneumococcal vaccine is indicated in children with DS even if it is not present in the routine immunization schedule of concerned country. For children less than 2 years it is better to give Prevnar 13® as Pneumovax® 23 despite covering more types of pneumococcal bacteria but it is not of the same efficacy of Prevnar 13® in children below the age of 2 years. Prevnar 13® can be given at 2, 4, 6, and 12 month of age and Pneumovax® 23 can be given at the age of 5 years [26].

Rotavirus can cause severe vomiting and diarrhea in children. Rota virus vaccine is considered now as one of the routine vaccinations in most countries. It should be given especially if the child has problems during feeding or with their gastrointestinal (digestive) system. There are two main types of Rota virus vaccine. One is given in a 2-doses series in infants and children (*e.g.* Rotarix which contains rotavirus strain of G1P) and another type which is given in 3 doses (*e.g.* RotaTeq which is pentavalent vaccine that contains five G1, G2, G3 and G4 serotypes). The first oral rotavirus vaccine is given before they are 14 weeks of age and their second oral dose is given before 24 weeks of age while the third dose (if given) should not be taken after 32 weeks of age [131].

Despite chicken pox usually resolve within one week, but serious complications that may need hospitalization can occur specially in immune compromised children as in children with DS who frequently have other skin disorders that may aggravate chicken pox. The chickenpox vaccine can be given from nine months of age and another booster dose can be given at the age of 4 years [132].

Meningococcal diseases are common among institutionalized people who carry a higher risk of meningococcal diseases than in normal population. Today, most children with DS live at home with their families and attending regular education system. However, this group of patients still carries a higher risk for meningococcal disease than normal children. Vaccines against meningococcal serogroup C are given in 3 doses at 2 month, 4 to 6 months and at 12 to 15 month of age. Annual influenza vaccine is advised for infants aged 6 months and over, children, adolescents and adults with DS [133].

CONCLUSION

Children with DS are more liable for recurrent infections than normal children and are more prone to more complications. Every effort should be done to minimize the risk of infection and to improve their immunity.

CONFLICT OF INTEREST

The authors confirm that this chapter contents have no conflict of interest.

ACKNOWLEDGEMENTS

Declared none.

REFERENCES

[1] Ram G, Chinen J. Infections and immunodeficiency in Down syndrome. Clin Exp Immunol 2011; 164(1): 9-16.
[http://dx.doi.org/10.1111/j.1365-2249.2011.04335.x] [PMID: 21352207]

[2] Sustrová M, Saríková V. [Down's syndrome--effect of increased gene expression in chromosome 21 on the function of the immune and nervous system]. Bratisl Lek Listy (Tlacene Vyd) 1997; 98(4): 221-8.
[PMID: 9264831]

[3] Kim YS, Cho KO, Lee HJ, Kim SY, Sato Y, Cho YJ. Down syndrome candidate region 1 increases the stability of the IkappaBalpha protein: implications for its anti-inflammatory effects. J Biol Chem 2006; 281(51): 39051-61.
[http://dx.doi.org/10.1074/jbc.M604659200] [PMID: 17062574]

[4] Gardiner K, Davisson M. The sequence of human chromosome 21 and implications for research into Down syndrome. Genome Biol 2000; 1(2) REVIEWS0002
[PMID: 11178230]

[5] Li C, Jin L, Bai Y, *et al.* Genome-wide expression analysis in Down syndrome: insight into immunodeficiency. PLoS One 2012; 7(11): e49130.
[http://dx.doi.org/10.1371/journal.pone.0049130] [PMID: 23155455]

[6] Gordon J, Manley NR. Mechanisms of thymus organogenesis and morphogenesis. Development 2011; 138(18): 3865-78.
[http://dx.doi.org/10.1242/dev.059998] [PMID: 21862553]

[7] Levin S, Schlesinger M, Handzel Z, *et al.* Thymic deficiency in Down's syndrome. Pediatrics 1979; 63(1): 80-7.
[PMID: 155804]

[8] Larocca LM, Lauriola L, Ranelletti FO, *et al.* Morphological and immunohistochemical study of Down syndrome thymus. Am J Med Genet Suppl 1990; 7: 225-30.
[PMID: 2149952]

[9] Murphy M, Friend DS, Pike-Nobile L, Epstein LB. Tumor necrosis factor-alpha and IFN-gamma expression in human thymus. Localization and overexpression in Down syndrome (trisomy 21). J Immunol 1992 Oct 1; 149(7): 2506-12.
[PMID: 1388194]

[10] Murphy M, Epstein LB. Down syndrome (DS) peripheral blood contains phenotypically mature CD3+TCR alpha, beta+ cells but abnormal proportions of TCR alpha, beta+, TCR gamma, delta+, and CD4+ CD45RA+ cells: evidence for an inefficient release of mature T cells by the DS thymus. Clin Immunol Immunopathol 1992; 62(2): 245-51.
[http://dx.doi.org/10.1016/0090-1229(92)90079-4] [PMID: 1530912]

[11] Roat E, Prada N, Lugli E, *et al.* Homeostatic cytokines and expansion of regulatory T cells accompany thymic impairment in children with Down syndrome. Rejuvenation Res 2008; 11(3): 573-83. [http://dx.doi.org/10.1089/rej.2007.0648] [PMID: 18386990]

[12] Guazzarotti L, Trabattoni D, Castelletti E, *et al.* T lymphocyte maturation is impaired in healthy young individuals carrying trisomy 21 (Down syndrome). Am J Intellect Dev Disabil 2009; 114(2): 100-9. [http://dx.doi.org/10.1352/2009.114.100-109] [PMID: 19391670]

[13] Ugazio AG. Down's syndrome: problems of immunodeficiency. Hum Genet Suppl 1981; 2: 33-9. [http://dx.doi.org/10.1007/978-3-642-68006-9_3] [PMID: 6218139]

[14] Roat E, Prada N, Lugli E, *et al.* Homeostatic cytokines and expansion of regulatory T cells accompany thymic impairment in children with Down syndrome. Rejuvenation Res 2008; 11(3): 573-83. [http://dx.doi.org/10.1089/rej.2007.0648] [PMID: 18386990]

[15] Wisniewski K, Cobill JM, Wilcox CB, Caspary EA, Williams DG, Wisniewski HM. T lymphocytes in patients with Down's syndrome. Biol Psychiatry 1979; 14(3): 463-71. [PMID: 157786]

[16] Abu Faddan N, Sayed D, Ghaleb F. T lymphocytes apoptosis and mitochondrial membrane potential in Down's syndrome. Fetal Pediatr Pathol 2011; 30(1): 45-52. [http://dx.doi.org/10.3109/15513815.2010.505626] [PMID: 21204666]

[17] Bloemers BL, Broers CJ, Bont L, Weijerman ME, Gemke RJ, van Furth AM. Increased risk of respiratory tract infections in children with Down syndrome: the consequence of an altered immune system. Microbes Infect 2010; 12(11): 799-808. [http://dx.doi.org/10.1016/j.micinf.2010.05.007] [PMID: 20685340]

[18] Epstein LB, Epstein CJ. T-lymphocyte function and sensitivity to interferon in trisomy 21. Cell Immunol 1980; 51(2): 303-18. [http://dx.doi.org/10.1016/0008-8749(80)90262-2] [PMID: 6154538]

[19] Nair MP, Schwartz SA. Association of decreased T-cell-mediated natural cytotoxicity and interferon production in Down's syndrome. Clin Immunol Immunopathol 1984; 33(3): 412-24. [http://dx.doi.org/10.1016/0090-1229(84)90312-X] [PMID: 6209046]

[20] Lin SJ, Wang JY, Klickstein LB, *et al.* Lack of age-associated LFA-1 up-regulation and impaired ICAM-1 binding in lymphocytes from patients with Down syndrome. Clin Exp Immunol 2001; 126(1): 54-63. [http://dx.doi.org/10.1046/j.1365-2249.2001.01660.x] [PMID: 11678899]

[21] Bloemers BL, van Bleek GM, Kimpen JL, Bont L. Distinct abnormalities in the innate immune system of children with Down syndrome. J Pediatr 2010 May; 156(5): 804-9. [http://dx.doi.org/10.1016/j.jpeds.2009.12.006] [PMID: 20172534]

[22] Elsayed SM, Elsayed GM. Phenotype of apoptotic lymphocytes in children with Down syndrome. Immun Ageing 2009 Mar 6; 6(2) [http://dx.doi.org/10.1186/1742-4933-6-2] [PMID: 19267926]

[23] Mauri C, Bosma A. Immune regulatory function of B cells. Annu Rev Immunol 2012; 30: 221-41. [http://dx.doi.org/10.1146/annurev-immunol-020711-074934] [PMID: 22224776]

[24] Cocchi G, Mastrocola M, Capelli M, Bastelli A, Vitali F, Corvaglia L. Immunological patterns in young children with Down syndrome: is there a temporal trend? Acta Paediatr 2007; 96(10): 1479-82. [http://dx.doi.org/10.1111/j.1651-2227.2007.00459.x] [PMID: 17727689]

[25] Annerén G, Magnusson CG, Lilja G, Nordvall SL. Abnormal serum IgG subclass pattern in children with Down's syndrome. Arch Dis Child 1992; 67(5): 628-31. [http://dx.doi.org/10.1136/adc.67.5.628] [PMID: 1534650]

[26] Costa-Carvalho BT, Martinez RM, Dias AT, *et al.* Antibody response to pneumococcal capsular polysaccharide vaccine in Down syndrome patients. Braz J Med Biol Res 2006; 39(12): 1587-92. [http://dx.doi.org/10.1590/S0100-879X2006001200010] [PMID: 17160268]

[27] Verstegen RH, Kusters MA, Gemen EF, DE Vries E. Down syndrome B-lymphocyte subpopulations, intrinsic defect or decreased T-lymphocyte help. Pediatr Res 2010; 67(5): 563-9. [http://dx.doi.org/10.1203/PDR.0b013e3181d4ecc1] [PMID: 20098344]

[28] Yamato F, Takaya J, Yasuhara A, Teraguchi M, Ikemoto Y, Kaneko K. Elevated intracellular calcium in neutrophils in patients with Down syndrome. Pediatr Int 2009; 51(4): 474-7. [http://dx.doi.org/10.1111/j.1442-200X.2008.02761.x] [PMID: 19400826]

[29] Gabbianelli R, Kantar A, Oggiano N, Fiorini R, Falcioni G, Giorgi PL. [Oxidative metabolism in polymorphonuclear granulocytes of children with trisomy 21]. Minerva Pediatr 1993; 45(12): 493-7. [PMID: 8145684]

[30] Seger R, Wildfeuer A, Buchinger G, *et al.* Defects in granulocyte function in various chromosome abnormalities (Down's-, Edwards'-, Cri-du-chat syndrome). Minerva Pediatr 1976 Feb 15; 54(4): 177-83.
[PMID: 176505]

[31] Barroeta O, Nungaray L, López-Osuna M, Armendares S, Salamanca F, Kretschmer RR. Defective monocyte chemotaxis in children with Down's syndrome. Pediatr Res 1983; 17(4): 292-5. [http://dx.doi.org/10.1203/00006450-198304000-00013] [PMID: 6222283]

[32] Novo E, García MI, Lavergne J. Nonspecific immunity in Down syndrome: a study of chemotaxis, phagocytosis, oxidative metabolism, and cell surface marker expression of polymorphonuclear cells. Am J Med Genet 1993; 46(4): 384-91. [http://dx.doi.org/10.1002/ajmg.1320460408] [PMID: 7689298]

[33] Rosner F, Kozinn PJ. Leucocyte function in Down's syndrome. Lancet 1972 Aug 5; 2(7771): 283-4. [http://dx.doi.org/10.1016/S0140-6736(72)91722-9] [PMID: 7689298]

[34] Costello C, Webber A. White cell function in Down's syndrome. Clin Genet 1976; 9(6): 603-5. [http://dx.doi.org/10.1111/j.1399-0004.1976.tb01619.x] [PMID: 132316]

[35] Yasui K, Shinozaki K, Nakazawa T, Agematsu K, Komiyama A. Presenility of granulocytes in Down syndrome individuals. Am J Med Genet 1999 Jun 11; 84(5): 406-12.

[36] Kusters MA, Verstegen RH, Gemen EF, de Vries E. Intrinsic defect of the immune system in children with Down syndrome: a review. Clin Exp Immunol 2009; 156(2): 189-93. [http://dx.doi.org/10.1111/j.1365-2249.2009.03890.x] [PMID: 19250275]

[37] Nurmi T, Huttunen K, Lassila O, *et al.* Natural killer cell function in trisomy-21 (Down's syndrome). Clin Exp Immunol 1982; 47(3): 735-41.

[PMID: 6177458]

[38] Brumbaugh DE, Accurso FJ. Persistent silent aspiration in a child with Trisomy 21. Curr Opinh normal memory counts and decreas Pediatr 2002; 14(2): 231-3. [http://dx.doi.org/10.1097/00008480-200204000-00015] [PMID: 11981296]

[39] Piatti G, Allegra L, Ambrosetti U, De Santi MM. Nasal ciliary function and ultrastructure in Down syndrome. Laryngoscope 2001; 111(7): 1227-30. [http://dx.doi.org/10.1097/00005537-200107000-00016] [PMID: 11568545]

[40] Kovesi T, Sinclair B, MacCormick J, Matzinger MA, Carpenter B. Primary ciliary dyskinesia associated with a novel microtubule defect in a child with Down's syndrome. Chest 2000; 117(4): 1207-9. [http://dx.doi.org/10.1378/chest.117.4.1207] [PMID: 10767266]

[41] Chaushu S, Chaushu G, Zigmond M, *et al.* Age-dependent deficiency in saliva and salivary antibodies secretion in Down's syndrome. Arch Oral Biol 2007; 52(11): 1088-96. [http://dx.doi.org/10.1016/j.archoralbio.2007.06.002] [PMID: 17658453]

[42] Chaushu S, Yefe Nof E, Becker A, Shapira J, Chaushu G. Parotid salivary immunoglobulins, recurrent respiratory tract infections and gingival health in institutionalized and non-institutionalized subjects with Down's syndrome. J Intellect Disabil Res 2003; 47(Pt 2): 101-7. [http://dx.doi.org/10.1046/j.1365-2788.2003.00446.x] [PMID: 12542575]

[43] Chaushu S, Yefenof E, Becker A, Shapira J, Chaushu G. Severe impairment of secretory Ig production in parotid saliva of Down Syndrome individuals. J Dent Res 2002; 81(5): 308-12. [http://dx.doi.org/10.1177/154405910208100504] [PMID: 12097442]

[44] Corsi MM, Ponti W, Venditti A, *et al.* Proapoptotic activated T-cells in the blood of children with Down's syndrome: relationship with dietary antigens and intestinal alterations. Int J Tissue React 2003; 25(3): 117-25. [PMID: 14756193]

[45] Lopez V, Ochs HD, Thuline HC, Davis SD, Wedgwood RJ. Defective antibody response to bacteriophage phichi 174 in Down syndrome. J Pediatr 1975; 86(2): 207-11. [http://dx.doi.org/10.1016/S0022-3476(75)80469-0] [PMID: 122905]

[46] Joshi AY, Abraham RS, Snyder MR, Boyce TG. Immune evaluation and vaccine responses in Down syndrome: evidence of immunodeficiency? Vaccine 2011 Jul 12; 29(31): 5040-6. [http://dx.doi.org/10.1016/j.vaccine.2011.04.060] [PMID: 21596078]

[47] Hawkes RA, Philbrook SC, Boughton CR. The response of institutionalized Down's syndrome subjects to enterovirus infections. J Hyg (Lond) 1980; 84(3): 433-41. [http://dx.doi.org/10.1017/S0022172400026978] [PMID: 6300224]

[48] Philip R, Berger AC, McManus NH, Warner NH, Peacock MA, Epstein LB. Abnormalities of the in vitro cellular and humoral responses to tetanus and influenza antigens with concomitant numerical alterations in lymphocyte subsets in Down syndrome (trisomy 21). J Immunol 1986; 136(5): 1661-7. [PMID: 2419411]

[49] Kusters MA, Gemen EF, Verstegen RH, Wever PC. Both normal memory counts and decreased naive cells favor intrinsic defect over early senescence of Down syndrome T lymphocytes. Pediatr Res 2010

May; 67(5): 557-62.
[http://dx.doi.org/10.1203/PDR.0b013e3181d4eca3] [PMID: 20098345]

[50] Seger R, Buchinger G, Ströder J. On the influence of age on immunity in Down's syndrome. Eur J Pediatr 1977 Jan 26; 124(2): 77-87.
[PMID: 137810]

[51] da Rosa Utiyama SR, Nisihara RM, Nass FR, Oliveira NP, Fiedler PT, de Messias-Reason IT. Autoantibodies in patients with Down syndrome: early senescence of the immune system or precocious markers for immunological diseases? J Paediatr Child Health 2008 Apr; 44(4): 182-6.2008 Apr;
[PMID: 17927730]

[52] Dyken ME, Lin-Dyken DC, Poulton S, Zimmerman MB, Sedars E. Prospective polysomnographic analysis of obstructive sleep apnea in down syndrome. Arch Pediatr Adolesc Med 2003; 157(7): 655-60.
[http://dx.doi.org/10.1001/archpedi.157.7.655] [PMID: 12860786]

[53] Bertrand P, Navarro H, Caussade S, Holmgren N, Sánchez I. Airway anomalies in children with Down syndrome: endoscopic findings. Pediatr Pulmonol 2003; 36(2): 137-41. INSERT FIGURE 001
[http://dx.doi.org/10.1002/ppul.10332] [PMID: 12833493]

[54] Aboussouan LS, O'Donovan PB, Moodie DS, Gragg LA, Stoller JK. Hypoplastic trachea in Down's syndrome. Am Rev Respir Dis 1993 Jan; 147(1): 72-5.
[http://dx.doi.org/10.1164/ajrccm/147.1.72]

[55] Cooney TP, Thurlbeck WM. Pulmonary hypoplasia in Down's syndrome. N Engl J Med 1982 Nov 4; 307(19): 1170-3.

[56] Pothos M. Aspiration: A Common Cause of Respiratory Problems in Down Syndrome Children. Pediatr Res 1999; 45: 130A-A.
[http://dx.doi.org/10.1203/00006450-199904020-00772]

[57] Shott SR. Down syndrome: common otolaryngoloic manifestations. Am J Med Genet C Semin Med Genet 2006 Aug 15; 142C(3): 131-40.
[http://dx.doi.org/10.1002/ajmg.c.30095]

[58] Al-Biltagi MA. Echocardiography in children with Down syndrome. World J Clin Pediatr 2013; 2(4): 36-45.
[http://dx.doi.org/10.5409/wjcp.v2.i4.36] [PMID: 25254173]

[59] Faria PF, Nicolau JA, Melek MZ, de Oliveira NdeS, Bermudez BE, Nisihara RM. Association between congenital heart defects and severe infections in children with Down syndrome. Rev Port Cardiol 2014; 33(1): 15-8.
[http://dx.doi.org/10.1016/j.repc.2013.05.008] [PMID: 24405557]

[60] Macchini F, Leva E, Torricelli M, Valadè A. Treating acid reflux disease in patients with Down syndrome: pharmacological and physiological approaches. Clin Exp Gastroenterol 2011; 4: 19-22.
[http://dx.doi.org/10.2147/CEG.S15872] [PMID: 21694868]

[61] Soto-Quintana M, Alvarez-Nava F, Rojas-Atencio A, *et al.* [Diminished zinc plasma concentrations and alterations in the number of lymphocyte subpopulations in Down's syndrome patients]. Invest Clin

2003; 44(1): 51-60.
[PMID: 12703183]

[62] Brigino EN, Good RA, Koutsonikolis A, Day NK, Kornfeld SJ. Normalization of cellular zinc levels in patients with Downs syndrome does not always correct low thymulin levels. Acta Paediatr 1996; 85(11): 1370-2.
[http://dx.doi.org/10.1111/j.1651-2227.1996.tb13929.x] [PMID: 8955470]

[63] Garrison MM, Jeffries H, Christakis DA. Risk of death for children with down syndrome and sepsis. J Pediatr 2005; 147(6): 748-52.
[http://dx.doi.org/10.1016/j.jpeds.2005.06.032] [PMID: 16356424]

[64] Selikowitz M. Health problems and health checks in school-aged children with Down syndrome. J Paediatr Child Health 1992; 28(5): 383-6.
[http://dx.doi.org/10.1111/j.1440-1754.1992.tb02697.x] [PMID: 1389451]

[65] Hilton JM, Fitzgerald DA, Cooper DM. Respiratory morbidity of hospitalized children with Trisomy 21. J Paediatr Child Health 1999; 35(4): 383-6.
[http://dx.doi.org/10.1046/j.1440-1754.1999.00386.x] [PMID: 10457298]

[66] Broers CJ, Gemke RJ, Weijerman ME, Kuik DJ, van Hoogstraten IM, van Furth AM. Frequency of lower respiratory tract infections in relation to adaptive immunity in children with Down syndrome compared to their healthy siblings. Acta Paediatr 2012; 101(8): 862-7.
[http://dx.doi.org/10.1111/j.1651-2227.2012.02696.x] [PMID: 22548641]

[67] Verstegen RH, van Gameren-Oosterom HB, Fekkes M, Dusseldorp E, de Vries E, van Wouwe JP. Significant impact of recurrent respiratory tract infections in children with Down syndrome. Child Care Health Dev 2013; 39(6): 801-9.
[http://dx.doi.org/10.1111/j.1365-2214.2012.01413.x] [PMID: 22774862]

[68] Maris M, Wojciechowski M, Van de Heyning P, Boudewyns A. A cross-sectional analysis of otitis media with effusion in children with Down syndrome. Eur J Pediatr 2014; 173(10): 1319-25.
[http://dx.doi.org/10.1007/s00431-014-2323-5] [PMID: 24816633]

[69] Iino Y, Imamura Y, Harigai S, Tanaka Y. Efficacy of tympanostomy tube insertion for otitis media with effusion in children with Down syndrome. Int J Pediatr Otorhinolaryngol 1999 Aug 5; 49(2): 143-9.
[http://dx.doi.org/10.1016/S0165-5876(99)00117-2] [PMID: 10504021]

[70] Glass RB, Yousefzadeh DK, Roizen NJ. Mastoid abnormalities in Down syndrome. Pediatr Radiol 1989; 19(5): 311-2.
[http://dx.doi.org/10.1007/BF02467300] [PMID: 2526944]

[71] Bacciu A, Pasanisi E, Vincenti V, *et al.* Surgical treatment of middle ear cholesteatoma in children with Down syndrome. Otol Neurotol 2005; 26(5): 1007-10.
[http://dx.doi.org/10.1097/01.mao.0000185042.46523.9b] [PMID: 16151350]

[72] Price DL, Orvidas LJ, Weaver AL, Farmer SA. Efficacy of adenoidectomy in the treatment of nasal and middle ear symptoms in children with Down syndrome. Int J Pediatr Otorhinolaryngol 2004; 68(1): 7-13.
[http://dx.doi.org/10.1016/j.ijporl.2003.08.053] [PMID: 14687681]

[73] Morais VM, Orsi AR, Maranhão FC, Castro TM, Castro KC, Silva DM. Prevalence of β-hemolytic Streptococcus in children with special health care needs. Braz J Otorhinolaryngol 2012; 78(5): 110-5. [http://dx.doi.org/10.5935/1808-8694.20120017] [PMID: 23108829]

[74] Cant AJ, Gibson PJ, West RJ. Bacterial tracheitis in Down's syndrome. Arch Dis Child 1987; 62(9): 962-3. [http://dx.doi.org/10.1136/adc.62.9.962] [PMID: 2960275]

[75] Bloemers BL, van Furth AM, Weijerman ME, *et al.* Down syndrome: a novel risk factor for respiratory syncytial virus bronchiolitis--a prospective birth-cohort study. Pediatrics 2007; 120(4): e1076-81. [http://dx.doi.org/10.1542/peds.2007-0788] [PMID: 17908728]

[76] Medrano López C, García-Guereta Silva L, Lirio Casero J, García Pérez J, Grupo CI. Grupo CIVIC, Grupo de Trabajo de Infecciones de la Sociedad Española de Cardiología Pediátrica y Cardiopatías Congénitas. [Respiratory infections, Down's syndrome and congenital heart disease: the CIVIC 21 study]. An Pediatr (Barc) 2009; 71(1): 38-46. [http://dx.doi.org/10.1016/j.anpedi.2008.11.007] [PMID: 19423411]

[77] Zachariah P, Ruttenber M, Simões EA. Down syndrome and hospitalizations due to respiratory syncytial virus: a population-based study. J Pediatr 2012; 160(5): 827-31.e1. [http://dx.doi.org/10.1016/j.jpeds.2011.11.004] [PMID: 22177993]

[78] Pérez-Padilla R, Fernández R, García-Sancho C, *et al.* Pandemic (H1N1) 2009 virus and Down syndrome patients. Emerg Infect Dis 2010; 16(8): 1312-4. [http://dx.doi.org/10.3201/eid1608.091931] [PMID: 20678334]

[79] Hull HF, Blumhagen JD, Benjamin D, Corey L. Herpes simplex viral pneumonitis in childhood. J Pediatr 1984; 104(2): 211-5. [http://dx.doi.org/10.1016/S0022-3476(84)80994-4] [PMID: 6319654]

[80] Orlicek SL, Walker MS, Kuhls TL. Severe *mycoplasma pneumonia* in young children with Down syndrome. Clin Pediatr (Phila) 1992; 31(7): 409-12. [http://dx.doi.org/10.1177/000992289203100706] [PMID: 1535577]

[81] Cassimos D, Bezirgiannidou Z, Pantelidou D, Christoforidis A, Chatzimichael A, Maritinis G. Warm autoimmune hemolytic anemia following recurrent *mycoplasma pneumonia* infections in a child with Down syndrome. Pediatr Hematol Oncol 2008; 25(7): 693-8. [http://dx.doi.org/10.1080/08880010802237492] [PMID: 18850483]

[82] Yoshida T, Asato Y, Kukita I, *et al.* A 7-year-old boy with mycoplasmal infection requiring extracorporeal membrane oxygenation. Eur J Pediatr 2003; 162(1): 44-6. [http://dx.doi.org/10.1007/s00431-002-1057-y] [PMID: 12486507]

[83] Ribeiro EL, Campos CdeC, Crespo AM, *et al.* [Detection of phospholipidolytic Candida albicans isolated from saliva of children with Down's syndrome]. Acta Med Port 2002; 15(3): 171-4. [PMID: 12379993]

[84] Ribeiro EL, Scroferneker ML, Cavalhaes MS, *et al.* Phenotypic aspects of oral strains of Candida albicans in children with Down's syndrome. Braz J Biol 2006; 66(3): 939-44. [http://dx.doi.org/10.1590/S1519-69842006000500020] [PMID: 17119842]

[85] Cichon P, Crawford L, Grimm WD. Early-onset periodontitis associated with Down's syndrome--clinical interventional study. Ann Periodontol 1998; 3(1): 370-80. [http://dx.doi.org/10.1902/annals.1998.3.1.370] [PMID: 9722720]

[86] Izumi Y, Sugiyama S, Shinozuka O, Yamazaki T, Ohyama T, Ishikawa I. Defective neutrophil chemotaxis in Down's syndrome patients and its relationship to periodontal destruction. J Periodontol 1989; 60(5): 238-42. [http://dx.doi.org/10.1902/jop.1989.60.5.238] [PMID: 2525619]

[87] Failla P, Pettinato R, Barone C, Romano C. Incidence of Helicobacter Pylori Antibodies in subjects with Down Syndrome. Downs Syndr Res Pract 1998; 5(3): 117-9. [http://dx.doi.org/10.3104/reports.85]

[88] Douraghi M, Goudarzi H, Rostami MN, Mirsamadi ES. Helicobacter pylori seropositivity in institutionalized children with Down syndrome. Pediatr Infect Dis J 2011; 30(12): 1123-4. [http://dx.doi.org/10.1097/INF.0b013e318227879f] [PMID: 22105426]

[89] Ferreira CT, Leite JC, Tanaguchi AN, Vieira SM, Pereira-Lima J, da Silveira TR. Seroprevalence of hepatitis a antibodies in a group of normal and Down syndrome children in Porto Alegre, southern Brazil. Braz J Infect Dis 2002; 6(5): 225-31. [http://dx.doi.org/10.1590/S1413-86702002000500003] [PMID: 12495604]

[90] Rua Armesto MJ, Ramírez Marín V, Onaindia Ercoreca MT, García Aguado J, Ruiz Moreno M. [Predisposition of Down syndrome to chronic infection with the hepatitis B virus]. An Esp Pediatr 1993; 38(6): 529-31. [PMID: 8368682]

[91] Nisihara R, De Bem RS, Negreiros PH, Utiyama SR, Oliveira NP, Amarante H. Low hepatitis B vaccine response in children with Down syndrome from Brazil. Child Care Health Dev 2013; 19 [http://dx.doi.org/10.1111/cch.12099] [PMID: 23952481]

[92] Miyoshi Y, Tajiri H, Okaniwa M, *et al.* Hepatitis C virus infection and interferon therapy in patients with Down syndrome. Pediatr Int 2008; 50(1): 7-11. [http://dx.doi.org/10.1111/j.1442-200X.2007.02515.x] [PMID: 18279197]

[93] Lewis ME, Gauderer MW, Blackhurst DW, Rogers RC, Cornett WR. Do patients with Down syndrome develop appendicitis? J Pediatr Surg 2011 Jan; 46(1): 197-9 . [http://dx.doi.org/10.1016/j.jpedsurg.2010.09.086.]

[94] Parsons C, Naqvi S, Wheeler R. Intra-thoracic appendicitis in a child with Down's syndrome. J Pediatr Surg 2013 Jun; 48(6): E29-31.

[95] Thekekara AG, Denham B, Duff DF. Eleven year review of infective endocarditis. Ir Med J 1994; 87(3): 80-2. [PMID: 8056546]

[96] Schmidt V, Wolter M, Lenschow U, Kienast W. [Lactobacillus paracasei endocarditis in an 18-year--old patient with trisomy 21, atrioventricular septal defect and Eisenmenger complex: therapeutic problems]. Klin Padiatr 2001; 213(1): 35-8. [http://dx.doi.org/10.1055/s-2001-11272] [PMID: 11225474]

[97] Cohen MI, Bush DM, Gaynor JW, Vetter VL, Tanel RE, Rhodes LA. Pediatric pacemaker infections:

twenty years of experience. J Thorac Cardiovasc Surg 2002; 124(4): 821-7.
[http://dx.doi.org/10.1067/mtc.2002.123643] [PMID: 12324742]

[98] Diab KA, Richani R, Al Kutoubi A, Mikati M, Dbaibo GS, Bitar FF. Cerebral mycotic aneurysm in a child with Down's syndrome: a unique association. J Child Neurol 2001; 16(11): 868-70.
[http://dx.doi.org/10.1177/088307380101601111405] [PMID: 11732778]

[99] Takasugi H, Maemoto T, Kitazawa K, Honda A. [A case of Down syndrome with moyamoya syndrome presenting extensive multiple cerebral infarction during measles infection]. No To Hattatsu 2000; 32(1): 39-43.
[PMID: 10655750]

[100] Cambonie G, Sarran N, Leboucq N, *et al.* [*Mycoplasma pneumoniae* meningoencephalitis]. Arch Pediatr 1999; 6(3): 275-8.
[http://dx.doi.org/10.1016/S0929-693X(99)80264-4] [PMID: 10191893]

[101] Sridhar A, Bhandari JK, Lewis G, Ganesan S, Parepalli S, Abulhoul L. Tuberculous radiculomyelitis presenting as urinary retention in a child with Down's syndrome. BMJ Case Rep 2012 ;2012. Apr 2; 2012: pii. bcr1020115005
[http://dx.doi.org/10.1136/bcr.10.2011.5005] [PMID: 22602831]

[102] Nakajima W, Ishida A, Takahashi M, Sato Y, Ito T, Takada G. Aseptic meningitis associated with cephalosporins in an infant with trisomy 21. J Child Neurol 2007; 22(6): 780-2.
[http://dx.doi.org/10.1177/0883073807304016] [PMID: 17641271]

[103] Fernández-Plaza S, Sevilla J, Contra T, Martín N, Madero L. [Acute leukemia in patients with Down syndrome]. An Pediatr (Barc) 2004; 61(6): 515-9.
[PMID: 15574252]

[104] Rabin KR, Smith J, Kozinetz CA. Myelosuppression and infectious complications in children with Down syndrome and acute lymphoblastic leukemia. Pediatr Blood Cancer 2012; 58(4): 633-5.
[http://dx.doi.org/10.1002/pbc.23371] [PMID: 22106003]

[105] Simon A, Völz S, Fleischhack G, *et al.* Human coronavirus OC43 pneumonia in a pediatric cancer patient with down syndrome and acute lymphoblastic leukemia. J Pediatr Hematol Oncol 2007; 29(6): 432-4.
[http://dx.doi.org/10.1097/MPH.0b013e31806451c1] [PMID: 17551411]

[106] Tran TH, Mitchell D, Dix D, *et al.* Infections in children with down syndrome and acute myeloid leukemia: a report from the Canadian infections in AML research group. Infect Agent Cancer 2013 Dec 2; 8(1): 47.
[http://dx.doi.org/10.1186/1750-9378-8-47]

[107] do Canto CL, Granato CF, Garcez E, *et al.* Cytomegalovirus infection in children with Down syndrome in a day-care center in Brazil. Rev Inst Med Trop Sao Paulo 2000; 42(4): 179-83.
[http://dx.doi.org/10.1590/S0036-46652000000400001] [PMID: 10968879]

[108] Higurashi M, Tada A, Miyahara S, Hirayama M. Chromosome damage in Down's syndrome induced by chickenpox infection. Pediatr Res 1976; 10(3): 189-97.
[http://dx.doi.org/10.1203/00006450-197603000-00009] [PMID: 129756]

[109] Gentile I, Altieri L, Lintas C, *et al.* Urinary polyomavirus infections in neurodevelopmental disorders.

Open J Psychiatr 2013; 3: 18-25.
[http://dx.doi.org/10.4236/ojpsych.2013.32A004]

[110] McNally RJ, Rankin J, Shirley MD, Rushton SP, Pless-Mulloli T. Space-time analysis of Down syndrome: results consistent with transient pre-disposing contagious agent. Int J Epidemiol 2008; 37(5): 1169-79.
[http://dx.doi.org/10.1093/ije/dyn083] [PMID: 18467377]

[111] Sever JL, Kapikian AZ, Finestone S, Purcell RH, Gilkeson MR. Hepatitis A and Down's syndrome: lack of an association. J Infect Dis 1976; 134(2): 198-200. g
[http://dx.doi.org/10.1093/infdis/134.2.198] [PMID: 135033]

[112] Madden DL, Matthew EB, Dietzman DE, *et al.* Hepatitis and Down's syndrome. Am J Ment Defic 1976; 80(4): 401-6.
[PMID: 129005]

[113] Pisacane A, Toscano E, Pirri I, *et al.* Down syndrome and breastfeeding. Acta Paediatr 2003; 92(12): 1479-81.
[http://dx.doi.org/10.1111/j.1651-2227.2003.tb00835.x] [PMID: 14971802]

[114] Vereen S, Gebretsadik T, Hartert TV, *et al.* Association between Breastfeeding and Severity of Acute Viral Respiratory Tract Infection. Pediatr Infect Dis J 2014 Sep; 33(9): 986-8..
[http://dx.doi.org/10.1097/INF.0000000000000364] [PMID: 24751863]

[115] Madan V, Williams J, Lear JT. Dermatological manifestations of Down's syndrome. Clin Exp Dermatol 2006; 31(5): 623-9.
[http://dx.doi.org/10.1111/j.1365-2230.2006.02164.x] [PMID: 16901300]

[116] Areias CM, Sampaio-Maia B, Guimaraes H, Melo P, Andrade D. Caries in Portuguese children with Down syndrome. Clinics (Sao Paulo) 2011; 66(7): 1183-6.
[http://dx.doi.org/10.1590/S1807-59322011000700010] [PMID: 21876971]

[117] Yi H, Lanctôt KL, Bont L, *et al.* CARESS investigators. Respiratory syncytial virus prophylaxis in Down syndrome: a prospective cohort study. Pediatrics 2014; 133(6): 1031-7.
[http://dx.doi.org/10.1542/peds.2013-3916] [PMID: 24799541]

[118] Zuccotti GV, Mameli C, Trabattoni D, *et al.* Immunomodulating activity of Pidotimod in children with Down syndrome. J Biol Regul Homeost Agents 2013; 27(1): 253-8.
[PMID: 23489705]

[119] Riboldi P, Gerosa M, Meroni PL. Pidotimod: a reappraisal. Int J Immunopathol Pharmacol 2009; 22(2): 255-62.
[PMID: 19505378]

[120] La Mantia I, Grillo C, Mattina T, *et al.* Prophylaxis with the novel immunomodulator pidotimod reduces the frequency and severity of upper respiratory tract infections in children with Down's syndrome. J Chemother 1999; 11(2): 126-30.
[http://dx.doi.org/10.1179/joc.1999.11.2.126] [PMID: 10326743]

[121] Whittingham S, Sharma DL. Levamisole: lack of immunopotentiation in a controlled trial. Med J Aust 1978 May 20; 1(10): 569-70.
[PMID: 150487]

[122] Lott IT. Antioxidants in Down syndrome. Biochim Biophys Acta 2012; 1822(5): 657-63. [http://dx.doi.org/10.1016/j.bbadis.2011.12.010] [PMID: 22206998]

[123] Magnusson CG, Nordvall SL, Annerén G. Differential effect of selenium supplementation on immunoglobulin levels in Down's syndrome. Acta Paediatr 1997; 86(12): 1385-6. [http://dx.doi.org/10.1111/j.1651-2227.1997.tb14923.x] [PMID: 9475325]

[124] Licastro F, Chiricolo M, Mocchegiani E, *et al.* Oral zinc supplementation in Down's syndrome subjects decreased infections and normalized some humoral and cellular immune parameters. J Intellect Disabil Res 1994; 38(Pt 2): 149-62. [http://dx.doi.org/10.1111/j.1365-2788.1994.tb00370.x] [PMID: 8193451]

[125] Colombo ML, Girardo E, Incarbone E, Conti R, Ricci BM, Maina D. [Vitamin C in children with trisomy 21]. Minerva Pediatr 1989; 41(4): 189-92. [PMID: 2528054]

[126] Gualandri W, Gualandri L, Demartini G, *et al.* Redox balance in patients with Down's syndrome before and after dietary supplementation with alpha-lipoic acid and L-cysteine. Int J Clin Pharmacol Res 2003; 23(1): 23-30. [PMID: 14621070]

[127] Kusters MA, Bok VL, Bolz WE, Huijskens EG, Peeters MF, de Vries E. Influenza A/H1N1 vaccination response is inadequate in down syndrome children when the latest cut-off values are used. Pediatr Infect Dis J 2012; 31(12): 1284-5. [http://dx.doi.org/10.1097/INF.0b013e3182737410] [PMID: 22986705]

[128] Nurmi T, Leinonen M, Häivä VM, Tiilikainen A, Kouvalainen K. Antibody response to pneumococcal vaccine in patients with trisomy-21 (Down's syndrome). Clin Exp Immunol 1982; 48(2): 485-90. [PMID: 6213331]

[129] Ferreira CT, Leite JC, Taniguchi A, Vieira SM, Pereira-Lima J, da Silveira TR. Immunogenicity and safety of an inactivated hepatitis A vaccine in children with Down syndrome. J Pediatr Gastroenterol Nutr 2004; 39(4): 337-40. [http://dx.doi.org/10.1097/00005176-200410000-00007] [PMID: 15448421]

[130] FCSD/DOWN ESPAÑA DOCUMENT. Vaccination schedule for people with Down's syndrome, 2012. Rev Med Int Sindr Down 2011; 15(3): 45-7. [http://dx.doi.org/10.1016/S2171-9748(11)70015-0]

[131] Pun SB. Rotavirus, vaccine and unanswered questions: a perspective from a least developed country. JNMA J Nepal Med Assoc 2013; 52(191): 534-7. p [PMID: 24907967]

[132] Thomas CA, Shwe T, Bixler D, *et al.* Two-Dose Varicella Vaccine Effectiveness and Rash Severity in Outbreaks of Varicella among Public School Students. Pediatr Infect Dis J 2014 Nov; 33(11): 1164-8. [http://dx.doi.org/10.1097/INF.0000000000000444] [PMID: 24911894]

[133] Hedari CP, Khinkarly RW, Dbaibo GS, *et al.* Meningococcal serogroups A, C, W-135, and Y tetanus toxoid conjugate vaccine: a new conjugate vaccine against invasive meningococcal disease. Infect Drug Resist 2014; 3(7): 85-99. eCollection 2014. Review. [http://dx.doi.org/10.2147/IDR.S36243] [PMID: 24729718]

CHAPTER 8

Update in Hematology and Oncology in Down Syndrome

Mohamed Ramadan El-Shanshory*

Hematology Unit, Faculty of Medicine, Tanta University, Egypt

Abstract: Down syndrome (DS) is commonly associated with hematological and oncologic disorders than non-syndromic children. Interpretation of the blood picture should be done with caution. Polycythemia and iron deficiency anemia (IDA); both are common in those children. Presence of IDA in DS children adds an extra load on them. Occurrence of transient abnormal myelopoiesis (TAM) in DS neonates is due to the effect of trisomy 21 on liver hematopoiesis with megakaryocyte – erythroid progenitor. Down syndrome children have a 500- fold increase in acute myeloblastic leukemia (AMKL) compared to the non-syndromic children. They also have increased risk for development of acute lymphoblastic leukemia (ALL) which affects 1 in 300 children with DS. At the same time; despite the high prevalence of leukemia's in DS children; the risk for the development of solid tumors is globally unexpected to be low. Several novel therapies will benefit many children with DS and ALL and other malignancies.

Keywords: Anemia, Angiogenesis-promoting protein vascular endothelial growth factor, Antigen-directed immune therapies, Blood picture, Children, Down syndrome, DSCR1, Hematological abnormalities, Iron deficiency, Leukemia, Liposomal formulations, Lymphoblastic, Myelodyplastic syndrome, Myeloid, Nephroblastoma, Neuroblastoma, Neutropenia, Polycythemia, Ruxolitinib, Transient abnormal Myelopoiesis.

1. INTRODUCTION

Hematological disorders are more common in children with Down syndrome (DS) than non-syndromic children. Evaluation and interpretation of blood picture in individuals with DS may need caution as it can cause some confusion. The blood cell counts (CBC) may reflect some abnormalities without an apparent reason as

* **Corresponding Author Mohamed Ramadan El-Shanshory:** Hematology Unit, Faculty of Medicine, Tanta University, Egypt; Tel: +201005680834; Email: elshanshory@gmail.Com

Mohammed Al-Biltagi (Ed)

well as the base lines of different parameters in the complete blood count may differ from the normal population. Some of these abnormalities resolve spontaneously and others persist throughout life. Such hematological abnormalities as increased mean corpuscular volume (MCV) can make the diagnosis of iron deficiency anemia difficult. Other abnormalities may include mild transient neutropenia, thrombocytopenia or thrombocytosis, as well as increased counts of circulating nucleated red cells with or without polycythemia [1]. At the same time; the risk of the development of acute lymphoblastic leukemia (ALL) increases up to 12 times in the age group between 5 years and 30 years and increases up to 40 times in children less than 5 years. The risk of the development of acute myeloid leukemia (AML) increases up to 150 times in children less than 5 years [2].

2. COMMON HEMATOLOGICAL ABNORMALITIES IN DS CHILDREN

2.1. Polycythemia

Sixty five percent of newborns with DS are presented by polycythemia which may or may not be associated with congenital heart diseases. This type of polycythemia is frequently not in need for treatment because of spontaneous resolution within few months. The treatment is limited to those with hyperviscosity syndrome. The development of polycythemia may be due to the increased erythropoietin levels in the setting of chronic intrauterine hypoxia. On the contrary, children with DS may present with iron deficiency anemia due to decrease dietary intake of iron because of delayed motor skills, hypotonia and dysphagia [2, 3].

2.2. Iron Deficiency Anemia (IDA)

There are few studies regarding IDA in DS. Children with DS have been associated with motor and cognitive developmental deficits. The presence of IDA in those children add an extra load on them, so screening for IDA is mandatory [4, 5]. The diagnosis of IDA in children is faced by the difficulty in screening of these children. Mean corpuscular volume (MCV) is usually high in children with DS, which is not related to Vitamin B12 or folic acid deficiencies [6]. Many researchers have documented erythrocyte macrocytosis in DS adults and children.

However; its clinical significance is still unclear. The explanation of macrocytosis could be that it is not a reflection of reduced red cell survival but may be related to altered folate remethylation pathway, secondary to increased cystathionine β-synthase (CBS) activity which is controlled by a gene present on chromosome 21 [7] As a result, macrocytosis makes characterization of IDA more difficult. This should be considered during evaluation of iron status of children with DS which should be monitored by both serial complete blood counts (CBCs) and iron studies with special emphasis upon serum ferritin.

2.3. Transient Abnormal Myelopoiesis (TAM)

The true incidence of transient abnormal myelopoiesis in DS is not actually known. Ten percent of neonates with DS are affected and about 10% of the fetuses may die intra uterine mostly due to TAM [7, 8]. The development of TAM in DS may be due to the effect of trisomy 21 on liver hematopoiesis together with megakaryocyte – erythroid progenitor frequency with common myeloid progenitor [7].

There are variable clinical presentations of TAM among the different cases with DS; where most cases are picked up during the routine testing by presence of circulating blast cells with or without leukocytosis [9]. Other cases may present with bleeding tendency, organ affections as, respiratory distress, hepatic dysfunction and/or pericardial effusion. Majority of TAM cases usually recover spontaneously within 3 months but, about 20-30% will develop acute myeloid leukemia of DS (ML-DS) [10, 11].

The diagnosis of TAM depends on the clinical manifestations and the presence of characteristic findings in the peripheral blood film; as nucleated red blood cell, thrombocytopenia or thrombocytosis, giant platelet and fragments of megakaryocyte with the characteristic basophilic immature blast cell. Blast cell in TAM undergo flow-cytometry express unique markers; as early myeloid (CD34, CD33), megakaryocyte (CD41, CD61), and erythroid (CD235a, glycophorin) markers (2). The differentiation between TAM and true AML is difficult, but TAM has usually a spontaneous resolving course. All neonates with DS and apparent leukemia who are well should initially be monitored for possible spontaneous recovery as only 20–30% of those with TAM subsequently develop AML [11], often after a period of myelodysplasia; although in TAM the abnormal clone seems to “burn out” [10].

GATA-1 mutations, a transcription factor mutation essential for the proper development of erythroid, megakaryocytic and basophilic cell lines, have been complicated with TAM and AML in DS [12]. Megakaryocyte transcription GATA1 is present in neonate with DS affected by TAM [13 - 17]. Although most children with TAM resolve spontaneously with 3 months, some cases may have a bad prognosis; especially cases with liver fibrosis due to release of megakaryocyte derived growth factor from blast cell and about 20% die from the disease. The use of low dose cytosine arabinoside (10-20 mg/day for up to 7 days) is indicated in symptomatic babies with elevated blast numbers or in presence of liver dysfunctions [18, 19].

2.4. Myelodysplastic Syndrome (MDS) and Down Syndrome

Myelodysplastic syndrome (MDS) is a clonal hematopoietic disorder with hypercellular or hypocellular bone marrow with cellular morphologic abnormalities [10, 19]. This disorder associated with peripheral blood cytopenia and is considered a premalignant condition. The development of clonal abnormally may result from hematopoietic stem cell genetic abnormalities or from its exposure to cytotoxic drugs, radiation, viral infection or chemical agents like benzene. Insecticide and fungicide may be possible factors for the development of MDS [20].

2.5. Acute Myeloblastic Leukemia (AML) in Down Syndrome

Down syndrome children have a 500- fold increase in AMKL compared to the non-syndromic children [12, 21 - 23]. AML is more common in children with DS with about 15% of cases of AML are encountered in DS. The most frequent French-American-British (FAB) subtype is acute megakaryocytic leukemia which represents more than 90% of cases of DS-AML [23 - 30]. Patients with DS develop the signs of MDS before the development of AML which referred as myeloid leukemia of DS. The molecular genetics of DS differ from those without DS. The common cytogenetic abnormalities associated with AML are trisomies 8,

11, and 21, dup(1p), del(6q), del(7p), dup(7q), and del(16q) [31].

GATA1 mutation is nearly present in all cases of DS, which is responsible for the proliferation to megakaryocyte. GATA1 mutations involve deletions, missense, nonsense, and splice site mutations at the exon 2/intron boundary with the end result of introducing early stop codons and the production of a shorter GATA1 protein [32]. Children with DS and AML unusually respond well to intensive chemotherapy. The need for aggressive cytotoxic chemotherapy has been questioned and debated worldwide. International trials are established with less intensive protocols and bone marrow transplantation (BMT) should no longer be necessary for any child with DS.

2.6. Acute Lymphoblastic Leukemia (ALL) in Down Syndrome

DS children have high risk for development of acute lymphoblastic leukemia (ALL). ALL affect 1 in 300 children with DS [33, 34]. The clinical manifestations in patients with DS-ALL don't differ from those with non-DS-ALL as regard to the age of presentation, and sex distribution (Table **1**). Also; there are no differences in the white blood cell counts (WBC) [35].

Table 1. Clinical and biological features of DS-ALL [53].

Cytogenetic features	• Almost exclusively B cell precursor immunophenotype • Heterogeneity - no DS ALL typical genetic abnormality as in DS myeloid leukemias • Decreased prevalence of favorable chromosomal aberrations of childhood ALL (ETV6-RUNX1, high hyperdiploid) • Decreased prevalence of unfavorable chromosomal aberrations of childhood ALL (BCR-ABL, AF4-MLL) • Aberrant expression of CRLF2 in 60% of DS-ALLs • Large proportion of cytogenetically normal ALL
Clinical features	• No Infant leukemia • High risk of relapse • High infectious associated therapy related mortality throughout treatment period

Immunophenotypic reports from patients with DS-ALL differ from those with non DS. Virtually all children DS-ALL display a B-cell precursor phenotype, with a rare mature B-cell and T-cell [36, 37]. At the same time; DS-ALL is cytogenetically distinct from non DS-ALL. DS-ALL are rarely hyperdiploid (51-67 chromosome) and seldom display Mixed Lineage Leukemia (MLL) gene rearrangements or t(9;22)(q34;q11)/BCR-ABL1 [38 - 40]. CRLF2 gene mutation at Xp22.33/Y11.32 is more prevalent in DS-ALL than non DS-ALL [41, 42].

In contrast to the excellent prognosis of the myeloid leukemia of DS, the prognosis of DS children -ALL is significantly worse than children without DS [43] and the outcome of DS-ALL is considered low compared with that with non DS-ALL [44 - 48]. At the same time; patients with DS-ALL had an poorer event-free survival (65·6% *vs*. 87·7% at 5 years) and overall survival (70·0% *vs*. 92·2%) compared with non-DS ALL. The increased treatment-linked mortality was mainly responsible for the poorer prognosis for DS-ALL due to treatment-related infections as well as a high relapse rate [44 - 48].

The causes of infectious toxicities in DS are multifactorial. Increased tendency for cellular apoptosis coupled with altered intracellular metabolism of certain drugs, such as methotrexate, lead to breakdown in cellular barriers and increased mucositis. Immunodeficiency, narrowed and hyper-reactive respiratory tract and congenital heart diseases increase the risk for respiratory as well as other infections. Children with DS develop serious generalized toxicity such as myelosuppression, mucositis, and hepatotoxicity after treatment with the antifolate agent, methotrexate, which implies that trisomy 21 cells have abnormal folate metabolism. The toxicity associated with the administration of methotrexate is the best-studied specific toxicity of a chemotherapeutic drug in DS [49]. Gene dosage effect of extra copies of the reduced folate carrier SLC19A1, located on chromosome 21, appears to cause increased intracellular accumulation of methotrexate in trisomy 21 cells [50]. This gene dosage effect may also explain the increased sensitivity of hyperdiploid ALL blasts, which uniformly carry 3 or 4 copies of chromosome 21. Biologically, these various leukemias are distinguished by under-representation of the frequent cytogenetic subgroups of childhood ALL and over demonstration of CRLF2-IL7R-JAK-STAT activating genetic aberrations.

A number of approaches can reduce the therapy related mortality. Reducing chemotherapy dose in patients with ETV6-RUNX1 or high hyperdiploidy DS-ALL or MRD negativity at the end of induction, and excessive toxicity should be considered. Careful surveillance should be done throughout therapy including maintenance period with intense monitoring/supervision during periods of prolonged neutropenia. At the same time; aggressive treatment of suspected infections even in absence of neutropenia or fever should be considered. Reducing chance of exposure to respiratory infections can be tried with immunization of family members and intimate contacts with Influenza vaccine. Antimicrobial prophylaxis for children with recurrent respiratory infections can also help to reduce these infections. Intravenous immunoglobulin therapy could be tried for children with low/normal or hypogammaglobulinemia [51].

The high relapse rate is another main risk factor for poor prognosis in this population. Minimal residual disease (MRD) is important risk factor for relapse in DS patients. Children with more MRD have a greater risk of relapse than those with less MRD. The prognosis after first relapse will depend on the site of relapse; time elapsed between diagnosis and relapse, the risk group classification at initial diagnosis, cytogenetics/genomic alterations and the immunophenotyping. Reducing the risk of relapse can be achieved by taking caution at reducing chemotherapy dosages in the absence of toxicity and by incorporating clinical trials with novel agents targeting unique biological features (*e.g.* JAK and mTOR inhibitors for CRLF2 expressing DS-ALL) [52]. Improvement in prognosis needs improved understanding of reasons of treatment failure and treatment-related mortality, integration of recent therapies targeting the distinctive biological features of DS-ALL, and improved supportive care procedures to decrease the risk of infection-related and treatment-related mortality.

2.6.1. Current Treatment Approaches in ALL

In an attempt to reduce excess treatment-associated morbidity and mortality, the current approach is to limit exposure to high doses of intravenous methotrexate by adopting a dose capping (500-1000 mg/m^2 with folinic acid rescue) or a cautious dose escalation strategy (starting dose, 500-2000 mg/m^2). No cranial radiotherapy will be done to patients with DS-ALL. NOPHO (Nordic), UKALL, and COG limit the use of anthracycline in induction to patients with a slow morphological marrow response (>25% blasts) at day 15 of a 3-drug regimen (steroid, vincristine, and pegylated asparaginase). DCOG (Dutch) and France Acute Lymphoblastic Leukemia (FRALLE) (French) groups avoid exposure to induction anthracyclines in all DS patients, whereas AIOEP-BFM (Italian-German consortium) gives 2 to 4 doses depending on karyotype and early MRD response, similar to patients with NDS-ALL. Whereas dexamethasone is given in induction to all DS patients in the United Kingdom, the COG gives it only to patients <10 years old and AIEOP-BFM (Italian-German consortium) gives it to patients with T-cell phenotype and a good response to prephase prednisolone. There are no planned alterations in maintenance therapy except in the United Kingdom and in DS-ALL patients in COG protocols, where the duration of maintenance has been shortened from 3 to 2 years for boys with DS-ALL and with a reduction in monthly vincristine/steroid pulses in COG protocols.

Interestingly, despite this variability in treatment plans, no significant differences in outcome were detected between the major therapeutic protocols of DS-ALL. Additional supportive care measures are recommended for DS-ALL patients ranging from antibiotic and antifungal prophylaxis during periods of neutropenia to intravenous immunoglobulin infusions in order to maintain IgG level above a defined threshold [38].

2.6.2. Novel Therapies in ALL

Many lines of therapy are tied in the treatment of ALL which will benefit patients with DS.

1. Antigen-directed immune therapies (*e.g.* Blinatumomab—bispecific anti-CD19 antibody or engineered autologous T cells) are exciting new technologies for therapy of B-cell precursor ALL [53].
2. JAK and mTOR inhibitors: Uniquely, 60% of DS-ALLs express the cytokine receptor CRLF2 that signals through JAK-STAT and mTOR pathways. Preclinical trials demonstrate activity of either JAK or mTOR inhibitors [54].
3. Ruxolitinib (a dual JAK1/JAK2 inhibitor) is approved for adults with myeloproliferative neoplasms, (provided that it is CRLF2 positive).
4. Liposomal formulations of standard cytotoxic agents used in the treatment of ALL such as daunomycin and vincristine offer the promise of improved therapeutic index leading to both improved outcomes and a reduction in toxicities in all children with ALL. Similarly, high-dose cytarabine, which is

usually tolerated by DS children treated for AML, may have a role in DS-ALL; however, to date, no data are available regarding the potential benefits of these agents in DS-ALL.

Improvement in outcomes for DS-ALL will only be realized from improved understanding of the reasons of treatment failure and TRM [38].

2.7. Down Syndrome and Solid Tumors

Despite the high prevalence of leukemia's in DS; the risk for the development of solid tumors is globally unexpected to be low. These include tumors affecting the central nervous system, peripheral nervous system (neuroblastoma), renal tissue (nephroblastoma), and tumors arising from the epithelial tissues [55]. But some reports demonstrate the high incidence of germ cell tumors [56], and testicular tumors in early life [57].

Now it appears that trisomy 21 provide a protection against solid tumors and increase susceptibility to leukemia. The mechanisms of DS resistance to the development of solid tumors depend upon the genetic abnormality observed in this syndrome. The one extra copy of Dscr1 (one out of the 231 genes present on chromosome 21 influenced by trisomy, with 3 copies instead of 2) is enough to extensively depress angiogenesis and tumor growth in mice, in addition to angiogenesis in human cells. The existence of its protein, DSCR1, is noted to be high in tissues obtained from people with DS as well as in a mouse model of the disease [58].

Some studies proved that DSCR1 works by repressing signaling by the angiogenesis-promoting protein vascular endothelial growth factor (VEGF). In a mouse model of DS, endothelial cells (which form blood vessel walls) showed impaired growth response to VEGF when they had an extra copy of Dscr1. An extra copy of another chromosome 21 gene, Dyrk1A, as well found to reduce cells' response to VEGF. According to researcher Judah Folkman, a well recognized pioneer scientist in the angiogenesis field; the cancer preventing effects in DS patients might present in the extra copy of chromosome 21. This chromosome includes genes that stop angiogenesis; formation of new blood vessels vital for tumor growth. Patients with DS have such a decreased risk for cancer because of the endostatin, which is an anti-angiogenic product formed inside the body. Endostatin is a fragment of collagen 18—whose gene is also located on chromosome 21. People with DS have almost doubled levels of endostatin because of the extra copy of the gene [59, 60].

CONCLUSION

Interpretation of CBC in children with DS must be taken with caution. Iron deficiency anemia is common in DS, but its diagnosis was masked by elevated MCV. The differentiation between TAM and true AML is difficult and follow up is essential. DS with MDS must be monitored for the high risk for development of AML. Despite the good prognosis observed in DS-AML; prognosis of DS-ALL is considered to be lower than that of non DS-ALL. TRM in DS with malignancies still represent a challenge in the prognosis.

CONFLICT OF INTEREST

The authors confirm that this chapter contents have no conflict of interest.

ACKNOWLEDGEMENTS

Declared none.

REFERENCES

[1] Watts TL, Murray NA, Roberts IA. Thrombopoietin has a primary role in the regulation of platelet production in preterm babies. Pediatr Res 1999; 46(1): 28-32. [http://dx.doi.org/10.1203/00006450-199907000-00005] [PMID: 10400130]

[2] Webb D, Roberts I, Vyas P. Haematology of Down syndrome. Arch Dis Child Fetal Neonatal Ed 2007; 92(6): F503-7. [http://dx.doi.org/10.1136/adc.2006.104638] [PMID: 17804520]

[3] Watts TL, Murray NA, Roberts IA. Thrombopoietin has a primary role in the regulation of platelet production in preterm babies. Pediatr Res 1999; 46(1): 28-32. [http://dx.doi.org/10.1203/00006450-199907000-00005] [PMID: 10400130]

[4] Petranovic D, Batinac T, Petranovic D, Ruzic A, Ruzic T. Iron deficiency anaemia influences cognitive functions. Med Hypotheses 2008; 70(1): 70-2. [http://dx.doi.org/10.1016/j.mehy.2007.04.029] [PMID: 17574345]

[5] Agaoglu L, Torun O, Unuvar E, Sefil Y, Demir D. "Effects of iron deficiency anemia on cognitive function in children," Arzneimittel-Forschung. Drug Res 2007; 57(6): 426-30. [http://dx.doi.org/10.1055/s-0031-1296691] [PMID: 17691592]

[6] Dixon NE, Crissman BG, Smith PB, Zimmerman SA, Worley G, Kishnani PS. Prevalence of iron deficiency in children with Down syndrome. J Pediatr 2010; 157(6): 967-971.e1. [http://dx.doi.org/10.1016/j.jpeds.2010.06.011] [PMID: 20650467]

[7] David O, Fiorucci GC, Tosi MT, *et al.* Hematological studies in children with Down syndrome. Pediatr Hematol Oncol 1996; 13(3): 271-5. [http://dx.doi.org/10.3109/08880019609030827] [PMID: 8735344]

[8] Henry E, Walker D, Wiedmeier SE, Christensen RD. . Hematological abnormalities during the first week of life among neonates with Down syndrome: data from a multihospital healthcare system. Am J Med Genet A 2007; 143A(1): 42-50. [PMID: 17163522]

[9] Webb D, Roberts I, Vyas P. Haematology of Down syndrome. Arch Dis Child Fetal Neonatal Ed 2007; 92(6): F503-7. [http://dx.doi.org/10.1136/adc.2006.104638] [PMID: 17804520]

[10] Massey GV, Zipursky A, Chang MN, *et al.* A prospective study of the natural history of transient leukemia (TL) in neonates with Down syndrome (DS): Children's Oncology Group (COG) study POG□9481. Blood , 2006 [Epub 2006 Feb 9.];107(12): 4613-3. [http://dx.doi.org/http://dx.doi.org/10.1182/blood-2005-06-2448] [PMID: 16469874]

[11] Zipursky A. Transient leukaemia--a benign form of leukaemia in newborn infants with trisomy 21. Br J Haematol 2003; 120(6): 930-8. [http://dx.doi.org/10.1046/j.1365-2141.2003.04229.x] [PMID: 12648061]

[12] Zipursky A, Poon A, Doyle J. Leukemia in Down syndrome: a review. Pediatr Hematol Oncol 1992; 9(2): 139-49. [http://dx.doi.org/10.3109/08880019209018329] [PMID: 1388043]

[13] Bain BJ. Transient leukaemia in newborn infants with Down's syndrome. Leuk Res 1994; 18(9): 723-4. [http://dx.doi.org/10.1016/0145-2126(94)90073-6] [PMID: 7934148]

[14] Tunstall-Pedoe O, Roy A, Karadimitris A, *et al.* Abnormalities in the myeloid progenitor compartment in Down syndrome fetal liver precede acquisition of GATA1 mutations. Blood 2008; 112(12): 4507-11. [http://dx.doi.org/10.1182/blood-2008-04-152967] [PMID: 18689547]

[15] Wechsler J, Greene M, McDevitt MA, *et al.* Acquired mutations in GATA1 in the megakaryoblastic leukemia of Down syndrome. Nat Genet , 2002 [Epub 2002 Aug 12];31(1): 148-52. [http://dx.doi.org/10.1038/ng955] [PMID: 12172547]

[16] Hitzler JK, Cheung J, Li Y, *et al.* GATA1 mutations in transient leukemia and acute megakaryoblastic leukemia of Down syndrome. Blood 2003; 101(11): 4301-4. [http://dx.doi.org/http://dx.doi.org/10.1182/blood-2003-01-0013] [PMID: 7934148]

[17] Groet J, McElwaine S, Spinelli M, *et al.* Acquired mutations in GATA1 in neonates with Down's syndrome with transient myeloid disorder. Lancet 2003; 361(9369): 1617-20. [http://dx.doi.org/10.1016/S0140-6736(03)13266-7] [PMID: 12747884]

[18] Rainis L, Bercovich D, Strehl S, *et al.* Mutations in exon 2 of GATA1 are early events in

megakaryocytic malignancies associated with trisomy 21. Blood 2003; 102(2): 981-6. [http://dx.doi.org/http://dx.doi.org/10.1182/blood-2002-11-3599] [PMID: 12649131]

[19] Ahmed M, Sternberg A, Hall G, *et al.* Natural history of GATA1 mutations in Down syndrome. Blood 2004; 103(7): 2480-9. [http://dx.doi.org/10.1182/blood-2003-10-3383] [PMID: 14656875]

[20] Besa EC. Myelodysplastic syndromes (refractory anemia). A perspective of the biologic, clinical, and therapeutic issues. Med Clin North Am 1992; 76(3): 599-617. [PMID: 1578959]

[21] Germing U, Kobbe G, Haas R, Gattermann N. Myelodysplastic syndromes: diagnosis, prognosis, and treatment. Dtsch Arztebl Int 2013; 110(46): 783-90. [http://dx.doi.org/10.3238/arztebl.2013.0783] [PMID: 24300826]

[22] Goldberg H, Lusk E, Moore J, Nowell PC, Besa EC. Survey of exposure to genotoxic agents in primary myelodysplastic syndrome: correlation with chromosome patterns and data on patients without hematological disease. Cancer Res 1990; 50(21): 6876-81. [PMID: 2208156]

[23] Creutzig U, Ritter J, Vormoor J, *et al.* Myelodysplasia and acute myelogenous leukemia in Down's syndrome. A report of 40 children of the AML-BFM Study Group. Leukemia 1996; 10(11): 1677-86. [PMID: 8892666]

[24] Lange BJ, Kobrinsky N, Barnard DR, *et al.* Distinctive demography, biology, and outcome of acute myeloid leukemia and myelodysplastic syndrome in children with Down syndrome: Children's Cancer Group Studies 2861 and 2891. Blood 1998; 91(2): 608-15. [PMID: 9427716]

[25] Ravindranath Y, Abella E, Krischer JP, *et al.* Acute myeloid leukemia (AML) in Down's syndrome is highly responsive to chemotherapy: experience on Pediatric Oncology Group AML Study 8498. Blood 1992; 80(9): 2210-4. [PMID: 1384797]

[26] Ravindranath Y, Yeager AM, Chang MN, *et al.* Autologous bone marrow transplantation *versus* intensive consolidation chemotherapy for acute myeloid leukemia in childhood. Pediatric Oncology Group. N Engl J Med 1996; 334(22): 1428-34. [http://dx.doi.org/ 10.1056/NEJM199605303342203] [PMID: 8618581]

[27] Lange BJ, Kobrinsky N, Barnard DR, *et al.* Distinctive demography, biology, and outcome of acute myeloid leukemia and myelodysplastic syndrome in children with Down syndrome: children's Cancer Group Studies 2861 and 2891. Blood 1998; 91(2): 608-15. [PMID: 9427716]

[28] Gamis AS, Woods WG, Alonzo TA, *et al.* Increased age at diagnosis has a significantly negative effect on outcome in children with Down syndrome and acute myeloid leukemia: a report from the Children's Cancer Group Study 2891. J Clin Oncol 2003; 21(18): 3415-22. [http://dx.doi.org/10.1200/JCO.2003.08.060] [PMID: 12885836]

[29] Creutzig U, Reinhardt D, Diekamp S, Dworzak M, Stary J, Zimmermann M. AML patients with Down syndrome have a high cure rate with AML-BFM therapy with reduced dose intensity. Leukemia 2005; 19: 1355-60.

[http://dx.doi.org/10.1038/sj.leu.2403814] [PMID: 15920490]

[30] Kudo K, Kojima S, Tabuchi K, *et al.* Prospective study of a pirarubicin, intermediate-dose cytarabine, and etoposide regimen in children with Down syndrome and acute myeloid leukemia: the Japanese Childhood AML Cooperative Study Group. J Clin Oncol 25(34): 5442-7.2007; [http://dx.doi.org/10.1200/JCO.2007.12.3687] [PMID: 1804882]

[31] Al-Ahmari A, Shah N, Sung L, Zipursky A, Hitzler J. Long-term results of an ultra low-dose cytarabine-based regimen for the treatment of acute megakaryoblastic leukaemia in children with Down syndrome. Br J Haematol 2006; 133(6): 646-8. [http://dx.doi.org/10.1111/j.1365-2141.2006.06097.x] [PMID: 16704441]

[32] Rao A, Hills RK, Stiller C, *et al.* Treatment for myeloid leukaemia of Down syndrome: population-based experience in the UK and results from the Medical Research Council AML 10 and AML 12 trials. Br J Haematol 2006; 132(5): 576-83. [http://dx.doi.org/10.1111/j.1365-2141.2005.05906.x] [PMID: 16445830]

[33] Forestier E, Izraeli S, Beverloo B, *et al.* Cytogenetic features of acute lymphoblastic and myeloid leukemias in pediatric patients with Down syndrome: an iBFM-SG study. Blood 2008; 111(3): 1575-83. [http://dx.doi.org/http://dx.doi.org/10.1182/blood-2007-09-114231] [PMID: 17971484]

[34] Wechsler J, Greene M, McDevitt MA, *et al.* Acquired mutations in GATA1 in the megakaryoblastic leukemia of Down syndrome. Nat Genet 2002; 32(1): 148-52. [http://dx.doi.org/10.1038/ng955] [PMID: 12172547]

[35] Hasle H, Clemmensen IH, Mikkelsen M. Risks of leukaemia and solid tumours in individuals with Down's syndrome. Lancet 2000; 355(9199): 165-9. [http://dx.doi.org/10.1016/S0140-6736(99)05264-2] [PMID: 10675114]

[36] Lange B. The management of neoplastic disorders of haematopoiesis in children with Down's syndrome. Br J Haematol 2000; 110(3): 512-24. [http://dx.doi.org/10.1046/j.1365-2141.2000.02027.x] [PMID: 10997960]

[37] Maloney KW. Acute lymphoblastic leukaemia in children with Down syndrome: an updated review. Br J Haematol 2011; 155(4): 420-5. [http://dx.doi.org/10.1111/j.1365-2141.2011.08846.x] [PMID: 21933171]

[38] Whitlock JA, Sather HN, Gaynon P, *et al.* Clinical characteristics and outcome of children with Down syndrome and acute lymphoblastic leukemia: a Children's Cancer Group study. Blood 2005; 106(13): 4043-9. [http://dx.doi.org/10.1182/blood-2003-10-3446] [PMID: 16109782]

[39] Chessells JM, Harrison G, Richards SM, *et al.* Down's syndrome and acute lymphoblastic leukaemia: clinical features and response to treatment. Arch Dis Child 2001; 85(4): 321-5. [http://dx.doi.org/10.1136/adc.85.4.321] [PMID: 11567943]

[40] Maloney KW, Carroll WL, Carroll AJ, *et al.* Down syndrome childhood acute lymphoblastic leukemia has a unique spectrum of sentinel cytogenetic lesions that influences treatment outcome: a report from the Children's Oncology Group. Blood 2010; 116(7): 1045-50. [http://dx.doi.org/10.1182/blood-2009-07-235291] [PMID: 20442364]

[41] Pui C-H, Raimondi SC, Borowitz MJ, *et al.* Immunophenotypes and karyotypes of leukemic cells in children with Down syndrome and acute lymphoblastic leukemia. J Clin Oncol 1993; 11(7): 1361-7. [PMID: 8315434]

[42] Lundin C, Hjorth L, Behrendtz M, *et al.* High frequency of BTG1 deletions in acute lymphoblastic leukemia in children with down syndrome. Genes Chromosomes Cancer 2012; 51(2): 196-206. [http://dx.doi.org/10.1002/gcc.20944] [PMID: 22072402]

[43] Bercovich D, Ganmore I, Scott LM, *et al.* Mutations of JAK2 in acute lymphoblastic leukaemias associated with Down's syndrome. Lancet 2008; 372(9648): 1484-92. [http://dx.doi.org/10.1016/S0140-6736(08)61341-0] [PMID: 18805579]

[44] Buitenkamp T, Izraeli S, Zimmermann M, *et al.* Acute lymphoblastic leukemia in children with Down syndrome: a report from the Ponte Di Legno Study Group. Blood 2014; 123(1): 70-7. [http://dx.doi.org/10.1182/blood-2013-06-509463] [PMID: 24222333]

[45] Russell LJ, Capasso M, Vater I, *et al.* Deregulated expression of cytokine receptor gene, CRLF2, is involved in lymphoid transformation in B-cell precursor acute lymphoblastic leukemia Blood 114(13): 2688-98.2009; [http://dx.doi.org/10.1182/blood-2009-03-208397] [PMID: 19641190]

[46] Zeller B, Gustafsson G, Forestier E, *et al.* Acute leukaemia in children with Down syndrome: a population-based Nordic study. Nordic study 2005; 128(6): 797-804. [http://dx.doi.org/10.1111/j.1365-2141.2005.05398.x] [PMID: 15755283]

[47] Robison LL, Nesbit ME Jr, Sather HN, *et al.* Down syndrome and acute leukemia in children: a 10-year retrospective survey from Childrens Cancer Study Group. J Pediatr 1984; 105(2): 235-42. [http://dx.doi.org/10.1016/S0022-3476(84)80119-5] [PMID: 6235337]

[48] Levitt GA, Stiller CA, Chessells JM. Prognosis of Down's syndrome with acute leukaemia. Arch Dis Child 1990; 65(2): 212-6. [http://dx.doi.org/10.1136/adc.65.2.212] [PMID: 2138446]

[49] Dördelmann M, Schrappe M, Reiter A, *et al.* Berlin-Frankfurt-Münster Group. Down's syndrome in childhood acute lymphoblastic leukemia: clinical characteristics and treatment outcome in four consecutive BFM trials. Leukemia 1998; 12(5): 645-51. [http://dx.doi.org/10.1038/sj.leu.2400989] [PMID: 9593260]

[50] Buitenkamp TD, Mathôt RA, de Haas V, Pieters R, Zwaan CM. Methotrexate-induced side effects are not due to differences in pharmacokinetics in children with Down syndrome and acute lymphoblastic leukemia. Haematologica 2010; 95(7): 1106-13. [http://dx.doi.org/10.3324/haematol.2009.019778] [PMID: 20418240]

[51] Taub JW, Ge Y. Down syndrome, drug metabolism and chromosome 21. Pediatr Blood Cancer 2005; 44(1): 33-9. [http://dx.doi.org/10.1002/pbc.20092] [PMID: 15390307]

[52] Patrick K, Wade R, Goulden N, *et al.* Outcome of Down syndrome associated acute lymphoblastic leukaemia treated on a contemporary protocol. Br J Haematol 2014; 165(4): 552-5. [http://dx.doi.org/10.1111/bjh.12739] [PMID: 24428704]

[53] Izraeli S, Vora A. How I treat ALL in Down's syndrome: pathobiology and management. Blood 2014;

123(1): 35-40.

[54] Handgretinger R, Zugmaier G, Henze G, Kreyenberg H, Lang P, von Stackelberg A. Complete remission after blinatumomab-induced donor T-cell activation in three pediatric patients with post-transplant relapsed acute lymphoblastic leukemia. Leukemia 2011; 25(1): 181-4. [http://dx.doi.org/10.1038/leu.2010.239] [PMID: 20944674]

[55] Maude SL, Tasian SK, Vincent T, *et al.* Targeting JAK1/2 and mTOR in murine xenograft models of Ph-like acute lymphoblastic leukemia. Blood 2012; 120(17): 3510-8. [http://dx.doi.org/10.1182/blood-2012-03-415448] [PMID: 22955920]

[56] Satgé D, Sommelet D, Geneix A, Nishi M, Malet P, Vekemans M. A tumor profile in Down syndrome. Am J Med Genet 1998; 78(3): 207-16. [http://dx.doi.org/10.1002/(SICI)1096-8628(19980707)78:3<207::AID-AJMG1>3.3.CO;2-Q] [PMID: 9677053]

[57] Satgé D, Sasco AJ, Cure H, Leduc B, Sommelet D, Vekemans MJ. An excess of testicular germ cell tumours in Down's syndrome: three case reports and a review of the literature. Cancer 1997; 80(5): 929-35. [PMID: 9307193]

[58] Chik K, Li C, Shing MM, Leung T, Yuen PM. Intracranial germ cell tumors in children with and without Down syndrome. J Pediatr Hematol Oncol 1999; 21(2): 149-51. [http://dx.doi.org/10.1097/00043426-199903000-00012] [PMID: 10206462]

[59] Baek KH, Zaslavsky A, Lynch RC, *et al.* Down syndrome suppression of tumor growth and the role of the calcineurin inhibitor DSCR1 Nature 2009; 459(7250): 1126-30. [http://dx.doi.org/10.1038/nature08062] [PMID: 19458618]

[60] Folkman J. Antiangiogenesis in cancer therapy-endostatin and its mechanisms of action. Exp Cell Res 2006; 312(5): 594-607. [http://dx.doi.org/10.1016/j.yexcr.2005.11.015] [PMID: 16376330]

CHAPTER 9

Neurological Manifestations of Down Syndrome

Ashraf El-Mitwalli*

Mansoura University, Egypt

Abstract: Down syndrome is the most common chromosomal abnormality. A variety of neurological manifestations including stroke, epilepsy, cervical spinal cord compression, and basal ganglia damage may complicate the syndrome. As the neurologists have little chance to see a good number of DS patients and hence their expertise in this field is lesser than psychiatrists, it is suggested that cooperation between both neurologists and psychiatrists especially the learning disability might lead to better outcome of neurological complications of DS. This chapter reviews the commonest neurological complications associated with DS.

Keywords: Alzheimer disease, Antiphospholipid antibodies, Atlanto-axial subluxation, Cerebral infarction, Cervical spinal cord compression, Children, Cognitive functions, Dementia, Down syndrome, EEG, Epilepsy, GABAergic transmission, Hypotonia, Intellectual disability, Memory, Mental retardation, Moyamoya disease, Pronoun comprehension, Protein C deficiency, Stroke, Trisomy 21.

1. INTRODUCTION

Trisomy 21 or Down syndrome (DS), is the most common chromosomal defect, its incidence in the United States is 1/733 live births [1]. In 1866 the British physician, John Langdon Down had described the condition of DS for the first time in a clinical lecture report entitled "Observation on the ethnic classification of Mongoloid idiots" [2]. Down syndrome has manifestations in many systems and is one of the major reasons for mental retardation. A variety of neurological manifestations including stroke, epilepsy, cervical spinal cord compression, and basal ganglia damage may complicate the syndrome [3]. All patients with DS

* **Corresponding Author Ashraf El-Mitwalli:** Mansoura University, Egypt; Mobile: 00201010113340; Email: metwally99@yahoo.com

Mohammed Al-Biltagi (Ed)

eventually develop neuropathologically Alzheimer's disease-like findings, and sometimes clinically associated with dementia [4, 5]. Diagnosis of epilepsy was confirmed in seven only cases in more than 4500 (0.2%) general referral of patients with DS suspected to have seizure disorders seen in neurology outpatient clinic by a consultant neurologist over a five-year period. Only one new, comorbid, diagnosis was made. Neurologists have little exposure to, and hence little chance to develop expertise in, the neurological complications of DS [6].

2. NEURO-ANATOMIC FUNCTIONS OF THE BRAIN IN DOWN SYNDROME

2.1. Gross Anatomy

Even when the measure is corrected for reduced body size, the brains of adults with DS are about 20% smaller than typically developing brains [7]. Brain changes, still incompletely understood, and fall into 2 categories. The first is a subtle developmental abnormality that results in lifelong mental retardation. The second is a less subtle, almost absolute predisposition to severe Alzheimer disease that commences at relatively young ages (forties, or even thirties) and results in demonstrable cognitive decline in these already impaired individuals [8]. Brains from DS patients are smaller than normal, often around 1,000 g in weight, with corresponding reductions in neuronal content. They show a characteristic rounding of contour and shortening in the anterior-posterior axis with a steeply rising, almost vertical occipital outline. A small superior temporal gyrus is also characteristic and the cerebellum and brainstem are also often disproportionately small. Subtle abnormalities such as focal heterotopias, polymicrogyria, and other abnormal convolutional patterns may also be found [9, 10]. All brain structures except for the parahippocampal gyrus are smaller in DS patients than in controls. The lateral and the third ventricles are larger in DS patients. Significant (non-zero) occipital petalia are found only among DS subjects. The volume of the frontal tips is larger in the right hemisphere in 69% of DS subjects and in 92% of controls. The volume of the occipital poles is greater on the left in 77% of DS subjects and in only 50% of controls. None of the group differences in petalia are significant. There is no relationship between the presence of petalia and handedness, and removal of left-handed subjects does not alter the results. Among the DS subjects, the age-related pyramis shrinkage is accompanied by reduction of the volumes of the cerebellar hemispheres and the caudate [11].

2.2. Microscopic Study

The most striking finding in young DS brains is apparent only with special Golgi preparations. Neuronal dendritic trees are normal in DS fetuses, but these fail to show the progressive increase in dendritic number and complexity that is seen in normal individuals from birth to young adulthood. This results in a striking "tree in winter" appearance of neuronal dendrites that persists into adulthood, and that immediately suggests a morphological substrate for mental retardation [12, 13]. In four old DS females with a mean age of 69 year, the total number of neurons and glial cells in the mediodorsal thalamic (MDT) nucleus was estimated and compared to six age- and sex-matched controls. Using the optical fractionator technique, The MDT nucleus was delineated on coronal sections, and cell numbers (large and small neurons, oligodendrocytes, and astrocytes) were estimated. The total neurons in the MDT nucleus in brains of the DS women was significantly lower compared with controls; 3.41×106 in DS and 5.97×106 in the controls, with no overlap (2p=0.004), large (projecting) and small (local inhibitory) neurons nearly affected equally. On the other hand, there were no significant difference in glial cell population of DS brains compared with controls. The basal ganglia were unaffected while the cortical structures of the same four DS brains were estimated to be half the normal size of controls with a reduction in cell numbers. The exact cause of reduced number of cells in MDT nucleus could not be determined but developmental delay, premature aging, and Alzheimer-like pathology could provide an evidence for a local reduction in neuron numbers in the MDT nucleus, which could affect the cognitive capacity of patients with DS [14].

2.3. Structural and Functional Neuroimaging

Early structural MRI reports suggested that total intracranial volume is smaller in DS, with the greatest volumetric differences in the cerebellum, brainstem, and frontal lobes [15]. Hippocampal volumes have been found to be smaller than for typically developing individuals [16]. A voxel-based morphometric analysis similarly showed decreased volume in the brainstem, cerebellum, cingulate gyrus, medial frontal lobe, superior temporal lobes, and hippocampi [17]. Adolescents with DS showed several regional grey matter GM concentration abnormalities compared to age-matched controls. In the adolescents with DS, there was an association between regional GM density and the neuropsychological measures. Short-term memory performances were correlated with superior temporal gyrus, the inferior parietal lobule, medial occipital lobe, cerebellum and insula. Long-term memory abilities were correlated with GM density in the lateral and medial temporal lobe regions, orbitofrontal cortex, and anterior cingulum and visuoperceptual abilities with GM density the left middle frontal gyrus. Regional grey matter density of the middle and inferior temporal gyrus and cerebellum was associated with linguistic measures. Results of this preliminary study showed that brain organization in DS is not always efficient [18]. A study of functional magnetic resonance imaging (fMRI) activation during passive story listening showed decreased activation in classical receptive language areas in DS compared with controls [19]. Neural activation during a semantic-classification/objec--recognition task in 13 persons with DS and 12 typically developing control participants (age range 12-26 years) was studied using fMRI. There were atypical patterns of brain activation for the individuals with DS. Correlating an index of visual spatial ability and brain activation regions showed a positive relationship between this index and the middle and dorsal frontal gyri in the individuals with DS and brain activation of the occipital and parietal lobes for the typically developing individuals. These findings supported the authors' hypothesis that persons with DS demonstrate atypical neural activation compared with typically developing individuals matched for chronological age [20]. Under connectivity and widespread increased synchrony between brain regions in DS patients were detected comparing fMRI scans of 15 individuals with DS to 14 typically developing control subjects while they viewed fifty minutes of cartoon video clips. Brain regions showing negative correlations were among the most strongly affected connections in the brain and were less anti-correlated. Increased correlation was observed between all of the studied distributed brain networks, subjects with the lowest performance intelligence quotient (IQ) showed the strongest internetwork correlation. A functional parcellation of the brain showed simplified network structure in DS organized by local connectivity. Despite increased interregional synchrony, inter-subject correlation to the cartoon stimuli was lower in DS, denoting that increased synchrony had a temporal pattern that was not in response to environmental stimuli, but idiosyncratic to each DS subject. These results suggest immature development of connectivity in DS with impaired ability to integrate information from distant brain regions into coherent distributed networks [21]. There was no relationship between total brain size and the cognitive variables but age-related decline in the DS subjects in general intelligence and basic linguistic skills was reported in correlating the size of brain regions that were significantly reduced in DS with performance on tests of intelligence and language. General intelligence and mastery of linguistic concepts correlated negatively with the volume of the parahippocampal gyrus. [11].

2.4. Electroencephalographic and Magnetoencephalography

An activation study using magnetoencephalography (MEG) indicated that different subjects with DS may differ in the ipsilateral *vs* contralateral response to a finger movement task [22]. Electroencephalographic (EEG) analysis has shown that the cortical sources of resting alpha and beta rhythms were lower in amplitude in central, parietal, occipital, and temporal regions in the DS than control subjects, whereas occipital delta cortical sources were higher in DS patients. A control analysis on absolute source values showed that they were globally larger in amplitude across several frequency bands in DS than control subjects. Decreased amplitude of synchronized alpha rhythms, suggesting impaired cortical neural synchronization [23]. The topology of the functional connectivity of DS patients is disrupted in the whole brain in alpha and theta bands, and especially in the left intra-hemispheric brain networks in upper alpha band in a study Using a nonlinear synchronization method, the functional brain connectivity (FBCs) of typically developing children and DS patients was computed. The global organization of the DS brain does not resemble a Small-World network, but it works as a random network [24]. In DS, individual alpha peak frequency was shifted to lower frequencies and correlated positively with Mini-Mental State examination and Wechsler Adult Intelligence Scale. Compared with controls, DS showed increased current source density (CSD) in: alpha-1, theta, and beta-1 classical bands and in individual alpha peak frequency

(IAF)-adjusted bands, while relative alpha-2 was decreased. There was a negative correlation between cognitive performance and theta/alpha CSD in the right posterior cingulate cortex and right frontal lobe. The relative alpha-2 correlated positively with cognitive tests. Increased CSD in DS, correlating with cognitive performance, for both slow and fast rhythms suggests involving of cortical and subcortical mechanisms. Exact/standard Low Resolution Electromagnetic Tomography (LORETA) might be useful for objective measure of cognitive decline in DS [25].

3. DOWN SYNDROME AND COGNITIVE FUNCTIONS

Down syndrome is the most common genetic cause of intellectual disabilities. DS is manifested by abnormalities in memory, learning, and language that lead to mild-to severe intellectual impairment [26, 27]. The cognitive phenotype in DS is characterized by impairments in explicit long-term memory morphosyntax, and verbal short-term memory. However, implicit long-term memory, visuospatial short-term memory, and associative learning functions are preserved. Seizures are associated with cognitive decline and seem to cause additional decline in cognitive functioning, particularly in people with DS and co morbid disorders such as autism. Hypothyroidism, hearing disorders and Vision can negatively impact cognitive functioning in people with DS [28].

Alterations in excitatory-inhibitory balance occur in DS and could be responsible for cognitive deficits observed through the life of all individuals carrying an extra copy of chromosome 21. Excess inhibition in the adult could produce synaptic plasticity deficits that may be a primary mechanism contributing to learning and memory impairments. γ-aminobutyric acid (GABA) is the major inhibitory neurotransmitter in the mature central nervous system that binds to GABA-benzodiazepine receptors have been extensively studied as targets for treatment of cognitive disorders, epilepsy, anxiety, sleep, and the induction of sedation. Molecules that are either inverse agonists of the GABA-benzodiazepine receptors or antagonists are able to reduce inhibitory GABAergic transmission. However modulating the excitatory-inhibitory balance towards increase of cognition without inducing seizures remains difficult particularly when using GABA antagonists. Inverse agonists selective for the alpha 5-subunit containing receptor can be used. Such inverse agonists, initially developed as cognitive enhancers for treatment of memory impairments, proved to be very efficient in reversing learning and memory deficits in a Down syndrome mouse model after acute treatment [29].

3.1. Assessment of Intellectual Disability

In patients with DS, the severity of intellectual disability and ageing are associated with acute neurological disease, visual impairment, and poor dental health [30]. People perceived variations in the facial appearance of 20 children with trisomy 21 influence how they are perceived in terms of intellectual disability, the more "trisomic" faces being rated as more intellectually disabled. These inferences were unrelated to individuals' actual test scores despite high degrees of inter-rater agreement which were also unrelated to perceived facial appearance. All these findings indicate that; in groups characterized by a genetic disorder such as trisomy 21 social inferences about intelligence based on facial appearance are unreliable [31]. Roberts and Richmond (2014) had tested preschool children with DS and typically developing children, age-matched on either non-verbal scores as a proxy for mental age (MA), or receptive language on a battery of behavioral measures that have been shown to depend on the hippocampus or the prefrontal cortex and eye-tracking. They concluded that, performance of preschool children with DS equivalently to MA-matched controls, suggesting that the cognitive delay and disability-specific memory deficits documented in adults with DS are not yet evident in preschoolers with DS, and likely emerge progressively with age. These results reinforce the idea that early childhood may be a critical time frame for targeted early intervention [32]. A hierarchical linear modeling was tried to examine the rate of change in performance in nonverbal cognitive abilities across adolescence for 20 males with DS on the subtests of the Leiter-R Brief IQ across four annual time points and to determine the relation between maternal IQ and level and rate of change in performance. There was no significant change in IQ (standard scores) with age in the sample, suggesting IQ stability during adolescence for individuals with DS, although several participants performed at floor level on the standard scores for the Leiter-R, limiting interpretation. Analysis of growth scores indicated significant gain in absolute nonverbal cognitive ability levels (growth score values) over time for the adolescents with DS, although the growth varied by subdomain. Maternal IQ did not explain variability in cognitive performance or change in that performance over time in a sample of adolescents with DS [33].

3.2. Memory Assessment

Down syndrome is associated with a specific verbal short-term memory (STM) deficit. A study explored the effects of grouping, semantic relations and visual presentation upon verbal STM recall performance in a group of 15 individuals with DS and 15 vocabulary-matched typically developing (TD) children. Participants were presented with memoranda in either a temporally grouped schedule, such that items were grouped as pairs, or in an equally spaced presentation schedule. The two items constituting each pair were either semantically related or unrelated. Performance across these conditions was compared in verbal or verbal plus visual presentation modes. Significant memory recall benefits were observed across populations as a result of temporal grouping, semantic relations and verbal and visual combined presentation. However, a reduced benefit of semantic relation in the DS group compared to the typically developed group indicated that those with DS were less influenced by long term memory (LTM) relational knowledge. In addition, those with DS only experienced a grouping benefit during verbal and visual combined presentation, in contrast to the TD group who experienced grouping benefits throughout. This indicates that individuals with DS are poorer at encoding temporal context for purely verbal memoranda. These findings were replicated in a follow-up experiment, aimed at aligning baseline performance in the two populations. This study provides encouraging evidence that, despite their difficulties in some areas, individuals with DS can benefit from the use of grouping and LTM knowledge to assist their verbal STM performance under certain circumstances [34].

3.3. Pronoun Comprehension

Using a manual picture selection task, the comprehension of different types of pronouns was examined in 14 -ranging from 10 to 34 years of age-Greek-speaking individuals with DS; a study examining pronoun comprehension in adolescents and adults with DS in comparison with typically developing (TD) children was conducted. Research questions are: Are some pronoun types more difficult than others for each of the two groups (DS and TD)? Is there a difference in performance between the two groups? Does performance correlate with chronological age in the DS group? The TD and DS groups were recruited and tested in pre-schools and schools/centers for individuals with learning disabilities, respectively. The DS group showed a significant positive correlation of age with performance, but only in structures that also presented difficulties to TD children. Structures that presented difficulties only to individuals with DS do not appear to be less problematic for older participants. The results provide support to the deviance hypothesis by suggesting that the syntactic deficit in the comprehension of pronouns in individuals with DS is present in individuals of a wide age range. At the same time, these findings suggest that some aspects of grammatical development in individuals with DS may continue even after adolescence and well into adulthood. The results can contribute towards more targeted intervention practices by increasing our knowledge of the behavioral phenotype of DS [35]. A Ts65Dn (TS) mouse model was used to evaluate the effect of the dual-specificity tyrosine-(Y)-phosphorylation regulated kinase 1A (DYRK1A) gene over expression on the behavioral and cognitive alterations as well as on several electrophysiological and neuromorphological properties proposed to underlie these deficits. The results revealed that normalization of the Dyrk1A copy number in TS mice improved reference and working memory based on the Morris water maze and contextual conditioning based on the fear conditioning test and rescued hippocampal long-term potentiation (LTP). Associated with these functional improvements, the proliferation and differentiation of hippocampal cells in the adult dentate gyrus (DG) and the density of GABAergic and glutamatergic synapse markers in the molecular layer of the hippocampus were restored with normalization of the Dyrk1A expression level in TS mice. These results suggest that Dyrk1A over expression is involved in some of the electrophysiological, neuromorphological and cognitive alterations, but not in the structural alterations found in DS, and suggest that pharmacological strategies targeting this gene may improve the treatment of DS-associated learning disabilities [36].

3.4. Dementia

There is a dramatic improvement in the life expectancy of people with DS.

Substantial increase in their longevity is mainly due to Improvements in the diagnosis and management of medical complications especially the neurological complications which are important in maintaining optimal cognitive functioning. Dementia resembling Alzheimer's disease (AD) is common in adults with DS. Early-onset dementia in adults with DS does not seem to be associated with atherosclerotic complications [28].

3.4.1. Prevalence

The prevalence of dementia increases with age in DS, it rises from approximately 15% after age 45 years to approximately 75% after age 65 years [28, 37]. While the association between early onset dementias such as AD and DS has been known for many years, there still remains considerable uncertainty regarding the clinical progression of comorbidities namely; visual impairment, hearing impairment, epilepsy, thyroid disorders and dementia [38]. By age 40 years, virtually all individuals with DS have the characteristic neuropathology of AD. The mortality rates in DS are increased, both during early and later stages of life, mortality risk remains higher in adults with DS compared with typically developing populations and the overall population of people with mental retardation. Causes of higher mortality rates later in life may be due to a number of factors, two of which are an increased risk for AD and an apparent tendency toward premature aging [39].

Comorbidities are more likely than their peers to experience other significant co-morbidities including mental health issues such as depression. A rebound in their functioning after a clear and sustained period of decline was noticed in three individuals with DS and dementia. It is hypothesized that this phenomenon is not actually a reversal of the expected dementia trajectory but is an undiagnosed depression exaggerating the true level of functional decline associated with the dementia. The identification and treatment of depressive symptoms may therefore increase the quality of life of some people with DS and dementia [40].

3.4.2. Predictor Biomarkers and Neuropathological Findings

The major neurological deficits that affect DS individuals are cognitive disability and neuropathological changes leading to an early onset of Alzheimer's disease

[41, 42]. Numerous systemic and cellular abnormalities in the DS nervous system have been reported, but other unknown factors could contribute to the range of neurological changes in DS [43]. In the DS adults brains, neuritic amyloid- ß (Aß) plaques - a characteristic neuropathological feature of AD- are a virtually certain finding [41, 44] and have been noted in some children with DS [45]. Cenini and colleagues analyzed the frontal cortex of DS subjects with or without significant AD pathology in comparison with age-matched controls, using a proteomics approach. The effects that age, DS, and AD neuropathology could have on protein expression levels have been investigated. Their results show overlapping and independent molecular pathways (including energy metabolism, oxidative damage, protein synthesis, and autophagy) contributing to DS, to aging, and to the presence of AD pathology in DS. Investigation of pathomechanisms involved in DS with AD may provide putative targets for therapeutic approaches to slow the development of AD [46].

Two out of 12 children with DS, (ages 8 and 9 years) had Aß plaques, and among those between the ages of 35 and 45 years, all had neuritic Aß plaques and other AD pathologies, such as glial activation and neurofibrillary tangles. Approximately 50 to 70% of individuals with DS develop dementia by age 60 to 70 years although the prediction of AD neuropathological changes at middle age is reported to be a virtual certainty in those with DS [47, 48]. Using Reversed phase High-performance liquid chromatography (RP-HPLC) with electrochemical detection, (nor) adrenergic (NA/A) and 3-Methoxy-4-hydroxyphenylglycol (MHPG), dopaminergic (DA, HVA, and DOPAC), and serotonergic (5-HT and 5-HIAA) compounds were quantified in the serum of DS subjects with Alzheimer's disease at baseline DS subjects without AD, non-demented DS individuals that converted to AD over time, and finally, healthy typically developed controls. Serum MHPG levels were significantly lower in demented and converted DS subjects compared to non-demented DS individuals and healthy controls. Those subjects with MHPG levels below median had a more than tenfold increased risk of developing dementia. Furthermore, significant correlations were observed between monoaminergic serum values and various probable behavioral and psychological signs and symptoms of dementia BPSD and progressive memory loss within each DS group, which considered a great potential as biomarker to monitor and predict conversion to AD in DS and demonstrating the need to develop a validated rating scale for BPSD in DS [49].

4. STROKE

Ischemic stroke is not rare in patients with DS, especially in association with congenital embolic cardiac disease [50]. Children with DS are at increased risk for cerebral infarction.

4.1. Arterial Stroke

The majority of strokes are secondary to cerebral embolism, originating from right-to-left shunting, atrioventricular canal defects, cardiac valvular abnormalities, or myocardial dysmotility. Cerebrovascular occlusion and stroke may be a consequence of increased susceptibility to bacterial infection, including meningitis, septicemia, and subacute bacterial endocarditis. Upper cervical subluxation, associated with atlantoaxial instability, can produce posterior cerebral circulation ischemia.

4.1.1. Congenital Heart Disorders

Down syndrome is major cause of congenital heart disease and the most frequent known cause of atrioventricular septal defects [51]. Congenital heart disorders such as tetralogy of Fallot, prosthetic valves, ventricular septal defect, rheumatic heart disease, bacterial endocarditic, atrial myxomas, and myocarditis may result in stroke. Strokes may occur from paradoxical embolization in association with patent foramen ovale [52].

4.1.2. Moyamoya Disease

Takeuchi and Shimizu 1957 were the first who described moyamoya arteriopathy in a case report from Japan [53]. The typical angiographic appearance of the small fragile basal collateral vessels prompted Suzuki and Takaku (1969) to use the Japanese word "moyamoya," meaning hazy, cloudy, or puff of smoke, to define the vasculopathy [54].

Moyamoya disease is a chronic occlusive cerebrovascular disorder characterized by progressive stenosis of the arteries of the circle of Willis. The process starts in the intracranial internal carotid arteries and progresses to involve the middle, anterior, and posterior cerebral arteries. Secondarily, small collateral vessels arise distal to stenosed or occluded vessels [55]. Moyamoya Figs. **(1a)**, **(1b)** and **(1c)** has been reported to occur more frequently in DS than the general pediatric population [56]. The first study to estimate the prevalence of DS in patients with moyamoya disease revealed 26-fold-greater prevalence of DS in patients with coexisting moyamoya disease compared with the prevalence of DS among live births (145 per 100,000) these findings suggest the need for a better understanding of the common pathophysiology of the two conditions [57]. Adults with moyamoya syndrome present with intraparenchymal, intraventricular, or subarachnoid hemorrhage as well as transient ischemic attack and stroke while the majority of children present with ischemic symptoms [58].

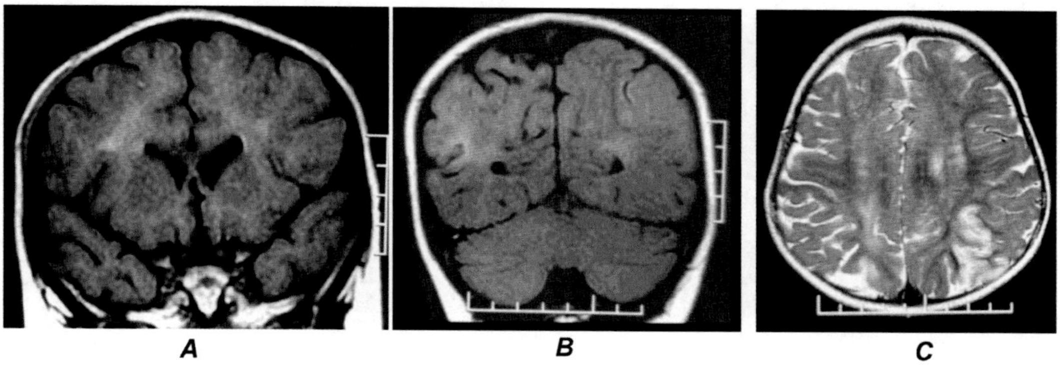

Fig. (1a). Brain magnetic resonance images (MRI) of a 5-year-old female patient with Down syndrome **(A)** and **(B)** Coronal flair image, **(C)** Axial T2 WI show periventricular white matter high signal denoting chronic ischemic changes. Prominent cortical sulci denote cortical atrophy.

Out of 19 patients with DS and moyamoya syndrome, 17 presented with transient ischemic episodes or cerebral infarction between 23 months and 15 years of age. an adult, aged 27 years, and a 13-year-old patient presented with an intracranial hemorrhage, The average age at onset in this series was 5 years [59]. A 20-month-old child with DS underscores the observation that cerebrovascular disease can occur earlier in life in children with DS than in those without DS. The structural defects associated with DS might create vulnerability for the development of ischemic cerebrovascular disease and, secondarily, moyamoya syndrome [60].

Moreover; perinatal cerebral infarct was presumed in a girl with trisomy 21 and bilateral moyamoya disease who presented, unusually, with the clinical, angiographic, and radiological features of moyamoya disease. Early diagnosis is important as moyamoya disease presenting in childhood is associated with a high rate of recurrent stroke and there is evidence that surgical revascularization can prevent further strokes [61].

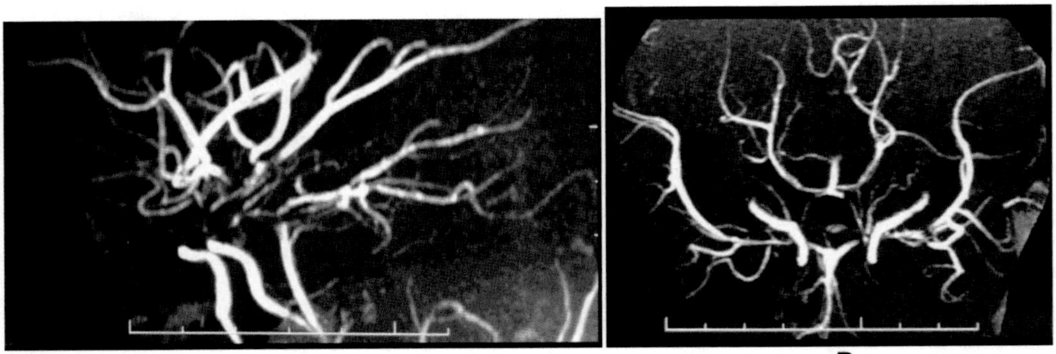

A B

Fig. (1b). Magnetic resonance angiogram (MRA) of the cerebral vessels using time of flight (TOF) of the same patient. (A) sagittal and **(B)** coronal views show loss of signal form of distal internal carotid arteries (ICAs) and the proximal parts of cerebral vessels bilaterally and non clearly visualized circle of Willis consistent with Moyamoya disease.

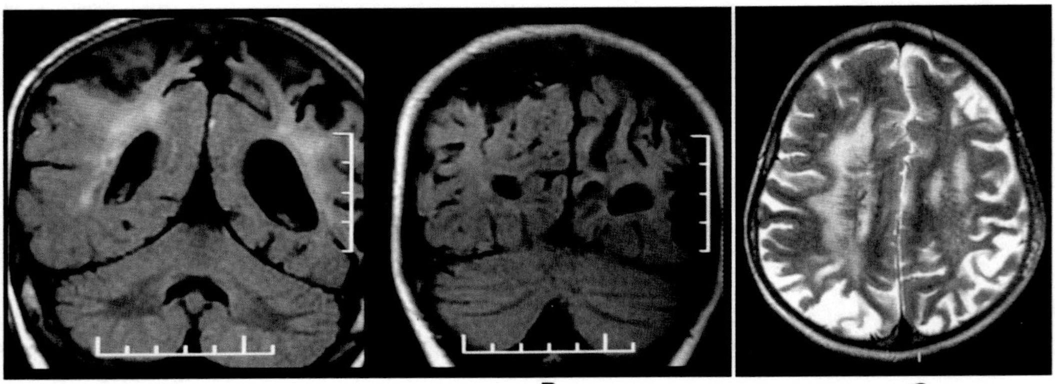

A B C

Fig. (1c). ***Follow up brain MRI after 2 years of the same patient.*** **(A)** and **(B)** Coronal flair image, **(C)** Axial T2 WI show progressive course of periventricular white matter high signal. More prominent cortical sulci and dilated both lateral ventricles denote progressive central and cortical brain atrophy.

Adel El-Badrawy [1], ***Ahmad El-Morsy*** [2] [1 Professor of Radiology, 2 Assistant Lecturer of Diagnostic and Intervention Radiology; Faculty of Medicine Mansoura University].

A 2-year-old boy with DS complicated by Moyamoya syndrome developed extensive multiple cerebral infarctions after status epilepticus on the third day of a measles infection. MR angiography revealed the occlusion of the terminal portion of the bilateral internal carotid artery and the basilar artery. Fever, dehydration, activation of coagulation associated with the infection, relatively decreased cerebral blood flow during status epilepticus, and central nervous invasion of the measles virus May have played a role in the development of the infarction. Moyamoya like cerebrovascular lesions occur more often and is more aggressive in children with DS than in the general pediatric population, and their clinical presentation is always the infarction type. In patients with DS complicated by Moyamoya syndrome, an early diagnosis and prevention of infarction are important [62].

4.1.3. Abnormalities of the Circle of Willis

Neuropathological investigation of a child with DS who did not have moyamoya syndrome showed significant structural abnormalities in vessels of the circle of Willis—irregular internal elastic membrane surrounding regions of marked endothelial hyperplasia, again suggesting a possible underlying structural change in the cerebral arteries of children with moyamoya syndrome and DS [63].

4.1.4. Infectious Diseases

Cerebral infarction may occur as a complication of infectious disease as acute infection with *Mycoplasma pneumonia*, infection with *Streptococcus oralis* (viridans subgroup), and bibasilar pneumonia. Selective IgG4 subclass deficiency may be associated risk factor. IgG4 subclass deficiency could conceivably play a role in the high frequency of para-infectious related stroke in this population [64]. A stroke was reported in a 2-year old Japanese boy; occurred soon after varicella infection. The laboratory examination revealed the presence of anticardiolipin antibodies and magnetic resonance (MR) angiography showed cranial vascular changes compatible with moyamoya syndrome [65].

4.1.5. Protein C Deficiency

Protein C deficiency; was reported in a child with moyamoya syndrome and DS who was admitted with recurrent strokes; his magnetic resonance imaging and magnetic resonance angiography findings confirmed the presence of occlusive cerebrovascular disease with basal collateral vessels. During the stroke, his protein C levels were significantly decreased. Complete clinical recovery was seen during follow-up. This suggests the possibility of a link between protein C deficiency and DS with moyamoya syndrome [66].

4.1.6. Antiphospholipid Antibodies

Down syndrome is characterized by immune system deficits with tendency to autoimmune phenomena. Two patients with DS and the primary antiphospholipid antibodies were described. One patient showed a vasculopathy similar to that previously described as Moyamoya. This report extends the scope of these observations and particularly draws out the potential role of antiphospholipid antibodies. Indeed antiphospholipid antibodies may well explain the well-known association of DS and stroke [67].

4.1.7. Cryptogenic Stroke

In rare cases, stroke etiology remains unexplained. A 19 year old girl with trisomy 21 with a 47XX+21 karyotype suffered from obesity, hypercholesterolemia and arterial hypertension who presented at age 11 years with a transient ischemic attack with left hemiparesis, and at age 17 years from an ischemic stroke in the territory of the right middle cerebral artery. Since blood coagulation studies, blood cultures, immunologic parameters, 24-h Holter monitoring, transthoracic and transesophageal echocardiography, magnetic resonance angiography of the extra- and intracranial vessels, thoracic and abdominal aorta and renal arteries did not provide any explanation for the stroke, implantation of a loop recorder is considered in order to detect episodes of clinically silent atrial fibrillation [68].

4.2. Venous Stroke

Venous thrombosis may be a cause of stroke in DS patients. A 25-year-old male with DS was hospitalized because of a generalized tonic–clonic seizure and prolonged postictal state. Cerebral magnetic resonance imaging (MRI) and MR venography revealed cerebral venous thrombosis. Investigations failed to reveal any cause for the venous thrombosis which may be an unusual cause of stroke in DS [69]. Another twenty-seven-year-old male with DS who presented with headache, vomiting and left hemiparesis, neuroimaging revealed cerebral venous thrombosis and anticoagulant treatment was started, and eventuated in a favorable clinical outcome [70]. Also, a twenty year old Hispanic male with DS presented with diminution of vision, progressively worsening headache and fundus examination revealed bilateral papilledema. Magnetic resonance venography showed thrombosis of left transverse and sigmoid sinuses. Catheter angiography angiogram showed a dural arteriovenous fistula in the wall of left transverse and sigmoid sinuses. The patient underwent Onyx endovascular embolization of the fistula, resulting in its angiographic obliteration, followed by resolution of his clinical signs and symptoms [71].

5. SPINAL CORD COMPRESSION

5.1. Atlanto-Axial Instability (Fig. 2: A, B and C)

Cervical spinal instability in association with DS has been first reported in 1961 [72]. Many patients with DS have greater than normal movement without clinical symptoms. Surgical stabilization for patients with the combination of radiographic abnormalities and clinical symptoms of myelopathy is recommended. The common clinical findings are brisk reflexes and or clonus, but symptoms may range from fatigability, gait disturbance, neck pain, torticollis, limited neck mobility, head tilt, incoordination, clumsiness, sensory deficits, spasticity, extensor plantar reflexes, posterior column symptoms, bowel or bladder dysfunction, or toe walking. Although acute neurological decline has been reported, most patients have long-standing symptoms prior to deterioration [73, 74]. Initial description of cervical spinal instability by Tishler and Martel (1965) proposed a possible etiology of ligamentous laxity to explain the increased motion [75]. Sherk and Nicholson (1969) suggested excessive motion may be due to inflammation instead [76]. The etiology remains unclear and they were limited to managing patients' symptoms [75]. Radiographic atlanto-axial instability in DS has been reported in 10% to 30% of patients [77]. Pueschel and Scola (1987) reported on 404 patients prospectively followed and noted a 14.6% rate of radiographic instability (atlanto-dental interval

[ADI] >4.5 mm, with only 1. 5% displaying symptoms and requiring surgery [78]. Comparing symptomatic and asymptomatic patients with radiographic instability, defined as ADI =4 mm and =2 mm of movement on dynamic radiographs; no difference was identified between the space available for the cord (SAC, distance between posterior dens and posterior arch of C1) or ADI between groups and patients were stable at 3 years of follow-up [79].

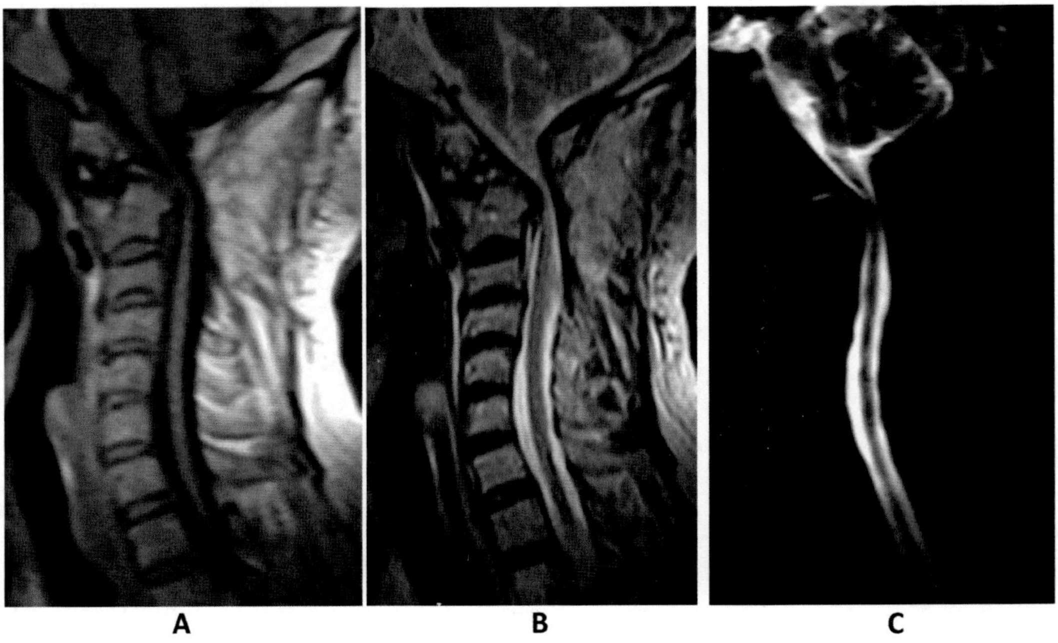

Fig. (2). A 45-year-old male patient with of Down syndrome. A) Sagittal T1 and B) Sagittal T2-weighted magnetic resonance images show atlanto-axial subluxation with subsequent severe canalstenosis and marked cord compression. C) MR myelogram shows complete obliteration of cerebrospinal fluid.
Adel El-Badrawy [1], ***Ahmad El-Morsy*** [2] [1 Professor of Radiology, 2 Assistant Lecturer of Diagnostic and Intervention Radiology; Faculty of Medicine Mansoura University].

In both neutral and flexed positions DS subjects showed a significant reduction of anterior subarachnoid space more in flexed position compared to healthy controls. The space available for cord and ligamentous thickness showed significant differences between DS subjects and healthy controls. In DS subjects with occipito-cervical instability, the anterior subarachnoidal space reduction was significantly reduced in flexed position. In DS subjects with asymptomatic cranio-cervical instability, anterior subarachnoidal evaluation and ligamentous status could add new information about the risk of spinal cord damage [80]. Early diagnosis of atlantoaxial instability (AAI) in pediatric is important for improved outcomes because of poor outcomes in progressed neurological symptoms. Conventional dynamic radiography of the cervical spine is associated with a potential risk of worsening neurological symptoms. The medical records of 50 patients (24 boys and 26 girls) with AAI associated with DS were retrospectively reviewed. Eleven had undergone and 4 had been scheduled for surgery. In addition to the atlas-dens interval (ADI) and space available for spinal cord (SAC), C1 inclination angle and C1/4 SAC ratio on lateral radiographs of the cervical spine in the neutral position were measured. Receiver operating characteristic (ROC) analysis of each index was performed to assess the diagnostic abilities of these indices to determine indication for surgery, and their diagnostic abilities were compared. The reproducibility of the two proposed indices was assessed. The discriminatory abilities of C1/4 SAC (AUC, 1.00) and C1 inclination angle (0.91) were comparable with those of ADI (0.98) and SAC (0.95). The diagnostic abilities of the two novel radiographic measurements were comparable with those of ADI and SAC. These novel measurements can be obtained safely on lateral radiographs of the cervical spine in the neutral position [81].

A functional unit formed by the occiput, the atlas (C1), and the axis (C2) assures a high degree of mobility of the upper cervical spine providing that strong ligaments keep these structures in place. Laxity of the ligaments in DS leads to instability of vertebral movement at the atlanto-axial junction. In individuals with DS, the excessive laxity of the posterior transverse ligament which attaches the odontoid bone to C1 appears to be the most common cause of atlanto-axial subluxation although there is no universal agreement on this point [82]. In addition, C-1 hypoplasia and occult spinal canal stenosis have been linked to the increased risk of compressive cervical myelopathy in individuals with DS.

5.2. Atlanto-Occipital Instability

Atlanto-occipital instability is a less well defined entity with DS and may be under diagnosed [83]. Out of 199 patients with DS; twelve (8.5%) had posterior occipital atlantal hypermobility. Many patients showed no changes or progression of their ratios with follow- up imaging and 66% of patients with excessive motion had neurological deficits, although none of them require surgical stabilization [84].

5.3. Other Spine Disorders

A higher incidence of degenerative changes in adulthood and a greater risk of developing symptomatic subaxial cervical spondylosis were reported in DS patients [85].

6. SLEEP

In typically developing children, sleep problems have been associated with day-time attentional difficulties. Children with developmental disabilities often suffer attention and sleep problems, yet their relationship is poorly understood. A study investigated this association was done. Actigraphy and pulse oximetry assessed sleep and sleep-disordered breathing respectively, and attention in school-aged children with DS and Williams syndrome (WS) was tested using a novel visual Continuous Performance Task (CPT). Attention deficits were evident in both DS and WS. In the TD group, higher scores on the CPT were related to better sleep quality, higher oxyhemoglobin saturation (SpO2), and fewer desaturation events. Sleep quality, duration, and SpO2 variables were not related to CPT performance for children with DS and WS [86].

7. EPILEPSY

Five to 13% of children with DS have seizures [87, 88]. The occurrence is bimodal with 40% having seizures before 1 year of age—generally west syndrome—and with 40% developing seizures after the third decade, mostly tonic– clonic or myoclonic seizures [89]. West syndrome (infantile spasms) is associated with electroencephalographic characteristics of idiopathic rather than symptomatic epilepsy. It appears that children with DS have better seizure control following the use of appropriate antiepileptic drugs compared to other patients with symptomatic infantile spasms, and early initiation of treatment may contribute to the prevention of late seizure development and better developmental outcome [87]. Cryptogenic epilepsy in DS may develop during the first year of life in the form of infantile spasms (IS), partial seizures (PS) or generalized seizures (GS). Electroclinical features of IS resemble those of idiopathic West syndrome, with a favorable response to treatment with adrenocorticotropic hormone. Patients experiencing PS and GS may be resistant to therapy with antiepileptic drugs [90]. The onset of Lennox–Gastaut syndrome in DS is usually later than seen in the typical population and may be associated with reflex seizures [91]. EEG findings do not correlate with outcome as there is a high rate of EEG abnormalities in DS without the evidence of clinical seizures [92]. EEG characteristics of seizures in adults with DS have included progressive slowing of background activity with frontal sharp and slow waves while generalized spike and slow wave discharges seen with those with myoclonic epilepsy [93].

Subjects with DS over age 45 years are more likely to develop dementia than those with seizures onset at younger ages [94]. Eighty four percent of demented individuals with DS develop seizures. The commonest seizure form associated with dementia in DS is the senile myoclonic epilepsy [95]. Some papers reported the development of adverse drug reactions in patients with DS during the treatment with antiepileptic drugs. Siniscalchi *et al.* reported a 17-year-old man with epilepsy and DS who experienced tremor during the treatment with a low dosage of sodium valproate. The Naranjo probability scale documented a possible association between tremor and sodium valproate. Sodium valproate was changed to lamotrigine with both a rapid improvement of tremor and an optimal control of symptoms. The development of tremor was probably through the decreased activity of GABAergic neurotransmission [96]. Down syndrome individuals are likely to present epigenetic aberrations. Epigenetic mechanisms, including DNA methylation and post-translational histone modifications, regulate gene expression and might play a crucial role in the development of the cognitive deficits in DS. Epigenetic marks are reversible, offering a huge therapeutic potential to alleviate or cure certain genetic deficits. Current epigenetic therapies are already used for cancer and epilepsy, and might provide novel possibilities for cognition-enhancing treatment in DS as well [97].

Adult patients with DS diagnosed with epilepsy are not routinely assessed for portosystemic venous shunts. Measuring ammonia levels in patients with DS the day after admission would help detect portosystemic shunts, even if the patients have been previously diagnosed with epilepsy. If ammonia levels fluctuate without any apparent cause after seizure, dynamic computed tomography should be performed, especially for patients with DS, whether or not they have been previously diagnosed with epilepsy [98].

8. HYPOTONIA

Children with DS usually show delayed motor development with independent walking and upright posture achieved 1 year later compared to infants with typical development [99, 100]. Almost all children with DS suffer from muscle hypotonia, due to this state of reduced muscle tone there is delay in developmental milestones, mastication problems (due to poor neuromuscular control), muscular weakness and dental anomalies are also of common occurrence in DS [101]. The hypotonia leads to difficulty in postural control so the individual with DS is focused on overcoming disturbed equilibrium compared to controls and this necessitates a different strategy in motor development [102]. The trunk control instability may be linked to atypical finger grasping patterns [103]. Among their several pathological traits, DS patients suffer from muscle hypotonia and an altered motor coordination, the most typical features being a slowed voluntary movement and a high error incidence in motion [104]. Subjects with DS appeared to show longer durations of execution across all of the standardized movements' tasks [105].

Motor control problems can be attributed mainly to the smaller cerebellum that is considered the source of the reduced muscle tone and the disturbances in postural and movement coordination [106]. As a complication of hypotonia, individuals with DS have inherent joint laxity resulting in disturbed gait stability and increased energetic costs for physical exertion [107]. The atypical gait patterns include decreased hip extension, increased hip abduction during the swing phase, and longer stance time. Hypotonia in DS is often associated with reduction of physical activity with the result of decreased bone mass accrual and predisposition to fractures [108]. The low levels of physical activity in DS result in a lower levels of lean mass, higher body mass index, and reduced bone mass-related parameters, which, in turn, may affect cardiovascular strength capacities [109]. The cerebellum appears to be the anatomic locus for hypotonia in DS, a structure which shows hypocellularity due to impairment in the periventricular and granular zones during fetal development [110]. Additionally, the cerebellum plays a major role in the regulation of motor learning and proprioceptive-motor control. Beyond its effect on motor functioning, disorganized cerebellar output may impair higher order functioning such as emotion and cognition [111, 112].

8.1. Mechanism

The mechanisms responsible for the overall motor dysfunction and muscle hypotonia in DS are still largely unknown; central activation and defective neuromuscular transmission are probably involved, but abnormal organization and function of myofiber components cannot be ruled out. It is worth noting that persons with DS undergo premature aging in multiple organs [113, 114]. These changes exhibit a decrement in muscle strength compared to euploid subjects as much as it occurs in aged *versus* healthy young subjects [115, 116]. A phosphorus magnetic resonance spectroscopy (31P -MRS) study was performed on the quadriceps muscle of 14 subjects with DS and 11 non-DS controls to investigate the post-exercise re-synthesis kinetics of phosphocreatine (PCr), which utilizes the mitochondrial respiratory function and yields a measure of muscle mitochondrial function *in vivo*. The PCr recovery rate constant was significantly reduced in adults with DS compared to non-DS controls who were matched for physical activity levels, these results suggest that the muscle mitochondrial function *in vivo* is impaired in subjects with DS [117].

Collagen molecules are formed by the assembly of three chains; alpha 1-3 are essential components for maintaining muscle integrity. The type VI collagen is crucial for skeletal as well as cardiac muscles. The COL a1 (VI) and a2 (VI) chains are encoded by genes located at the chromosome 21 and are expected to have higher dosage in individuals with DS. Target genetic loci were studied by DNA sequence analysis. In the studied population, rs2270668 was found to be non-polymorphic. rs2270669 showed significant association of the "C" allele and "CC" genotype with DS probands having Muscle hypotonia. rs2270669 may induce functional and structural alterations in the COL a3 (VI). Interaction of COLa3 (VI) with different proteins, crucial for muscle integrity, was also noticed. This study on COL6A3 with DS related Muscle hypotonia thus indicates that rs2270669 "C" could be a risk factor for DS related Muscle hypotonia [118].

In vitro muscle contractile experiments of soleus muscles from male Ts65Dn mouse model and wild-type (WT) colony controls revealed normal force generation of non-fatigued Ts65Dn soleus, but a significant reduction in force was noticed during recovery from fatiguing contractions compared with WT muscle. Protein expression of copper-zinc superoxide dismutase (SOD1), was significantly increased in Ts65Dn soleus. There was non-significant difference in Non-triplicated antioxidant protein expression between groups. Protein oxidation was twenty percent greater in Ts65Dn animals but Lipid peroxidation was unaltered compared with controls. Citrate synthase was similar between groups but Cytochrome-c oxidase expression was significantly lower in Ts65Dn muscle. Numerous pathways alterations in Ts65Dn muscle including glucose and fat metabolism, proteolysis, neuromuscular transmission, and ATP biosynthesis [119]. By combining morphometry and immunocytochemistry at transmission electron microscopy, the fine structure of skeletal fibers of the quadriceps femoris muscle of the Ts65Dn mouse was analyzed in adult (12 months) and aging (19 months) animals and their age-matched euploid controls. Results revealed structural alterations of myonuclei reminiscent and mitochondria of those observed in age-related sarcopenia, finding supports the hypothesis that trisomy leads to an early aging of skeletal muscle consistent with the multi-systemic premature aging typical of DS [120].

8.2. Management

Thirty children (8-10 years old) with DS were randomized to receive a designed physical therapy program (control group), or to receive the same program given to the control group in addition to whole-body vibration training (study group). Both groups received the treatment sessions three times per week for 6 successive months. Measurement of muscle strength of the knee flexors and extensors by using a handheld dynamometer and stability indices by using the Biodex Stability System was done before and after the 6 months of the treatment program. A significant improvement in stability indices and muscle strength after treatment was demonstrated in each group, with significantly greater improvements seen in the study group. They concluded that, whole-body vibration may be a useful technique to improve balance and muscle strength in children with DS [121].

CONCLUSION

Down syndrome has manifestations in many systems and is one of the major reasons for mental retardation. It may be associated with a variety of neurological complications including stroke, epileptic seizures, cervical spinal cord compression, and basal ganglia damage.

CONFLICT OF INTEREST

The authors confirm that this chapter contents have no conflict of interest.

ACKNOWLEDGEMENTS

I express my warm thanks to Dr. Adel El-Badrawy (professor of radiology) and Dr. Ahmad El-Morsy (assistant Lecturer of Diagnostic and Intervention Radiology); Faculty of Medicine Mansoura University for providing me with the radiologic figures used in this chapter.

REFERENCES

[1] Centers for Disease Control and Prevention (CDC). Improved national prevalence estimates for 18 selected major birth defects--United States, 1999-2001. MMWR Morb Mortal Wkly Rep 2006; 54(51): 1301-5.
[PMID: 16397457]

[2] Down JLH. Observations on an ethnic classification of idiots. London hospital reports 1866; 3: pp. (1866)259-62.

[3] Lev N, Melamed E. [Neurological complications in Down's Syndrome]. Harefuah 2002; 141(9): 820-823, 857.
[PMID: 12362489]

[4] Berg JM, Karlinsky H, Holland AJ, Eds. Alzheimer disease, Down syndrome, and their relationship. Oxford: Oxford University Press 1993.

[5] Mann DM. Down's syndrome and Alzheimer's disease. In: Esiri MM, Trojanowski JQ, Lee VM, Eds. The neuropathology of dementia. (2nd ed.) Cambridge: Cambridge University Press 2004; pp. 207-26.
[http://dx.doi.org/10.1017/CBO9780511526886.011]

[6] Larner AJ. Down syndrome in the neurology clinic: Too much? Too little? Too late? Downs Syndr Res Pract 2007; 12(1): 69-71.
[http://dx.doi.org/10.3104/reports.2011] [PMID: 17692191]

[7] Kemper TL. Down syndrome. In: Peters A, Jones EJ, Eds. Cerebral cortex. Plenum Press Kluwer

Academic 1991.
[http://dx.doi.org/10.1007/978-1-4615-6622-9_12]

[8] Mrak RE, Griffin WS. Trisomy 21 and the brain. J Neuropathol Exp Neurol 2004; 63(7): 679-85. [PMID: 15290893]

[9] Shaw CM. Correlates of mental retardation and structural changes of the brain. Brain Dev 1987; 9(1): 1-8.
[http://dx.doi.org/10.1016/S0387-7604(87)80002-5] [PMID: 2955713]

[10] Coyle JT, Oster-Granite ML, Gearhart JD. The neurobiologic consequences of Down syndrome. Brain Res Bull 1986; 16(6): 773-87.
[http://dx.doi.org/10.1016/0361-9230(86)90074-2] [PMID: 2875770]

[11] Raz N, Torres IJ, Briggs SD, *et al.* Selective neuroanatomic abnormalities in Down's syndrome and their cognitive correlates: evidence from MRI morphometry. Neurology 1995; 45(2): 356-66.
[http://dx.doi.org/10.1212/WNL.45.2.356] [PMID: 7854539]

[12] Takashima S, Becker LE, Armstrong DL, Chan F. Abnormal neuronal development in the visual cortex of the human fetus and infant with Down's syndrome. A quantitative and qualitative Golgi study. Brain Res 1981; 23;225(1): 1-21.
[http://dx.doi.org/10.1016/0006-8993(81)90314-0] [PMID: 6457667]

[13] Takashima S, Iida K, Mito T, Arima M. Dendritic and histochemical development and ageing in patients with Down's syndrome. J Intellect Disabil Res 1994; 38(Pt 3): 265-73.
[http://dx.doi.org/10.1111/j.1365-2788.1994.tb00394.x] [PMID: 8061472]

[14] Karlsen AS, Korbo S, Uylings HB, Pakkenberg B. A stereological study of the mediodorsal thalamic nucleus in Down syndrome. Neuroscience 2014; 279(279): 253-9.
[http://dx.doi.org/10.1016/j.neuroscience.2014.08.046] [PMID: 25220902]

[15] Aylward EH, Li Q, Honeycutt NA, *et al.* MRI volumes of the hippocampus and amygdala in adults with Down's syndrome with and without dementia. Am J Psychiatry 1999; 156(4): 564-8.
[PMID: 10200735]

[16] Pinter JD, Brown WE, Eliez S, Schmitt JE, Capone GT, Reiss AL. Amygdala and hippocampal volumes in children with Down syndrome: a high-resolution MRI study. Neurology 2001; 10;56(7): 972-4.
[http://dx.doi.org/10.1212/WNL.56.7.972] [PMID: 11294940]

[17] White NS, Alkire MT, Haier RJ. A voxel-based morphometric study of nondemented adults with Down Syndrome. Neuroimage 2003; 20(1): 393-403.
[http://dx.doi.org/10.1016/S1053-8119(03)00273-8] [PMID: 14527599]

[18] Menghini D, Costanzo F, Vicari S. Relationship between brain and cognitive processes in Down syndrome. Behav Genet 2011; 41(3): 381-93.
[http://dx.doi.org/10.1007/s10519-011-9448-3] [PMID: 21279430]

[19] Losin EA, Rivera SM, O'Hare ED, Sowell ER, Pinter JD. Abnormal fMRI activation pattern during story listening in individuals with Down syndrome. Am J Intellect Dev Disabil 2009; 114(5): 369-80.
[http://dx.doi.org/10.1352/1944-7558-114.5.369] [PMID: 19928018]

[20] Jacola LM, Byars AW, Chalfonte-Evans M, *et al.* Functional magnetic resonance imaging of cognitive

processing in young adults with Down syndrome. Am J Intellect Dev Disabil 2011; 116(5): 344-59. [http://dx.doi.org/10.1352/1944-7558-116.5.344] [PMID: 21905803]

[21] Anderson JS, Nielsen JA, Ferguson MA, *et al.* Abnormal brain synchrony in Down Syndrome. Neuroimage Clin 2013; 2: 703-15. [http://dx.doi.org/10.1016/j.nicl.2013.05.006] [PMID: 24179822]

[22] Virji-Babul N, Moiseev A, Moiseeva N, Sun W, Ribary U, Lott I. Altered brain dynamics during voluntary movement in individuals with Down syndrome. Neuroreport 2011; 11;22(7): 358-64. [http://dx.doi.org/10.1097/WNR.0b013e328346a1a0] [PMID: 21464774]

[23] Babiloni C, Albertini G, Onorati P, *et al.* Cortical sources of EEG rhythms are abnormal in down syndrome. Clin Neurophysiol 2010; 121(8): 1205-12. [http://dx.doi.org/10.1016/j.clinph.2010.02.155] [PMID: 20362500]

[24] Ahmadlou M, Gharib M, Hemmati S, Vameghi R, Sajedi F. Disrupted small-world brain network in children with Down Syndrome. Clin Neurophysiol 2013; 124(9): 1755-64. [http://dx.doi.org/10.1016/j.clinph.2013.03.004] [PMID: 23583023]

[25] Velikova S, Magnani G, Arcari C, *et al.* Cognitive impairment and EEG background activity in adults with Down's syndrome: a topographic study. Hum Brain Mapp 2011; 32(5): 716-29. [http://dx.doi.org/10.1002/hbm.21061] [PMID: 21484947]

[26] Nelson L, Johnson JK, Freedman M, *et al.* Learning and memory as a function of age in Down syndrome: a study using animal-based tasks. Prog Neuropsychopharmacol Biol Psychiatry 2005; 29(3): 443-53. [http://dx.doi.org/10.1016/j.pnpbp.2004.12.009] [PMID: 15795053]

[27] Dierssen M, Herault Y, Estivill X. Aneuploidy: from a physiological mechanism of variance to Down syndrome. Physiol Rev 2009; 89(3): 887-920. [http://dx.doi.org/10.1152/physrev.00032.2007] [PMID: 19584316]

[28] Lott IT, Dierssen M. Cognitive deficits and associated neurological complications in individuals with Down's syndrome. Lancet Neurol 2010; 9(6): 623-33. [http://dx.doi.org/10.1016/S1474-4422(10)70112-5] [PMID: 20494326]

[29] Potier MC, Braudeau J, Dauphinot L, Delatour B. Reducing GABAergic inhibition restores cognitive functions in a mouse model of Down syndrome. CNS Neurol Disord Drug Targets 2014; 13(1): 8-15. [http://dx.doi.org/10.2174/18715273113126660185] [PMID: 24152333.]

[30] Määttä T, Kaski M, Taanila A, Keinänen-Kiukaanniemi S, Iivanainen M. Sensory impairments and health concerns related to the degree of intellectual disability in people with Down syndrome. Downs Syndr Res Pract 2006; 11(2): 78-83. [http://dx.doi.org/10.3104/reports.317] [PMID: 17048801]

[31] Enea-Drapeau C, Huguet P, Carlier M. Misleading face-based judgment of cognitive level in intellectual disability: the case of trisomy 21 (Down syndrome). Res Dev Disabil 2014; 35(12): 3598-605. [http://dx.doi.org/10.1016/j.ridd.2014.09.003] [PMID: 25244694]

[32] Roberts LV, Richmond JL. Preschoolers with Down syndrome do not yet show the learning and memory impairments seen in adults with Down syndrome. Dev Sci 2014; 5

[http://dx.doi.org/10.1111/desc.12225] [PMID: 25283764]

[33] Channell MM, Thurman AJ, Kover ST, Abbeduto L. Patterns of change in nonverbal cognition in adolescents with Down syndrome. Res Dev Disabil 2014; 35(11): 2933-41. [http://dx.doi.org/10.1016/j.ridd.2014.07.014] [PMID: 25112795]

[34] Smith E, Jarrold C. Grouping, semantic relation and imagery effects in individuals with Down syndrome. Res Dev Disabil 2014; 35(11): 3162-74. [http://dx.doi.org/10.1016/j.ridd.2014.07.061] [PMID: 25151606]

[35] Sanoudaki E, Varlokosta S. Pronoun comprehension in individuals with Down syndrome: the role of age. Int J Lang Commun Disord 2014; 2 [http://dx.doi.org/10.1111/1460-6984.12122] [PMID: 25180983]

[36] García-Cerro S, Martínez P, Vidal V, *et al.* Overexpression of Dyrk1A is implicated in several cognitive, electrophysiological and neuromorphological alterations found in a mouse model of Down syndrome. PLoS One 2014 Sep 4; 9(9): e106572. [http://dx.doi.org/10.1371/journal.pone.0106572] [PMID: 25188425]

[37] Coppus A, Evenhuis H, Verberne GJ, *et al.* Dementia and mortality in persons with Down's syndrome. J Intellect Disabil Res 2006; 50(Pt 10): 768-77. [http://dx.doi.org/10.1111/j.1365-2788.2006.00842.x] [PMID: 16961706]

[38] Glasson EJ, Dye DE, Bittles AH. The triple challenges associated with age-related comorbidities in Down syndrome. J Intellect Disabil Res 2014; 58(4): 393-8. [http://dx.doi.org/10.1111/jir.12026] [PMID: 23510031]

[39] Zigman WB, Lott IT. Alzheimer's disease in Down syndrome: neurobiology and risk. Ment Retard Dev Disabil Res Rev 2007; 13(3): 237-46. [http://dx.doi.org/10.1002/mrdd.20163] [PMID: 17910085]

[40] Wark S, Hussain R, Parmenter T. Down syndrome and dementia: Is depression a confounder for accurate diagnosis and treatment? J Intellect Disabil 2014; 18(4): 305-14. [http://dx.doi.org/10.1177/1744629514552152] [PMID: 25249377]

[41] Burger PC, Vogel FS. The development of the pathologic changes of Alzheimer's disease and senile dementia in patients with Down's syndrome. Am J Pathol 1973; 73(2): 457-76. [PMID: 4271339]

[42] Wisniewski KE, Dalton AJ, McLachlan C, Wen GY, Wisniewski HM. Alzheimer's disease in Down's syndrome: clinicopathologic studies. Neurology 1985; 35(7): 957-61. [http://dx.doi.org/10.1212/WNL.35.7.957] [PMID: 3159974]

[43] Galdzicki Z, Siarey RJ. Understanding mental retardation in Down's syndrome using trisomy 16 mouse models. Genes Brain Behav 2003; 2(3): 167-78. [http://dx.doi.org/10.1034/j.1601-183X.2003.00024.x] [PMID: 12931790]

[44] Leverenz JB, Raskind MA. Early amyloid deposition in the medial temporal lobe of young Down syndrome patients: a regional quantitative analysis. Exp Neurol 1998; 150(2): 296-304. [http://dx.doi.org/10.1006/exnr.1997.6777] [PMID: 9527899]

[45] Olson MI, Shaw CM. Presenile dementia and Alzheimer's disease in mongolism. Brain 1969; 92(1): 147-56.

[http://dx.doi.org/10.1093/brain/92.1.147] [PMID: 4237656]

[46] Cenini G, Fiorini A, Sultana R, *et al.* An investigation of the molecular mechanisms engaged before and after the development of Alzheimer disease neuropathology in Down syndrome: a proteomics approach. Free Radic Biol Med 2014; 76: 89-95. [http://dx.doi.org/10.1016/j.freeradbiomed.2014.08.006] [PMID: 25151119]

[47] Janicki MP, Dalton AJ. Prevalence of dementia and impact on intellectual disability services. Ment Retard 2000; 38(3): 276-88. [http://dx.doi.org/10.1352/0047-6765(2000)038<0276:PODAIO>2.0.CO;2] [PMID: 10900935]

[48] Lott IT, Head E. Down syndrome and Alzheimer's disease: a link between development and aging. Ment Retard Dev Disabil Res Rev 2001; 7(3): 172-8. [http://dx.doi.org/10.1002/mrdd.1025] [PMID: 11553933]

[49] Dekker AD, Coppus AM, Vermeiren Y, *et al.* Serum MHPG Strongly Predicts Conversion to Alzheimer's Disease in Behaviorally Characterized Subjects with Down Syndrome. J Alzheimers Dis 2015; 1;43(3): 871-91. [http://dx.doi.org/10.3233/JAD-140783] [PMID: 25125467]

[50] Freeman SB, Taft LF, Dooley KJ, *et al.* Population-based study of congenital heart defects in Down syndrome. Am J Med Genet 1998; 80(3): 213-7. [http://dx.doi.org/10.1002/(SICI)1096-8628(19981116)80:3<213::AID-AJMG6>3.0.CO;2-8] [PMID: 9843040]

[51] Barlow GM, Chen XN, Shi ZY, *et al.* Down syndrome congenital heart disease: a narrowed region and a candidate gene Genet Med 2001; 3(2): 91-101. [http://dx.doi.org/10.1097/00125817-200103000-00002] [PMID: 11280955]

[52] Liebeskind DS, Saver JL. Etiology and management of stroke in children. In: Alexander MJ, Spetzler RF, Eds. Pediatric Neurovascular Disease: Surgical, Endovascular, and Medical Management. New York, NY: Thieme 2006; pp. 35-51.

[53] Takeuchi K, Shimizu K. Hypoplasia of the bilateral internal carotid arteries. Brain Nerve (Tokyo) 1957; 9: 37-43.

[54] Suzuki J, Takaku A. Cerebrovascular "moyamoya" disease. Disease showing abnormal net-like vessels in base of brain. Arch Neurol 1969; 20(3): 288-99. [http://dx.doi.org/10.1001/archneur.1969.00480090076012] [PMID: 5775283]

[55] Ueki K, Meyer FB, Mellinger JF. Moyamoya disease: the disorder and surgical treatment. Mayo Clin Proc 1994; 69(8): 749-57. [http://dx.doi.org/10.1016/S0025-6196(12)61094-5] [PMID: 8035631]

[56] Fukushima Y, Kondo Y, Kuroki Y, *et al.* Are Down syndrome patients predisposed to Moyamoya disease? Eur J Pediatr 1986; 144(5): 516-7. [http://dx.doi.org/10.1007/BF00441756] [PMID: 2937636]

[57] Kainth DS, Chaudhry SA, Kainth HS, Suri FK, Qureshi AI. Prevalence and characteristics of concurrent down syndrome in patients with moyamoya disease. Neurosurgery 2013; 72(2): 210-5. [http://dx.doi.org/10.1227/NEU.0b013e31827b9beb] [PMID: 23149966]

[58] Nishimoto A, Ueta K, Onbe H. Cooperative study on moyamoya disease in Japan. In: Abstracts of the

10th Meeting on Surgery for Stroke.; 1981; Tokyo, Japan: Nyuuronsha. 53-8.

[59] Fukuyama Y, Osawa M, Kanai N. Moyamoya disease (syndrome) and the Down syndrome. Brain Dev 1992; 14(4): 254-6. [http://dx.doi.org/10.1016/S0387-7604(12)80242-7] [PMID: 1443408]

[60] Dai AI, Shaikh ZA, Cohen ME. Early-onset Moyamoya syndrome in a patient with Down syndrome: case report and review of the literature. J Child Neurol 2000; 15(10): 696-9. [http://dx.doi.org/10.1177/088307380001501012] [PMID: 11063086]

[61] Pysden K, Fallon P, Moorthy B, Ganesan V. Presumed perinatal stroke in a child with Down syndrome and moyamoya disease. Dev Med Child Neurol 2010; 52(2): 212-4. [http://dx.doi.org/10.1111/j.1469-8749.2009.03377.x] [PMID: 19583743]

[62] Takasugi H, Maemoto T, Kitazawa K, Honda A. [A case of Down syndrome with moyamoya syndrome presenting extensive multiple cerebral infarction during measles infection]. No To Hattatsu 2000; 32(1): 39-43. [PMID: 10655750]

[63] Mito T, Becker LE. Vascular dysplasia in Down syndrome: a possible relationship to moyamoya disease. Brain Dev 1992; 14(4): 248-51. [http://dx.doi.org/10.1016/S0387-7604(12)80239-7] [PMID: 1443405]

[64] Pavone P, Falsaperla R, De Silva K, *et al.* Down syndrome and arterial ischemic stroke in childhood: a potential immunologic link with selective IgG4 subclass deficiency. Eur J Paediatr Neurol 2014; 18(4): 520-5. [http://dx.doi.org/10.1016/j.ejpn.2014.02.004] [PMID: 24613243]

[65] Morino M, Yamano H, Sasaki N. Role of varicella virus and anticardiolipin antibodies in the development of stroke in a patient with Down syndrome associated with Moyamoya syndrome. Pediatr Int 2009; 51(2): 300-2. [http://dx.doi.org/10.1111/j.1442-200X.2009.02805.x] [PMID: 19379264]

[66] Gururaj A, Hardy D, Al-Gazali LI, Sztriha L, Roos A, Nork M. Are the strokes in moyamoya syndrome associated with Down syndrome due to protein C deficiency? Brain Dev 2002; 24(7): 719-22. [http://dx.doi.org/10.1016/S0387-7604(02)00075-X] [PMID: 12427521]

[67] Gatenby P, Tucko R, Andrews C, O'Neil R. Antiphospholipid antibodies and stroke in Down syndrome. Lupus 2003; 12(1): 58-62. [http://dx.doi.org/10.1191/0961203303lu240cr] [PMID: 12587828]

[68] Stöllberger C, Weiss S, Zlabinger G, Finsterer J. Cryptogenic embolic stroke in a girl with a trisomy 21 mosaic. Acta Neurol Belg 2012; 112(2): 203-4. [http://dx.doi.org/10.1007/s13760-012-0010-8] [PMID: 22426657]

[69] Tarlaci S, Sagduyu A. Cerebral venous thrombosis in Down's syndrome. Clin Neurol Neurosurg 2001; 103(4): 242-4. [http://dx.doi.org/10.1016/S0303-8467(01)00147-0] [PMID: 11714571]

[70] Garzón Ruiz J, Fajardo-Picó E, Aguilar-García J, Ruiz-Guerrero C, Miranda Matilla RM, Iribarren-Marín MA. Discussion and review of the literature following the case of a young man with Down's

syndrome and cerebral venous thrombosis. Rev Med Int Sindr Down 2011; 15(3): 37-40. [http://dx.doi.org/10.1016/S2171-9748(11)70013-7]

[71] Kim JD, Crockett C, Diaz O, Lee AG, Miller NR. Down but not out. Surv Ophthalmol 2013; 58(6): 644-51. [http://dx.doi.org/10.1016/j.survophthal.2012.10.005] [PMID: 23453400]

[72] Spitzer R, Rabinowitch JY, Wybar KC. A study of the abnormalities of the skull, teeth and lenses in Mongolism. Can Med Assoc J 1961; 18;84(11): 567-72. [PMID: 20326668]

[73] Selby KA, Newton RW, Gupta S, Hunt L. Clinical predictors and radiological reliability in atlantoaxial subluxation in Down's syndrome. Arch Dis Child 1991; 66(7): 876-8. [http://dx.doi.org/10.1136/adc.66.7.876] [PMID: 1830735]

[74] American Academy of Pediatrics Committee on Sports Medicine and Fitness. Atlantoaxial instability in Down syndrome: subject review. Pediatrics 1995; 96(1 Pt 1): 151-4. [PMID: 7596705]

[75] Tishler J, Martel W. Dislocation of the atlas in Mongolism: preliminary report. Radiology 1965; 84: 904-6. [http://dx.doi.org/10.1148/84.5.904] [PMID: 14282702]

[76] Sherk HH, Nicholson JT. Rotatory atlanto-axial dislocation associated with ossiculum terminale and mongolism. A case report. J Bone Joint Surg Am 1969; 51(5): 957-64. [PMID: 4240092]

[77] Roy M, Baxter M, Roy A. Atlantoaxial instability in Down syndrome--guidelines for screening and detection. J R Soc Med 1990; 83(7): 433-5. [PMID: 2144323]

[78] Pueschel SM, Scola FH. Atlantoaxial instability in individuals with Down syndrome: epidemiologic, radiographic, and clinical studies. Pediatrics 1987; 80(4): 555-60. [PMID: 2958770]

[79] Ferguson RL, Putney ME, Allen BL Jr. Comparison of neurologic deficits with atlanto-dens intervals in patients with Down syndrome. J Spinal Disord 1997; 10(3): 246-52. [http://dx.doi.org/10.1097/00002517-199706000-00011] [PMID: 9213282]

[80] Romano A, Albertini G, Guida D, *et al.* Cervical Flexion-Extension MRI Study in Down Syndrome. Indian J Pediatr 2014; 2 [http://dx.doi.org/10.1007/s12098-014-1549-6] [PMID: 25175489]

[81] Nakamura N, Inaba Y, Oba M, *et al.* Novel Two Radiographic Measurements for Atlantoaxial Instability in Down Syndrome Children. Spine (Phila Pa 1976) 2014 Sep 29.; [PMID: 25271511]

[82] Merrick J, Ezra E, Josef B, Hendel D, Steinberg DM, Wientroub S. Musculoskeletal problems in Down Syndrome European Paediatric Orthopaedic Society Survey: the Israeli sample. J Pediatr Orthop B 2000; 9(3): 185-92. [http://dx.doi.org/10.1097/01202412-200006000-00008] [PMID: 10904905]

[83] Hwang SW, Jea A. A review of the neurological and neurosurgical implications of Down syndrome in

children. Clin Pediatr (Phila) 2013; 52(9): 845-56.
[http://dx.doi.org/10.1177/0009922813491311] [PMID: 23743011]

[84] Parfenchuck TA, Bertrand SL, Powers MJ, Drvaric DM, Pueschel SM, Roberts JM. Posterior occipitoatlantal hypermobility in Down syndrome: an analysis of 199 patients. J Pediatr Orthop 1994; 14(3): 304-8.
[http://dx.doi.org/10.1097/01241398-199405000-00006] [PMID: 8006159]

[85] Bosma GP, van Buchem MA, Voormolen JH, van Biezen FC, Brouwer OF. Cervical spondylarthrotic myelopathy with early onset in Down's syndrome: five cases and a review of the literature. J Intellect Disabil Res 1999; 43(Pt 4): 283-8.
[http://dx.doi.org/10.1046/j.1365-2788.1999.00212.x] [PMID: 10466866]

[86] Ashworth A, Hill CM, Karmiloff-Smith A, Dimitriou D. The Importance of Sleep: Attentional Problems in School-Aged Children With Down Syndrome and Williams Syndrome. Behav Sleep Med 2014; 15: 1-17.
[http://dx.doi.org/10.1080/15402002.2014.940107] [PMID: 25127421]

[87] Arya R, Kabra M, Gulati S. Epilepsy in children with Down syndrome. Epileptic Disord 2011; 13(1): 1-7.
[http://dx.doi.org/10.1684/epd.2011.0415] [PMID: 21398208]

[88] Lujić L, Bosnjak VM, Delin S, Duranović V, Krakar G. Infantile spasms in children with Down syndrome. Coll Antropol 2011; 35 (Suppl. 1): 213-8.
[PMID: 21648336]

[89] Pueschel SM, Louis S, McKnight P. Seizure disorders in Down syndrome. Arch Neurol 1991; 48(3): 318-20.
[http://dx.doi.org/10.1001/archneur.1991.00530150088024] [PMID: 1825777]

[90] Verrotti A, Cusmai R, Nicita F, *et al.* Electroclinical features and long-term outcome of cryptogenic epilepsy in children with Down syndrome. J Pediatr 2013; 163(6): 1754-8.
[http://dx.doi.org/10.1016/j.jpeds.2013.07.022] [PMID: 23992680]

[91] Ferlazzo E, Adjien CK, Guerrini R, *et al.* Lennox-Gastaut syndrome with late-onset and prominent reflex seizures in trisomy 21 patients. Epilepsia 2009; 50(6): 1587-95.
[http://dx.doi.org/10.1111/j.1528-1167.2008.01944.x] [PMID: 19187280]

[92] Smigielska-Kuzia J, Sobaniec W, Kułak W, Boćkowski L. Clinical and EEG features of epilepsy in children and adolescents in Down syndrome. J Child Neurol 2009; 24(4): 416-20.
[http://dx.doi.org/10.1177/0883073808324542] [PMID: 19339285]

[93] Vignoli A, Zambrelli E, Chiesa V, *et al.* Epilepsy in adult patients with Down syndrome: a clinical-video EEG study. Epileptic Disord 2011; 13(2): 125-32.
[http://dx.doi.org/10.1684/epd.2011.0426] [PMID: 21561839]

[94] Menéndez M. Down syndrome, Alzheimer's disease and seizures. Brain Dev 2005; 27(4): 246-52.
[http://dx.doi.org/10.1016/j.braindev.2004.07.008] [PMID: 15862185]

[95] De Simone R, Puig XS, Gélisse P, Crespel A, Genton P. Senile myoclonic epilepsy: delineation of a common condition associated with Alzheimer's disease in Down syndrome. Seizure 2010; 19(7): 383-9.

[http://dx.doi.org/10.1016/j.seizure.2010.04.008] [PMID: 20598585]

[96] Siniscalchi A, Gallelli L, Loizzo S, Tiziana A, Russo E, De Sarro G. Sodium valproate induced tremor in a patient with epilepsy and Down's syndrome Curr Drug Saf 2013yes;; 8(1): 69-71. [http://dx.doi.org/10.2174/15748863113080100010] [PMID: 23656451]

[97] Dekker AD, De Deyn PP, Rots MG. Epigenetics: the neglected key to minimize learning and memory deficits in Down syndrome. Neurosci Biobehav Rev 2014; 45: 72-84. [http://dx.doi.org/10.1016/j.neubiorev.2014.05.004] [PMID: 24858130]

[98] Inokuchi R, Nakamura K, Mizuno N, *et al.* Adult-onset seizures in a patient with Down syndrome and portosystemic shunt. Brain Dev 2014; 36(7): 626-9. [http://dx.doi.org/10.1016/j.braindev.2013.08.007] [PMID: 24035599]

[99] Palisano RJ, Walter SD, Russell DJ, *et al.* Gross motor function of children with down syndrome: creation of motor growth curves. Arch Phys Med Rehabil 2001; 82(4): 494-500. [http://dx.doi.org/10.1053/apmr.2001.21956] [PMID: 11295010]

[100] Pereira K, Basso RP, Lindquist AR, da Silva LG, Tudella E. Infants with Down syndrome: percentage and age for acquisition of gross motor skills. Res Dev Disabil 2013; 34(3): 894-901. [http://dx.doi.org/10.1016/j.ridd.2012.11.021] [PMID: 23291506]

[101] Faulks D, Collado V, Mazille MN, Veyrune JL, Hennequin M. Masticatory dysfunction in persons with Down's syndrome. Part 1: aetiology and incidence. J Oral Rehabil 2008; 35(11): 854-62. [http://dx.doi.org/10.1111/j.1365-2842.2008.01877.x] [PMID: 18702629]

[102] Rigoldi C, Galli M, Mainardi L, Crivellini M, Albertini G. Postural control in children, teenagers and adults with Down syndrome. Res Dev Disabil 2011; 32(1): 170-5. [http://dx.doi.org/10.1016/j.ridd.2010.09.007] [PMID: 20933364]

[103] Jover M, Ayoun C, Berton C, Carlier M. Specific grasp characteristics of children with trisomy 21. Dev Psychobiol 2010; 52(8): 782-93. [http://dx.doi.org/10.1002/dev.20474] [PMID: 20564329]

[104] Latash ML, Kang N, Patterson D. Finger coordination in persons with Down syndrome: atypical patterns of coordination and the effects of practice. Exp Brain Res 2002; 146(3): 345-55. [http://dx.doi.org/10.1007/s00221-002-1189-3] [PMID: 12232691]

[105] Galli M, Cimolin V, Patti P, *et al.* Quantifying established clinical assessment measures using 3D-movement analysis in individuals with Down syndrome. Disabil Rehabil 2010; 32(21): 1768-74. [http://dx.doi.org/10.3109/09638281003734367] [PMID: 20353361]

[106] Shumway-Cook A, Woollacott MH. Dynamics of postural control in the child with Down syndrome. Phys Ther 1985; 65(9): 1315-22. [PMID: 3162178]

[107] Agiovlasitis S, McCubbin JA, Yun J, Pavol MJ, Widrick JJ. Economy and preferred speed of walking in adults with and without Down syndrome. Adapt Phys Activ Q 2009; 26(2): 118-30. [PMID: 19478345]

[108] Hawli Y, Nasrallah M, El-Hajj Fuleihan G. Endocrine and musculoskeletal abnormalities in patients with Down syndrome. Nat Rev Endocrinol 2009; 5(6): 327-34. [http://dx.doi.org/10.1038/nrendo.2009.80] [PMID: 19421241]

[109] Gonzalez-Aguero A, Vicente-Rodriguez G, Moreno LA, Guerra-Balic M, Ara I, Casajus JA. Health related physical fitness in Scand J. Med Sci Sports 2010; 20(5): 716-24. [http://dx.doi.org/10.1111/j.1600-0838.2010.01120.x]

[110] Guidi S, Ciani E, Bonasoni P, Santini D, Bartesaghi R. Widespread proliferation impairment and hypocellularity in the cerebellum of fetuses with down syndrome. Brain Pathol 2011; 21(4): 361-73. [http://dx.doi.org/10.1111/j.1750-3639.2010.00459.x] [PMID: 21040072]

[111] Schmahmann JD. Disorders of the cerebellum: ataxia, dysmetria of thought, and the cerebellar cognitive affective syndrome. J Neuropsychiatry Clin Neurosci 2004; 16(3): 367-78. [http://dx.doi.org/10.1176/jnp.16.3.367] [PMID: 15377747]

[112] Teipel SJ, Alexander GE, Schapiro MB, Moller HJ, Rapoport SI, Hampel H. Age-related cortical grey matter reductions in non-demented Down's syndrome adults determined by MRI with voxel-based morphometry. Brain 2004; 127(Pt 4): 811-24.. [http://dx.doi.org/10.1093/brain/awh101] [PMID: 14985261]

[113] Roth GM, Sun B, Greensite FS, Lott IT, Dietrich RB. Premature aging in persons with Down syndrome: MR findings. AJNR Am J Neuroradiol 1996; 17(7): 1283-9. [PMID: 8871713]

[114] Nakamura E, Tanaka S. Biological ages of adult men and women with Down's syndrome and its changes with aging. Mech Ageing Dev 1998; 15(105): 1-2. [http://dx.doi.org/10.1016/S0047-6374] [PMID: 9922121]

[115] Overend TJ, Cunningham DA, Kramer JF, Lefcoe MS, Paterson DH. Knee extensor and knee flexor strength: cross-sectional area ratios in young and elderly men. J Gerontol 1992; 47(6): M204-10. [http://dx.doi.org/10.1093/geronj/47.6.M204] [PMID: 1430855]

[116] Angelopoulou N, Matziari C, Tsimaras V, Sakadamis A, Souftas V, Mandroukas K. Bone mineral density and muscle strength in young men with mental retardation (with and without Down syndrome). Calcif Tissue Int 2000; 66(3): 176-80. [http://dx.doi.org/10.1007/s002230010035] [PMID: 10666490]

[117] Phillips AC, Sleigh A, McAllister CJ, *et al.* Defective mitochondrial function *in vivo* in skeletal muscle in adults with Down's syndrome: a 31P-MRS study. PLoS One 2013; 8(12): e84031.. [http://dx.doi.org/10.1371/journal.pone.0084031.] [PMID: 24391872]

[118] Dey A, Bhowmik K, Chatterjee A, Chakrabarty PB, Sinha S, Mukhopadhyay K. Down Syndrome Related Muscle Hypotonia: Association with COL6A3 Functional SNP rs2270669. Front Genet 2013; 22;4(57) [http://dx.doi.org/10.3389/fgene.2013.00057.] [PMID: 23626599.]

[119] Cowley PM, Keslacy S, Middleton FA, *et al.* Functional and biochemical characterization of soleus muscle in Down syndrome mice: insight into the muscle dysfunction seen in the human condition. Am J Physiol Regul Integr Comp Physiol 2012; 15;303(12): R1251-60. [http://dx.doi.org/10.1152/ajpregu.00312.2012] [PMID: 23115123]

[120] Cisterna B, Costanzo M, Scherini E, Zancanaro C, Malatesta M. Ultrastructural features of skeletal muscle in adult and aging Ts65Dn mice, a murine model of Down syndrome. Muscles Ligaments Tendons J 2014; 24;3(4): 287-94.

[PMID: 24596692.]

[121] Eid MA. Effect of Whole-Body Vibration Training on Standing Balance and Muscle Strength in Children with Down Syndrome. Am J Phys Med Rehabil 2014; 8 [http://dx.doi.org/10.1097/PHM.0000000000000224] [PMID: 25299536]

CHAPTER 10

Psychological Change in Down Syndrome Children and Adolescents

Mohammed Al-Biltagi[1,*], Fu Yong Jiao[2], Vivian Song[3], Feilan Lv[3], April Wang[3], Guoyan Lee[3]

[1] *Pediatric Department, Faculty of Medicine, Tanta University, Egypt*

[2] *Shaanxi Provincial People's Hospital, China*

[3] *Pediatric Department, Shaanxi Provincial People's Hospital, China*

Abstract: Children and adolescents with DS are exposed to significant physical, sexual and emotional developmental changes. They also often have some psychiatric problems as externalizing disorders, depression, anxiety and/or obsessive-compulsive disorder.

They also suffer from behavior and psychosocial problems in the process of their growth, such as expressing their feelings, learning problems as their shortage of language and cognition. Children with DS are amenable for good education and they can enter a special education school for special education, so that training of their fine motor, gross motor and intellectual abilities is helpful to improve their development.

They can be encouraged to improve body functions and accentuating gaining more functional proficiencies that facilitate improving participation in age-suitable activities. Early detection and proper treatment of emotional, psychiatric or developmental disorders ensure good prognosis.

Keywords: Abuse, Academic achievements, Anxiety, Articulation, Behavioral, Children, Communication, Depression, Developmental, Down syndrome, Education, Early Stimulation Emotional, Grammar, Mental, Obsessive-compulsive disorder, Phenotypes, Psychological, Sexual, Speech, Talking.

* **Corresponding Author Dr. Mohammed Al-Biltagi:** Pediatric Department, Faculty of Medicine, Tanta University, Egypt; Tel: (+973)39545472; Fax: (+973) 1759 0495; Email: mbelrem@hotmail.com

Mohammed Al-Biltagi (Ed)

1. INTRODUCTION

In general, adolescence stage is defined by quick change from dependence to independence. They start to feel their need for being somewhat free in travelling; running money, choosing friends and freedom interests, looking out their personal daily needs. They start to prepare themselves to leave the family home by 18 years of age. This period shows also significant physical, sexual and emotional developmental changes. The same changes are also observed in children and adolescents with Down syndrome (DS); when they show considerable growth in all era of development during their adolescence and into early adult life. They behave in an essentially similar way to other teenagers and should be recognized as such. They keep on developing their fundamental abilities and experiences in speech, language, literacy and numeracy and teaching process. They commonly demonstrate psychiatric problems as externalizing disorders, depression, anxiety and obsessive-compulsive disorder. They suffer also from behavior and psychosocial problems in the process of their growth, such as expressing their feelings, learning problems as their shortage of language and cognition. These issues are reflected on the concepts of academic achievement, psychosocial stress emotional challenges, behavioral disorders, communication disorders and development of autism. All problems above will be aggravated by negative behaviors and emotion of parents or others and also evoked by some strange things such as moving house. Understanding social development in this category of children will help to develop effective interventions and teaching strategies [1].

2. MENTAL DEVELOPMENT

Down syndrome is the main genetic reason of mental retardation and patients with DS demonstrate marked psychopathologic changes (18-23%). Over expression of genes present on chromosome 21 induces change in biological stability state in the DS brain to a new less functional condition causing variable degrees of mental retardation. The expression variability caused by this gene-dosage imbalance may initially stimulate brain functional variability at cellular level, as primary phenotypes, and lastly stimulate neuromorphological changes and cognitive deficits as resultant phenotypes. Identification of over expressed trisomic genes in the brain and their function, their over expression-induced effects on regulation of neurological development, their downstream effects, their interaction with other proteins, and their role in regulatory and metabolic pathways is providing us with a clearer vision about the origin of the mental retardation (MR) in DS. Children with DS have a delayed and sub mental development (Oligophrenia) as a cardinal sign of the syndrome with a variable degree of mental retardation from mild to profound. Their Intelligence Quotient (IQ) is usually between 25 and 50 with more gaps between them and their peers and their IQ will go lower with advancing age. This difference in IQ level is mainly due to heterogeneity of phenotyping. The low IQ observed in DS is recognized by delay in development, impaired language skills, deficits in memory and other cognitive function abnormalities. Individuals with mosaic forms of DS have been found to score 10–30 points higher on IQ measures than those with trisomy 21, and have demonstrated normal visual perceptual skills. Language development is often delayed or impaired in people with DS; they understand more than they can verbalize [2]. They also show a decrease of cognitive functions related to ageing and is characterized by declining in memory, language and other cognitive functions. The linguistic development in DS progresses differently along unique developmental trajectories. Thus, for example, morphosyntax defects, especially in production, is more obvious in adolescence than in early childhood and lexicon is usually better conserved in all ages (at least in comprehension) [3, 4].

They are usually able to sit after one full year of life, and sometimes walking will be delayed till the age of 3 years. Children with higher IQ can learn to read and to do simple manual work while children with lower IQ will have more difficulty in language and self-reliance. However, training can improve their abilities to do more work regardless of their sub-mental abilities. This sub mental development observed in DS is related to occurrence of errors in neurodevelopment during fetal stage of the central nervous system (CNS) development. There is reduction in the total number of neurons throughout several cortical areas, abnormalities within the neurons themselves, and abnormalities in the ability of the neurons to communicate with each other with reduction in the neuronal density in cortical areas and decreased dendritic arborization. The cerebral cortex is the most affected area of the brain. Reduction in the number of neurons, existence of dendritic spines, and poor synaptic connections contribute to difficulties in cognitive and learning processes (*e.g.* attention, information processing, integration, short- and long-term memory, and language skills) [5].

There is decrease in brain weight and volume, with reduction in cerebellum, brain stem structures, hippocampus, frontal and temporal lobes size, and atypical cortical surface features, including the superior temporal gyrus in subjects with DS [6]. MRI studies showed decreased cerebellar gray and white tissue volumes, decreased white matter in the superior temporal sulcus, but increased temporal lobe white matter. There is also an enlargement in parahippocampal volume and quite conserved lenticular nuclei, basal ganglia, and occipital lobe volumes [7]. The existence of these anomalies from an early age implies that fetal or early postnatal developmental variations may trigger this noted model of neuroanatomic anomalies and perhaps may induce the unique cognitive and developmental defects seen in patients with DS [8]. Functional MRI showed higher regional connectivity in a ventral brain system involving the amygdala/anterior temporal region and the ventral aspect of both the anterior cingulate and frontal cortices. It showed also lower functional connectivity identified in dorsal executive networks involving dorsal prefrontal and anterior cingulate cortices and posterior insula. There is also under development of connectivity in DS with reduced capability to integrate and assimilate information from distant brain regions into coherent disseminated networks [9]. This distinctive functional organization with system-specific anomalies is associated with reduced adaptive efficiency and can be used as a marker of the brain functional anomaly [10].

3. BEHAVIOR PHENOTYPES IN DOWN'S SYNDROME

Children with DS -especially teenagers- have more behavior problems than non syndromic children, in particular attention deficit, noncompliance, thought disorder, and social withdrawal. However when compared with the majority of children with other intellectual disabilities; children with DS are at lesser risk for major psychopathology. There is variability in behavioral phenotypes in individuals with DS. This variability result from the interaction of different factors including over expression of interacting gene alleles and environmental factors as health, educational, and housing conditions of persons with DS. The genetic factor is related to differential over expression of the interacting gene alleles in various tissues at diverse times, and restrained by differences in alleles on other chromosomes, instead of with a single, malfunctioning gene. Inconsistency in expression during fetal development may influence the developing brain structure, or affect vital times of brain development, to create selectively declined cognitive functioning. The following action of such genes may influence other features of physiological and behavioral function [11].

There are two main behavioral phenotypes of DS "primary" and "secondary" phenotypes. The primary phenotype results from genetic and biological effects related to trisomy 21 and are straightforwardly connected to basic characteristics of the syndrome that occur directly from the atypically emerging physiology and neurodevelopment associated with trisomy 21. Examples of primary phenotypes are verbal processing deficits (which are related to uncharacteristic brain development and a lesser planum temporal) and motor and articulatory deficits in expressive language (which are connected to structural variations in the development of the oral cavity). The secondary Phenotypes are features that result indirectly from interfacing between two or more primary phenotypic features. For example; gestures advantage in children with DS which one of the important methods of communication results indirectly from interaction of visual processing strengths (due to sparing of occipital and temporal gray matter) and social associated strengths in early development in the population [12].

Some of DS behavioral phenotypes are already developing in infants and toddlers, including developing comparative potencies in some aspects of visual processing, receptive language and nonverbal social functioning, and comparative limitations in gross motor skills and expressive language skills [8]. Infant and children with DS have a major tardiness in nonverbal cognitive development associated with additional, certain deficits in speech, language production, and auditory short-term memory, but less adaptive behavior disorders than persons with other cognitive disabilities [11]. Pre-school children with DS are found to have good-imitato--poor-talker profile However, only the superior bodily imitation capability looks to be syndrome-specific. The percent of children with DS who develop expressive language weaknesses increases as they grow up, getting older and as their mental ages (MAs) is increasing. Expressive defects also became more frequent as children grow and increase in mental ages. They also have a decline in their speed of social development with increasing chronological age [13].

However, some children with DS may have comparative steadiness in the speed at which they gain adaptive and cognitive skills. This deceleration of development may be caused by slow speed of brain myelination during this developmental period [14]. Presence of certain adaptive profiles, variations based on level of development, and flat rates during the early and middle childhood years in children with DS may finally induce development of more specific training programs to improve the adaptive skills - a goal of special importance in view of the role that adaptive behavior participates in the long-standing modification and success of individuals with mental retardation including DS [15].

Adolescents with DS have a higher problem behavior score than adolescents without DS. In one survey; about 51% of adolescents with DS have problem scores in the clinical or borderline range on 1 or more Child Behavior Checklist subscales; which is more than twice as high as adolescents without DS. They have nearly twice time more internalizing behavior problems than their counterparts without DS. The highest problem scores in adolescents with DS were observed on the social problems and thought problems subscales. Being a male and having more severe mental disabilities are two important factors associated with more behavioral problems [16]. Elder DS adolescents may have reduced externalizing features and subtle raises in withdrawal [17]. Externalizing behaviors (dominant, opposing/refusing, impulsiveness, inattention and increased motor activity) are markedly more frequent in the 5-10 years age group, while internalizing behaviors (shy/insecure, low self confidence, decreased motor activity) are more widespread in adolescents and adults (10-30 years) [18].

Disruptive behavior disorders such as attention-deficit/hyperactivity disorder, conduct disorder, oppositional defiant disorder, and aggressive behavior are responsible for the majority of the behavior disorders in DS persons under 20 years of age. On the other hand, aggressive behavior, major depressive disorder, and stereotypic behavior are the most frequent abnormal behavior encountered in DS cases over the age of 20 [3]. Autism is another psychiatric disorder that may be comorbid with DS. Autism is 10 times more prevalent in DS children than in the general population, but diagnosis of associated autism in DS with marked intellectual disability is a real challenge. DS children with comorbid autism have considerably diminished brain functions than non-autistic DS children. However, the defects in the main era of social reciprocity and communication, and the limited and repetitive interests are not entirely clarified by the more severe cognitive impairment. This autism phenotype in DS children which involves a raised risk for seizures may signify an extensive loss of functional connectivity in the brain [19]. The autistic phenotype in DS is manifested by a distinctive pattern of stereotypies, anxiety and social withdrawal. However, there may be an overlap of autism and obsessive compulsive behavior. Diagnosis of autism in DS is difficult, an important bias resulting from the existence of strong stereotypes as regards the perceived behavior of subjects with DS. Although children with DS tend to be considered sociable, good humored and friendly; they are also perceived as stubborn, resistant to change, and showing obsessive personality traits. As a result, parents are more likely to under-report social deficit items, whereas professionals tend to attribute pervasive behaviors to the chromosomal abnormality and to intellectual disability (ID), rather than to co morbidity with autism [20]. Co morbidity of autistic manifestations in DS hindered their gaining of adaptive skills more frequently than did the presence of DS alone [21].

4. ACADEMIC ACHIEVEMENTS OF YOUNG PEOPLE WITH DOWN SYNDROME

Despite being suffering from delay in mental development and physical development, children with DS often have the ability to have good education and training. The misperception that school-age children with DS always function at the trainable (non-educable) level at the time they enter kindergarten, or will assuredly function at the trainable level later in their schooling, continues to restrict their educational opportunities. There is clear evidence that an acceptable level of educable performance can be achieved [22].

Children with DS have increased rate of hearing loss, impaired auditory processing and auditory skills. They frequently have considerable speech and language delay so they have to depend on non-verbal skills such as gesture. However, they have a good visual processing and adequate auditory memory skills which can be used to improve their learning abilities. Children with DS syndrome usually have relatively good communication skills and are devoted to interact and cooperate socially exactly from infancy. They can comprehend more than they can speak, and their verbal language is not obvious. They have unique trouble with learning grammar and with developing obvious language [23].

4.1. Factors Affecting Academic Achievements in Down Syndrome

There are different factors that control the educational achievement in children with DS. These factors include the chronological age of the child at the time of the school entry, the child mental age, the gender, the attendance at mainstream school, the degree of the child attentiveness, the mother's actual coping pattern, and the father's internal position of control. The children's mental age score is most powerfully correlated with the educational achievements scores [24]. The lower chronological age at the child entry to the school and the attendance at mainstream school are associated with greater progress of the child academic achievements. Attendance to mainstream school has a moderate useful outcome on academic attainments index throughout the school skills in the children, separately from level of degree of intellectual impairment. The achievements of teenagers with DS educated in mainstream classrooms showed more continuous improvement and progress in communication skills and have less behavioral difficulties than those attended special education classrooms [25]. The higher the mental age of the child and the higher the mother's actual coping pattern; the higher is the child attention abilities and hence the child academic achievements. The father's internal position of control is another important factor for the child academic attainments. Proper home literacy environments provided by the parents markedly help children with DS to achieve some advanced literacy talents than what is predicted for their mental age, emphasizing the significance of early reading enhancement and encouragement for this population [26]. Motivation has an important implication for subsequent education competence, despite being difficult in children with DS. However, early mastery encouragement is important for the afterward attainment and has significant effects for the focus of early interventions. Perseverance in early childhood is correlated with the academic skills in adolescence, even when the effects of cognitive capability at the younger age are controlled [27]. Recreational orientation and informal play contacts with other children both improve significantly the child's school social life and hence his academic achievements [28]. Females show more favorable course than males with DS as regard to their educational achievement. However, the degree of intellectual deterioration is undoubtedly the most important predictor of satisfactory academic achievements. Proper education of children with DS can promote their learning, help them to achieve better state, and in some ways they can do it as good as their peers, at the same time, we should care about their psychological development, they like all people need to be loved, and needs to be respected [29].

Providing an environment with maximum support is clearly vital for proper cognitive development of DS children. The number of DS children who are taught in ordinary school is continuing to increase over the last 20 years. Every DS child is unique and has his own potentiality and unique learning requirements. It is vital to set up the support for the learning mechanism to evade the various learning difficulties and to help them in maximizing their developmental capabilities. It is essential to supply them with proper support to evade failure, predominantly during the early stages of learning. It is also advised that the DS child joins a mainstream classroom and contribute, with the proper support, in the whole class on a more ordinary basis. By this way; DS children will have less improper behavior in the whole class setting in comparison to individual and group settings [30].

4.2. Items of Academic Achievements in Down Syndrome

All the items of academic achievement are affected in a variable degree in children with DS. This variability is related to some extent to the areas of relative strengths and weakness of some developmental skills in children with DS *e.g.* as mentioned before developing comparative potencies in some features of visual processing, receptive language and nonverbal social functioning, and comparative limitations in gross motor skills and expressive language skills.

4.2.1. Talking, Speech and Articulation

Once DS children are able to talk, they can have appropriate speech and language skills. They have almost similar assortment of communicative activities like everybody else, especially with proper encouragement and sensitive support from at home, at school and in the community [31]. The majority of DS children usually delay to start talking. However, DS infants may babble normally, but they usually have difficulty to say single words as early or as clearly as their normally developing peers. The usual age for the first spoken word is about 18 months and for the first ten words, the average is about 27 months [23]. Similar to the other kids, DS children usually start to combine two words together when they are able to vocabulary produce about 50 different words. This is usually gained by about 37 months on average. After this primary progression; the rate will be stable but slow and they start to use 3-4 word sentences and to learn the grammatical rules and diverse sentence structures [32]. Considerable tardiness in speech and language skills will influence their development during their elementary school years. DS children are more probable to be understood if they use only two and three word statements, because of the increased chance of producing more clear words enough for them to be recognized [33].

The spoken words of many DS children and teenagers are not constantly simply understood, in particular when they talk with strangers due the poor speech clarity as well as their characteristic telegraphic style. Teenagers often have the ability to read at a higher level than that expected from their general cognitive and language abilities. Those who have not acquired adequate reading success in their primary years may have considerable improvement during their teenage years. Some teenagers will start their secondary school education capable to read and write at a typical 8-9 year level at 11 years of age. This is somewhat a competent level of reading and writing skills and they will be capable to record their work and to write short texts [34].

However, speech production in DS has major impairment in spoken language. These impairments are due to a combination of delayed development and errors not seen in typical development. Delayed (*i.e.* developmental) and disordered (*i.e.* non-developmental) styles are obvious by about 3 years of age, although DS-related disorders possibly become visible earlier, even in infant babbling. Fluency and prosody have marked deterioration. There is also marked limitations of intelligibility [35]. Articulation disorder includes one or a few sound errors, and should be differentiated from dysarthria which results from muscle weakness, and apraxia which results from muscle discoordination. In articulation disorders; the sounds can be substituted, left off, added or changed which make it difficult to be understood by the others. Articulation disorders arise from anatomical variation in the mouth, chronic ear infections or effusion, or other associated health disorders that disrupt speech development. The rate of stuttering and/or cluttering in DS is about 10%-45%, compared with about 1% in the typical children [36].

Phonological mechanism disorder is linked to understanding and the ability to use the regulations of speech production. With growth of children, they start to know how to manage the sounds of speech. They listen to the sounds around them, accumulating them and storing each in their mind. When they start to have their own speech; they rely on the stored sound (s), along with the regulations they learned through listening to mature speech, and start to produce sounds by themselves. Children with phonological mechanism disorder display trouble in categorizing and managing the sounds and in understanding the regulations that control their sound production. The rate of occurrence of phonological mechanism disorders is notably elevated in DS children than non-syndromic children. They demonstrate an elevated rate of occurrence of simpler phonotactic styles than the later acquired complex ones. Some phonological mechanism disorders may be detected only in children with DS [37, 38].

Studies of speech disfluency showed that stuttering and/or cluttering are very common in DS to reach a rate of 10 to 45% [39, 40]. They have impaired productivity in both semantic and phonological tasks, which is understood as a reflection of the inefficient retrieval strategies. They create fewer clusters in phonological task. Reduced productivity in semantic/ phonological fluency is mostly related to abnormal processing [41].

4.2.2. Grammar and Sentence Structures

Learning grammar is a real challenge to children and adolescents with DS. Most of them find more difficulties to learn the grammar of their language than vocabulary. This difficulty could result from their poor ability of auditory processing and auditory memory [42]. Once babies have mastered 50 words (usually at 19 months), they start to combine two words together to intercommunicate using a wide range of meaning. However, they do not maintain the same rate of progress in grammar when their language vocabulary achieves 300 words. Beside their limited comprehension abilities of grammar, they usually have a delay in their grammar production [31]. However, children with a productive vocabulary of 300 words or less have very limited grammatical capabilities. Thus, this vocabulary volume is a critical accumulation essential for proper development of productive grammar [43]. Advancement in sentence production and in complex grammar learning may be impaired by a weakness and rustiness in short-term memory. Children prefer to communicate using keywords rather than complete sentences. Teenagers and adults may still communicate with short, telegraphic sentences. However, certain intervention programs can help them to improve their grammatical abilities [44].

4.2.3. Number Skills for Individuals with Down Syndrome

The numbering and mathematics skills show significant variability among children and adults with DS. While some children DS find number difficult, others may enjoy mathematics. The chronological age, and the receptive grammar ability, the schooling history and the gender are more significantly correlated with numerical ability than vocabulary knowledge in children with DS.

They usually show some delay in their numbering achievements as compared to their peers and only count using rote learning. This delay results from the associated tardiness in language learning, tardiness in development of auditory short term memory and because of their restricted skills in handling or playing with objects. However, they have potencies in their visual learning. Strengthening the children visual learning promotes their learning and can help their progression in stages similar to the normally developing kids, though frequently with additional steps and practice required at each stage.

With focused language teaching, repetition and visual teaching methods, they can learn the language for numbers and mathematics. DS pupil is competent enough to work within the ordinary classroom and contribute, with the proper support, in the whole class 'mental mathematics' session and plenary on a more regular basis [30, 45].

5. PSYCHOSOCIAL PROBLEMS IN CHILDREN AND ADOLESCENTS WITH DS

Patients with DS are more prone for major psychopathologic disorders (18-23%). They also often have psychiatric problems such as externalizing disorders as well as depression, anxiety and obsessive-compulsive disorder. They are more liable to more psychosocial stress, additional family stress and disturbances, emotional challenges, behavioral disorders, and communication disorders. They are also at increased risk to develop autism [3].

5.1. Psychosocial Stress

Adolescents with DS have many challenges facing them, which have the potential to create stress. This stress results from the different mental health issues as they are more liable to different metal disorders as eating disorders, conduct disorders, as well as depression. It also results from their feeling of being dissimilar with non-acceptance by their school peers which could be aggravated by unexpected change or loss in personal relationship. Adolescence also adds more challenges for persons with DS. Due to lower metabolic rate and lower activity levels, there are increased risk of obesity, social isolation and depression. Changes in school from primary to secondary; pending family move, developmental tasks such as identity formation, low self-esteem issues, concerns about the appearance, issues related to dating and sexual relationships, the individual health, school scores, concerns about employment, work and educational plans; and physical changes which happen during puberty including sleep apnea effects, and commencement of pubertal changes and menses, are other stressors. These are the risk factors to trigger symptoms of depression and further impair the quality of life. Sleep apnea has also been related to impaired school achievement [46 - 48].

These emotional challenges often present with added stress and difficult presentation with impairment or even loss of functional talents including speech, toilet control, and sleep. Adult with DS are more prone to behavioral problems, and mood disorders such as depression [49]. It is difficult for children and adolescents with DS to clearly express their feelings of being stressed and to expose their thoughts and feelings through the usual channels because of their intellectual disability. Self-talking is a frequent behavior in young children and has a vital task in the progress of advanced-level thinking and self-directed skills. Self-talking can be adaptive and can help them to appraise their past experiences, create plans, be able to do various experiments with alternatives, convey their feelings that they are not able to express in other ways, and amuse themselves. It can also indicate an underlying pathology. Self-talking can help to detect hidden psychological disorders as anxiety, depression, physical discomfort or other type of illness. Self-talking should be encouraged making it socially acceptable. Different strategies can help to alleviate this stress. Their stresses should be figured out, and listed and then these children should be helped to cope with the stress [50, 51].

5.2. Family Stress

Having children with intellectual disability is stressful for most parents. Mothers of children with DS, find it more difficult to accept that their children have this disorder. Specific behavior problems associated with the behavioral phenotype of DS also influence the level of maternal stress [52]. The cognitive-linguistic and behavioral scenarios noted in early development in DS children may share in the changes in maternal stress levels experienced all over these early years [53].

There are different factors that affect the maternal and the paternal stress level for having a child with DS. The mother response will depend on maternal education level, socio-economical status, presence of marital problems, lack of acceptance of having a child with DS, the children's behavioral difficulties, the child excitability and self-sufficiency, everyday functioning, the children current health status, children's care-giving difficulties, the degree of intellectual disability and the spousal support. The mother stress can be decrease with use of acceptance, religious and optimist coping styles. The father degree of stress is related to the marital relationship, paternal age, and the child's behavior problems. Consequently, it is apparent that the families who have children with DS need social and psychological support to overcome their feelings of hopelessness. Early assessment of these stressors is required to reduce undesirable effects on the child's development and on family life style. Emerging directed and time-sensitive family treatment strategies for families of DS children is important to improve behavior management skills for their child and their own psychological well-being. It is of the utmost importance to emphasize that the family should not neglect their other kids or the other spouse, as preservation of the family integrity is of crucial importance to all, including DS children. Parents should never feel enforced to dedicate all their extra time to their child with DS [54 - 57].

5.3. Emotional Challenges

Although children with DS are well known to be temperamentally "easy" and sociable, they also suffer behavior disorders. Affective development is vital for social and behavioral competency. Emotional experience of children with DS influences their emotional regulation and that their emotional experience/ expression may not be as flat or mild as previously suggested. Children with DS have troubles in interpreting their social and emotional needs, expressing and communicating about their social experiences and emotional feelings, understanding their mental states such as wishes and beliefs in self and others; and, controlling and working on cognitions and emotions in an adaptive way. They have significantly more frustration than their peers and they utilize a restricted range of strategies to deal with frustration [58]. They have unstable emotion in the process of learning difficult things and strict upbringing by parents. They also have significantly poorer emotion-recognition ability than in the typically developing children particularly for fearful expressions due to presence of specific deficits in socio-cognitive functioning as well as their morphological differences in the facial expressions and their biochemical and neurological anomalies [59]. Lack of proper labeling emotions in DS children may hamper their achievement of emotional language referring to their own internal states. However, recent studies showed that children with DS have no significant differences from others at recognizing emotions [60]. They are more sensitive and caring than many of their peers at all ages. Significant life accidents and events such as loss or separation of one of the family members may induce reduction of proper behavior at school or work.

5.4. Behavioral Disorders

Despite that behavior disorders are very frequent in pediatric age (10% of children), but these disorders are more widespread in DS children (about 33% of DS children). These behavior disorders can be severe enough to be identified by a professional or may be subtle and might not be identified, but still result in difficulties for the children and their families. The behavioral disorders noted in DS children are usually similar to those observed in the typically developing children. However, they may occur at older age and persist for somewhat longer time. For example, temper tantrums are characteristically frequent in 2-3 year old children, but for a DS child, they may start at 3-4 years. However, about 6 out of 10 of DS children have no behavior difficulties. At the same time, 12 – 14% comes with major behavioral disorders, but generally, DS children present with less behavior problems than other kid of similar age with a comparable degree of learning difficulty which results from a reason other than DS. They have troubles in controlling impulses as they frequently don't observe the "stop signs" that notify them not to perform in certain ways. They also have problem in communicating with others as they cannot express their feelings and ideas or understand others easily, so they become easily frustrated. Meanwhile, they have troubles relating to other children and adults. Many of them are social and friendly; but frequently, they may not know how to play competently with peers. This can load more stress on the children and induces misbehavior. Children with DS have problems in managing frustration. Many of them have difficulties to relax and feel better when frustrations arise. This can further deteriorate behavior problems as (oppositional behavior). DS Children are usually brilliant at distracting parents or teachers when they are facing a difficult duty [61, 62].

Children with DS may struggle to pay attention. However, this doesn't necessarily mean that they suffer from Attention Deficit-Hyperactivity Disorder (ADHD). Actually; they are at less risk of ADHD than in typical children. However, this struggling may be a result of the child try to communicate something with the others [63]. They may also suffer from obsessive/compulsive behaviors which may appear very simple and clear (The child may always want the same chair) or may occur as a subtle repetitive, appearing as habits like dangling beads or belts when not involved directly in an activity. This kind of behavior is noted more frequently in younger DS children. While the number of compulsive behaviors in DS children is similar to those in typical children with the same mental age, the frequency and severity of the behavior is frequently more. Increased degrees of restlessness and worry may induce the child or adult to behave in a very inflexible style [64, 65].

5.5. Communication Disorders

Children with DS are not able to fully express their whole feelings, emotional challenges, emotional distress, sadness, and irritability, and even their blessing feelings due to difficult communication as a result of speech and language problem due to poor quality and articulation problems. The associated mental retardation combined with perceptual disturbances can cause delays in language development. Children with DS have deficits in the verbal mode and speech intelligibility that are generally compensated by the use of gestures and vocalizations. The verbal unintelligibility does not limit their communicative attempts and the social-interactive language is usually strength for children with DS, since they present high rates of intentional communication with predominance of comments and acknowledgment. The parents and caregivers' motivation concerning the child's communication possibilities is as important as the knowledge of the family social and economic conditions [66, 67].

5.6. Development of Autism

Despite being affectionate, cheerful, friendly, clownish, playful, good-natured, and the special strength in social interaction in DS; more recent study shows that an important minority of DS children also meets up the diagnostic features for an autistic spectrum disorder (ASD). DS Children are a greater risk to have autism relative to the general population, in whom the risk is about 1%. Autism risk in children with DS is 10 times more often than in the general population [68]. Diagnosis of associated autism in DS children with serious intellectual impairment is a true challenge. They have atypical autistic unique profile compared with individuals with idiopathic ASD. This atypical symptomatic profile results from the more significantly impaired brain function observed in DS children with autism than DS children without autism. Children with DS and autistic features are found to have increased volumes of white matter in the cerebellum and in the brainstem, which are significantly associated with a higher frequency of stereotypies. They also have great risk for convulsions that may specify an extensive loss of functional connectivity in the brain [19, 69].

The autistic profile in DS is distinguished by a typical model of stereotypies, anxiety and social withdrawal. They are more liable to have emotional symptoms, conduct problems and hyperactivity. They also have considerably increased incidence of behavioral disorders than children with DS only. An important bias in diagnosing autism in children with DS is resulting from the existence of strong stereotypes as regards the perceived behavior in DS. Although children with DS tend to be considered sociable, good humored and friendly, they are also perceived as stubborn, resistant to change, and showing obsessive personality traits. This results in underreporting of the autistic features by their parents. Early recognition of autism features is essential for proper intervention. However, the atypical pattern of autism features in this group may influence its detection and delay the achievement of proper interventions [20, 70].

5.7. Development of Depression

Depression is one of the most frequently diagnosed psychiatric disorders for persons with mental retardation especially those with DS and often goes unrecognized or untreated. There are different factors that increase the vulnerability of Teens and adults with DS to have depression. Changing the safety of the surrounding environment is an important stressful factor that may trigger depression *e.g.* changes in staff or classmates, moving from school to school; moving away of grandparents, going away to college; unbearable grief and mourning such as losing of a loved one *etc*. Presence of co morbidities such as obstructive sleep apnea syndrome (OSAS) may have a contributing role to this phenomenon. Being more sensitive to situations that are distinctive to their abnormal culture is another causal factor. Isolation and loneliness of DS children and adolescents can be both reasons and results of depression. They are also as at risk to mental diseases [71].

Detection of depression in DS children, teens and young adults is tricky, complex and often delayed or missed. This difficulty results from impaired verbal ability, conceptual thinking, and overall cognitive functioning. Also many of the diagnostic tools used to diagnose depression rely on standard diagnostic criteria developed by the American Psychiatric Association which is based upon the self-report of subjective feelings (such as verbal expressions of sadness or worthlessness); making these tools of limited diagnostic value. Diagnosis may also be complicated by other medical conditions which have symptoms that can mimic depression such as hypothyroidism, and vitamin B12 deficiency. Good prognosis and higher treatment success rate occur with early and proper diagnosis and effective treatment of depression in individuals with DS. Sympathy, family counseling and encouragement, understanding and support from experts concerned in the clinical care of the person with DS can significantly improve treatment success rate [72, 73].

5.8. Physical Abuse

Down syndrome is usually coupled with mild to moderate intellectual impairment. This may make them more susceptible to abuse, harm, and other types of injuries. Children with mental retardation including those with DS are more reliant on their care providers, less concerned with others, and are more probable to withhold any abuse they suffer inside themselves. The child abuse could be physical, emotional or due to neglect. Physical abuse includes physical injury or harm to the child. It may be the outcome of an on purpose trial to hurt the child, but could also a consequence of severe discipline and try to control the child, such as using a belt on a child, or physical penalty that is unsuitable to the child's age, mental or physical status. The perpetrator could be a family member, acquaintances, strangers, institutional personnel, and care givers. A lot of the physically abusive parents and caregivers claim that what they did was just simply a form of discipline and ways to push the children to learn how to behave. Child neglect is a very common form of child abuse where the family fails to supply for a child's fundamental requirements, whether it be satisfactory food, clothing, hygiene, or supervision. Sometimes this type of neglect is difficult to be discovered. Parents' mental problems, shortage of parenting expertise, socioeconomic status, stress, lack of support, and alcohol or drug addiction are significant risk factors for the child abuse [74, 75].

It is difficult to discover child abuse because their mental retardation is affecting their perceptions. They may also not realize when somebody wants to hurt them physically. However, careful observation of any change in the child behavior can detect occurrence of the child abuse. A change in the child behavior is one of the first signs of abuse. Frequently the DS adult or child will imitate the abuse they receive. Abused children with DS often repeat what is said to them. By observing the changes in behavior, aspects of abuse may unhide what would have remained hidden. The abused child may have a feeling of being shocked, disbelief, or denial of the abuse occurred with strong emotions of fear, anger, and confusion, guilt, humiliation and grief. To avoid such forms of abuse, the child should know how to keep away from unsafe circumstances and preserve his or her self-esteem. The child should acquire the proper assertive and self assured behaviors and when and how to identify threats. He/she should learn also to be accompanied by somebody while going out rather than going alone. They also need to learn how to respond to strangers and to recognize and learn rules about giving out personal information such as his or her full name and address. In case of family related abuse, the family should receive support to develop parenting skills and to learn how to control their emotions. Parenting classes, books, and seminars can provide adequate information and training [76 - 78].

6. PSYCHOLOGY OF SEX AND LOVE IN ADOLESCENTS WITH DS

Sexual activity in mentally or physically disabled people has a lot of troubles and insufficiencies, if not with complete rejection, the end result being that young disabled people are frequently relegated to a destiny of loneliness, isolation and abandon. This is even more obvious with mental retardation [79]. Fortunately, there is marked improvement and change in the life of teenagers with DS with increased inclusion into society. They usually mature physically and hormonally the same way as the general population and have normal development in the exercise of their sexuality. They have the same feelings, desires and requirements for emotional and physical nearness and intimacy as their compeers. However, they frequently enface important difficulties in their autonomy and in school. They need careful interventions to make their social interaction the best possible. Their pubertal development is usually normal and they usually are satisfied with their body image with future perspectives of working, finding a partner, and living a normal life of getting married and having children [80]. They have similar emotional changes typical of adolescence found in their compeers, and may be exaggerated by social factors. Any adolescent who lives in the society, goes to school and is exposed to media unavoidably develops the knowledge of sexuality.

Children with DS usually have a prolonged time of dependence on the parents and caregivers to meet up their emotional, social, and physical requirements and needs, including individual care and hygiene. This can delay their own feeling of body possession and to discriminate between the public and private, and the sexual and nonsexual parts of the body. It can be hard for them to realize the various social conditions as regard to the appropriate social, emotional, and physical restrictions, including the difference between public and private time for activities especially sexual activities such as masturbation. This point is very important to be elaborated because it is an important factor particularly for exposing those children and adolescents to sexual activities; partially due to their social loneliness and reliance on adults for assistance and guidance. To prevent sexual abuse in this susceptible age group, the parents should start setting up early privacy behaviors and habits such as closing bathroom doors behind them, going to the toilet on their own instead of going in a group, and dressing with the curtains drawn. It is also important for the parents to help those children and adolescents to develop social skills and to build at the same time safe boundaries and to differentiate between good touch–bad touch concept and when to say firmly "no" to an unaccepted contact or sexual advance. Educating the children about privacy and how to protect themselves can start in nursery school or first grade. Sex education and support for adolescent with DS will help to avoid sexual abuse [81]. Factors that increase the risk of sexual abuse are the degree of the mental disability, loneliness and frustration, multiple living conditions and temporary caregivers, some of whom may be pedophiles. Rape or incest had been documented in one third of mildly mentally disabled persons and one fourth of moderately mentally disabled persons. Loneliness and frustration may enforce anyone to allow any kind of personal attention whether it is negative or positive [82].

About 50% of DS women are fertile and capable to be pregnant with 35 - 50% of the off spring having the possibility to born with DS or other developmental disabilities. Also; there are some reported cases of fertility in men with DS; but it is not known if their offspring are more likely to have DS or not. This chance of being able to be pregnant elaborates the needs to use contraception. Any means of contraception can be used without additional medical risk. However, the ideal method depends on the personal preference, the capability to use the contraceptive efficiently and the possible adverse effects. Many scientists prefer tubal ligation that can be done without additional risk for DS women who have stable medical status. Contraception must constantly be used, except if a couple takes a decision for parenthood. Over half the care-givers may prefer to go thought that sterilization. However, DS woman should be included as much as possible in decision-making [83, 84].

7. DIAGNOSIS AND ASSESSMENT OF PSYCHOSOCIAL AND DEVELOPMENTAL PROBLEMS IN ADOLESCENTS WITH DS

Proper and comprehensive diagnosis and assessment of psychological and developmental problems in children and adolescents with DS need multi-disciplinary approach that help to define and illustrate troubles that can guide to reach the most suitable intervention service for the child and family. A precise evaluation of cognitive functioning is vital for adequate outcome and intervention planning. The pediatrician should suspect, screen, and is able to detect the presence of any of these problem and refer to local Child and Family Centre when appropriate and be able to conduct feedback to the parents. The assessment will identify most data when it is performed in a organized and comprehensive way. The physician should review the records/history of the child for any significant history of behavior, education or developmental problems including family medical/mental health history and interview the child developmental parameters with the parent/guardian and relationship of the child with others at school. The history should include, psychosexual history, any remarkable life events, especially loss, abuse, and changes in placement or care-givers and the maximum level of functioning that the child achieved. Any personality and behavior changes preceding the development of the psychiatric diseases must be recognized.

The family history includes history of intellectual or psychiatric illness, neurological disorders (*e.g.* epilepsy or dementia) or other related illness (such as organic diseases). The history also should include the level of family's management and behavior towards the child with DS. Forensic history of the family is important such as past and present history of legal troubles both in patients and in their friends and relatives. Then; a thorough medical/physical examination including developmental neurological evaluation should be conducted. Then psychological and mental evaluation is performed either with a psychologist or with the help of screening questionnaires; including cognitive evaluation, adaptive functioning evaluation, mental health evaluation, and communication evaluation and screening for presence of any restrictive behaviors, interests and activities. Then the physician should perform evaluation of social competence & functioning as well as evaluation of the family functioning.

Evaluation of the child's cognitive functioning is of paramount importance and every possible effort should be done to get accurate estimate of it. This will helps to provide a framework for the interpretation of all of the other qualitative and quantitative observations as well as a framework for decisions on intervention and teaching strategies and help to identify the area of strengths and the possible services that can be provided. A social worker should assess any relevant psychosocial issues and concerns; through a family visit where data are collected directly from the patient himself and from accompanying family members or agency staff. Data about personal income, talents, the accessibility of financial, teaching, and leisure resources in the society; and the network of family, peers, and society supports are significant items.

8. MANAGEMENT OF PSYCHOSOCIAL AND DEVELOPMENTAL PROBLEMS IN ADOLESCENTS WITH DS

Early intervention with multidisciplinary approaches including and proper medical management for different health aspects associated with DS, speech therapy, physiotherapy, and occupational therapy will notably improve the long term prognosis as compared to other genetic causes of intellectual impairments in children. It should be noted that prevention of psychosocial and developmental disorders starts at birth and the parents have to to be prepared to positive and constructive child-rearing approaches from infancy. Presence of significant behavior problems in children or adolescents with DS necessitates professional help. Various strategies for behavior management strategies are present such as self-instruction, proper constructive strengthening, and other behavior modification strategies. An intimate complementary collaboration of the psychotherapist, counselor, school team, parents, and other caregivers will distinctly benefit the DS child. If presence of certain psychiatric disorder is confirmed; then the child/adolescent will need specific psychotropic medications and/or psychotherapy as well as parental counseling. These behavior or psychiatric disorders should be treated effectively and early as possible to help them to have proper communication with people and to enjoy good quality of life [85]. Here; there are a number of considerations that will result in improved mental health in DS children/adolescents.

8.1. Early Stimulation or Intervention

Early intervention can help children with DS to learn how to live and work like normal. It involves different activities planned to improve a young child's progress and development, directly through structured experiences and/or indirectly *via* affecting the care giving environment. Early intervention assure that families with DS children obtain resources and supports that help them in enhance their child's physical, cognitive, and social/emotional progress and development while considering the differences among the families and communities. Early intervention emphasize and set down learning of certain behaviors that influence the rest of development during the vital times of the early years when a child is most reactive to learning experiences. Early correction of any wrong environmental factors like depriving or improper nurturing has a significant influence on the mental development and level of learning. Both significantly impact the level to which the child achieves his/her full potential. A realistic but optimistic approach should be followed by the attending physicians, care providers and the parents in their managements with kids with DS. The earlier the initiation of the stimulation therapy, the better will be the developmental quotients (DQ). An early intervention program is not only helpful in reduction of further costs of rehabilitation and special schools but it also reduces the parental stress and frustration. These interventions are also helpful in decreasing the behavioral problems. It provides a chance to meet other parents coping with similar situations, and share experiences. Most of these children are able to attain daily skills such as feeding, washing, dressing, and toileting. They gradually learn to talk, read and write. They attain appropriate social skills; learn self discipline and self regulation with proper training, which can reduce the burden on parents. Early and appropriate intervention, friendly environment, positive and encouraging parental or caretaker attitude builds their confidence, and help the children to grow healthily [86, 87]. However, there are many factors hinder the success of early intervention program. These factors include both environmental and patients factors. Environmental factors include low parental education level and joblessness, broken family life, unsteady and disordered childcare practices, financial and psychological dependence, increased degrees of life stress and social separation, poor parental spirits and emotional withdrawal and problems in care-giving. Child factors include different child vulnerabilities (*e.g.* temperament, illness, sex) [88]. The contribution of parents in early developmental intervention (EDI) is vital in gaining positive outcomes, which can be enhanced by implementing EDI *via* home visits by a parent trainer [89].

8.2. Education and Opportunities

Despite wide variations in the needs of children with DS, most of them can be in the normal school till the age of 6 years. After the age of 6 years, children with border line intelligence can join mainstream integrated schools while children with mildly and moderately low IQ need to go to the special schools having special educators. Many children with DS can acquire accepted academic skills in reading and number, and benefit from an educational curriculum. They will have rapid progress if they are socially included and accepted in the mainstream integrated schools; benefiting from age appropriate role models and from the benefits of feeling that they are parts of the ordinary community. This approach will give them more self-confidence, self identity and self esteem. However, to achieve this desired effect, the whole school community should be caring and supportive to all its members [90 - 92].

After a smooth transition into adolescence, according to their mental abilities, they can join part time jobs in certain employment centre. Occupational therapy can improve and polish their skills. Adolescent and adults with high functioning abilities can successfully engage themselves in various hobbies, recreational activities and sports. Adolescents with enhanced cognitive and motor functions contribute more frequently in activities and report more satisfaction and social engagement with these activities. Children with DS are amenable for good education and they can enter a special education school for special education, so that the fine motor, gross motor and intellectual training can started since early infancy to improve their development and are very helpful. They can be encouraged to improve body functions and accentuating gaining functional talents that allow improved contribution in age-suitable activities [93 - 95].

8.3. The Role of Dietary Supplements and Drugs in Cognitive Improvement

Vasoactive Intestinal Peptide (VIP) is a neuropeptide critical for the mental development and the brain. The VIP blood level was found to be high in neonates with DS. Blockade the physiological action of VIP during embryogenesis is associated with development of postnatal hypotonia, growth restriction and developmental delay. So, up-regulation of VIP levels in DS may be a try to balance for the loss of neuronal function, which may clarify the elevated levels of VIP. VIP motivates astrocytes to secrete neurotrophic factors, as Activity Dependent Neuroprotective Protein (ADNP) and Activity Dependent Neurotrophic Factor (ADNF), which have been confirmed to have neuroprotective effects. Active fragments of ADNP and ADNF, NAPVSIPQ (NAP) and SALLRSIPA (SAL) correspondingly, have a therapeutic potential to improve developmental delay and learning defects. Addition of SAL or NAP to DS cortical neurons causes a double increase in neuronal survival rates in addition to a decline in degenerative morphological changes [96 - 99].

Fluoxetine is a selective serotonin reuptake inhibitor; capable for complete restoring neurogenesis and dendritic development in the Ts65Dn mouse model of DS. Treatment with fluoxetine can save the granule neurons and correct neuronal maturation and connectivity. These effects suggest fluoxetine as a drug of choice to improve the major defects in the DS brain and, possibly, the mental retardation [100]. Targeting β2 adrenergic receptors is a successful approach to restore synaptic plasticity and cognitive function in the mouse model of DS. Taking into account its frequent use in humans and encouraging impacts on cognition in Ts65Dn mice, formoterol or similar β2 adrenergic receptor agonists which is able to cross the blood brain barrier might be a good candidate for clinical studies to enhance the cognitive function in DS persons [101]. Over expression of HSA21 homologous genes in DS is associated with strong visuo-spatial cognitive changes, related to hippocampal dysfunction. Normalization of the expression levels of Dyrk1A (Dual specificity tyrosine-phosphorylation-regulated kinase 1A), a target gene for DS, may mend the hippocampal deficits in Ts65Dn mice [102]. Epigallocatechin gallate, a green tea polyphenol, that modulates DYRK1A functioning is proved to be helpful in enhancement of cognitive performance in DS patients [103]. The N-methyl-D-aspartate (NMDA) receptor uncompetitive antagonist, memantine hydrochloride (memantine), is able to improve learning/ memory and save one type of hippocampus synaptic plasticity dysfunction in the best-studied mouse model of DS [104]. The use of folinic acid or antioxidants in DS patients is not supported by scientific evidence and do not improve the cognitive performance in such patients. Treatment of trisomic mice with the acetylcholinesterase inhibitor galantamine resulted in a major enhancement in olfactory learning. The olfactory learning can be a sensitive measure to evaluate defects in associative learning in mouse models of DS. Galantamine has a potential therapeutic effects to enhance the cognitive capabilities in DS persons [105].

8.4. Treatment of Inappropriate Sexual and Social Behaviors

If the child or adolescent with DS exposed to improper sexual and social acts; an incorporated treatment plan should be delivered in cooperation with the psychologist and special educator, traditional psychotherapy with a private psychologist, and vigorous social skills training done by a female professional (if the patient is female) in the victim's home and in community settings. The earlier the treatment; the greater the chance of successful treatment and recovery from child abuse, as well as the greater the chance to breaking the cycle of abuse and learn how to heal. Individual psychotherapy is frequently utilized to treat most cases of childhood abuse. However, group psychotherapy is very essential for victims of child abuse as it helps abused children to work together on different topics. The family also may need to have a family therapy were a child-centered session will be performed to engage everyone involved with the plan of care, concentrating on the proper parent-child relations, and elaborating and meeting any needs that may arise outside of the planned psychotherapy program.

Medications are sometimes needed during management of child abuse to decrease the symptoms of anxiety and depression to permit the child to contribute fully in his/her treatment [106].

CONCLUSION

Children and adolescents with DS are exposed to various, physical, sexual, emotional, developmental and psychological problems. Early identification and management of these problems provide good prognosis and ensure better quality of life for this group of population.

CONFLICT OF INTEREST

The authors confirm that this chapter contents have no conflict of interest.

ACKNOWLEDGEMENTS

Declared none.

REFERENCES

[1] Campbell C, Landry O, Russo N, Flores H, Jacques S, Burack JA. Cognitive flexibility among individuals with Down syndrome: assessing the influence of verbal and nonverbal abilities. Am J Intellect Dev Disabil 2013; 118(3): 193-200.
[http://dx.doi.org/10.1352/1944-7558-118.3.193] [PMID: 23734614]

[2] Rachidi M, Lopes C, Delezoide AL, Delabar JM. C21orf5, a human candidate gene for brain abnormalities and mental retardation in Down syndrome. Cytogenet Genome Res 2006; 112(1-2): 16-22.
[http://dx.doi.org/10.1159/000087509] [PMID: 16276086]

[3] Vicari S, Pontillo M, Armando M. Neurodevelopmental and psychiatric issues in Down's syndrome: assessment and intervention. Psychiatr Genet 2013; 23(3): 95-107.
[http://dx.doi.org/10.1097/YPG.0b013e32835fe426] [PMID: 23492931]

[4] Martin GE, Klusek J, Estigarribia B, Roberts JE. Language Characteristics of Individuals with Down Syndrome. Top Lang Disord 2009; 29(2): 112-32.
[http://dx.doi.org/10.1097/TLD.0b013e3181a71fe1] [PMID: 20428477]

[5] Pulsifer MB. The neuropsychology of mental retardation. J Int Neuropsychol Soc 1996; 2(2): 159-76.
[http://dx.doi.org/10.1017/S1355617700001016] [PMID: 9375201]

[6] Galdzicki Z, Siarey RJ. Understanding mental retardation in Down's syndrome using trisomy 16 mouse models. Genes Brain Behav 2003; 2(3): 167-78.
[http://dx.doi.org/10.1034/j.1601-183X.2003.00024.x] [PMID: 12931790]

[7] Koran ME, Hohman TJ, Edwards CM, *et al.* Differences in age-related effects on brain volume in Down syndrome as compared to Williams syndrome and typical development. J Neurodev Disord 2014; 6(1): 8.
[http://dx.doi.org/10.1186/1866-1955-6-8] [PMID: 24713364]

[8] Pinter JD, Eliez S, Schmitt JE, Capone GT, Reiss AL. Neuroanatomy of Down's syndrome: a high-resolution MRI study. Am J Psychiatry 2001; 158(10): 1659-65.
[http://dx.doi.org/10.1176/appi.ajp.158.10.1659] [PMID: 11578999]

[9] Anderson JS, Nielsen JA, Ferguson MA, *et al.* Abnormal brain synchrony in Down Syndrome. Neuroimage Clin 2013; 2: 703-15.
[http://dx.doi.org/10.1016/j.nicl.2013.05.006] [PMID: 24179822]

[10] Pujol J, del Hoyo L, Blanco-Hinojo L, *et al.* Anomalous brain functional connectivity contributing to poor adaptive behavior in Down syndrome. Cortex 2015; 64(64C): 148-56.
[http://dx.doi.org/10.1016/j.cortex.2014.10.012] [PMID: 25461715]

[11] Chapman RS, Hesketh LJ. Behavioral phenotype of individuals with Down syndrome. Ment Retard Dev Disabil Res Rev 2000; 6(2): 84-95.
[http://dx.doi.org/10.1002/1098-2779(2000)6:2<84::AID-MRDD2>3.0.CO;2-P] [PMID: 10899801]

[12] Frangou S, Aylward E, Warren A, Sharma T, Barta P, Pearlson G. Small planum temporale volume in Down's syndrome: a volumetric MRI study. Am J Psychiatry 1997; 154(10): 1424-9.
[http://dx.doi.org/10.1176/ajp.154.10.1424] [PMID: 9326826]

[13] Vanvuchelen M, Feys H, De Weerdt W. Is the good-imitator-poor-talker profile syndrome-specific in Down syndrome?: evidence from standardised imitation and language measures. Res Dev Disabil 2011; 32(1): 148-57.
[http://dx.doi.org/10.1016/j.ridd.2010.09.010] [PMID: 20926249]

[14] Koo BK, Blaser S, Harwood-Nash D, Becker LE, Murphy EG. Magnetic resonance imaging evaluation of delayed myelination in Down syndrome: a case report and review of the literature. J Child Neurol 1992; 7(4): 417-21.
[http://dx.doi.org/10.1177/088307389200700417] [PMID: 1469252]

[15] Dykens EM, Hodapp RM, Evans DW. Profiles and development of adaptive behavior in children with Down syndrome. Downs Syndr Res Pract 2006; 9(3): 45-50.
[http://dx.doi.org/10.3104/reprints.293] [PMID: 16869374]

[16] van Gameren-Oosterom HB, Fekkes M, van Wouwe JP, Detmar SB, Oudesluys-Murphy AM, Verkerk PH. Problem behavior of individuals with Down syndrome in a nationwide cohort assessed in late adolescence. J Pediatr 2013; 163(5): 1396-401.
[http://dx.doi.org/10.1016/j.jpeds.2013.06.054] [PMID: 23916224]

[17] Dykens EM, Shah B, Sagun J, Beck T, King BH. Maladaptive behaviour in children and adolescents with Down's syndrome. J Intellect Disabil Res 2002; 46(Pt 6): 484-92.
[http://dx.doi.org/10.1046/j.1365-2788.2002.00431.x] [PMID: 12354319]

[18] Nicham R, Weitzdörfer R, Hauser E, *et al.* Spectrum of cognitive, behavioural and emotional problems in children and young adults with Down syndrome. J Neural Transm Suppl 2003; (67): 173-91.
[http://dx.doi.org/10.1007/978-3-7091-6721-2_16] [PMID: 15068250]

[19] Molloy CA, Murray DS, Kinsman A, *et al.* Differences in the clinical presentation of Trisomy 21 with and without autism. J Intellect Disabil Res 2009; 53(2): 143-51.
[http://dx.doi.org/10.1111/j.1365-2788.2008.01138.x] [PMID: 19198037]

[20] Dressler A, Perelli V, Bozza M, Bargagna S. The autistic phenotype in Down syndrome: differences in adaptive behaviour *versus* Down syndrome alone and autistic disorder alone. Funct Neurol 2011; 26(3): 151-8.
[PMID: 22152436]

[21] Kent L, Evans J, Paul M, Sharp M. Comorbidity of autistic spectrum disorders in children with Down syndrome. Dev Med Child Neurol 1999; 41(3): 153-8.
[http://dx.doi.org/10.1017/S001216229900033X] [PMID: 10210247]

[22] Rynders JE, Horrobin JM. Always trainable? never educable? Updating educational expectations concerning children with Down syndrome. Am J Ment Retard 1990; 95(1): 77-83.
[PMID: 2143660]

[23] Rutter T, Buckley SJ. The acquisition of grammatical morphemes in children with Down syndrome. Downs Syndr Res Pract 1994; 2(2): 76-82.
[http://dx.doi.org/10.3104/reports.34]

[24] Sloper P, Cunningham C, Turner S, Knussen C. Factors related to the academic attainments of children with Down's syndrome. Br J Educ Psychol 1990; 60(Pt 3): 284-98.
[http://dx.doi.org/10.1111/j.2044-8279.1990.tb00945.x] [PMID: 2150752]

[25] Buckley S, Bird G, Sacks B, Archer T. A comparison of mainstream and special education for teenagers with Down syndrome: implications for parents and teachers. Downs Syndr Res Pract 2006; 9(3): 54-67.
[http://dx.doi.org/10.3104/reports.295] [PMID: 16869376]

[26] Ricci L. Home literacy environments, interest in reading and emergent literacy skills of children with Down syndrome *versus* typical children. J Intellect Disabil Res 2011; 55(6): 596-609.
[http://dx.doi.org/10.1111/j.1365-2788.2011.01415.x] [PMID: 21435070]

[27] Gilmore L, Cuskelly M. A longitudinal study of motivation and competence in children with Down syndrome: early childhood to early adolescence. J Intellect Disabil Res 2009; 53(5): 484-92.
[http://dx.doi.org/10.1111/j.1365-2788.2009.01166.x] [PMID: 19302472]

[28] Sloper P, Turner S, Knussen C, Cunningham C. Social life of school children with Down's syndrome. Child Care Health Dev 1990; 16(4): 235-51.
[http://dx.doi.org/10.1111/j.1365-2214.1990.tb00658.x] [PMID: 2143704]

[29] Turner S, Alborz A, Gayle V. Predictors of academic attainments of young people with Down's syndrome. J Intellect Disabil Res 2008; 52(Pt 5): 380-92.
[http://dx.doi.org/10.1111/j.1365-2788.2007.01038.x] [PMID: 18205756]

[30] Germain R. A 'positive' approach to supporting a pupil with Down syndrome during 'dedicated numeracy time'? Downs Syndr Res Pract 2002; 8(2): 53-8.
[http://dx.doi.org/10.3104/case-studies.130] [PMID: 12407969]

[31] Buckley SJ. Improving the speech and language skills of children and teenagers with Down syndrome Down Syndrome News and Update 1999; 1(3): 111-28.

[http://dx.doi.org/10.3104/practice.146]

[32] Oliver B, Buckley SJ. The language development of children with Down syndrome: First words to two-word phrases. Downs Syndr Res Pract 1994; 2(2): 71-5.
[http://dx.doi.org/10.3104/reports.33]

[33] Stoel-Gammon C. Phonological development in Down syndrome. Ment Retard Dev Disabil Res Rev 1997; 3: 300-6.
[http://dx.doi.org/10.1002/(SICI)1098-2779(1997)3:4<300::AID-MRDD4>3.0.CO;2-R]

[34] Burgoyne K, Duff FJ, Clarke PJ, Buckley S, Snowling MJ, Hulme C. Efficacy of a reading and language intervention for children with Down syndrome: a randomized controlled trial. J Child Psychol Psychiatry 2012; 53(10): 1044-53.
[http://dx.doi.org/10.1111/j.1469-7610.2012.02557.x] [PMID: 22533801]

[35] Ray D. Speech Impairment in Down Syndrome: A Review. J Speech Lang Hear Res 2013; 56(1): 178-210.
[http://dx.doi.org/10.1044/1092-4388(2012/12-0148] [PMID: 23275397]

[36] Van Borsel J. Articulation in Down's syndrome adolescents and adults. Eur J Disord Commun 1996; 31(4): 415-44.
[http://dx.doi.org/10.3109/13682829609031330] [PMID: 9059573]

[37] Rupela V, Manjula R. Phonotactic patterns in the speech of children with Down syndrome. Clin Linguist Phon 2007; 21(8): 605-22.
[http://dx.doi.org/10.1080/02699200701416784] [PMID: 17653970]

[38] Rupela V, Manjula R, Velleman SL. Phonological processes in Kannada-speaking adolescents with Down syndrome. Clin Linguist Phon 2010; 24(6): 431-50.
[http://dx.doi.org/10.3109/02699200903450164] [PMID: 20136507]

[39] Van Borsel J, Vandermeulen A. Cluttering in Down syndrome. Folia Phoniatr Logop 2008; 60(6): 312-7.
[http://dx.doi.org/10.1159/000170081] [PMID: 19011303]

[40] Howell P. Speech control in children with Down syndrome. Downs Syndr Res Pract 2010; 12(2): 98-102.
[http://dx.doi.org/10.3104/reviews.2095]

[41] Nash HM, Snowling MJ. Semantic and phonological fluency in children with Down syndrome: atypical organization of language or less efficient retrieval strategies? Cogn Neuropsychol 2008; 25(5): 690-703.
[http://dx.doi.org/10.1080/02643290802274064] [PMID: 18642139]

[42] Bates E, Goodman JC. On the Inseparability of Grammar and the Lexicon: Evidence from Acquisition, Aphasia and Real-time Processing. Lang Cogn Process 1997; 12(5-6): 507-84.
[http://dx.doi.org/10.1080/016909697386628]

[43] Bates E, Marchman V, Thal D, *et al.* Developmental and stylistic variation in the composition of early vocabulary. J Child Lang 1994; 21(1): 85-123.
[http://dx.doi.org/10.1017/S0305000900008680] [PMID: 8006096]

[44] Sepúlveda EM, López-Villaseñor ML, Heinze EG. Can individuals with Down syndrome improve

their grammar? Int J Lang Commun Disord 2013; 48(3): 343-9.
[http://dx.doi.org/10.1111/1460-6984.12002] [PMID: 23650890]

[45] Nye J, Clibbens J, Bird G. Numerical ability, general ability and language in children with Down syndrome. Downs Syndr Res Pract 1995; 3(3): 92-102.
[http://dx.doi.org/10.3104/reports.55]

[46] Stein DS, Munir KM, Karweck AJ, Davidson EJ, Stein MT. Developmental regression, depression, and psychosocial stress in an adolescent with Down syndrome. J Dev Behav Pediatr 2013; 34(3): 216-8.
[http://dx.doi.org/10.1097/DBP.0b013e31828b2b42] [PMID: 23572173]

[47] Petersen AC, Compas BE, Brooks-Gunn J, Stemmler M, Ey S, Grant KE. Depression in adolescence. Am Psychol 1993; 48(2): 155-68.
[http://dx.doi.org/10.1037/0003-066X.48.2.155] [PMID: 8442570]

[48] Crabtree VM, Varni JW, Gozal D. Health-related quality of life and depressive symptoms in children with suspected sleep-disordered breathing. Sleep 2004; 27(2): 1131-8.
[PMID: 15532207]

[49] Capone G, Goyal P, Ares W, Lannigan E. Neurobehavioral disorders in children, adolescents, and young adults with Down syndrome. Am J Med Genet C Semin Med Genet 2004; 142C(3): 158-72.
[http://dx.doi.org/10.1002/ajmg.c.30097] [PMID: 16838318]

[50] Ploeg Booth KV. Health disparities and intellectual disabilities: lessons from individuals with Down syndrome. Dev Disabil Res Rev 2011; 17(1): 32-5.
[http://dx.doi.org/10.1002/ddrr.136] [PMID: 22447753]

[51] Glenn SM, Cunningham CC. Parents' reports of young people with Down syndrome talking out loud to themselves. Ment Retard 2000; 38(6): 498-505.
[http://dx.doi.org/10.1352/0047-6765(2000)038<0498:PROYPW>2.0.CO;2] [PMID: 11126073]

[52] Gosch A. [Maternal stress among mothers of children with Williams-Beuren syndrome, Down's syndrome and mental retardation of non-syndromal etiology in comparison to mothers of non-disabled children]. Z Kinder Jugendpsychiatr Psychother 2001; 29(4): 285-95.
[http://dx.doi.org/10.1024//1422-4917.29.4.285] [PMID: 11763608]

[53] Most DE, Fidler DJ, Booth-LaForce C, Kelly J. Stress trajectories in mothers of young children with Down syndrome. J Intellect Disabil Res 2006; 50(Pt 7): 501-14.
[http://dx.doi.org/10.1111/j.1365-2788.2006.00796.x] [PMID: 16774635]

[54] Yildirim A, Yildirim MS. Hopelessness of mothers who have children with Down syndrome. Genet Couns 2010; 21(4): 375-80.
[PMID: 21290966]

[55] Bourke J, Ricciardo B, Bebbington A, *et al.* Physical and mental health in mothers of children with Down syndrome. J Pediatr 2008; 153(3): 320-6.
[http://dx.doi.org/10.1016/j.jpeds.2008.02.047] [PMID: 18534233]

[56] Stores R, Stores G, Fellows B, Buckley S. Daytime behaviour problems and maternal stress in children with Down's syndrome, their siblings, and non-intellectually disabled and other intellectually disabled peers. J Intellect Disabil Res 1998; 42(Pt 3): 228-37.

[http://dx.doi.org/10.1046/j.1365-2788.1998.00123.x] [PMID: 9678407]

[57] Norizan A, Shamsuddin K. Predictors of parenting stress among Malaysian mothers of children with Down syndrome. J Intellect Disabil Res 2010; 54(11): 992-1003. [http://dx.doi.org/10.1111/j.1365-2788.2010.01324.x] [PMID: 20868445]

[58] Jahromi LB, Gulsrud A, Kasari C. Emotional competence in children with Down syndrome: negativity and regulation. Am J Ment Retard 2008; 113(1): 32-43. [http://dx.doi.org/10.1352/0895-8017(2008)113[32:ECICWD]2.0.CO;2] [PMID: 18173298]

[59] Williams KR, Wishart JG, Pitcairn TK, Willis DS. Emotion recognition by children with Down syndrome: investigation of specific impairments and error patterns. Am J Ment Retard 2005; 110(5): 378-92. [http://dx.doi.org/10.1352/0895-8017(2005)110[378:ERBCWD]2.0.CO;2] [PMID: 16080776]

[60] Pochon R, Declercq C. Emotion recognition by children with Down syndrome: a longitudinal study. J Intellect Dev Disabil 2013; 38(4): 332-43. [http://dx.doi.org/10.3109/13668250.2013.826346] [PMID: 24279786]

[61] Cuskelly M, Dadds M. Behavioural problems in children with Down's syndrome and their siblings. J Child Psychol Psychiatry 1992; 33(4): 749-61. [http://dx.doi.org/10.1111/j.1469-7610.1992.tb00910.x] [PMID: 1534811]

[62] Clark D, Wilson GN. Behavioral assessment of children with Down syndrome using the Reiss psychopathology scale. Am J Med Genet A 1992; 118A(3): 210-6. [http://dx.doi.org/10.1002/ajmg.a.20007] [PMID: 12673649]

[63] Feeley KM, Jones EA. Addressing challenging behaviour in children with Down syndrome: the use of applied behaviour analysis for assessment and intervention. Downs Syndr Res Pract 2006; 11(2): 64-77. [http://dx.doi.org/10.3104/perspectives.316] [PMID: 17048800]

[64] Sutor B, Hansen MR, Black JL. Obsessive compulsive disorder treatment in patients with Down syndrome: a case series. Downs Syndr Res Pract 2006; 10(1): 1-3. [http://dx.doi.org/10.3104/case-studies.299] [PMID: 16869367]

[65] Evans DW, Gray FL. Compulsive-like behavior in individuals with Down syndrome: its relation to mental age level, adaptive and maladaptive behavior. Child Dev 2000; 71(2): 288-300. [http://dx.doi.org/10.1111/1467-8624.00144] [PMID: 10834464]

[66] Cleland J, Wood S, Hardcastle W, Wishart J, Timmins C. Relationship between speech, oromotor, language and cognitive abilities in children with Down's syndrome. Int J Lang Commun Disord 2010; 45(1): 83-95. [http://dx.doi.org/10.3109/13682820902745453] [PMID: 19821789]

[67] Porto-Cunha E, Limongi SC. Communicative performance of children with Down syndrome in two different situations. Pro Fono 2010; 22(3): 251-6. [http://dx.doi.org/10.1590/S0104-56872010000300016] [PMID: 21103714]

[68] Ji NY, Capone GT, Kaufmann WE. Autism spectrum disorder in Down syndrome: cluster analysis of Aberrant Behaviour Checklist data supports diagnosis. J Intellect Disabil Res 2011; 55(11): 1064-77. [http://dx.doi.org/10.1111/j.1365-2788.2011.01465.x] [PMID: 21883598]

[69] Carter JC, Capone GT, Kaufmann WE. Neuroanatomic correlates of autism and stereotypy in children with Down syndrome. Neuroreport 2008; 19(6): 653-6.
[http://dx.doi.org/10.1097/WNR.0b013e3282faa8d8] [PMID: 18382280]

[70] Warner G, Moss J, Smith P, Howlin P. Autism characteristics and behavioural disturbances in ~ 500 children with Down's syndrome in England and Wales. Autism Res 2014; 7(4): 433-41.
[http://dx.doi.org/10.1002/aur.1371] [PMID: 24664986]

[71] Capone GT, Aidikoff JM, Taylor K, Rykiel N. Adolescents and young adults with Down syndrome presenting to a medical clinic with depression: co-morbid obstructive sleep apnea. Am J Med Genet A 2013; 161A(9): 2188-96.
[http://dx.doi.org/10.1002/ajmg.a.36052] [PMID: 23913657]

[72] Ramstad K, Loge JH, Sponheim E. Depression and Down syndrome. Tidsskr Nor Laegeforen 1998; 118(14): 2153-4.
[PMID: 9656809]

[73] Cooper SA, Collacott RA. Clinical features and diagnostic criteria of depression in Down's syndrome. Br J Psychiatry 1994; 165(3): 399-403.
[http://dx.doi.org/10.1192/bjp.165.3.399] [PMID: 7994516]

[74] Motzkau E. Abused--tortured--neglected. Tracking down child abuse (interview by Sabine Riem). MMW Fortschr Med 2001; 143(49-50): 10.
[PMID: 11808440]

[75] Mossakowska B. Medical observations on child abuse. Child Abuse Negl 1996; 20(2): 141-3.
[http://dx.doi.org/10.1016/0145-2134(95)00123-9] [PMID: 8838410]

[76] Thorpe EL, Zuckerbraun NS, Wolford JE, Berger RP. Missed opportunities to diagnose child physical abuse. Pediatr Emerg Care 2014; 30(11): 771-6.
[http://dx.doi.org/10.1097/PEC.0000000000000257] [PMID: 25343739]

[77] Chang L, Dong M, Yu R, Sun C, Zeng L. [Current status and associated risk factors of child abuse on children aged 7-12 in rural areas of Ningxia]. Zhonghua Liu Xing Bing Xue Za Zhi 2014; 35(8): 913-6.
[PMID: 25376682]

[78] Klevens J, Barnett SB, Florence C, Moore D. Exploring policies for the reduction of child physical abuse and neglect. Child Abuse Negl 2014; 40: 1-11.
[http://dx.doi.org/10.1016/j.chiabu.2014.07.013] [PMID: 25376682]

[79] La Grutta S, Lo Baido R, Calì A, Sarno I, Trombini E, Roccella M. People with Down's sindrome: adolescence and the journey towards adulthood. Minerva Pediatr 2009; 61(3): 305-21.
[PMID: 19461574]

[80] Bononi BM, Sant'Anna MJ, de Oliveira AC, *et al.* Sexuality and persons with Down syndrome. A study from Brazil. Int J Adolesc Med Health 2009; 21(3): 319-26.
[http://dx.doi.org/10.1515/IJAMH.2009.21.3.319] [PMID: 20014635]

[81] Barg E, Bury M, Marczyk T, Pałac K, Wirth M. [Psychosexual problem in young people with Down syndrome in parents' opinions - personal experience]. Pediatr Endocrinol Diabetes Metab 2008; 14(4): 225-30.

[PMID: 19239790]

[82] Van Dyke DC, McBrien DM, Sherbondy A. Issues of sexuality in Down syndrome. Downs Syndr Res Pract 1995; 3(2): 65-9.
[http://dx.doi.org/10.3104/reviews.53]

[83] Shepperdson B. The control of sexuality in young people with Down's syndrome. Child Care Health Dev 1995; 21(5): 333-49.
[http://dx.doi.org/10.1111/j.1365-2214.1995.tb00762.x] [PMID: 8529295]

[84] Ross WT, Olsen M. Care of the adult patient with Down syndrome. South Med J 2014; 107(11): 715-21.
[http://dx.doi.org/10.14423/SMJ.0000000000000193] [PMID: 25365441]

[85] Pueschel SM. Towards optimal mental health of persons with Down syndrome. Downs Syndr Res Pract 1998; 5(1): 43-6.
[http://dx.doi.org/10.3104/reviews.75] [PMID: 10890860]

[86] Wallander JL, Biasini FJ, Thorsten V, *et al.* Dose of early intervention treatment during children's first 36 months of life is associated with developmental outcomes: an observational cohort study in three low/low-middle income countries. BMC Pediatr 2014; 14: 281.
[http://dx.doi.org/10.1186/1471-2431-14-281] [PMID: 25344731]

[87] Fuengfoo A, Sakulnoom K. Clinical abnormalities, early intervention program of Down syndrome children: Queen Sirikit National Institute of Child Health experience. J Med Assoc Thai 2014; 97 (Suppl. 6): S152-8.
[PMID: 25391188]

[88] Mahoney G, Boyce G, Fewell RR, Spker D, Wheeden CA. The relationship of parent–child interaction to the effectiveness of early intervention services for at-risk children and children with disabilities. Top Early Child Spec Educ 1998; 18: 5-17.
[http://dx.doi.org/10.1177/027112149801800104]

[89] Pelchat D, Ricard N, Lefebvre H. [Parents' adaptation to a delayed developmental child. Effects of a family early intervention program]. Infirm Que 2001; 9(2): 14-24.
[PMID: 12942806]

[90] van Wouwe JP, van Gameren-Oosterom HB, Verkerk PH, van Dommelen P, Fekkes M. Mainstream and special school attendance among a Dutch cohort of children with Down Syndrome. PLoS One 2014; 9(3): e91737.
[http://dx.doi.org/10.1371/journal.pone.0091737] [PMID: 24638156]

[91] Daunhauer LA, Fidler DJ, Will E. School function in students with Down syndrome. Am J Occup Ther 2014; 68(2): 167-76.
[http://dx.doi.org/10.5014/ajot.2014.009274] [PMID: 24581403]

[92] De Graaf G, Van Hove G, Haveman M. A quantitative assessment of educational integration of students with Down syndrome in the Netherlands. J Intellect Disabil Res 2014; 58(7): 625-36.
[http://dx.doi.org/10.1111/jir.12060] [PMID: 23796135]

[93] Daunhauer LA, Fidler DJ. The down syndrome behavioral phenotype: implications for practice and research in occupational therapy. Occup Ther Health Care 2011; 25(1): 7-25.

[http://dx.doi.org/10.3109/07380577.2010.535601] [PMID: 23898980]

[94] Wuang Y, Su CY. Patterns of participation and enjoyment in adolescents with Down syndrome. Res Dev Disabil 2012; 33(3): 841-8.
[http://dx.doi.org/10.1016/j.ridd.2011.12.008] [PMID: 22245731]

[95] Rihtman T, Tekuzener E, Parush S, Tenenbaum A, Bachrach SJ, Ornoy A. Are the cognitive functions of children with Down syndrome related to their participation? Dev Med Child Neurol 2010; 52(1): 72-8.
[http://dx.doi.org/10.1111/j.1469-8749.2009.03356.x] [PMID: 19758365]

[96] Brenneman DE, Spong CY, Hauser JM, *et al.* Protective peptides that are orally active and mechanistically nonchiral. J Pharmacol Exp Ther 2004; 309(3): 1190-7.
[http://dx.doi.org/10.1124/jpet.103.063891] [PMID: 15007105]

[97] Incerti M, Horowitz K, Roberson R, *et al.* Prenatal treatment prevents learning deficit in Down syndrome model. PLoS One 2012; 7(11): e50724.
[http://dx.doi.org/10.1371/journal.pone.0050724] [PMID: 23209818]

[98] Incerti M, Toso L, Vink J, *et al.* Prevention of learning deficit in a Down syndrome model. Obstet Gynecol 2011; 117(2 Pt 1): 354-61.
[http://dx.doi.org/10.1097/AOG.0b013e3182051ca5] [PMID: 21252750]

[99] Busciglio J, Pelsman A, Helguera P, *et al.* NAP and ADNF-9 protect normal and Down's syndrome cortical neurons from oxidative damage and apoptosis. Curr Pharm Des 2007; 13(11): 1091-8.
[http://dx.doi.org/10.2174/138161207780618957] [PMID: 17430172]

[100] Guidi S, Stagni F, Bianchi P, *et al.* Early pharmacotherapy with fluoxetine rescues dendritic pathology in the Ts65Dn mouse model of down syndrome. Brain Pathol 2013; 23(2): 129-43.
[http://dx.doi.org/10.1111/j.1750-3639.2012.00624.x] [PMID: 22817700]

[101] Dang V, Medina B, Das D, *et al.* Formoterol, a long-acting β2 adrenergic agonist, improves cognitive function and promotes dendritic complexity in a mouse model of Down syndrome. Biol Psychiatry 2014; 75(3): 179-88.
[http://dx.doi.org/10.1016/j.biopsych.2013.05.024] [PMID: 23827853]

[102] Altafaj X, Martín ED, Ortiz-Abalia J, *et al.* Normalization of Dyrk1A expression by AAV2/1-shDyrk1A attenuates hippocampal-dependent defects in the Ts65Dn mouse model of Down syndrome. Neurobiol Dis 2013; 52: 117-27.
[http://dx.doi.org/10.1016/j.nbd.2012.11.017] [PMID: 23220201]

[103] de la Torre R, Dierssen M. Therapeutic approaches in the improvement of cognitive performance in Down syndrome: past, present, and future. Prog Brain Res 2012; 197: 1-14.
[http://dx.doi.org/10.1016/B978-0-444-54299-1.00001-7] [PMID: 22541285]

[104] Boada R, Hutaff-Lee C, Schrader A, *et al.* Antagonism of NMDA receptors as a potential treatment for Down syndrome: a pilot randomized controlled trial. Transl Psychiatry 2012; 2: e141.
[http://dx.doi.org/10.1038/tp.2012.66] [PMID: 22806212]

[105] de Souza FM, Busquet N, Blatner M, Maclean KN, Restrepo D. Galantamine improves olfactory learning in the Ts65Dn mouse model of Down syndrome. Sci Rep 2011; 1: 137.
[http://dx.doi.org/10.1038/srep00137] [PMID: 22355654]

[106] Treatment of Child Abuse Reece Robert Hanson Rochelle Sargent John. Treatment of Child Abuse 392pp £50 Johns Hopkins University Press 9781421412733 142141273X. Emerg Nurse 2015; 22(10): 13.
[http://dx.doi.org/10.7748/en.22.10.13.s17]

CHAPTER 11

Anesthesia in Down Syndrome Children

Mohammed Al-Biltagi[1,*], Hasan Alasy[1], Avijit Gaikwad[2]

[1] *Pediatric Department, Faculty of Medicine, Tanta University, Egypt*

[2] *American Mission Hospital, Bahrain. M.D,DNB University of Mumbai; India*

Abstract: Down syndrome (DS) Children are more liable for frequent sedation and anesthesia either for imaging procedure or for surgical intervention. They have many risk factors that increase the anesthesia related complications. These risk factors include cardiac, esophageal, gastrointestinal or urinary tracts, eyes, ears, and joints anomalies. There is also an increased risk of infection due to immune deficiency. Proper preoperative, operative and post operative management are mandatory to decrease the anesthesia-related complications. In this chapter; these co morbidities and the factors that increase the risk of complications during anesthesia will be addressed, as well as pre-operative, intraoperative and post-operative management will be discussed.

Keywords: Anesthesia, Atropine, Cardiac, Children, Cognitive, Down syndrome, Ears, Epilepsy, Esophageal, Eyes, Gastrointestinal, joints anomalies, Mental retardation, Operative, Post operative, Preoperative, Sedation, Sleep apnea, Trisomy, Urinary tracts.

1. INTRODUCTION

Sedation and anesthesia are frequently needed for children with Down syndrome (DS); either for imaging procedure or for surgical intervention. Infants and children with DS have more frequent congenital anomalies than non-syndromic children. About 50% of these children have major cardiac anomalies that may require early surgical intervention. Other major anomalies that may involve esophageal, gastrointestinal or urinary tracts, eyes, ears, and joints may also need early intervention. Proper sedation and anesthesia are needed to carry on with imaging and surgical correction of these anomalies [1]. Anesthetic care for

* **Corresponding Author Dr. Mohammed Al-Biltagi:** Pediatric Department, Faculty of Medicine, Tanta University, Egypt; Tel: (+973)39545472; Fax: (+973) 1759 0495; Email: mbelrem@hotmail.com

children with DS may be a real challenge even for the most well experienced anesthesiologist. This challenge arises from the increased frequency of numerous functional co-morbidities that are frequently encountered in these children. These co morbidities can affect any system and organ ranging from unnoticed condition *e.g.* hypersensitivity to atropine; to a serious medical problem *e.g.* complex congenital heart diseases. These augmented with the characteristics emotional, psychological and mental problems of children with DS and their inability to recognize their sickness increase the difficulties that meet the anesthesiologist when dealing with them and conducting preoperative risk evaluation, perioperative management, and maintenance of their vital organ functions. During sedation or anesthesia; they are more liable to have difficult airways, altered respiratory mechanics, problems related to gastric reflux, cardiovascular compromise and neuromuscular disorders. Knowledge of these frequent disorders can assist anesthesiologist to arrange safer practice in DS people.

2. ASSOCIATED CO MORBIDITIES THAT COULD INCREASE ANESTHESIA RISKS AND COMPLICATIONS

2.1. Cognitive, Cerebral and Neurologic Problems in DS children

Neurological disorders in children with DS are relatively common. These disorders could be anatomical or functional including disordered neurotransmission. People with DS have structural abnormalities in the nerve cells including the neuronal axis, cerebellum and central structures with alterations of the neurotransmission system, and vulnerability of the cholinergic and noradrenergic systems [2]. They have decreased pain perception due to the raised levels of opioid peptides in the frontal cortex of these people which explains the increased pain threshold in DS patients. Peripheral somatosensory hypofunction including transmission of painful stimuli is another cause of decreased pain perception. This altered pain tolerance, and the incapacity to give a qualitative and quantitative pain description cause difficulty in measuring pain in children with DS [3]. Variable degrees of mild to moderate mental retardation (IQ between 20 and 70) with inadequate understanding in contrast to the normal children of similar age in addition to severe learning difficulties; are observed in these children. Many of them may have lack of cooperation due to fear, anxiety, and incapacity to communicate rather than due to the degree of mental retardation. They also may show a tendency towards hyperactivity [4].

Children with DS have impaired expressive communication capabilities, but they have relatively more developed receptive communication skills. Thus, they can feel the nervousness and anxiety in their caregivers, and will respond to what they feel. Expressive language development is often delayed or impaired in children with DS as they understand more than they can verbalize. Proper communication is essential for comfortable transition of the patients into unfamiliar environments or scenarios. Difficult communication observed in children with DS may increase their anxiety & agitation before anesthesia and they may have some difficulties describing pain & other symptoms. Yoshikawa *et al.* found that the risk of hypoxemia and delayed recovery after midazolam administration is increased in children with DS, or mental retardation. Patients with mental retardation may show vigorous treatment-refusal actions. Anxiety & agitation can lead to unsafe behavior and possible injuries to patient, family, or health care providers. They may have marked sympathetic nervous system stimulation and possible "fight or flight" body reaction that may take part in anesthetic complications [5]. Lack of adequate communication impairs the ability of children with DS to describe their feelings with pain, nausea and other symptoms that may have. This may increases the risk of misdiagnosis of anesthesia related complications and hence inadequate treatment [6].

Epilepsy can occur in 5-10% of children with DS. These children are at increased risk of missing scheduled anticonvulsants during the home-to-hospital transition, including when being admitted for procedures requiring anesthesia. This may contribute to breakthrough seizures because of lowered anticonvulsant levels [7]. At the same time; epileptic seizures can occur during anesthesia. Some of the used general anesthesia medication can induce epilepsy as sevoflurane and enflurane. Sevoflurane is considered as the gold standard for inhalation induction anesthesia in children. Nevertheless; high concentrations of sevoflurane can induce epileptiform electroencephalographic signs in both children and adults in the form of polymorphic spike-wave, polyspike-wave and periodic epileptiform discharges that come before electroencephalographic or actual clinical seizure [8]. Enflurane is also able to provoke seizures and is used to stimulate epileptic foci during epilepsy surgery. Enflurane-induced EEG abnormalities a can persist for several days after anesthesia exposure and can provoke occurrence of delayed seizures. Similarly, Ketamine reduces the threshold for fits in epileptic patients. Fentanyl is an opioid utilized in induction of general anesthesia. It can also induce myoclonic activity by blocking of cortical inhibitory pathways and permit the lower cerebral structures to release unsuppressed excitability [9]. Continuous intravenous infusion of tramadol was reported to induce seizures in children in some cases [10].

Some antiepileptic drugs (AED) may cause coagulation disturbances and even bleeding during the perioperative phase of epilepsy surgery. Care must be considered in children taking AEDs who will be subjected to complex brain epilepsy surgery due to the risk of major blood loss [11]. In the same way, some antiepileptics may increase the body resistance to the effect of some non-depolarising muscle relaxants used during general anesthesia. Chronic phenytoin therapy can induce resistance to vecuronium. Clonazepam and zonisamide can increase phenytoin blood level and hence they might be also cofactors in resistance to vecuronium. At least one week of phenytoin treatment is needed to produce this effect. The mechanism of resistance is not fully known but may be related to inhibition of the exaggerated rise in serum potassium after succinylcholine intake. Another possible mechanism is through hepatic microsomal enzyme induction as a result of the prolonged treatment with phenytoin or carbamazepine that probably induces increased hepatic metabolism and inactivation of the non-depolarizing neuromuscular blockers casing shortened duration of neuromuscular blockade. Therefore, patients undergoing chronic anticonvulsant therapy should be paid more attention because they have resistance to neuromuscular blocking drugs [12, 13].

There were some old studies which showed altered atropine sensitivity in children with DS. Both overstated mydriatic response to ocular atropine and raised response of heart rate to parental atropine are well recognized. However, other studies failed to show the cardiovascular response and no recent studies confirmed this altered response. However, even there is raised incidence of atropine hypersensitivity, it is recommended to utilize vagolytic dose of atropine as these patients have reduced sympathetic activity [14]. At the same time; atropine should be given with extreme precaution if the patients are treated with digoxin for heart failure to avoid atrial fibrillation [15]. Children with DS have reduced CNS catecholamine levels which are accompanied with decrease in minimum alveolar concentration (MAC) of inhaled anesthetic agents and hence they need less requirements of volatile anesthetic agent compared with normal patients. DS children are more liable to deeper states of anesthesia obtained with similar MAC of inhaled anesthetic agents than non-syndromic children. They lack also the increase of plasma Dopamine- α- hydroxylase that usually occurs following stressful situations in contrast to the typically normal children or other mentally retarded children [14].

2.2. Sleep Apnea & Airway Obstruction

Children with DS frequently have sleep apnea syndrome both obstructive and central which increase the risk of hypoxemia, and hypoventilation during natural sleep states. At the same time, obstructive sleep apnea syndrome (OSAS) may contribute to unexplained pulmonary hypertension seen in children with DS. Chronic airway obstruction may lead to pulmonary artery hypertension (PAH) that is more likely to develop in premature infants or children with DS and cardiac anomalies. Many factors may contribute to development of sleep apnea including central hypoventilation, low tone of oral muscles & upper airway muscles, poor coordination of swallowing/breathing, narrowed airways, larger tongue, enlarged tonsils & adenoids. Polysomnography may be useful and is currently considered the gold standard for objectively assessing sleep disorders; but not routinely indicated in OSAS [16, 17].

DS children with OSA are more prone to airway obstruction with increased incidence of perioperative complications when undergoing surgery under sedation or general anesthesia [18]. These complications may comprise hypoxemia, myocardial injury, cardiac arrhythmias, unexpected admission to the ICU, life threatening obstructive scenarios, and even sudden unexpected death. These complications may be related to the interaction between widespread sedative and analgesic drugs utilized for anesthesia and OSA. During anesthesia; these children lose the defensive airway reflexes (like the gag reflex and cough reflex) and the muscle tone, which makes airway tissues to collapse briefly close and compromise the already compromised airway predisposing them to numerous complications. Other complications may arise from difficulties met during airway management. Absence of identification of OSA and, hence, poor perioperative preparation is also cited as a reason of raised undesirable events in this population [19]. Other co morbidities frequently encountered in children with DS such as systolic or diastolic myocardial dysfunction, insulin resistance, pulmonary hypertension, and cardiac arrhythmias result in more difficult perioperative management of these children [20]. Any child with DS should be suspected to have OSA and every effort should be done to rule it out. Otherwise, anesthetic preparation should include the assumption that some degree of obstruction may be encountered during most anesthetics, and pulmonary hypertension may also be present.

2.3. Airway and Respiratory Compromise

Children with DS frequently have abnormal lungs structures and functions with reduced alveolar complexity. The lungs may have a sponge-like appearance due to the enlargement of alveoli and terminal bronchioles that is accompanied by a decrease in the overall number of alveoli and reduction in airway branching with disturbance of alveolar multiplication [21]. Alveolar hypoplasia is a common finding in DS which could be one of the reasons of decreased cardio-respiratory capacity that is frequently seen in children with DS and manifested by lower levels of peak oxygen uptake (peak VO_2) consistent with low levels of cardiovascular fitness compared with non-syndromic children. The hypoplastic lung tissue observed in children with DS predisposes the lung to be more prone to mechanical stress, with additional probability for distension of peripheral air spaces or development of interstitial emphysema, following artificial inflation of the lungs during surgery and this is possible to be the reason of postoperative respiratory failure [22]. There is also reduced mucociliary clearance in children with DS due to both a primitive defect of cilia as well as recurrent respiratory tract infections that cause changes in mucus properties, such as in rheological parameters [23]. Persistence of antenatal double capillary network around the alveoli to the post natal life is also observed in these children [24].

Congenital upper airways anomalies are common in children with DS and are strongly associated with cardiovascular anomalies. These anomalies may be stenotic anomalies [*e.g.* tracheal stenosis, hourglass trachea,and midtracheal absence], anomalies that cause collapse [laryngomalacia,tracheomalacia, and bronchomalacia], tracheoesophageal fistula, or branching anomalies. Vascular ring can also cause compression of the large airways *e.g.* aberrant innominate artery in patients with DS [25]. DS children have narrower airways than other children. This results from generalized reduction of the diameter of the tracheal lumens. Tracheal stenosis is of particular importance during endotracheal intubation. In congenital tracheal stenosis, there is absence of the membranous portion of the trachea with fusion of the posterior aspect of tracheal cartilage with loss of the C-shaped picture of normal cartilage of the trachea. Anomalies of this cartilage can involve the tracheal cartilaginous sleeves, predisposing to obstruction and crusting, and complete tracheal rings, in which the trachea is formed of several or more complete rings of cartilage with a reduced diameter. Other types of tracheal stenosis include hourglass trachea, and midtracheal absence of the tracheal pars membranacea. However, despite being infrequent, tracheal stenosis is clinically significant as a reason for difficult intubation in DS children [26].

DS Children typically have microbrachycephaly, short neck, microglossia, mandibular hypoplasia, prominent tongue, narrow nasopharynx, subglottic stenosis, and smaller glottic and tracheal diameters than their peers without DS. The generalized hypotonia and ligamentous laxity cause hypotonia of the pharyngeal muscles and cervical spine instability. Lingual tonsillar hypertrophy (LTH) is a quite uncommon form of lymphoid hyperplasia, but it might induce life-threatening airway obstruction in DS children [27]. Because of all these factors; endotracheal intubation may be difficult with increased frequency of post extubation stridor due to subglottic stenosis and tracheomalacia. The percent of hard intubation in DS children was expected in one study to be about 4.62%. Intubation's difficulty rose with decreasing age of non-Down patients. The risk of difficult intubation in those patients was, regardless of age, almost 27% more than in non-Downs. However, DS appears to be significant only in the age group between one month and one year. Smaller endotracheal tubes may be indicated when undergoing endotracheal intubation for anesthesia [28]. At the same time, children with DS are more liable to frequent respiratory infections due to relative both cell and antibody-mediated immunodeficiency combined with reduced mucociliary clearance and the frequent presence of congenital heart disease. All these factors increase the morality rate in children with DS due to respiratory infections, about 124 times greater than that of the non-DS children. Adequate management of respiratory infections should be done before presenting for surgery [29]. Alveolar hypoplasia, over distension of air spaces, interstitial emphysema and alveolar septitis are principal factors for postoperative respiratory failure in DS as the reduced alveolar surface area and loss of capillary surface area may aggravate pre-existing pulmonary hypertension [30]. Interstitial lung disease is another possible reason for prolonged postoperative desaturation in children with DS [31].

2.4. Cardiovascular Compromise

Congenital heart disease during anesthesia for both cardiac and non-cardiac surgery add various physiological and functional abnormalities and create a severe challenge for anesthesia with elevated risk of perioperative morbidity and mortality relative to the other children [32]. Congenital heart defects occur in about 40-60% of children with DS. Atrio-ventricular septal defect (AVSD) is the most frequent cardiac anomaly and ventricular septal defect (VSD) comes second to it. Excessive blood flow through large cardiac defects to the pulmonary vasculature may result in congestive heart failure or induce poor pulmonary function, small airway obstruction, obstruction of the left main-stem bronchus, increased interstitial/alveolar lung water, and vascular obstructive disease. Intra-cardiac shunts may increase the risk of air embolism through the intravenous line inserted during anesthesia which could increase myocardial or cerebral ischemia. Hypercyanotic spells may happen in children with intra-cardiac shunts with reversal of the shunt due to development of increased pulmonary vascular resistance which may develop in children with DS due to volume overload or even independent of cardiac anomalies [33]. Development of shunt reversal and Eisenmenger's syndrome is related to the elevated mortality rates during anesthesia. Pulmonary vascular disease may also develop even without cardiac anomalies as a result of chronic pulmonary hypoxaemia resulting from frequent pulmonary infections, hypoventilation due to muscle hypotonia and obstructive sleep apnoea [34]. Patients with pulmonary hypertension have high morbidity and mortality rates during anesthesia and surgery due to occurrence of right ventricular failure, arrhythmias, postoperative hypoxemia, and myocardial ischemia [35].

Temporary or permanent rise in pulmonary vascular resistance (PVR) can jeopardize the perioperative care of many infants with CHD such as endocardial cushion defects, ventricular septal defects, patent ductus arteriosus, and aortic outflow anomalies, which are frequent in DS children than among others. Shunt reversal can occur during anesthesia due to increase pulmonary vascular (PVR) resistance and decrease systemic vascular resistance (SVR) due to anesthetic consequences of elevated airway pressures. At the same time; hypercyanotic spells during anesthesia may arise from surgical manipulation, dynamic obstruction of the right ventricular outflow track, reduced pulmonary blood flow related to hypovolemia, elevated airway pressures, or reduced SVR [36, 37].

Children who previously subjected to corrective cardiac surgery may still at risk of increase the anesthesia related complications. Residual defects if present may result in limitation of physical activity. Intra-cardiac fibrosis following corrective cardiac surgery may increase risk of atrial rhythm anomalies *e.g.* after correction of transposition of great vessels (TGA) with an atrial baffle [38]. Furthermore, anomalies of the cardiac valves, especially mitral valve prolapse (MVP), present in about half of DS adolescents and adults. Cardiac valve disorders can influence the hemodynamic stability during anesthesia, such as heart rate and rhythm, blood pressure, as well as pulmonary blood pressure. If valvular cardiac disease is suspected, the anesthesiologist must be informed prior to sedation or anesthesia [39].

Up to 57% of people with DS with or without congenital heart diseases, however, may exhibit bradycardia and hypotension during anesthetic induction with sevoflurane or sedation compared with 12% of non-syndromic patients. This slowing may even proceed to the point of asystole and even cardiac arrest. Children with DS are most likely liable to have bradycardia with anesthesia than adults, but the risk is important all over the age ranges. Though there is often minor hemodynamic effect of bradycardia during sevoflurane induction in DS, it can be accompanied with severe hypotension in some patients with a rate-dependent cardiac output, mainly if other drugs such as dexmedetomidine are utilized. The phenomenon of the induction-associated bradycardia arises independently of presence or absence of clinically evident structural heart defects which signifies the role of other responsible factors. Very slow heart rates may be partially responsible for the hemodynamic sequelae and hypotension, which could affect delivery of oxygen to vital organs [40].

Children with DS may have cardiac dysfunctions even without structural cardiac diseases [41]. However, Recalde *et al.* found an enlarged cell size and a decreased number of cardiac muscle fibers/unit area which might clarify occurrence of cardiac dysfunctions [42]. Another study showed that DS patients without structural heart disease develop left ventricular hyperkinesia, which is related to the reduced after load [43]. Decreased heart rate and hypotensive responses to sympatho-excitatory stimuli were observed in DS patients, denoting decreased sympathetic nervous system activity in such patients [44].Vascular access may be difficult and a real challenge to the anesthesiologist due to small size of the vessel and less supportive tissue; obesity or xerodermia which can jeopardize the release of anesthesia and pain medications.

2.5. Gastrointestinal Considerations

Gastrointestinal problems are common in children with DS, including gastro-esophageal reflux, pyloric stenosis, duodenal atresia, tracheo-esophageal fistula, imperforate anus, and Hirschsprung disease. Newborns with DS have up to a 12% prevalence of various gastrointestinal atresias, which usually necessitate surgery within the first few days of life. Duodenal atresia is 300 times more frequent in DS children than in the general population. Celiac disease is more prevalent in children with DS (7 to 16%) which may need strict lifelong dietary adherence in order to prevent small bowel mucosal damage [45, 46].

Gastro-esophageal reflux disease (GERD) is more common in DS children and should be assessed before any surgery. It could present with vomiting; symptoms of esophagitis as chest pain, anemia and irritability; respiratory manifestations as apnea, coughing, wheezing and/or even symptoms of aspiration pneumonia.

Gastroesophageal reflux has significant concern particularly during anesthesia, as it raises the hazard of aspiration during anesthesia because sedation and anesthesia suppress the normal protective airways reflexes such as cough and gagging reflexes as well as the swallowing actions. Aspiration occurring during anesthesia induction or emergence periods (going to sleep and waking) may take part in airway irritation, inflammation and even predispose to infection and airway obstruction, including life threatening airway spasms. To prevent aspiration during anesthesia, the child should fast for an adequate time prior to anesthesia and sedation. The necessary fasting duration vary according to the age of the child and the nature of ingested food or liquids. Modified rapid sequence induction may be utilized together with the agents to raise the gastric pH and reduce the aspiration risk during anesthesia [47, 48].

2.6. Autoimmunity and Endocrinal Considerations

Autoimmune diseases are common in children with DS and become increasingly frequent as the children grow older. These autoimmune diseases include celiac disease, celiac-like enteropathy, hemolytic anemia, diabetes and show cellular immunity response against peripheral nerve antigen and basic myeloprotein, and serum autoantibodies against many other tissue antigens. Clinical and subclinical thyroid dysfunction is frequent in DS patients and the risk increases with age. Hypothyroidism may be seen in as many as 10 to 50% of patients with DS and the clinical pictures ranges from subclinical to overt hypothyroidism. On the other hand; despite hyperthyroidism is less frequent than hypothyroidism but it is more prevalent in patients with DS than non syndromic patients. Hypothyroidism may develop in DS due to impaired development of the thyroid gland and may become clinically manifested when thyroiditis is superimposed on a pre-existing diminished thyroid reserve. Autoimmune thyroiditis is the most frequent disorder and appears to affect 39% of adult patients with DS [49, 50]. Hypothyroidism results in significant defects in normal physiology. Impairment of myocardial functions; reduced hypoxic and hypercapnic ventilatory responses; unusual baroreceptor function; and decreases in plasma volume may all occur. Additionally, the association of anemia, hypoglycemia, hyponatremia, reduced free water excretion, and deteriorated hepatic drug metabolism may all negatively affect the responses to anesthesia [51, 52]. Hypothyroid patients are more liable to hypothermia with possible delayed recovery from anesthesia related to the thyroid condition of these patients. Though the effect of neuromuscular blocking drugs is not lengthened in this category of patients they may have late recovery results from hypothermia or other factors related to hypothyroidism [53]. Preoperative detection of hypothyroidism is necessary for the secured anesthetic administration of these patients. Elective surgeries must not be performed in presence of untreated hypothyroidism.

Autoimmune thyroid disease may be associated with diabetes mellitus as a part of the generalized autoimmune disorder in patients with DS. Type 1 diabetes mellitus is present in up to 10.6% in patients with DS which is higher than in non syndromic population [54]. Continuous supplementation with exogenous insulin is required due to their inability to produce insulin themselves. The insulin dosage required is individual-specific and may change dramatically during the perioperative period. These diabetic patients are at increased risk of metabolic derangement including hypoglycemia and diabetic ketoacidosis [55]. Despite the infants with DS have lower curves for both height and weight compared with the rest of the population; however, they start to be overweight by the age of 2 to 3 years which may reach 50% of individuals with DS by adulthood. Obesity is co-factor contributes in worsening diabetes, sleep apnea, pulmonary hypertension and adds airway, ventilatory, and positioning challenges during aesthesia [56]. Obese children not only have anesthesia-relevant co-existing diseases that are, asthma and hypertension, but also have a higher incidence of anesthesia-related complication [57].

2.7. Hematological Considerations

Down syndrome is accompanied with numerous hematological problems happening at various ages. Newborns with DS may have transient asymptomatic blood count disorders such as neutrophilia, thrombocytopenia and polycythemia. In the first two months of life, about 3-10% of DS infants have transient myeloproliferative disease (TMD). Though most cases have a spontaneous regression, TMD can be lethal or lead to later regression to myeloid leukemia in about 20% of DS children (DS ML). DS ML has unique clinical and biological characteristics with increased sensitivity to chemotherapy and a good prognosis.

At the same time; DS children also have high risk of developing acute lymphoblastic leukemia (ALL) which is characterized by being having heterogeneous pattern of genetic features and by an increased rate of treatment-induced toxicities [58].

DS children have a higher incidence of polycythemia than control children; with levels of haematocrit values could reach 70%. Polycythemia may complicate some types of congenital heart defects but the majority of children with DS who develop polycythemia don't have an associated structural heart defect. Haematocrit values greater than 80% imply the need for immediate phlebotomy to prevent circulatory failure [59]. Children with polycythemia younger than 5 yr are at high risk of hyper viscosity which may precipitate cerebral vein and sinus thrombosis. Presence of dehydration, fever, and iron deficiency anemia increase this risk. Preoperative intravenous fluid therapy may help to decrease the risk [60].

2.8. Musculoskeletal Considerations

Children with DS have generalized hypotonia and poor muscle tone especially in the early years of life. This could cause laxity of different joints including finger, thumb, elbow and/or knee. However, laxities of the transverse ligament that support atlanto-axial and atlanto-occipital joints are of particular importance as laxities of these joints place them to a higher risk for catastrophic spinal cord injury. Atlanto-axial unsteadiness is seen in about 15% of patients with DS and up to 20 % of children with DS have radiographic evidence of atlanto-axial instability (AAI) as defined by presence of an atlanto-axial gap of 4-0 mm or more between the anterior arch of the atlas and odontoid process of the axis for children below the age of 8 years and a gap of 3 mm or less in children over 8 years old. On the other hand; only approximately 1% of all patients with DS will exhibit any symptoms including easy fatigability, torticollis, and varying signs of spinal cord compression as difficult walking, unusual gait, neck pain restricting neck mobility, in-coordination and awkwardness, sensory defects, spasticity, hyper-reflexia and presence of bladder and bowel dysfunction. The symptoms may develop gradually over months or years, or acutely after specific trauma [61, 62].

Manipulations of the head and neck during anesthesia to open obstructive airways and inserting airway devices, including endotracheal tubes, are common practices during nearly every sedation and anesthetic. These manipulations can be very dangerous and predispose to spinal cord injury which is important complicating realities of anesthesia for such cohort of patients [63, 64]. However; keeping a neutral head and neck position during airway instrumentation or intubation is generally adequate to avoid spinal cord injury, but such positioning can hamper the anesthesiologist's capability to effectively intubate [65].

3. PRE OPERATIVE MANAGEMENT

Preoperative evaluation and preparation of children with DS is of paramount importance to identify a wide variety of coexisting conditions and congenital problems prior to anesthesia, and to assess an individual's plan of care and to put an appropriate anesthesiologic strategy for each patient to avoid or at least to decrease the possible anesthesia/surgery-related morbidity and mortality risks. The risks are frequently hard to evaluate in these patients but possibly relays on the seriousness of the cardiac lesion, pulmonary lesion, seriousness of systemic diseases, occurrence of other anomalies, age of the child, type of the procedure, and the condition of the pulmonary vasculature. Meticulous attention should be paid to assess the cardiovascular status, respiratory system, the airway, the endocrine condition, the musculoskeletal system especially the atlanto-axial joint, hematological abnormalities and gastroesophageal reflux. The anesthesiologist should take adequate past medical and surgical histories, such as structural heart anomalies, hard intubation, rheumatic fever, or malignant hyperthermia which could result in serious consequences even if being asymptomatic - that could have direct influence on the anesthetic safety. The history should include any regular medications that could impede any drug therapy or could affect the choice of anesthetic induction agent. Many DS children have congenital heart diseases and receive numerous medications such as aspirin, angiotensin converting enzyme (ACE) inhibitors, diuretics, and anti-arrhythmic.

Successful history taking and examination depends on the age of the patients, the severity of physical disability, how much the child is cooperative, the degree of impairment of the learning disability, his ability to understand as well as the ability of the anesthesiologist to explain what will occur in a language suitable to the child. Presence of the parents or the care-giver will significantly help in calming the child as well as conduction of smooth thorough examination. Situations that affect vision or hearing will additionally impair the already impaired communication that characterizes people with DS. This will increase the child anxiety, agitation and behavioral problem which also may complicate history taking and proper examination. Presence of the parents can help to conduct clear explanation of the anesthetic procedure. Play therapists may also take part in calming the child and ensure smooth induction of anesthesia. A pre-anesthesia informed consent should be taken and signed by the parents or guardian prior to the procedure after enough explanation and proper understanding of the procedure and the related risks. However, the consent may be provided by two health professionals.

Congenital heart anomalies are common in DS children that need a high index of suspicion. Preoperative evaluation of the cardiac condition for children with DS is important even if asymptomatic. Congenital heart anomalies may present impaired growth and failure to thrive, difficult breathing and easily fatigability with efforts, or unexplained fainting. Clinical examination may reveal presence of central cyanosis, blue or pale clubbing of the fingers or toes, signs of respiratory distress, or hepatomegaly. Cardiac examination may reveal signs of cardiomegaly with displaced cardiac apex, and/or presence of cardiac murmur, probably accompanied with 'thrill'. It is also important to detect any residual lesion from a previous corrective cardiac surgery that could increase the anesthetic risk before enrollment into anesthesia. Conduction abnormalities could also result from a corrective cardiac surgery for atrioventricular canal, Fallot tetralogy, and some types of ventricular defects [38]. Pre anesthetic recognition of these residual lesions helps to minimize the anesthetic and surgical risk and decreases the procedure related morbidity and mortality rates. A comprehensive cardiovascular examination, ECG, and preferably a referral to a cardiologist together with echocardiography examination could be done in all DS children before surgery. Biltagi *et al.* had recommended doing an echocardiographic examination before involvement in cardiac or major non-cardiac surgery [41]. Preoperative antibiotic prophylaxis against infective endocarditis is required prior to any surgery in some

DS children even following successful repair of the cardiac defects as in case of valve replacement; aortic valvotomy, pulmonary valvotomy, resection of aortic coarctation, correction of Fallot tetralogy. It is also indicated if there is residual valve regurgitation more than grade I, presence of any shunt (except an atrial septal defect); congenital heart disease surgery within the past 6 months, or previous history of endocarditis [14]. Pre-operative evaluation of the pulmonary pressure is very important to avoid pulmonary hypertensive crisis during surgery.

Children with DS may suffer presence of polycythemia (haematocrit value is more than 70%) especially in presence of cyanotic congenital heart diseases (CHD) or chronic lung pathology. Manifestations of hyperviscosity comprise headache, tiredness, weakness, numbness, dizziness, and impaired mental state. The symptoms are mainly frequent with haematocrit value more than 65%. The major adverse effects of polycythemia include reduced cardiopulmonary reserve, raised systemic vascular resistance due to increased blood viscosity, increased risk of cerebral, pulmonary or renal thrombosis especially with dehydration, plus increased risk of coagulopathy. Phlebotomy may be needed if haematocrit value is more than 80%, otherwise there is chances of circulatory failure [58, 66]. Sufficient perioperative hydration is mandatory in children having cyanotic CHD; so preoperative fasting must be reduced as far as possible (plain fluids till 2 hours prior to surgery in infants 0-12 months; plain fluids till 4 hours preoperatively in children 12 months or older) or an intravenous fluid infusion can be initiated. However, children with DS are more liable to volume overload especially if there is left to right intra-cardiac shunt (*e.g.* VSD) or valvular defect which may end with congestive heart failure. Meticulous care should be given during intravenous fluid administration [67].

Meticulous attention should be directed to the airway and should be adequately examined and properly evaluated preoperatively. Endo-tracheal intubation may be difficult and could be a real challenge to the anesthesiologist. Children with DS usually have a narrowed airway, a small mouth, an enlarged tongue, enlarged tonsils and adenoids, a high arched palate, a short and broad neck, small or fused teeth, and pharyngeal muscle hypotonia. All these factors may cause upper airway obstruction and a small trachea which may require an endo-tracheal tube with two sizes smaller than predicted to avoid potential airway trauma [26]. The frequency of airway obstruction and difficult intubation in DS children was found to be 1.83% and 0.54% correspondingly [68].

If there is a history of obstructive sleep apnea, the children may have obstructive airway disorders when sleeping and will be particularly liable to airway obstruction under the effect of sedation and anesthesia which impair the protective airway reflexes (like the cough reflex and gag reflex) and decrease the muscle tone, thereby causing airway tissues to be collapsible and briefly close. The airway tissues in DS children are already liable to collapse during normal sleep states; so, loss of protective airway reflexes under anesthesia is a warranty of obstruction. Routine sleep studies are not necessary indicated prior to sedation or anesthesia. However, if the child will have complex surgical procedures involving airway tissues or if already had a previous history of obstructive problems during anesthesia, a polysomnography study before anesthesia or sedation is recommended. Anesthesiologists should be able to alleviate any airway obstruction encountered by different methods, including intubation. In rare circumstances, cricothyrotomy may be essential to ensure an open airway [69, 70]. A tracheal tube with small lumen may be required due to possible presence of sub-glottic stenosis. A laryngeal mask airway (LMA) has been used successfully in a DS child suffering from atlanto-axial dislocation [27]. A thorough pre-operative respiratory assessment is essential for successful intraoperative course.

The anesthesiologist should be aware of the neurological manifestations of atlantoaxial instability and should be able to assess and document their presence. The anesthesiologist should inform the parents or guardians about the possible risk related to manipulation of the head and neck during the anesthetic procedures and the possible neurologic deficit and injury that could occur and require further management [63]. All DS children should have adequate preoperative neurologic screening and evaluation by the operating surgeon. A cervical roentgenogram in the lateral, extension, and flexion positions is recommended if atlantoaxial joint instability is suspected. Presence of any abnormality requires full investigations prior to surgery. Some authors have advised cervical spine radiographs before any elective surgery in any child with DS. However, the radiographs of the cervical spine are untrustworthy for identification of atlanto-axial subluxation in DS children, and no reliable clinical predictor could be identified and at this time;

there is no agreement in the literature to recommend whether every DS patient should be screened radiologically before an anesthetic/surgical procedure [71, 72].

Patient positioning and manual handling also need to be taken into account. The neck should be maintained in a neutral position which can be achieved by placement of soft collar after induction of anesthesia to avoid extreme flexion, extension or rotation of the neck during the procedure. It is better to leave the collar in place after the procedure to remind the caring staff about the possibility of occurrence of cervical injury and myelopathy and to take care while transferring the child to the postoperative care unit. If there is any sign of cervical myelopathy present before the procedure, consultation with neurosurgeon or orthopedic surgeon should be done and the elective procedure could be postponed until proper addressing of cervical spine stability is done [4].

Thyroid functions should be assessed prior to the procedure and both hypothyroidism of hyperthyroidism should be adequately controlled before elective surgery. Deranged thyroid physiology warrants optimal preoperative preparation. Hypothyroidism may precipitate hypothermia and ultimately may be a causative factor of delay recovery from anesthesia. Oral supplemental therapy is to be given before elective surgery [73]. For emergency surgery; intravenous thyroid hormones with hydrocortisone should be given to prevent myxedema coma. In hyperthyroidism; thyroid storm can occur during intraoperative and postoperative period in inadequately prepared surgical patients [74]. Aspiration during anesthesia could occur to due to presence of gastro-esophageal reflux disease which is common in DS children. They may present with frequent vomiting, reflux of gastric content and sometimes aspiration may lead to aspiration pneumonia. To prevent such reflux, H_2-receptor blockers or non-particulate antacid like sodium citrate *etc.* may be used to decrease the PH in the stomach. Rapid sequence intubation with Sellick maneuver is also helpful [75]. For proper preoperative evaluation of children with DS, some laboratory investigations may be needs. Preoperative diagnostic and laboratory assessments rely on the patient's medical condition, previous history and the nature of the surgical procedures. These investigations are summarized in Table **1**.

Table 1. Shows pre-anesthetic investigations that could be needed in a child with DS.

1- Haematological profile: CBC, bleeding time, clotting time, partial thromboplastin time and prothrombin time, platelet count and hematocrit value.
2- Serum Biochemistry: live function tests, kidney function tests, glucose, electrolytes *etc.*
3- Arterial blood gases (if not available from previous evaluation).
4. Urine analysis
5- Digoxin level; if the child will do cardiac surgery and will need cardiopulmonary bypass (CPB). Rebound elevation of digoxin level and increased sensitivity to its effect were reported after CPC.
6- Sickling test: sickling test should be done when suitable as hypothermia, acidosis, and anemia can induce sickling and crises may occur following CPB and the bypass circuit due to decreased perfusion.
7- Immunological Profile: thyroid function tests, and viral markers
8- The ECG to evaluate rate, rhythm, ventricular strain (ST-T changes), and to detect presence of cardiac hypertrophy.
9- Radiograph of head, neck and chest. The chest X-ray can assess the cardiac size, exclude presence of atelectasis, acute respiratory infection, or elevated hemidiaphragms. X-ray head and neck assesses the atlanto-axial joint. Neck CT or MRI may be requested when clinically indicated.
10- Ultrasonography to evaluate the abdomen
11- Echocardiography (if not performed recently) is usually sufficient to evaluate most of CHD.

Generally, all cardiac medicines should be given as usual on the morning of surgery. However, some anesthetists choose to skip ACE inhibitors to prevent significant hypotension during induction of anesthesia. If the children are on aspirin therapy as prevention of intra-cardiac shunt thrombosis, they must keep using it. Children on warfarin therapy require hospital admission to monitor anticoagulation and to start intravenous heparin before surgery [76]. Pre-anesthetic medication is generally required in children and infants over six months of age as crying and generalized emotional upset deteriorate oxygenation and increase shunting in case of CHD. However, intramuscular pre-medications are better to be avoided to decrease pain-associated stress and better to give the medicines through the mouth, nose or rectum. Oral premedications include use of midazolam (dormicum) 0.5-0.75 mg/kg or diazepam (valium) 0.15 mg/kg plus meperidine 1.5 mg/kg. Nasal midazolam 0.2-0.3 mg/kg or rectal methohexital 25 mg/kg can be used. For parenteral premedication, morphine 0.1-0.2 mg/kg plus pentobarbital 2 mg/kg and scopolamine 0.01 mg/kg can be used. Rectal diclofenac suppository (12.5 mg or 25 mg) can be used as pre emptive analgesia provided that there is no contraindication of its use [77].

4. INTRA-OPERATIVE MANAGEMENT

With proper pre-medication; the child arrive the operating suite in a quiet, or sleeping state which permits to choice the suitable anesthetic induction technique (*e.g.* inhalation of sevoflurane or halothane, intramuscular ketamine, or insertion of an intravenous catheter and use of narcotics, propofol, or barbiturates). The parents have important role in keeping the child calm and quite. Throughout preparation and intake of the induction of anesthesia, titration of the sedatives administered for anxiolysis should be done slowly to reach the required effect otherwise; anxiolytic sedative should not be used at all. Pre-oxygenation with 100% oxygen till the exhaled or end tidal oxygen is at least 90% can be done using CPAP at 10 cm H_2O for 3 to 5 min with the patient in a 25° head-up position [78].

Particular induction techniques may be needed according to the cardiac condition, the child's general health and the presence or absence of gastroesophageal reflux. The speed of induction is affected by the presence of an intra-cardiac or extra-cardiac shunt with a quicker induction using a volatile agent in children with a left-to-right shunt due to increased pulmonary blood flow and the lungs trap even more anesthetic drugs and have an elevated anesthetic concentration. On the other hand, right to left shunt prolongs inhalation induction due to bypassing the lungs, though prolongation is merely moderate. In the right to left shunt, the concentration of anesthetic in the blood coming from the lungs will be diluted by the blood coming directly through the shunt from the right side of the heart to the left side, causing lower concentration of anesthetic in the blood leaving the heart and hence the induction will be slow. This is particularly evident with insoluble anesthetic gases as nitrous oxide and less obvious with the more soluble gases. The desire to raise the concentration too fast in children with right to left shunts should be cautiously controlled. It is also possible to change the shunting direction during use of a volatile inhalation anesthetic. When venous access is difficult especially in infants and young children, mild gaseous induction, using a cupped hand and T piece, with either halothane or sevoflurane in oxygen, frequently permits soft unconsciousness and separation from the parent. It is also reported that there is less need for volatile anesthetic agents than in normal patients which should be considered during anesthesia. Since there is low immunity in such type of patients possibly due to thymus dependent immune-suppression, proper aseptic precautions should be taken for securing the intravenous lines. If central venous line is required; it should be removed as early as possible after surgery together with proper care of peripheral line which should also be removed as early as possible to reduce the chance of nosocomial infection. Intravenous fluid should be used with due precaution especially in those having pulmonary vascular disease. Meticulous care should be directed not to allow air in the intravenous line especially in presence of intra-cardiac shunt to avoid possible occurrence of myocardial or cerebral ischemia. Monitoring of central venous pressure (CVP) & urine output are helpful in such patients. The systemic arterial pressure should be maintained because systemic perfusion will affect the pulmonary blood flow and oxygenation in such patients. The child should be monitored for heart rate, blood pressure, oxygen saturation, capnography and temperature. The degree of intraoperative monitoring depends on the type of surgery and associated co-morbidities in any given patient. Invasive arterial blood pressure (BP) monitoring may be needed if noninvasive BP monitoring is incorrect or unfeasible due to associated morbid obesity. Arterial blood gases can be examined repeatedly to sustain metabolic control as required. Capnography will distinguish severe changes in pulmonary blood flow and cardiac output. Transesophageal echocardiography (TEE) will help in monitoring the cardiac functions intraoperative, particularly during the cardiac surgeries. Any drugs that might increase pulmonary vascular resistance (PVR) and worsen systemic oxygenation should be avoided. Any events that decrease the myocardial contractility and may deteriorate the systemic perfusion and exaggerate the heart failure must be avoided. Apart from these measures proper warming arrangement should be ready to prevent intraoperative hypothermia [14, 66, 79, 80].

Awareness of the anesthesiologist with the anatomical changes and adequate technical maneuvers are of paramount importance, especially in the case of oropharyngeal surgeries. The success of the procedure is based on the anticipation of possible problems and on the adequate interaction between the surgical and anesthetic teams. If the cervical malformation is the cause of cervical instability, with the consequent risk of nerve lesion, avoiding cervical mobilization, not only during airway management, but also during positioning of the patient and the surgery, can prevent this complication. Restriction of the cervical movement and associated abnormalities may hamper the ability to access the airways, complicating the anesthetic-surgical procedure especially during laryngoscopy, intubation, and positioning of the patient for the surgery. Although ventilation with a face mask is usually easy in those patients, the access to the airways represents a great challenge and requires previous planning. Mccoys/Truptis blade can be used to intubate patient in neutral position. The anesthesiologist and surgeon should be extremely careful to avoid inappropriate cervical movements while positioning to prevent neurological damage. If the anesthetic plan includes tracheal intubation in DS children, we should select appropriate size of tracheal tube. Because of the general reduction in the diameter of the tracheal lumen in children with DS; it is recommended to start initial intubation with a tracheal tube that is two -sizes smaller than that usually utilized as determined by the standard formula. The successful use of tracheal intubation with fibrobronchoscopy and of the laryngeal mask has been reported. Fibrobronchoscopy is considered the safest technique. Awake intubation using fibrobronchoscopy have been used successfully by some anesthesiologists, but this technique requires the patient's cooperation, which is not always feasible, especially in children or patients with behavioral changes. Laryngeal mask is an easy option, and it has been used successfully in some patients who are difficult to ventilate after anesthetic induction [26, 81 - 84].

When intubation is expected to be difficult; the anesthesiologist may keep the infant spontaneously breathing and view the larynx under deep inhalational anesthesia or he/she can confirm that ventilation easily assisted by hand, administer a muscle relaxant and then view the larynx. In any child with serious abnormal facial anatomy, the safest approach is to maintain spontaneous ventilation. However, a range of approaches is available if visualization of larynx remains difficult or impossible. The anesthesiologist can insert laryngeal mask airway to provide a patent airway, and to deliver anesthetic agents, and can insert a conduit through which a fiber-optic laryngoscope may be inserted to view the larynx, then a stiff enough guide wire (stylet) may be passed into the trachea followed by removal of the fiber-optic laryngoscope and laryngeal mask airway and insertion of endotracheal tube over the wire into the trachea. Instead, with spontaneous ventilation, an endotracheal tube is cut to length, positioned as a nasopharyngeal airway, and anesthesia continued through one nostril while intubation is done with the fiber-optic laryngoscope through the other. There are several other manners of management that have been described. The Glidescope® Cobalt has a camera included in a reusable handle with a single-use blade bent at 60°. It offers visualization of the laryngeal anatomy on a separate screen. This device can be utilized under direct vision passing *via* centre of the tongue with the head in the neutral position; thus providing a glottic view without the alignment of oral, pharyngeal, and tracheal axes; and preventing neurological injury due to cervical movement [85]. The Airtraq® is a single use indirect laryngoscope which assists to direct the tip of the endotracheal tube into the glottic opening under direct visual control [86]. Once the airway has been secured, ventilation is then adjusted to keep normocapnia, thus preventing vasodilatation and excessive blood loss from the surgery site. Neuromuscular monitor is useful to titer the muscle relaxant dose and reversing the effect [87, 88].

Intra-operative increase in pulmonary vascular resistance (PVR) and development of pulmonary hypertensive crisis can occur in children with CHD and left-to-right shunt which causes reversal of the shunt and development of cyanosis and possibly acidosis. In this situation, immediate measures should be taken to reverse pulmonary hypertension including increasing the PaO_2 and decreasing the $PaCO_2$ (but avoid over distension of the lungs which can also increase PVR. In addition, intravenous fluids should be administered to increase preload. Sodium bicarbonate can reverse any acidosis that may have developed. Phenylephrine can be given to increase the systemic vascular resistance (SVR), and opioids can reduce sympathetic outflow to the pulmonary bed and decrease PVR. Forceful hyperventilation without positive end-expiratory pressure (PEEP) is one of the most effective methods existing to decrease PVR. Acidosis, hypoxia, hypercarbia, increased airway pressure and sympathetic stimulation can be precipitating factors [89]. On the other hand, if the infant with DS will have pulmonary artery banding to decrease the pulmonary flow in cases of severe left-to-right shunt, It is advisable to evade hyperoxia and hyperventilation to prevent rising pulmonary blood flow even more than baseline [90].

Pain-killers should be provided before the child wakes up. Intraoperative and postoperative analgesia must be offered preferably with non-opioid analgesics. If the anesthesiologist is in need to use opioid, he should select ultrashort-acting opioids such as remifentanil. Other ways of pain relief, including regional blocks, must be attempted when feasible, although anatomic restrictions can be a true challenging. Rarely, infiltrating the surgical incision site with local anesthetics is a suitable method to diminish the requirement for postoperative use of opioid analgesia. At the end of surgery, careful assessment for the return of protective airway reflexes and recovery of muscle strength after reversal of neuromuscular blocking agents should be done before tracheal extubation. Tracheal extubation should not be done except when the patient is entirely awake and can follow simple instructions [19].

5. POST-OPERATIVE MANAGEMENT

As any child, children with DS will kept in the recovery room for smooth transition from general anesthesia to the full awake state where the endotracheal tube is removed; breathing treatment can be given as needed; and pain management is given as required. The child should be kept under strict monitoring till he/she is discharged to a regular hospital bed as DS children have a considerably elevated prevalence of complications like airway obstruction, pneumothorax, pleural effusions, and infections in the early postoperative period than non-DS children. There is a tendency for prolonged period of mechanical ventilation in those children [91]. The child will need to be closely observed for any airway obstruction. Adequate pain control should be done the same way of pain management of their age-matched counterparts without DS. Sufficient pain killers should be prescribed to remain the children calm and relaxed as they may not be able to communicate for their pain or discomfort because of their learning disability. It must be put into consideration the patient's ability to request pain medications or to use a patient-controlled analgesia button. If opioids have to be used we should avoid any degree of hypercarbia in the patient who has episodes of intraoperative pulmonary hypertensive crises [92]. If a nerve-block technique will be done as a method of pain management; we should consider the degree of cooperation of the child; otherwise, it is better to incorporate it during a general anesthesia [93]. As the child will be agitated from unfamiliar environment, a family member or care give is better to accompany him/her. Presence of familiar face of a parent or care-giver as the child awakes; will help to sooth him/her and to prevent the patient from possibly injuring him/herself (*i.e.* pulling out the IV, falling out of bed, eating something they should not). Presence of family member with the children will also decrease the chance of their dissatisfaction with the anesthesia [94]. If no family member will be available, a sitter should be assigned to the child for close monitoring and observation and to prevent self-injury and will help the post-anesthetic recovery practitioner to provide improved child care.

The child should be monitored intimately in the recovery room till complete recovery from anesthesia. Apnea and airway obstruction are very common in children with DS. Decreased SpO_2 can be caused by occlusion of the upper respiratory tract following opioid drug overdose, or deep sedation; transient glossoptosis caused by decreased tone or swelling; or due to the use of instruments such as those used for maintaining mouth opening during oral manipulations [95]. Prolonged desaturation can occur due to atelectasis after general anesthesia or due to undiagnosed interstitial lung diseases. Alveolar hypoplasia, over distension of air spaces, interstitial emphysema and alveolar septitis are principal factors for the possible occurrence of postoperative respiratory failure in DS. The lesser alveolar surface area with decrease of capillary surface area may aggravate pre-existing pulmonary hypertension [31].

Hypotonia may also influence the capability to preserve an opened airway. It can be controlled by easy airway maneuvers like head tilt, chin lift or jaw thrust; or proper positioning of the child in the lateral position to preserve patency of the airway. If atlanto-axial instability is assumed or present, only the jaw thrust maneuver is allowed Use of airway appliances (oropharyngeal or nasopharyngeal airway) may be useful. However, their use will rely on the degree of consciousness of the child. It is better to leave the child to wear cervical collar to remind the health care providers to be more careful while manipulating the child. Post-extubation stridor and croup is more common in children with DS and estimated to be 1.8% of the operated children.

If the child had difficulty during intubation, extubation should be done very carefully and in a very organized condition; same like what was done in difficult intubation. The croup can be managed by inhalation of humidified oxygen, nebulised racemic epinephrine (400 mcg/kg – max. dose 5 mg) and intravenous dexamethasone (250 mcg/kg is given as initial dose followed by 100 mcg/kg/6hrs for 3 doses). If nebulised epinephrine is used, the child should be monitored by ECG for risk of development of arrhythmia and tachycardia. Epinephrine should be stopped if the child developed tachycardia with heart rate more than 200/min or if any arrhythmia occurs [31].

Elevation of pulmonary artery pressure and development of pulmonary hypertensive crises may occur especially with tracheal suctioning and the weaning from the respirator and could be resistant to therapy [96]. However, infants operated on before the age of 6 months are unlikely to develop pulmonary hypertensive crises during the postoperative period. Inhaled nitric oxide is very effective in management of such crises [97]. Care should be oriented against development of postoperative renal failure which may need either haemodialysis or peritoneal dialysis. It could result from development of cardio-renal syndrome or from previous use of anti-congestive medications. Infection is also a common problem in post-operative phase in DS children most probably due to impaired immune responses. These children have also increased prevalence of autoimmunity, including hypothyroidism. Postoperative isolated thrombocytopenia, thrombocytosis and numerous other hematological disorders are frequently encountered in DS children [98].

Late complications can also occur after repeated anesthesia. Human studies suggest that multiple anesthetics prior to age 4 may be associated with learning difficulties. Exposure less than 2 hours did not appear to be linked to learning problems. Most of the surgical procedures that children with DS are in need to (*e.g.* ear tubes, tonsillectomy) usually last less than 60 minutes. However, delay surgery (and anesthesia) should be avoided when medically necessary as there is no clear evidence that anesthetics are unsafe for children [99].

CONCLUSION

Sedation and anesthesia are frequently needed for children with DS; either for imaging procedure or for surgical intervention. Anesthetic care for children with DS may be a real challenge even for the most well experienced anesthesiologist.

This challenge arises from the increased frequency of numerous functional co morbidities that are frequently encountered in these children. During sedation or anesthesia; they are more liable to have difficult airway, altered respiratory mechanics, problems related to gastric reflux, cardiovascular compromise and neuromuscular problems. Orientation with these frequent problems can help anesthesiologist to arrange safer practice in DS people.

CONFLICT OF INTEREST

The authors confirm that this chapter contents have no conflict of interest.

ACKNOWLEDGEMENTS

Declared none.

REFERENCES

[1] Hoffman JI, Kaplan S. The incidence of congenital heart disease. J Am Coll Cardiol 2002; 39(12): 1890-900.
[http://dx.doi.org/10.1016/S0735-1097(02)01886-7] [PMID: 12084585]

[2] Bhattacharyya A, Svendsen CN. Human neural stem cells: a new tool for studying cortical development in Down's syndrome. Genes Brain Behav 2003; 2(3): 179-86.
[http://dx.doi.org/10.1034/j.1601-183X.2003.00025.x] [PMID: 12931791]

[3] Brandt BR. Pain in Down's syndrome. Lancet 2001; 357(9261): 1041-2.
[http://dx.doi.org/10.1016/S0140-6736(05)71612-3] [PMID: 11293619]

[4] Ihringer K, Russ N, Walther A, Schiff JH. [Anesthesiological considerations for patients with trisomy 21 (Down syndrome)]. Anaesthesist 2013; 62(5): 407-19.
[http://dx.doi.org/10.1007/s00101-013-2170-1] [PMID: 23657534]

[5] Yoshikawa F, Tamaki Y, Okumura H, *et al.* Risk factors with intravenous sedation for patients with disabilities. Anesth Prog 2013; 60(4): 153-61. [INSERT FIGURE 002].
[http://dx.doi.org/10.2344/0003-3006-60.4.153] [PMID: 24423418]

[6] Khin Hla T, Hegarty M, Russell P, Drake-Brockman TF, Ramgolam A, von Ungern-Sternberg BS. Perception of pediatric pain: a comparison of postoperative pain assessments between child, parent, nurse, and independent observer. Paediatr Anaesth 2014; 24(11): 1127-31.
[http://dx.doi.org/10.1111/pan.12484] [PMID: 25074484]

[7] Jones CT, Raman VT, DeVries S, Cole JW, Kelleher KJ, Tobias JD. Optimizing Anticonvulsant Administration for Children Before Anesthesia: A Quality Improvement Project. Pediatr Neurol 2014 Nov; 51(5): 632-40.
[http://dx.doi.org/10.1016/j.pediatrneurol.2014.07.029] [PMID: 25193412]

[8] Gibert S, Sabourdin N, Louvet N, *et al.* Epileptogenic effect of sevoflurane: determination of the

minimal alveolar concentration of sevoflurane associated with major epileptoid signs in children. Anesthesiology 2012; 117(6): 1253-61.
[http://dx.doi.org/10.1097/ALN.0b013e318273e272] [PMID: 23103557]

[9] Kerz T, Jantzen JP. A myoclonic seizure during propofol-alfentanil anesthesia? 1992 Jul; 41(7): 426-30.
[PMID: 1497134]

[10] Li X, Zuo Y, Dai Y. Children's seizures caused by continuous intravenous infusion of tramadol analgesia: two rare case reports. Paediatr Anaesth 2012; 22(3): 308-9.
[http://dx.doi.org/10.1111/j.1460-9592.2011.03765.x] [PMID: 22272680]

[11] Manohar C, Avitsian R, Lozano S, Gonzalez-Martinez J, Cata JP. The effect of antiepileptic drugs on coagulation and bleeding in the perioperative period of epilepsy surgery: the Cleveland Clinic experience. J Clin Neurosci 2011; 18(9): 1180-4.
[http://dx.doi.org/10.1016/j.jocn.2011.02.018] [PMID: 21757355]

[12] Kira S. [Resistance to vecuronium induced muscle relaxation in a patient with mental retardation receiving phenytoin for chronic anticonvulsant therapy]. Masui 2011; 60(1): 80-3.
[PMID: 21348254]

[13] Chowdhury L, Laha A, Chaudhuri T, Chatterjee S. Chronic phenytoin therapy-induced vecuronium resistance. Indian J Pharmacol 2011; 43(2): 214-5.
[http://dx.doi.org/10.4103/0253-7613.77378] [PMID: 21572664]

[14] Bhattarai B, Kulkarni AH, Rao ST, Mairpadi A. Anesthetic consideration in downs syndrome--a review. Nepal Med Coll J 2008; 10(3): 199-203.
[PMID: 19253867]

[15] Kumar S, Verma VK, Kumar A, *et al.* Anesthetic consideration in Patients of Down s Syndrome. Journal of Evolution of Medical and Dental Sciences 2014; 3(28)(14): 7715-21.

[16] Roland PS, Rosenfeld RM, Brooks LJ, *et al.* American Academy of Otolaryngology—Head and Neck Surgery Foundation. Clinical practice guideline: Polysomnography for sleep-disordered breathing prior to tonsillectomy in children. Otolaryngol Head Neck Surg 2011; 145(1) (Suppl.): S1-S15.
[http://dx.doi.org/10.1177/0194599811409837] [PMID: 21676944]

[17] Luscri N, Tobias JD. Monitored anesthesia care with a combination of ketamine and dexmedetomidine during magnetic resonance imaging in three children with trisomy 21 and obstructive sleep apnea. Paediatr Anaesth 2006; 16(7): 782-6.
[http://dx.doi.org/10.1111/j.1460-9592.2006.01857.x] [PMID: 16879522]

[18] Rahimi E, Mariappan R, Tharmaradinam S, Manninen P, Venkatraghavan L. Perioperative management and complications in patients with obstructive sleep apnea undergoing transsphenoidal surgery: Our institutional experience. J Anaesthesiol Clin Pharmacol 2014; 30(3): 351-4.
[http://dx.doi.org/10.4103/0970-9185.137266] [PMID: 25190942]

[19] Adesanya AO, Lee W, Greilich NB, Joshi GP. Perioperative management of obstructive sleep apnea. Chest 2010; 138(6): 1489-98.
[http://dx.doi.org/10.1378/chest.10-1108] [PMID: 21138886]

[20] McNicholas WT, Ryan S. Obstructive sleep apnoea syndrome: translating science to clinical practice.

Respirology 2006; 11(2): 136-44.
[http://dx.doi.org/10.1111/j.1440-1843.2006.00824.x] [PMID: 16548897]

[21] Schloo BL, Vawter GF, Reid LM. Down syndrome: patterns of disturbed lung growth. Hum Pathol 1991; 22(9): 919-23.
[http://dx.doi.org/10.1016/0046-8177(91)90183-P] [PMID: 1833304]

[22] Fernhall B, Pitetti KH, Rimmer JH, *et al.* Cardiorespiratory capacity of individuals with mental retardation including Down syndrome. Med Sci Sports Exerc 1996; 28(3): 366-71.
[PMID: 8776225]

[23] Piatti G, Allegra L, Ambrosetti U, De Santi MM. Nasal ciliary function and ultrastructure in Down syndrome. Laryngoscope 2001; 111(7): 1227-30.
[http://dx.doi.org/10.1097/00005537-200107000-00016] [PMID: 11568545]

[24] Cooney TP, Wentworth PJ, Thurlbeck WM. Diminished radial count is found only postnatally in Down's syndrome. Pediatr Pulmonol 1988; 5(4): 204-9.
[http://dx.doi.org/10.1002/ppul.1950050405] [PMID: 2976929]

[25] Van Cleve SN, Cohen WI. Part I: clinical practice guidelines for children with Down syndrome from birth to 12 years. J Pediatr Health Care 2006; 20(1): 47-54.
[PMID: 16399479]

[26] Shott SR. Down syndrome: analysis of airway size and a guide for appropriate intubation. Laryngoscope 2000; 110(4): 585-92.
[http://dx.doi.org/10.1097/00005537-200004000-00010] [PMID: 10764002]

[27] Nakazawa K, Ikeda D, Ishikawa S, Makita K. A case of difficult airway due to lingual tonsillar hypertrophy in a patient with Down's syndrome. Anesth Analg 2003; 97(3): 704-5.
[http://dx.doi.org/10.1213/01.ANE.0000074347.64382.A4] [PMID: 12933389]

[28] Bevilacqua S, Nicolini A, Del Sarto P, *et al.* [Difficult intubation in paediatric cardiac surgery. Significance of age. Association with Down's syndrome]. Minerva Anestesiol 1996; 62(7-8): 259-64.
[PMID: 8999376]

[29] Hartley B, Newton M, Albert A. Down's syndrome and anaesthesia. Paediatr Anaesth 1998; 8(2): 182-3.
[PMID: 9549752]

[30] Yamaki S, Horiuchi T, Takahashi T. Pulmonary changes in congenital heart disease with Down's syndrome: their significance as a cause of postoperative respiratory failure. Thorax 1985; 40(5): 380-6.
[http://dx.doi.org/10.1136/thx.40.5.380] [PMID: 3161204]

[31] Sinha R, Thangaswamy CR, Muthiah T, Chandra P, Subramaniam R. Prolonged postoperative desaturation in a child with Down syndrome and atrial septal defect. Indian J Anaesth 2011; 55(6): 608-10.
[http://dx.doi.org/10.4103/0019-5049.90619] [PMID: 22223907]

[32] Ramamoorthy C, Haberkern CM, Bhananker SM. Anesthesia-related cardiac arrest in children with heart disease: data from the Pediatric Perioperative Cardiac Arrest (POCA) registry. Anesth Analg 2010 May 1; 110(5): 1376-82.
[PMID: 20103543]

[33] Simić D, Djukic M, Budić I, Milojević I, Strajina V. [Anaesthesia for noncardiac surgery in children with congenital heart disease]. Srp Arh Celok Lek 2011; 139(1-2): 107-15. [http://dx.doi.org/10.2298/SARH1102107S] [PMID: 21568092]

[34] Lake CL. Anesthesia for noncardiac surgery in children with congenital heart disease. Anestesiología 2004; 27(1): 63-6.

[35] McGlothlin D, Ivascu N, Heerdt PM. Anesthesia and pulmonary hypertension. Prog Cardiovasc Dis 2012; 55(2): 199-217. [http://dx.doi.org/10.1016/j.pcad.2012.08.002] [PMID: 23009916]

[36] Subramaniam K, Yared JP. Management of pulmonary hypertension in the operating room. Semin Cardiothorac Vasc Anesth 2007; 11(2): 119-36. [http://dx.doi.org/10.1177/1089253207301733] [PMID: 17536116]

[37] Hosseinian L. Pulmonary hypertension and noncardiac surgery: implications for the anesthesiologist. J Cardiothorac Vasc Anesth 2014; 28(4): 1076-86. [http://dx.doi.org/10.1053/j.jvca.2013.11.017] [PMID: 24675000]

[38] Finesilver C. A new age for childhood diseases. Down syndrome. RN 2002; 65(11): 43-8. [PMID: 12465526]

[39] Pueschel SM, Werner JC. Mitral valve prolapse in persons with Down syndrome. Res Dev Disabil 1994; 15(2): 91-7. [http://dx.doi.org/10.1016/0891-4222(94)90015-9] [PMID: 8085032]

[40] Kraemer FW, Stricker PA, Gurnaney HG, *et al.* Bradycardia during induction of anesthesia with sevoflurane in children with Down syndrome. Anesth Analg 2010; 111(5): 1259-63. [http://dx.doi.org/10.1213/ANE.0b013e3181f2eacf] [PMID: 20736433]

[41] Al-Biltagi M. Echocardiography in children with Down syndrome. World J Clin Pediatr 2013 Nov 8; 2(4): 36-45. [http://dx.doi.org/10.5409/wjcp.v2.i4.36] [PMID: 25254173]

[42] Recalde AL, Landing BH, Lipsey AI. Increased cardiac muscle fiber size and reduced cell number in Down syndrome: heart muscle cell number in Down syndrome. Pediatr Pathol 1986; 6(1): 47-53. [http://dx.doi.org/10.3109/15513818609025924] [PMID: 2950384]

[43] Russo MG, Pacileo G, Marino B, *et al.* Echocardiographic evaluation of left ventricular systolic function in the Down syndrome. Am J Cardiol 1998; 81(10): 1215-7. [http://dx.doi.org/10.1016/S0002-9149(98)00094-0] [PMID: 9604950]

[44] O'Driscoll DM, Horne RS, Davey MJ, *et al.* Cardiac and sympathetic activation are reduced in children with Down syndrome and sleep disordered breathing. Sleep 2012; 35(9): 1269-75. [http://dx.doi.org/10.5665/sleep.2084] [PMID: 22942505]

[45] American Academy of Pediatrics. Committee on Genetics. American Academy of Pediatrics: Health supervision for children with Down syndrome. Pediatrics 2001; 107(2): 442-9. [http://dx.doi.org/10.1542/peds.107.2.442] [PMID: 11158488]

[46] Van Riper M, Cohen WI. Caring for children with Down syndrome and their families. J Pediatr Health Care 2001; 15(3): 123-31. [http://dx.doi.org/10.1067/mph.2001.110627] [PMID: 11353361]

[47] Cohen WI. Healthcare Guidelines for child with downs syndrome. Downs Syndr Q 1996; 12: 1-11.

[48] Moore SW. Down syndrome and the enteric nervous system. Pediatr Surg Int 2008; 24(8): 873-83. [http://dx.doi.org/10.1007/s00383-008-2188-7] [PMID: 18633623]

[49] Dayal D, Jain P, Panigrahi I, Bhattacharya A, Sachdeva N. Thyroid dysfunction in Indian children with down syndrome. Indian Pediatr 2014 Sep; 51(9): 751-2. [http://dx.doi.org/10.1007/s13312-014-0495-8] [PMID: 25228616]

[50] King K, O'Gorman C, Gallagher S. Thyroid dysfunction in children with Down syndrome: a literature review. Ir J Med Sci 2014; 183(1): 1-6. [http://dx.doi.org/10.1007/s11845-013-0994-y] [PMID: 23934377]

[51] Prasher VP. Down syndrome and thyroid disorders: a review. Downs Syndr Res Pract 1999; 6(1): 25-42. [http://dx.doi.org/10.3104/reviews.95] [PMID: 10890245]

[52] Murkin JM. Anesthesia and hypothyroidism: a review of thyroxine physiology, pharmacology, and anesthetic implications. Anesth Analg 1982; 61(4): 371-83. [http://dx.doi.org/10.1213/00000539-198204000-00012] [PMID: 7039417]

[53] Mizuno J, Nakayama Y, Dohi T, Tokioka H. [A case of hypothyroidism found by delayed awakening after the operation]. Masui 2000; 49(3): 305-8. [PMID: 10752328]

[54] Herbst A, Kiess W. [Type 1 diabetes mellitus. Perioperative management of children and adolescents]. Anaesthesist 2007; 56(5): 454-60. [http://dx.doi.org/10.1007/s00101-007-1168-y] [PMID: 17364186]

[55] Anwar AJ, Walker JD, Frier BM. Type 1 diabetes mellitus and Down's syndrome: prevalence, management and diabetic complications. Diabet Med 1998; 15(2): 160-3. [http://dx.doi.org/10.1002/(SICI)1096-9136(199802)15:2<160::AID-DIA537>3.0.CO;2-J] [PMID: 9507919]

[56] H Aburawi E, Nagelkerke N, Deeb A, Abdulla S, Abdulrazzaq YM. National Growth Charts for United Arab Emirates Children With Down Syndrome From Birth to 15 Years of Age. J Epidemiol 2014; 6 [http://dx.doi.org/10.2188/jea.JE20130081]

[57] Baines D. Anaesthetic considerations for the obese child. Paediatr Respir Rev 2011; 12(2): 144-7. [http://dx.doi.org/10.1016/j.prrv.2010.10.002] [PMID: 21458744]

[58] Bruwier A, Chantrain CF. Hematological disorders and leukemia in children with Down syndrome. Eur J Pediatr 2012; 171(9): 1301-7. [http://dx.doi.org/10.1007/s00431-011-1624-1] [PMID: 22113227]

[59] Bull MJ. Committee on Genetics. Health supervision for children with Down syndrome. Pediatrics 2011; 128(2): 393-406. [http://dx.doi.org/10.1542/peds.2011-1605] [PMID: 21788214]

[60] Menghraj SJ. Anaesthetic considerations in children with congenital heart disease undergoing non-cardiac surgery. Indian J Anaesth 2012; 56(5): 491-5. [http://dx.doi.org/10.4103/0019-5049.103969] [PMID: 23293389]

[61] Cohen WI. Atlantoaxial instability. What's next? Arch Pediatr Adolesc Med 1998; 152(2): 119-22. [http://dx.doi.org/10.1001/archpedi.152.2.119] [PMID: 9491035]

[62] Pueschel SM. Should children with Down syndrome be screened for atlantoaxial instability? Arch Pediatr Adolesc Med 1998; 152(2): 123-5. [http://dx.doi.org/10.1001/archpedi.152.2.123] [PMID: 9491036]

[63] Harley EH, Collins MD. Neurologic sequelae secondary to atlantoaxial instability in Down syndrome. Implications in otolaryngologic surgery. Arch Otolaryngol Head Neck Surg 1994; 120(2): 159-65. [http://dx.doi.org/10.1001/archotol.1994.01880260031007] [PMID: 8297573]

[64] Dedlow ER, Siddiqi S, Fillipps DJ, Kelly MN, Nackashi JA, Tuli SY. Symptomatic atlantoaxial instability in an adolescent with trisomy 21 (Down's syndrome). Clin Pediatr (Phila) 2013; 52(7): 633-8. [http://dx.doi.org/10.1177/0009922813482178] [PMID: 23564301]

[65] Meitzner MC, Skurnowicz JA. Anesthetic considerations for patients with Down syndrome. AANA J 2005; 73(2): 103-7. [PMID: 15835829]

[66] Lack CL. Anesthesia for noncardiac surgery in children with congenital heart disease. Revista Mexicana de Anestesiología 2004; 27(1): 63-6.

[67] Kawai T, Wada Y, Enmoto T, *et al.* Comparison of hemodynamic data before and after corrective surgery for Down's syndrome and ventricular septal defect. Heart Vessels 1995; 10(3): 154-7. [http://dx.doi.org/10.1007/BF01744483] [PMID: 7673086]

[68] Borland LM, Colligan J, Brandom BW. Frequency of anesthesia-related complications in children with Down syndrome under general anesthesia for noncardiac procedures. Paediatr Anaesth 2004; 14(9): 733-8. [http://dx.doi.org/10.1111/j.1460-9592.2004.01329.x] [PMID: 15330954]

[69] Clarke RW. Ear, nose and throat problems in children with Down syndrome. Br J Hosp Med (Lond) 2005; 66(9): 504-6. [http://dx.doi.org/10.12968/hmed.2005.66.9.19700] [PMID: 16200785]

[70] Ng A, Vas L, Goel S. Difficult paediatric intubation when fibreoptic laryngoscopy fails. Paediatr Anaesth 2002; 12(9): 801-5. [http://dx.doi.org/10.1046/j.1460-9592.2002.00925.x] [PMID: 12519141]

[71] Uno K, Kataoka O, Shiba R. Occipitoatlantal and occipitoaxial hypermobility in Down syndrome. Spine (Phila Pa 1976) 1996 Jun 15; 21(12): 1430-4. [http://dx.doi.org/10.1097/00007632-199606150-00006] [PMID: 8792519]

[72] Selby KA, Newton RW, Gupta S, Hunt L. Clinical predictors and radiological reliability in atlantoaxial subluxation in Down's syndrome. Arch Dis Child 1991; 66(7): 876-8. [http://dx.doi.org/10.1136/adc.66.7.876] [PMID: 1830735]

[73] Bajwa SJ, Sehgal V. Anesthesia and thyroid surgery: The never ending challenges. Indian J Endocrinol Metab 2013; 17(2): 228-34. [http://dx.doi.org/10.4103/2230-8210.109671] [PMID: 23776893]

[74] Aderinto-Adike AO, Quigley EM. Gastrointestinal motility problems in critical care: a clinical perspective. J Dig Dis 2014; 15(7): 335-44.
[http://dx.doi.org/10.1111/1751-2980.12147] [PMID: 24673805]

[75] Neuhaus D, Schmitz A, Gerber A, Weiss M. Controlled rapid sequence induction and intubation - an analysis of 1001 children. Paediatr Anaesth 2013; 23(8): 734-40.
[http://dx.doi.org/10.1111/pan.12213] [PMID: 23763293]

[76] White MC. Approach to managing children with heart disease for noncardiac surgery. Paediatr Anaesth 2011; 21(5): 522-9.
[http://dx.doi.org/10.1111/j.1460-9592.2010.03416.x] [PMID: 20880154]

[77] Frascaroli G, Fucà A, Buda S, Gargiulo G, Pace C. [Anesthesia for non-cardiac surgery in children with congenital heart diseases]. Minerva Anestesiol 2003; 69(5): 460-7.
[PMID: 12768185]

[78] Delay JM, Sebbane M, Jung B, *et al.* The effectiveness of noninvasive positive pressure ventilation to enhance preoxygenation in morbidly obese patients: a randomized controlled study. Anesth Analg 2008; 107(5): 1707-13.
[http://dx.doi.org/10.1213/ane.0b013e318183909b] [PMID: 18931236]

[79] Kobel M, Creighton RE, Steward DJ. Anaesthetic considerations in Down's syndrome: experience with 100 patients and a review of the literature. Can Anaesth Soc J 1982; 29(6): 593-9.
[http://dx.doi.org/10.1007/BF03007747] [PMID: 6215973]

[80] Levin S, Schlesinger M, Handzel Z, *et al.* Thymic deficiency in Down's syndrome. Pediatrics 1979; 63(1): 80-7.
[PMID: 155804]

[81] Nargozian C. The airway in patients with craniofacial abnormalities. Paediatr Anaesth 2004; 14(1): 53-9.
[http://dx.doi.org/10.1046/j.1460-9592.2003.01200.x] [PMID: 14717875]

[82] Manivel S, Prasad R, Jacob R. Anesthetic management of a child with Klippel-Feil syndrome in the radiology suite. Paediatr Anaesth 2005; 15(2): 171-2.
[http://dx.doi.org/10.1111/j.1460-9592.2005.01492.x] [PMID: 15675938]

[83] Naguib M, Farag H. Ibrahim A el-W. Anaesthetic considerations in Klippel-Feil syndrome. Can Anaesth Soc J 1986; 33(1): 66-70.
[http://dx.doi.org/10.1007/BF03010911] [PMID: 3948050]

[84] Cakmakkaya OS, Kaya G, Altintas F, Bakan M, Yildirim A. Anesthetic management of a child with Arnold-Chiari malformation and Klippel-Feil syndrome. Paediatr Anaesth 2006; 16(3): 355-6.
[http://dx.doi.org/10.1111/j.1460-9592.2005.01795.x] [PMID: 16490108]

[85] Redel A, Karademir F, Schlitterlau A, *et al.* Validation of the GlideScope video laryngoscope in pediatric patients. Paediatr Anaesth 2009; 19(7): 667-71.
[http://dx.doi.org/10.1111/j.1460-9592.2009.03046.x] [PMID: 19638111]

[86] Vlatten A, Soder C. Airtraq optical laryngoscope intubation in a 5-month-old infant with a difficult airway because of Robin Sequence. Paediatr Anaesth 2009; 19(7): 699-700.
[http://dx.doi.org/10.1111/j.1460-9592.2009.03038.x] [PMID: 19638117]

[87] Dubreuil M, Ecoffey C. Laryngeal mask guided tracheal intubation in paediatricanaesthesia. Paediatr Anaesth 1992; 2: 344.

[88] Patil AD, Nandi A, Sathe V. Anaesthesia for a Child with Down syndrome Undergoing Cleft Palate Repair and Review of Anaesthesia Management of Other Associated Congenital Syndromes. IOSR Journal of Dental and Medical Sciences 2014; 13(2): 32-9.

[89] Saji T. Clinical characteristics of pulmonary arterial hypertension associated with Down syndrome. Pediatr Int 2014; 56(3): 297-303.
[http://dx.doi.org/10.1111/ped.12349] [PMID: 24689825]

[90] Smolinsky AK, Shinfeld A, Paret G, *et al.* End-tidal CO2 levels are a reliable indicator of band tightness in pulmonary artery banding. Ann Thorac Surg 1995; 60(6) (Suppl.): S523-4.
[http://dx.doi.org/10.1016/0003-4975(95)00852-7] [PMID: 8604925]

[91] Desai AR, Branco RG, Comitis GA, *et al.* Early postoperative outcomes following surgical repair of complete atrioventricular septal defects: is down syndrome a risk factor? Pediatr Crit Care Med 2014; 15(1): 35-41.
[http://dx.doi.org/10.1097/PCC.0000000000000004] [PMID: 24201860]

[92] Van Driest SL, Shah A, Marshall MD, *et al.* Opioid use after cardiac surgery in children with Down syndrome. Pediatr Crit Care Med 2013; 14(9): 862-8.
[http://dx.doi.org/10.1097/PCC.0b013e31829f5d9d] [PMID: 23962833]

[93] Tsang R, Checchia PA. Defining adequate pain control in the child with Down syndrome: are we treating perception or reality? Pediatr Crit Care Med 2013; 14(9): 899-900.
[http://dx.doi.org/10.1097/PCC.0b013e3182a54dd3] [PMID: 24226557]

[94] Schiff JH, Russ N, Ihringer K, Heal C, Martin E, Walther A. Pediatric patients with disabilities - assessment of satisfaction with anesthesia. Paediatr Anaesth 2012; 22(11): 1117-23.
[http://dx.doi.org/10.1111/j.1460-9592.2012.03886.x] [PMID: 22738165]

[95] Infosino A. Pediatric upper airway and congenital anomalies. Anesthesiol Clin North America 2002; 20(4): 747-66.
[http://dx.doi.org/10.1016/S0889-8537(02)00018-4] [PMID: 12512261]

[96] Soneda J, Ban T, Okamoto Y, Matsuda K, Sakamoto K, Yamada T. [Severe postoperative pulmonary hypertensive crisis in a case of ventricular septal defect with Down's syndrome]. Nippon Kyobu Geka Gakkai Zasshi 1989; 37(6): 1247-50.
[PMID: 2530290]

[97] Seale A, Shinebourne EA. Cardiac problems in Down syndrome. Curr Paediatr 2004; 14: 33-8.
[http://dx.doi.org/10.1016/j.cupe.2003.09.005]

[98] Tóth R, Szántó P, Prodán Z, *et al.* Down syndrome and postoperative complications after paediatric cardiac surgery: a propensity-matched analysis. Interact Cardiovasc Thorac Surg 2013; 17(4): 691-7.
[http://dx.doi.org/10.1093/icvts/ivt267] [PMID: 23832837]

[99] Flick RP, Katusic SK, Colligan RC, *et al.* Cognitive and behavioral outcomes after early exposure to anesthesia and surgery Pediatrics 2011; 128(5): e1053-61.
[http://dx.doi.org/10.1542/peds.2011-0351] [PMID: 21969289]

CHAPTER 12

Dental Problems in Down Syndrome Children

Mohammed Al-Biltagi[1,*], Ahmed Kamal Saeed[2], John Jacob Meakkara[3], Vikas Raj Somarajan[3]

[1] *Pediatric Department, Faculty of Medicine, Tanta University, Egypt*

[2] *Ministry of Health, Kingdom of Bahrain*

[3] *International Hospital of Bahrain, Kingdom of Bahrain.*

Abstract: Down syndrome (DS) is a common malformation affecting the whole body with a unique craniofacial and distinctive oral feature and anomalies. These dental anomalies and the associated systemic manifestations of children with DS pose real challenges to the dentist as well as the pediatrician which necessitate a multidisciplinary team to be involved in taking care of children with this syndrome. It is important that the dentist can recognize the types of structural soft tissue and dental abnormalities which are part of the classic features and developmental prototype of D children. The dentist should also be able to detect and to appropriately manage these problems through an integrated team work including the family and the child primary physician. Good oral hygiene and healthy dental life are of paramount importance for an integrated health and better quality of life for such children.

Keywords: Anodontia, Bruxism, Children, Craniofacial, Down syndrome, Gingiva, Gingivitis, Halitosis, Hypotonia, Oral health, Occlusion, Oligodontia, Palate, Periodontitis, Periodontal disease, Taurodontism, Teeth, Tongue, Tracheoesophageal fistula, Tooth agenesis.

1. INTRODUCTION

Down's syndrome (which is also known as trisomy 21, trisomy G, and mongolism) is a systemic disorder occurs as a result of genetic alteration due to triplication of human autosomal chromosome 21 with a frequency of 1/800-1000 live births in different populations. It is the commonest of all malformation

* **Corresponding Author Dr. Mohammed Al-Biltagi:** Associate Professor of Pediatrics, Pediatric Department, Faculty of Medicine, Tanta University, Egypt; Tel: (+973)39545472; Fax: (+973) 1759 0495; Email: mbelrem@hotmail.com

syndromes that affect human beings [1]. It has certain characteristics that affect the whole body including generalized hypotonia, mental retardation, and unique craniofacial and distinctive oral features, regardless of race or ethnicity. Both the dental anomalies and the associated systemic manifestations of children with DS pose real challenges to the dentist as well as the pediatrician which necessitate a multidisciplinary team to be involved in taking care of these children. It is important that the dentist can recognize the types of structural soft tissue and dental abnormalities which are part of the classic features and developmental prototype of D children. An Oral Health Care provider should be aware of all the underlying medical conditions of his patient, the complications that he/she can come across in future, and what precautions one should take to avoid any adverse events in the clinic. Understanding patients' medical condition helps the dentist to start preventive measures early. However, professional care alone is not sufficient enough for good and adequate oral health; support from the parents and (primary) care-givers is of crucial importance [2]. In this chapter; we will discuss the oro-cranial changes, the patho-mechanism, the magnitude and the types of dental problems in children with DS (teeth, gingiva, tongue, palate and occlusion). Clinical significance and management of Dental problems in children with DS as well as proper home care and prevention of these problems will be discussed.

2. CRANIO-FACIAL CHANGES IN CHILDREN WITH DS

Several oro-facial features are characteristic of people with DS. These changes could affect both hard tissues and soft tissues and can affect feeding, chewing, swallowing, and speech.

2.1. Hard Tissues Changes

These features include an overall reduction in head size, short neck together with a modification of head shape; and a relatively concave facial profile. There is a decrease in the interorbital distance, small palpebral fissures, upper slanting of the eyes with epicanthic folds, ocular hypotelorism, strabismus and prominent forehead [3]. With the reduced head size of children with DS, there is also lesser brain size than non-syndromic children with diminution of parietal cortex, and the temporal lobe which occur as a result of improper neural development associated with DS [4]. The mid-facial zone may be less developed, impacting the look of the lips, tongue and palate. There is also hypoplasia of the middle third of the face with poorly developed paranasal air sinuses, with depressed nasal bridge; decreased nasal protrusion, small nose producing an inclined forehead and a flat face with smaller ears. Maxillary development is deficient in vertical height which induces over closure of the mandible and thus protruding the lower arch anteriorly comparative to the upper [5].

The lower third of the face is also reduced with mandibular prognathism. The mandible is smaller (micrognathia) than non-syndromic children. The maxilla, the nasal bridge, and the mid-face bones are less developed than in the normal population, inducing a prognathic occlusal relation, small oral cavity and broader alveolar ridges. The palate, though being of average size, may seem highly arched and narrow. This misleading look is due to the abnormal thickening of the sides of the hard palate. This thickness limits the space amount the tongue can take up in the mouth and influences the capability to talk and chew. Underdevelopment of the mid-face reduces the size and deepness of the palate [6].

There is reduction of the anterior skull base and anterior-posterior cranial base lengths are shorter with a backward inclination of the posterior cranial base in DS children than non syndromic children that cause protrusion and proclination of lower incisors and class III malocclusion. There is also hypoplasia of maxilla and mandible with a retrognathic maxilla and shorter effective length, and increased lower facial height with an increment in the mandibular plane angle, smaller mandibular ramus and body, a tendency to skeletal open bite and a hyperdivergent mandible. Bimaxillary dental protrusion may present in DS children with prominent lips and a reduced nasolabial angle [7].

There are controversial data about the palatal morphology in children with DS. The palate is frequently described as high-arched with narrow palatal vault. Other findings suggest that the palate in DS subjects is generally smaller. Objective evaluation confirmed that the palatals vault in DS is smaller than in normal subjects. The palatal dimensions in DS are in lower depth, and shorter in height. Early hypotonia in DS and lingual diastasis were recognized as an etiological factor of specific palatal morphology with soft tissue prominence along the palatal surfaces of the maxillary dental arch giving the palatal vault an elliptic paraboloid shape. Such a type of palate has been described as shelf-like or stair palate. Lingual diastasis is frequently found in persons with DS and it contributes to the characteristic shape of the palatal vault. In lingual diastasis; a midline prominence of the tongue appears during contractions due to insufficiency of transversal fibers of the genioglossus muscle and insufficiency of the lingual fibrous septum. As a result, the hypotonic tongue is unable to contribute in remodeling of the palatal vault giving the characteristic stair palate. Age changes of palatal shape can lead to a higher frequency of so-called V-shaped palate in children of school age [8, 9]. However; Skrinjarić *et al.* showed no considerable dissimilarity in dental arch morphology between DS patients and non-syndromic subjects. They showed that a specific type of shelf-like palate is dominant during the early years of growth and development and that the increased rate of shelf-like palate is declining by age. They suggested that palatal vault shape is affected by age-related modifications. These changes can be attributed to the increased tonus and function of the tongue and orofacial musculature, which leads to reshaping of the palatal vault in DS patients [10]. Increases in incidence of bifid uvula, submucous cleft and cleft palate with and without cleft lip may present in some children with DS [11].

The teeth in children with DS show total mineralization, but with a huge difference in the eruption pattern, though it keeps a definite resemblance in the order and symmetry. At the same times, congenital anomalies of teeth are extremely frequent affecting both in the primary and permanent teeth in DS children with an incidence five times more than in the normal population including microdontia, hypoplasia, partial anodontia, oligodontia, taurodontism, periodontal disease, and tooth agenesis. Differences in tooth number and shape are the most frequent dental disorders associated with DS. Absence of the lateral incisors is the most common anomaly affecting the primary dentition while absent third molars, second premolars and lateral incisors is the most common anomaly affecting the permanent dentition in this sequence. There is also an increased incidence of congenitally absent teeth in both the primary and permanent dentitions. Agenesis happened more often in the mandible than in the maxilla and most frequently on the left side. Tooth eruption may occur late, and happen in an abnormal order. It can occur 2 to 3 years later than the child's normal eruption pattern. Occasionally, the full deciduous dentition may not occur till the age of 5 years. Over-impacted primary teeth are also frequent. There is an increased rate of over-retained teeth, tooth size reduction, reduced root lengths, changes in tooth shape, excessive tooth wear and hypodontia. Peg laterals, enamel hypo-calcification, shovel-shaped incisors and taurodontic teeth are frequently noted. Association of concomitant hypodontia and supernumeraries was described in some cases with DS [12, 13]. True generalized microdontia is common in permanent teeth in DS individuals. Clinical crowns are commonly conical, small, and short. The reduced crown size of the permanent teeth is associated with reduced both enamel and dentine thickness [14, 15]. The enamel hypoplasia and hypocalcification affect both primary and permanent dentitions. Except for mandibular first premolar, crown and root lengths of permanent teeth are shorter than normal and taurodontism is a common observation in DS persons (Fig. **1**). Taurodontism associated with abnormally short root can decrease the degree of periodontal attachment and increase incidence of tooth mobility frequently seen in DS persons [16].

Numerous occlusion elements are observed with increased rate of malalignment; malocclusion; anterior proclination; open bite; and anterior/posterior cross bite [17]. There is an increased rate of malalignments in both the primary and permanent dentition in children with DS compared with the other non-syndromic children. The most common malalignment in the deciduous dentition in DS children were mesiopalatal, mesiolingual, and mesiovestibular. In the permanent dentition, the most common malalignments are distopalatal or distolingual. Anterior and posterior crowding is also frequently seen in DS individuals. Crowding is common, especially in maxilla, due to underdevelopment [18]. There is an increased frequency of canine impaction (15%), and upper canine/first premolar transposition (15%) in DS individuals, which is mostly due to genetic anomaly and represents another phenotypic expression of DS [19]. The unique craniofacial phenotype of DS subjects can be recognized before birth, by intrauterine ultrasonographic evaluation of facial morphology which is at present a helpful diagnostic tool [20]. Postnatal assessment of these features can be done by conventional anthropometry, or by digital, computerized instruments including optical instruments which allow fast data collection in those children [21].

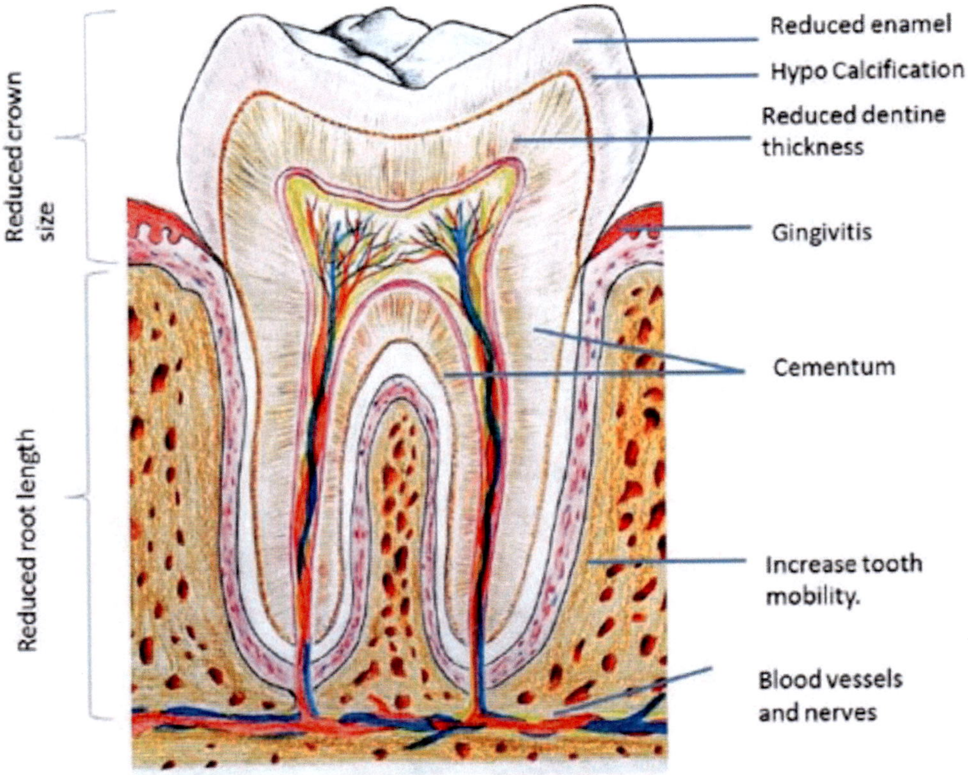

Fig.(1). Showed Down syndrome tooth with reduced crown sized, reduced root length, educed enamel with *hypoplasia*, hypo calcification, reduced dentine thickness, increased incidence of gingivitis and increased tooth mobility.

2.2. Soft Tissues Changes

The chewing, mastication and facial expression muscles of are weak and hypotonic, with some laxity of the temporomandibular joint ligaments. Hypotonia of the lips and cheeks muscle participates in the imbalance of forces on the teeth, with the force of the tongue being of more effect. The lips may grow large and thick. There is also significantly smaller and acute nasolabial angle and protruded and prominent upper and lower lips in children with DS than non-syndromic children [7]. However, more obtuse nasolabial angle was reported in some Sudanese cases which could be due to ethnic differences [22]. Fissured lips are caused by chronic mouth breathing. Hypotonia causes also mouth droop and protrusion of the lower lip. Chronic mouth opening will increase drooling which in turn contributes to development of angular cheilitis. Lingual cracks and fissures usually develop and increase with age due to frictional movement against teeth, diastema, tongue thrusting, tongue sucking, clenching or enlarged tongue. Geographic tongue is frequently seen in DS individuals. Tongue may also have bilateral, unilateral or isolated oval depression and is frequently described as raised white scalloped border [23, 24]. Fissuring of both tongue can cause food impaction and may contribute to halitosis. The tongue is protruded and often located between the dental arches and up against the palate. The tongue is actually normal size but appears large due to the relatively small size mouth cavity with shallow roof. Tongue protrusion and thrusting during drinking, eating, and speaking is reported in the presence of a hypotonic tongue especially when the child is fatigued or in a relaxed state [24].

Generalized hypotonia is one of the characteristic features of DS. It is particularly expressed during the early age of postnatal development. Hypotonia affects the orofacial muscles *e.g.* orbicularis, zygomatic, masseter, and temporalis muscles; as well as tongue participates in impaired oral seal, weak sucking, improper tongue control, and troubles with jaw stability. It has also an important influence on the shaping of palatal morphology. It lets the jaw to fall and the tongue to go forward, producing the distinctive mouth posture. The reduced tongue activity, impaired tongue control, and limited tongue motion caused by the short and narrow palate result in swallowing disorders during drinking and eating and can affect speaking in DS children [25]. Persistent mouth opening occurs as a result of the relatively large tongue compared with the reduced oral cavity and protruded tongue. It occurs also due to the hypotonic orofacial muscles and the associated upper airway obstruction as a result of adenoidal hypertrophy or smaller nasal passages, and obligatory mouth breathing. Hypertrophied lingual tonsils were reported as a cause of upper airway obstruction and mouth breathing [26].

Persistent mouth opening may cause drooling, chapped lower lip, and angular cheilitis or infectious lesion at the corner of the mouth (Fig. **2**). The oral mucosa is thin due to reduced salivary flow rate. Drooling in DS individual is unlikely to be due to hypersalivation, since they demonstrated a reduced stimulated parotid salivary flow rate [27]. Children with DS frequently have an exaggerated gag reflex due to the tongue position, in addition to anxiety related to any oral stimulation. Computerized anthropometry can be performed to quantitatively examine the characteristic facial features of DS patients [28].

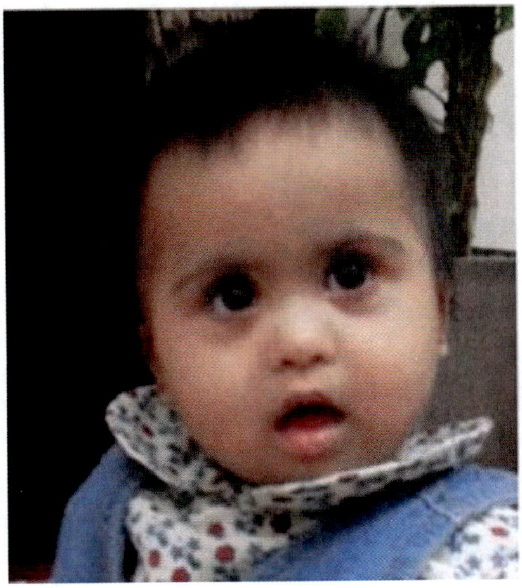

Fig. (2). Persistent mouth opening with drooling, and relatively wide tongue.

3. MAGNITUDE OF DENTAL PROBLEMS IN CHILDREN WITH DS

Dental problem that encountered in children with DS can affect teeth, gingiva, tongue, palate and occlusion. Table **1** summarizes these problems.

Table 1. Unpleasant odours in some industries.

Organ	Problem
General	Reduced oral cavity, open- mouth and mouth- breathing, lack of muscle tone, drooling, bruxism, halitosis, atlanto axial instability.
Maxilla & Mandible	Maxillary hypoplasia; poorly developed para-nasal air sinuses; bimaxillary dental protrusion smaller mandibular ramus and body; hyperdivergent mandible; mandibular prognathism; micrognathia; prognathic occlusal relationship, broader alveolar ridges.
Lips	Angular cheilitis, prominent lips, reduced nasolabial angle, chapped lower lip, perleche, commissural fissures, cleft lip
Tongue	Lingual collapses, geographic tongue, fissured tongue, lingual diastasis, relative macroglossia, hypertrophy of tongue papilla, lingual tonsillar hypertrophy, forward position of the tongue, tongue protrusion, absent changes of the lingual maturation, mucormycosis of the tongue

(Table 1) contd.....

Organ	Problem
Periodontal & Gingival diseases	Marginal gingival inflammation, acute and subacute necrotizing gingivitis, severe chronic periodontitis, gingival recession, increased pocket depth, alveolar bone loss, gingival suppuration or even abscesses, furcation involvement in the molars, increased tooth mobility, attrition, erosion, periodontitis, aggressive periodontitis
Teeth abnormalities	Delayed teething (Both primary and permanent teeth), microdontia, hypoplasia, partial anodontia, oligodontia, taurodontism, tooth agenesis, high incidence of impacted teeth, tooth size reduction, reduced root lengths, changes in tooth shape, excessive tooth wear, enamel hypo-calcification, concomitant hypodontia & supernumeraries, conical crown, reduced crown size of the permanent teeth, reduced enamel and dentine thickness, enamel hypoplasia and hypocalcification, increase incidence of tooth mobility.
Occlusion Disorders	higher frequency of malalignment, malocclusion, anterior proclination, open bite, and anterior/posterior cross bite, crowding, class III Skeletal pattern and malocclusion
Palate	High-arched with narrow palatal vault, V-shaped palate, shelf-like palate, bifid uvula, sub mucous or complete cleft palate,

3.1. Periodontal and Gingival Diseases (Figs. 3 & 4)

Periodontal disease in DS population seems to be a more common and serious problem than non syndromic children and caries has a wide range of presentation; from nondestructive to destructive forms. It occurs commonly due to the poor oral hygiene and the competitive antagonism between cariogenic bacteria and those present in periodontium with pathological changes. Poor oral hygiene commonly observed in DS children can precipitate and manifest as marginal gingival inflammation, acute and subacute necrotizing gingivitis, advanced chronic periodontitis, loss of attachment in form of gingival recession and increased pocket depth, alveolar bone loss, suppuration or even abscesses, furcation involvement in the molars, increased tooth mobility, and even loss of teeth. Attrition and erosion are significantly more frequent in DS than the non-DS patients [29, 30]. Periodontal disease prevalence in DS population is between 58% and 96% for persons younger than 35 years of age. Some races may have increased risk of periodontitis than the others. Adding the genetic disorder of DS to African-Americans race imposes additional risks for periodontitis [31].

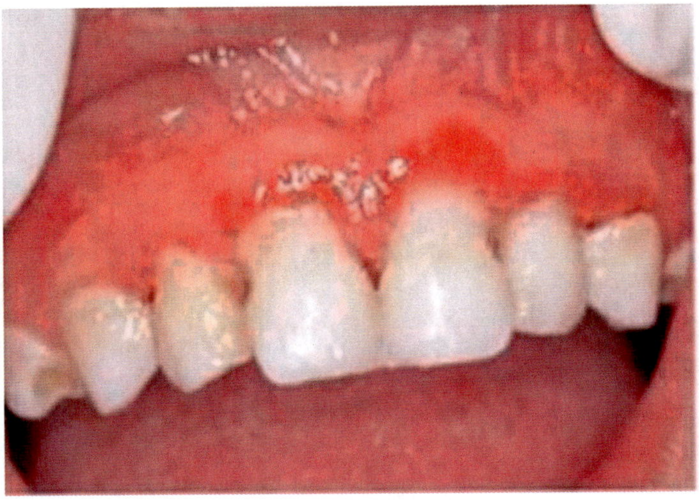

Fig. (3). Gingivitis of the anterior teeth due to improper oral hygiene measures as a result of constant presence of plaques leading to gum inflammation and possible progression to periodontitis.

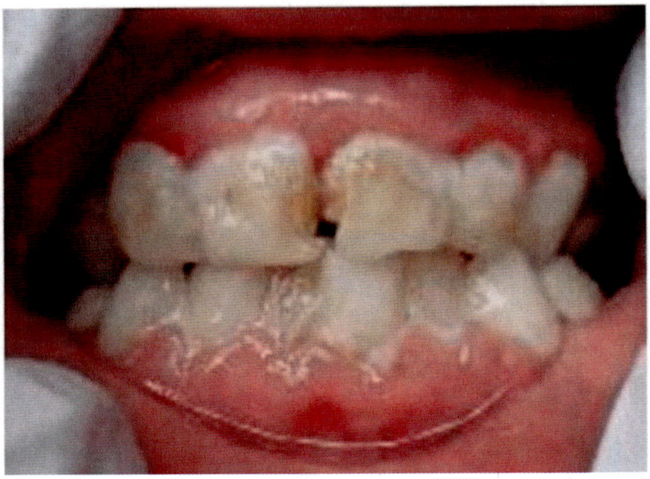

Fig. (4). Gingivitis of the anterior teeth due to improper oral hygiene measures as a result of constant presence of plaques leading to gum inflammation and possible progression to periodontitis.

The increased prevalence of periodontitis in children with DS is related to the increased prevalence of hypodontia, which entails dental instability due to the loss of contact points. Meanwhile; increased prevalence of fused molar roots in DS patients (65.1% in the maxilla and 40.5% in the mandible) as compared to normal subjects (40.5% in the maxilla and 21.1% in the mandible), suggesting that such a high prevalence of molars with fused roots may also be a reason participating in the high prevalence of periodontal disease in DS subjects. Studies have shown an increased prevalence of fused molar roots in DS patients (65.1% in the maxilla and 40.5% in the mandible) as compared to normal subjects (40.5% in the maxilla and 21.1% in the mandible), suggesting that such a high prevalence of molars with fused roots may also be a factor contributing to the high prevalence of periodontal disease in DS subjects. However, both prevalence and degree of periodontal disease among DS persons is improving due to the better dental care available now to this cohort of people since their early life [32, 33].

The extent and severity of gingivitis and the extent of periodontitis mainly located on the lower incisors are greater in the group with DS than in otherwise normal, age-matched control groups [34]. The periodontium is less intact in persons with DS than non-syndromic persons. Early features of periodontitis are commonly observed as early as 11 yr of age in DS children. The mandibular anterior region is the first region to be affected. Greater incidence in the anterior mandibular and posterior maxillary region with periodontal disease is occasionally present in DS children below the age of six, which results in the loss of teeth, usually lower central incisors [35]. Deep pockets are more frequent with rapidly progressing periodontal disease observed in DS group than in the control group [29].

Juvenile periodontitis which is frequently seen in DS children characterizes by young age of onset, severe destruction of periodontal tissues and typical pathogenesis mechanism [36]. Aggressive periodontitis is cauterized by its early-onset, destructive nature of the disease with increased rate of periodontal progression and distinctive clinical features. Colonization by *Actinobacillus actinomycetemcomitans* and *Fusobacterium nucleatum* are strongly related to the onset of gingival inflammation in DS children below the age of 5 years while colonization by *Prevotella intermedia*, *Actinobacillus actinomycetemcomitans*, *Selenomonas sputigena*, and *Streptococcus mitis* in DS is related to development of gingivitis at puberty. There is also a moderate relationship between dental plaque and the severity of gingivitis [37]. Diagnosis of this disease depends on the characteristic clinical, immunologic, microbiologic and genetic profile of the patients. BANA test is used for detection of certain enzymatic activity of bacteria implicated in periodontal disease. It depends on presence of periodontal pathogenic bacteria that generate enzymes able to hydrolyze the synthetic material

N-benzoyl-DL-argininenaphthylamide (BANA). DS Children have an age-dependant increase in the BANA test score. On the other hand, the BANA test score in normal children is not age-dependant but is considerably elevated than that observed in DS children [38]. Oral infections, mainly acute infections, can extend to extra-oral regions and cause severe medical complications, and even mortality. Therefore, rapid diagnosis and adequate treatment are of major importance [39].

3.2. Tongue and Lip Disorders

The frequency of angular cheilitis (angular stomatitis, perleche, commissural fissures) looks to be high in DS persons. Fissures of the lips and angular cheilitis occur in at least 25% of DS patients. A study done in Iran 2007 involving 100 children with DS; showed that fissured tongue was present in 28%, hypertrophy of tongue papilla in 22%, cheilitis in 13%, and geographic tongue in 4% of the group [40, 41]. Lingual collapses are also noted more in DS children than non-syndromic children. Hypertrophy of the lingual tonsils is more frequent in patients with DS than in controls, with increasing frequency with increasing age. C-spine radiograph is usually performed in such children and is proved to be useful in discovering this hypertrophy [42, 43]. Gisel *et al.* found that forward placement of the tongue in the mouth is the most frequent tongue position observed in DS children. They observed also absence of the typical maturational changes that usually observed in normal children of similar age [44]. Oral load with Candida albicans is frequent in DS children. They are notably more heavily colonized by C. albicans than the controls. This extensive colonization with C. albicans is mostly related to abnormalities of the immune response in DS children [45]. However, localized invasive lingual mucormycosis is extremely rare but reported in a 4-month-old immune compromised girl with DS who was admitted in the hospital for severe acute gastroenteritis. She had localized bluish-black discoloration of the oral mucosa and tongue [46].

3.3. Hypodontia (Fig. 5)

Hypodontia is a developmental missing of one or more of primary or permanent teeth as result of failure of teeth development excluding the third molar teeth. It is either syndromic or non-syndromic. Down syndrome is the most frequent genetic reason of hypodontia with approximately 10 times prevalence of missing teeth in the DS persons more than observed in the controls [47]. The prevalence of hypodontia in DS is about 90% if the third molars are considered and between 30% and 60% when the third molars are not considered in the analysis. A very high prevalence of total agenesis of all third molars has also been described. Suri *et al.* reported that the affected subject has 4.74 as an average number of missing teeth when third molars are considered, and 2.78 when third molars are not considered. It is more common and extensive in the females than males with DS. The most commonly affected teeth are (in a descending frequency) maxillary and mandibular third molars followed by maxillary lateral incisors, then mandibular second premolars, then mandibular incisors, then maxillary second premolars and lastly maxillary second molars [48]. In contrast to the general population, bilateral hypodontia is more frequent than unilateral hypodontia in DS children [49].

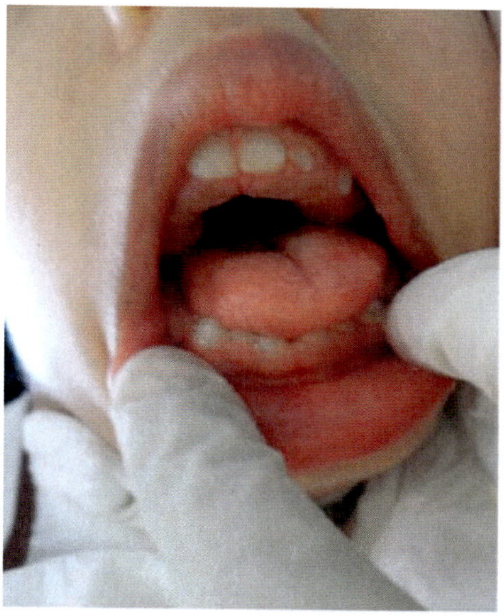

Fig. (5). A 5 year old child who has hypodontia, no canine erupted and even the erupted central and lateral incisors are small and irregular. Observe also the relatively large tongue and the narrow palate.

3.4. Dental Caries (Fig. 6)

Down syndrome children presented lower caries rates as proved by many studies. Macho *et al.* showed that a considerably higher number of DS children (72%)

within the caries-free group in Portuguese children *versus* non DS siblings (46%). This confirms that that DS children have lesser caries prevalence rate [50].This low prevalence may be related to the increased parents' concern about oral health care in DS children, which is reflected in by increasing frequency of dental clinic visits, as well as due to the increased rate of microdontia, hypodontia, and bruxism prevalence, less exposure time to the environmental cariogens, higher salivary pH and bicarbonate levels, spaced dentition, shallow fissures of the teeth, and delayed tooth eruption [51].

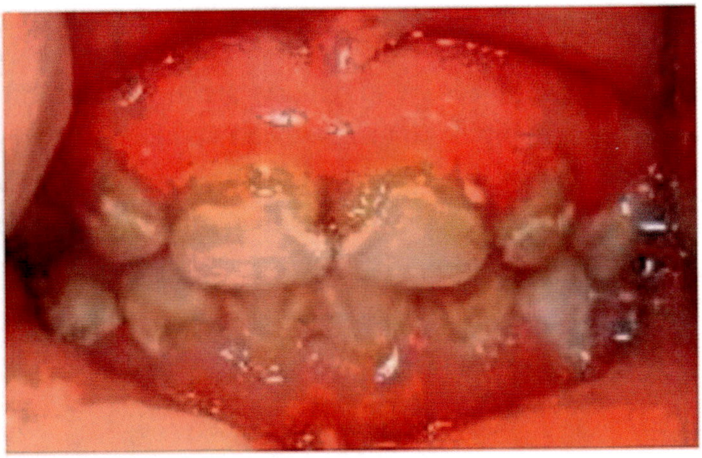

Fig. (6). Shows initial dental caries due to poor oral hygiene. There is initial decalcification in the cervical region of the tooth.

The different salivary electrolytes composition and the more alkaline pH observed in DS children, is an important factor contributing in the reported lesser caries prevalence [52]. Also, lee *et al.* found that low caries incidence in DS children is probably related to immune protection induced by the high salivary *S. mutans* specific IgA levels [53]. However, Mathias *et al.* reported that children with DS have higher Modified Gingival Index (MGI), and lower Simplified Oral Hygiene Index (OHI-S) than the control children [54]. After, correcting for the age of teeth eruption, there was small or no considerable difference in caries rates in DS children than non syndromic children. However, much lower caries-free rate was reported by Asokan *et al.* from India and Oredugba from Nigeria. This lower caries-free rate could be attributed to inabilities of people with disabilities from certain countries to have adequate access to oral health services and to find a dentist. This also indicate the caries-free rate depends on many factors including the age of the patients, as well as the socioeconomic standards of the family and the availability of medical care access in the community [55, 56].

3.5. Sleep Bruxism

Sleep bruxism (SB) is defined as a para-functional behavior sleep disorder of the mandible, characterized by forceful clenching and/or grinding of the occlusal surfaces of the teeth. Bruxism may occur as a result of masticatory neuromuscular system immaturity in younger kids with a rate ranges between 7% and 88% in children. They usually begin to brux at about four to eight years of age and the incidence reaches its higher rate between 10 and 14 years of age, after that; it started to decrease. The prevalence of bruxism was found to be higher in boys and girls with DS when compared with children without DS with a rate reaching up to 42% [57]. However, a more recent study by Miamoto *et al.* showed that the prevalence of bruxism in individuals with DS was similar to that found in individuals without cognitive impairment (approximately 24%). Presence of sucking habits, posterior cross bite and tooth wear facets usually increases the risk of having sleep bruxism [58].

3.6. Disorders of Feedings and Deglutition

Feeding problems are common in children with DS which could affect about 80% of them due to delayed development of motor coordination. There is a delayed development of oral-motor function in DS children delayed beyond that usually expected for the same age and follows an irregular pathway. The abnormal oral structure and physiology together with orofacial dysfunctions result in feeding, chewing and swallowing impairment [59]. DS Children have inadequate chewing movements due to tongue and jaw dysfunction and are unable to maintain a smooth sequence of feeding actions [60]. All the chewing parameters including; masticatory time, number of masticatory cycles, number of open masticatory cycles, chewing frequency, and number of food refusals are significantly impaired compare to the healthy children [61]. Delayed introduction of solid food is a common practice in children with DS which add more deleterious effects to oral motor development. Children with DS have a similar chewing rate comparable to that of normal children but with significantly prolonged chewing duration per bite of food [62]. At the same time, swallowing is also impaired in DS children. The oral phase of swallowing may be impacted by oral hypersensitivity which can interfere with the child acceptance of textured foods. A disordered pharyngeal phase of swallowing is also common with abnormal pharyngeal movements during swallowing, and frequent aspiration. Silent aspiration is a real trouble present in DS population with liquid or semi liquid food. It contributes to high incidence of pulmonary infections [63].

4. PATHOMECHANISM OF DENTAL PROBLEMS IN CHILDREN WITH DS

The increased incidence of the oral and dental problems in children with DS is due to a number of interacting factors including local oro-dental factors, systemic factors and social and emotional factors affecting dental care. Fig. (7) summarizes these factors.

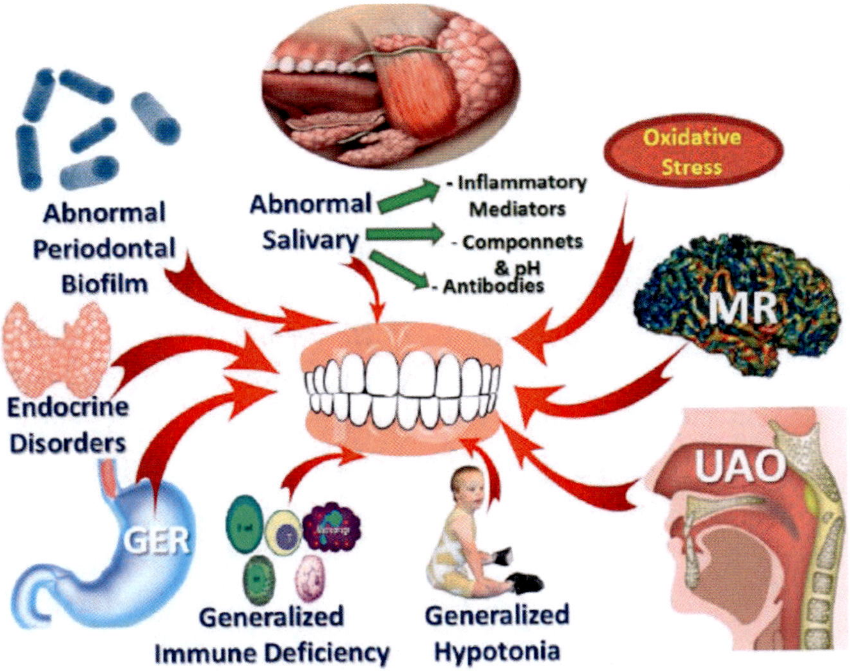

Fig. (7). Showed the local and systemic factors that affect oro-dental changes in children with Down syndrome; increased oxidative stress, Abnormal salivary inflammatory mediators , abnormal salivary chemical composition including PH, proteins *etc*; abnormal salivary antibodies composition; abnormal periodontal biofilm. Systemic factors include; mental retardation; Upper airway obstruction; generalized hypotonia and ligamentous laxity , Generalized immune deficiency; endocrinal problems including hypothyroidism.

4.1. Local Factors

There are many local factors in the teeth and oral cavity that increase the risk of oro-dental diseases in children with DS.

4.1.1. Decreased Total Antioxidant Capacity

DS persons are suffering from increased oxidative stress level they exposed to throughout their lifetime. This level will also increase in response to exposure infection or disease as a result of alteration of the antioxidants levels. Meanwhile, DS children have considerably lesser salivary total antioxidant capacity [64]. Saliva itself is vital for oral resistance against infections. So; reduction of the salivary secretion may increase rate of dental caries, and can induce oral mucosal alterations, change in sense of taste, difficulty in swallowing, as well as oral pain.

The production of reactive oxygen species (ROS) is elevated in cultured fibroblasts obtained from gingiva of DS patients. The salivary secretion in children with DS is lesser than that of normal children and even goes further lower with increasing age compared with the younger age. Saliva of DS children has significantly higher sialic acid levels than non-syndromic children [65]. The level of elevation of salivary of sialic acid can be a useful index of the severity of periodontal disease [66].

The 8-hydroxy-2'-deoxyguanosine (8-OHdG) is the result of DNA oxidation as is used as a valuable biomarker of oxidative stress. Komatsu *et al.* found an important positive correlations between the levels of salivary 8-OHdG and gingival index observed in DS individuals. This positive correlation indicates the role oxidative stress in production of the clinical features of DS, mainly the progressive periodontitis that is observed mainly in early ageing [67]. There is also increasing iron-dependant H_2O_2 generation in gingival fibroblasts in children with DS. This could be a factor involved in progressive periodontitis in DS [68].

4.1.2. Abnormal Salivary Inflammatory Mediators

Down syndrome may be associated with differential modification of genetic expression associated with proinflammatory and anti-inflammatory responses in periodontal disease. This modification mounts excessive host inflammatory responses and initiates exaggerated inflammatory responses upon periodontal infection. Cavalcante *et al.* found decreased expression of IL-10 associated with a probable raise of signal transducer and activator of transcription 3 (STAT3) activation (increase of STAT3 and reduction of suppressor of cytokine signaling 3 [SOCS3] mRNA) which denotes an significant modification of the immune response, with decrease of anti-inflammatory and increase of proinflammatory mediators. This modification may be linked to the increased rate and severity of periodontitis in DS individuals [69]. Tsilingaridis *et al.* showed that persons with DS have elevated levels of T-helper 1 (Th1)-, Th2- and Th17-related cytokines with a changed relation between Th1 cytokine, IFN-γ and Th2 cytokine, IL-4, in the gingival crevicular fluid compared to controls [70].

4.1.3. Salivary Chemical Composition

Salivary composition may differ in proteins and electrolyte contents in DS children than controls. Siqueira *et al.* showed that protein and sodium concentration were higher in the group with DS compared to the control group. On the other hand, the flow rate, pH, amylase and peroxidase activities and potassium concentration were lower in those with DS compared to those children in the control group [71]. However, Siqueira *et al.* in a previous study showed that children with DS demonstrated higher buffer capacity than the controls in the pH ranges. This better buffer capacity observed in DS children supports the results observed in several studies which found the low dental caries in persons with DS [72].

4.1.4. Abnormal Salivary Antibodies Composition

Saliva is a combination of salivary glands secretion and transudate from the capillaries under the oral mucosa, the so-called crevicular fluid that continually flows from the crevice between the gum margin and the teeth. The crevicular fluid contains a number of immunoglobulins mainly secretory immunoglobulin A (Ig

A) beside a number of other classes of immunoglobulins [73]. Cogulu *et al.* found a significantly higher levels of salivary secretory IgA in DS children than the control which may play a role in protection against dental caries [74]. Previously, Lee *et al.* found that salivary *S. mutans* (serotype g and c) specific IgA levels were considerably elevated in DS children than in the normal children [53]. Other Salivary immunoglobulins classes IgM, and IgG showed no difference between healthy children and those with DS but IgG1 was found to be higher in children with DS than normal children [75]. However, Chaushu *et al.* showed significantly diminished secretion rates of parotid salivary IgA and IgG by 83% in DS individuals [76]. Meanwhile; Bachrach *et al.* found normal rate of the antimicrobial peptide LL-37 secretion in DS children. This peptide is one component of the innate immune system and has a defensive role against periodontitis [77].

4.1.5. Abnormal Microscopic Periodontal, Gingival and Dental Ultra-Structures

Persons with DS suffering from gingivitis have elevated levels of salivary matrix metalloproteinases (MMPs) in gingival crevicular fluid with a changed relationship between MMP-8 and tissue inhibitor of matrix metalloproteinase (TIMP-2) which may deteriorate the periodontal tissue turnover. Salivary MMPs and especially their ratios and combinations are potential candidates in the detection of advanced periodontitis [78]. Gingival fibroblasts cellular motility is a vital event for healing of wound and regeneration of periodontal tissues. Murakami *et al.* found that the cellular motility of gingival fibroblasts in individuals with DS was significantly impaired compared with controls. They explained this difference by invasion of these cells by *Porphyromonas gingivalis* is a periodontal pathogen able to invade host cells, resulting in periodontal destruction. These bacteria degrade paxillin, and result in impairment of cellular motility and likely prevent wound healing and the regeneration of periodontal tissues [79]. There is also a concomitant hyperinnervation of the gingival sensory component in DS patients. This hyperinnervation contributes to gingival inflammation in these patients and releases certain chemical transmitters from these nerves that might be responsible for the inflammatory reaction. In addition, capillary fragility of gingival tissues was suggested to be related to the initiation and progression of DS periodontitis [80, 81].

Keinan *et al.* showed that mineralization of the enamel of the mesial cusps in DS children is significantly lesser than that of the controls. The teeth growth and mineralization of all cusps in DS were also affected which indicate occurrence of prenatal growth insults in fetal DS that also cause permanent effects in the developing primary teeth and even can be identified in later life [82]. Zilberman *et al.* showed significant decrease of enamel height and dentin thickness in children with DS compared with the control due to decreased proliferation during tooth germ formation [83]. Children with DS showed a transient increase in mitotic activity of developing enamel organs at the early phase of gestation, which continues during the initial stages of mineralization of the primary teeth. The initial increase will be followed by the generally recognized retardation in growth, manifested by smaller permanent teeth [84]. The root canals of these teeth are somewhat simple and showed a considerable diminution in root and crown length due to slowing of the mitotic cycle and rate of cell proliferation [16].

4.1.6. Abnormal Periodontal Biofilm

The composition of dentogingival microbial biofilm is fundamental and essential for initiation, development and progression of periodontal disease independently of immunological alterations associated with DS. Most of microbial biofilm species found in individuals with DS are similar to non-DS subjects. However, Khocht *et al.* found higher proportions of *Selenomonas noxia*, *Propionibacterium acnes*, *Streptococcus gordonii*, *Streptococcus mitis*, and *Streptococcus oralis* in microbial biofilm obtained from DS persons as compared with non-DS persons [85]. Martinez-Martinez *et al.* found that *Tannerella forsythia* was the most common organism isolated from subgingival dental plaque in subjects with DS with or without periodontitis followed by *Treponema denticola* and *Porphyromonas gingivalis*. *Pg fimA type I* was the most frequent *Porphyromonas gingivalis* genotype isolated [86]. However, *Aggregatibacter actinomycetemcomitans* was more common in the subgingival plaque of children with DS, than in healthy children. They may acquire infection with these bacteria as early as 5 years of age [87].

4.2. Systemic Factors Affecting Dental Care

Down syndrome is a condition that affects the whole body. The systemic changes that occur in children with DS have many implications for oral condition of those children. These changes include mental retardation, generalized hypotonia and joint laxity, generalized immune deficiency state, upper airway obstruction with or without obstructive sleep apnea.

4.2.1. Mental Retardation

All children with DS have low IQ and delayed mental development typically in the mild to moderate range of cognitive disability. These mentally disabled children have more prevalent and severe oral disease a when compared to the general population. Mental impairment associated with DS is a significant factor affecting oral hygiene and probably has a great impact on periodontal health, in addition to oral bacterial ecosystem. They suffer poor periodontal health and oral cleanliness due to the lower physical abilities, mental power and manual dexterity of these individuals compared to the non-syndromic children and consequently they have many difficulties in tooth brushing, cleaning and flossing, limited understanding on the importance of oral health management, difficulties in communicating their needs and a fear of oral health procedures. The frequency of dental decay among mentally disabled individuals may reach up to 84.6% [88]. However, DS children are usually passive, have innate gullibility, real warmness regard to other people, fond of music, gentleness, endurance and tolerance, with absolute honesty. All these distinguishing features make providing supervised oral hygiene care possible [89]. People with DS may complain also from impairment of the vision. This visual impairment, together with the poor dental health and acute neurological disease are directly correlated with the severity of intellectual disability and ageing [90].

4.2.2. Generalized Hypotonia and Ligamentous Laxity

Hypotonia is a frequent finding in DS children especially in the early years of life. Hypotonia is a major factor in the failure of proper development of the midface in individuals with DS. It also induces poor neuromotor control, and weakness or perioral muscle and tongue muscles which impairs oral functions as tongue protrusion, sucking, mastication, and swallowing. Hypotonia of buccal muscles may also cause less competent chewing with more leftover food on the teeth after eating; increasing the incidence of decay, periodontal, and gingival diseases. Although the degree of tone tends to improve somewhat with age, some persons may have significant ligamentous and joint laxity, which results in instability of the joints. The majority of cases are asymptomatic with symptomatic disease occurring in 1% to 2%, particularly as the result of an accident. It is particularly important in management of children with DS especially with general anesthesia for the need of proper anatomical positioning, and provides sufficient head support in the dental chair, when rendering dental care to such individuals to avoid cervical cord injury [1, 91].

4.2.3. Generalized Immune Deficiency

DS children may have an increased incidence of dental infections, including gingivitis and periodontitis, with increasing severity and duration of the disease, which are somewhat due to immune deficiencies. The DS associated immune system abnormalities include: mild to moderate T and B cell lymphopenia, with significant reduction of naive lymphocytes, weakened mitogen-induced T cell proliferation, decreased specific antibody responses to immunizations and impaired neutrophil chemotaxis. Metabolic or nutritional factors frequently encountered in DS mainly zinc deficiency; are important causes of secondary immunodeficiency [92]. The neutrophils have less segmented nuclei and shorter half-life of circulating cells in children with DS than control children. In addition, these neutrophils have defective chemotaxis which significantly correlated with the progression of periodontitis including bone loss in DS patients [93]. At the same time, the phagocytic ability and intracellular killing capacity of these cells are significantly impaired in DS children. There is also depleted thymocytes number in the DS thymus and a diminished proportion of mature T cells [94].

4.2.4. Endocrinal Problems

There are a wide range of autoimmune disorders observed in DS, most commonly thyroid gland disorders. Hypothyroidism is a frequent disorder in DS children and the incidence and risk for thyroid disease is gradually increasing with age. About

0.7% of DS newborns have persistent primary congenital hypothyroidism. On the other side, 12% of DS adults have hypothyroidism [95]. The thyroid hormones are vital for maintaining adequate cellular metabolic rate *via* controlling thermoregulation and calorigenesis; the metabolism of carbohydrates, fats, and proteins; and oxygen utilization. Thyroid hormones also work in synergy with epinephrine and increase tissue sensitivity to catecholamines. The oral cavity is negatively affected by either decrease or increase thyroid hormones. Thyroxin deficiency can induce many oral findings as macroglossia, impaired taste sensation, delayed tooth eruption, poor periodontal health, altered tooth shape and impaired wound healing (Fig. **8**). Classic manifestations of hypothyroidism involve apathy, fatigue, cold intolerance, skin changes like dryness and hair loss, constipation, weight gain, muscle pain, and bradycardia. Manifestations of hyperthyroidism include anxiety, irritability, tremors, heat intolerance, excessive sweating, frequent loose bowel motions, and tachycardia [96].

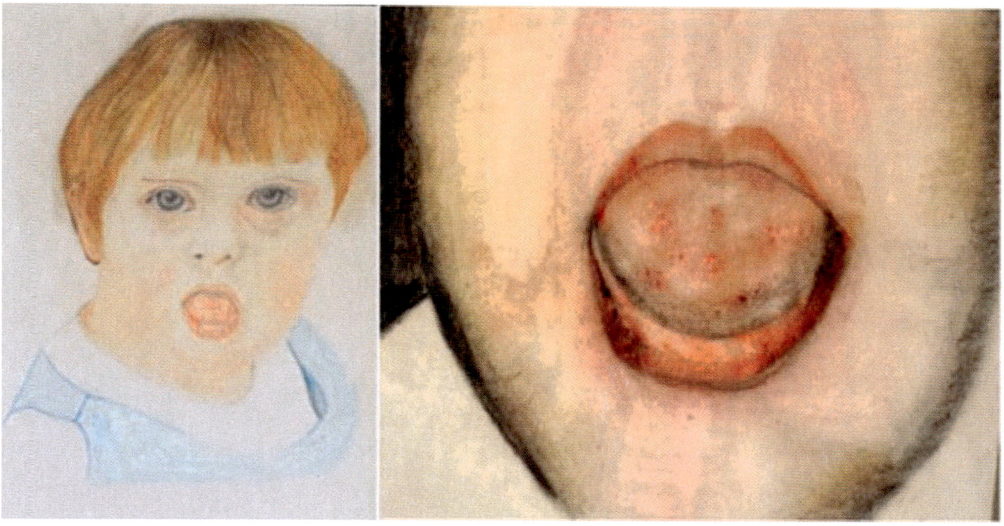

Fig. (8). A diagram showed a DS adolescent with hypothyroidism and the characteristic macroglossia.

Early hypothyroidism in infancy causes a distinct clinical condition known as cretinism with characteristic thick lips, macroglossia, malocclusion and delayed teeth eruption. Macroglossia results from increased accumulation of mucopolysaccharides as glycosaminoglycans due to their impaired breakdown. Severe degrees of hypothyroidism have deleterious effects on dental development and teeth eruption. It results in prolonged impaction of the primary teeth, suboptimal growth of the maxilla and mandible with a significant decrease in the dimensions of the facial complex, and absent coordination between mandibular growth and dental development [97]. The patients may have also superficial and internal changes in the enamel, dentin, and cement of intact and carious teeth and the resistance of dental tissue depends on the homogeneous structure of enamel and dentin [98].

There is an increased risk of diabetes in children with DS, particularly in young age which occurs in about 22% of DS children by 2 years of age, compared with only 7% in children without DS [99]. This is because the phosphofructokinase gene (PKF) which is a gene related to diabetes mellitus and obesity in persons with DS; is situated in the 21q22.3 region [100]. Autoimmunity is another reason for increased incidence of diabetes in children with DS especially at older age. Type 1 diabetes can cause difficulties in dental treatment due to generalized immune deficiency. Diminished production of T cells and B cells and reduced polymorphonuclear neutrophils will cause increased incidence of gum infection leading to early loss of tooth due to periodontitis. Diabetes can induce numerous oral disorders as dry mouth, burning sensation in the mouth or tongue, increased incidence of candidal infection, progressive periodontitis, oral neuropathies, parotid enlargement, sialosis, and impaired wound healing. Patients with uncontrolled diabetes are at higher risk of periodontitis with increased possibility for systemic exposure to periodontal bacteria and increased proinflammatory mediators associated with periodontitis [101].

4.2.5. Hematological Disorders

Hematological disorders are quit common in neonates and children with DS with several hematological problems occurring at different ages. Transient asymptomatic blood count abnormalities such as neutrophilia, thrombocytopenia and polycythemia may present in the neonatal period. About 3-10% of DS infants may develop transient myeloproliferative disease within 1-2 months of life [102]. Chromosome 21 has an important role in leukemogenesis and several genes on chromosome 21 have been disrupted in leukemia. Triplication of this chromosome increases risk of leukemia in children with DS. The risk of acute lymphoblastic leukaemia is about 12-fold in DS person between 5-30 years but increases to about approximately 40-fold in DS children below 5 years of age who have also 150-fold increased risk of acute myeloid leukaemia [103, 104]. Leukemia may have numerous buccal findings due to infiltration oral structures such as the gingiva and bone with the malignant cells. The manifestations also may result from myelophthisic effects of the disease as anemia, bleeding tendency, and increased susceptibility to infection; and may result from the effects of anti-leukemic treatment. Chemotherapeutic medications may cause myelosuppression which may induce acute exacerbation of chronic periodontal conditions. The oral findings of leukemia include oral candidiasis, mucosal pallor, gingival bleeding, oral mucosal petechiae, and ecchymosis due to thrombocytopenia, platelet defects, increased capillary fragility, and coagulation factors abnormalities [105]. Children with leukemia are at high risk for dental caries. Meanwhile, oral granulocyte numbers is a useful noninvasive tool for monitoring the onset and recovery of chemotherapy-induced myelosuppression and granulocytopenia in patients with leukemia [106].

4.2.6. Gastro Esophageal Reflux Disease

Gastrointestinal diseases are common in Down syndrome, occurring mainly in early infancy and often need therapy. Gastroesophageal reflux disease is the most frequent motility disorders observed in DS. It may often be misdiagnosed, because of its atypical presentation and because of the patients' difficulty in expressing themselves. This usually delays the diagnosis and hinders its clinical assessment and management [107]. The increased incidence of reflux in DS is due to various pathological abnormalities in the nervous system of patients with DS as a result of reduced neuronal migration or due to failure of the typical dendritic development and maturation within nervous system [108]. Gastroesophageal reflux increases the incidence of tooth wear, mainly dental erosion by 2-folds in children with DS. Most DS children who suffer gastric reflux and vomiting have severe to very severe teeth wear [109].

4.3. Social and Emotional Factors Affecting Dental Care

Mothers of children with DS tend to hold themselves accountable for their children's health status. However, many mothers encountered some difficulties in caring for their children's oral health. These difficulties are mostly related to financial constraints, time, and access to healthcare referral services hamper the search for specialized dental care for individuals with special needs. The family income and the availability of transportation may be real barriers to oral health care [110]. Other pressing medical problems may enforce the parents to wait till the child becomes more mature to visit the dentist.

5. CLINICAL SIGNIFICANCE OF DENTAL PROBLEMS IN CHILDREN WITH DS

The oral health is a clue about the overall general health and the healthy tooth is the window for a healthy person. Most children with DS have other concomitant medical problems as cardiac, immunologic, hematologic and respiratory problems. Impaired oral health can negatively impact these associated disorders.

5.1. Cardiac Disorders

Congenital heart diseases (CHDs) occur in 40-60% of children with DS. *Streptococcus viridans* (*s.mutans, s.mitior*) is the commonest microorganism for infective endocarditis isolated in more than 60% of the patients with positive blood culture. Consequently, it is mandatory for these children to maintain their oral health [111]. Preprocedural antibiotic prophylaxis against infective endocarditis is mandatory and should be assessed and followed for those with unrepaired cyanotic or potentially-cyanotic congenital heart diseases, artificial valves, previous history of infective endocarditis (IE), and those with cardiac transplantation. The procedures that need infective endocarditis prophylaxis include any procedure that involves handling gingival tissue or periapical region and perforation of the oral mucosa, such as during subgingival scaling, dental extractions, suture removal, rubber dam matrix placement, and placing of orthodontic bands. Antibiotic prophylaxis is not recommended any more for patients with other types of congenital heart defects or who have had complete surgical repair [112]. Stressful situations during dental treatment can induce cyanosis and hypoxia in children with unrepaired cyanotic CHD. Stress should be avoided or minimized as possible by proper sedation and reduction of anxiety.

Post-procedural bleeding is common in children with cyanotic heart diseases [113]. Presence of heart failure may raise the risk of general anesthesia and its complications. All these factors can potentially prevent the oral health providers to smoothly deliver the primary care [114].

Eisenmenger syndrome is a serious complication of some CHDs such as large atrial or ventricular septal defects. The cardiac structural changes associated with Eisenmenger syndrome may prevent the use of conscious sedation and increase the risk of bacterial endocarditis. DS patients suffering from this condition need particular concerns in delivering the dental care to avoid additional medical complications or emergencies such as infection, cyanotic spells, and thromboembolim because of the increased perioperative risks even for non-cardiac surgery, such as dental extractions. A prophylactic antibiotic protocol is advised for patients with Eisenmenger syndrome who will undergo any procedure that results in a transient bacteremia. Hence careful cardiac assessment may be indicated before some dental procedures; cooperation with a cardiologist is mandatory to guarantee a complete and comprehensive pre-operative work up [115].

5.2. Generalized Hypotonia and Joint Laxity

DS children have ligamentous laxity, joint hypermobility and hypotonia manifested in different ways. Musculoskeletal defects like hypermobility and joint dislocations are important factors to be considered while doing treatments on a dental chair. Dentist might come across jaw dislocation due to hypermobility of the jaw joint [116]. While treating the patient on a dental chair, proper support should be given to the atlanto-occipital joint area to prevent dislocations. Care must be given especially while extending the neck as injury can happen with hyperextension or major flexion of the neck or upper spine, which can result in irreversible damage to the spinal cord [117]. Screening for atlantooccipital joint instability should be done before any treatments on a dental chair. Cervical radiograph is recommended for children with DS at 3 years of age and must be repeated prior to the commencement and at the end of puberty to assess the occurrence of atlantoaxial instability [118].

Both the anesthesiologist and the dentist should be alert to this risk during handling the patient's neck. An alternative choice is to place the patient's arms extended around the head in to prevent sudden head movements if restraint is required [119].

5.3. Respiratory Tract Infections and Obstruction

Periodontal and gingival infections are relatively common in children with DS. These infections may serve as septic foci and may precipitate increased frequency of upper respiratory tract infections. Recurrent upper respiratory tract infections can lead to lymphadenopathy or adenoid enlargement. A dentist should be able to identify these problems and to do appropriate referral when needed. It is also important to be alert to the increased rate of sleep apnea and upper airway obstruction which may reach up to 31% in children with DS. The reduced airway size in addition to hypotonia, glossoptosis, hypopharyngeal collapse, recurrent adenoid and tonsillar hypertrophy, enlarged lingual tonsils, and relative macroglossia expose these patients to the increased risk of obstructive sleep apnea (OSA). If left untreated, OSA can additionally increase the degree of developmental delay and cause pulmonary hypertension and even congestive heart failure. Manifestations of OSA involve snoring, agitated sleep and unusual sleeping positions [42, 120]. Airway management in children with DS may be challenging because of the patient's lack of cooperation with airway management and underlying complications. Difficult intubation may become a real challenge during general anesthesia for a dental procedure [25]. Meticulous intubation and intimate monitoring of the airway are essential to avoid obstructions due to structural problems, such as short neck and rib anomalies. Proper position and adequate care of the patient's head during intubation and measures should prevent most spinal nerve injuries and potential paralysis in these patients, since many of them have atlantoaxial instability and hypotonia [121].

5.4. Endocrinal Disorders

The increased incidence of endocrinal disorders in children with DS imposes extra-burdens on the treating dentist. The dentist should be able to recognize signs of hypothyroidism and to ensure that the patient gets appropriate medical care prior to any dental procedures. This is because patients with hypothyroidism are more liable to increased depressant effects of opioid analgesics, or anxiolytic agents on the central nervous system increasing the risk of respiratory depression. Therefore use of these medications should be done with more care [96]. In severe hypothyroidism, the use of depressants to central nervous system, sedatives, or narcotic analgesics must be evaded or given in a reduced dose, because of the increased risk of respiratory depression. Sedation and analgesia are advised to be under the care of pain specialist [122].

Periodontitis and other oral infection can induce insulin resistance, deteriorate the diabetes control and make it more difficult. So, dentist should implement a preventive protocol; relieve any symptoms related to diabetic oral manifestations; and provide immediate primary care to treat dental pain and recognized dental infections [101]. The dentist also should be able to detect diabetic manifestations, assess the diabetic risk, detect signs of inadequate diabetes control, and recognize the challenges of "tight control" with insulin regarding to hypoglycemia when encounters a child with DS. It is advised that the dentist gets a detailed patient's medical history including the medications. It is better to consults the patient's physician to evaluate the patient's glycemic control, and to make sure that the patient's blood glucose levels and dietary intake are monitored before treatment. The dentist also should discuss any oral manifestation with the primary physician in charge for the patient's care. Patients with well-controlled diabetes can be treated in a similar way to the healthy patients. Treatment of periodontal diseases should be regarded as an essential and fundamental part of the patient's general healthcare plan [123].

5.5. Hematological Disorders

DS children with hematologic disorders need a professional dental care and follow-up incorporated into their medical follow-up. Meticulous oral health care is essential to decrease the rate and severity of oral consequences of the treatment protocol. This is of utmost importance to prevent and early treat any complications during subsequent treatment. The main role of the dentist is to preserve most favorable oral health during cancer therapy, to handle any oral adverse effects that may complicate the cancer therapy, and to emphasize the patient and parents' education concerning the significance of maximum oral care to reduce oral problems/discomfort associated with treatment [124]. There is no justification to stop oral hygiene during the treatment of children with leukemia. In patients who are able to maintain oral hygiene, they should continue the hygienic procedures to avoid the development of oral problems without increasing the risk of infection. Mild localized intraoral bleeding can usually be stopped using topical hemostatic agents such as fibrin glue or gelatin sponge [125]. Decontamination of the oral cavity will reduce the severity of mucositis and prevent oral microbial colonization. Fluoride supplements and neutral fluoride rinses or gels are indicated to prevent caries because of the elevated risk of dental caries in leukemic children [126].

5.6. Gastro Esophageal Reflux

Acidic oral environment associated with gastro esophageal reflux induces high levels of tooth wear. Educational programs should be developed to increase awareness of the caregivers and health professionals about this problem. Gastro esophageal reflux is usually silent in children with DS and should be suspected in presence of tooth wear. When dentists observe presence of tooth wear, they should refer the patient to a gastroenterologist for further evaluation to minimize the dental destruction and dentinal hypersensitivity which can promote and improve the patient's general health [109].

5.7. Injuries and Abuse

Children with DS like any child with mental disabilities are more liable to falls or accidents with oral trauma and injuries which may require immediate professional attention. Child physical abuse is also more common in this group of children than in the general population and often presents with oral trauma. If a child abuse or neglect is suspected, the dentist has to contact the concerned local authorities [127].

5.8. Mental Retardation

Children with DS are frequently suffering from the stigma of previously taken impression and stereotype image about their mental impairment despite that their mental retardation is usually of a mild or moderate degree, and they often have a wide range of comprehensive and performance abilities. The clinician should carefully assess the potentials of every child independently and organize the treatment plans accordingly [15].

6. MANAGEMENT OF DENTAL PROBLEMS IN CHILDREN WITH DS

The objectives of dental management in children with DS are the same as that of normal children by providing a comprehensive treatment as possible through some adaptation according to each individual's condition. Cosmetic dentistry, orthodontics, prosthodontics, and reconstructive oral surgery can be offered for those children with the availability of more extensive treatment options today [51].

Management of the commonly encountered periodontal disease needs adequate home care. However, the intellectual deterioration and reduced manual dexterity observed in DS children can hamper adequate home management. Flossing may be so difficult for such patients and instruction how to use the floss holder may be helpful. Recent automatic tooth brushing and flossing aids available in the markets may also be of great help. Proper education and training of the parents and/or caregiver about appropriate home care is compulsory. They should fully understand the significance of correct daily home care because the DS child may be unwilling to use tooth brushing. Moreover, the age at which a DS child can take care of his/her own teeth and oral health may be much delayed than that of normal children [128].

6.1. Communication Between Children With DS and Dentist

Children with DS have variable degrees of mental disability from mild to moderate that restricts their capability to study, learn, communicate, and adjust to their environment. The dentist needs to develop a form of adequate communication skills to gain their confidence; to develop a co-operative relationship with the child; and to ease both their examination and the needed procedure. First; the dentist should discuss with the parent or caregiver to verify the patient's intellectual and functional capabilities, and then clarify each procedure at a degree the child can understand. The dentist should communicate directly with the child and must be able to explain and spend adequate time in demonstrating different techniques and instruments he will use. The dentist should use simple words, uncomplicated instructions, and repeat them frequently to compensate for any short-term memory defects. Most children with DS can cope with the daily dental care with slightly prolonged time and adjustment. The scheduled time is better to be early in the morning as both the child and the dentist are more rested. Early appointments ensure that everybody is attentive and alert and that waiting time is minimized. The first appointments should be for orientation only, for full medical history intake, evaluating the general condition of the child and for planning the dental management [129].

Oral care environment should be with few distractions reducing the needless sights, sounds, or other stimuli that might irritate the child and make it difficult for the child to cooperate. Soft music may help to comfort the child during treatment. If the child resist treatment, it is wise that the dentist sooth him; lets him/her to feel comfortable and reward the child when cooperates. The dentist should not use restriction procedures except when absolutely indicated to protect both the patient and staff during dental procedures. Immobilization should be done only after obtaining permission from the patient's legal guardian with the least restrictive method that will permit providing safe care without causing any physical harm or undue discomfort [130].

6.2. Prevention and Management of Dental Caries (Fig. 9)

Proper oral hygiene education is mandatory in children with DS. Topical and systemic fluorides have a lot of benefits in protecting against dental caries. Occlusal sealants are also recommended when indicated. Due to the delay in permanent teeth eruption and the high incidence of anodontia and hypodontia, proper treatment of any decay in the primary dentition is a must. It is vital to preserve the primary dentition as long as possible [131]. Prolonged nursing should be avoided at night and to put only formula, breast milk or water in bottle. Extended use of a bottle or a no-spill sippy cup with any liquid other than water may result in cavities. Once the primary teeth erupted, teeth brushing should be started and the infant should be checked by a dentist at the age of 6 months. Fluoride supplements can be started once indicated. The child should be instructed not to use personnel utensils to avoid acquiring cavity-causing germs from the others [132].

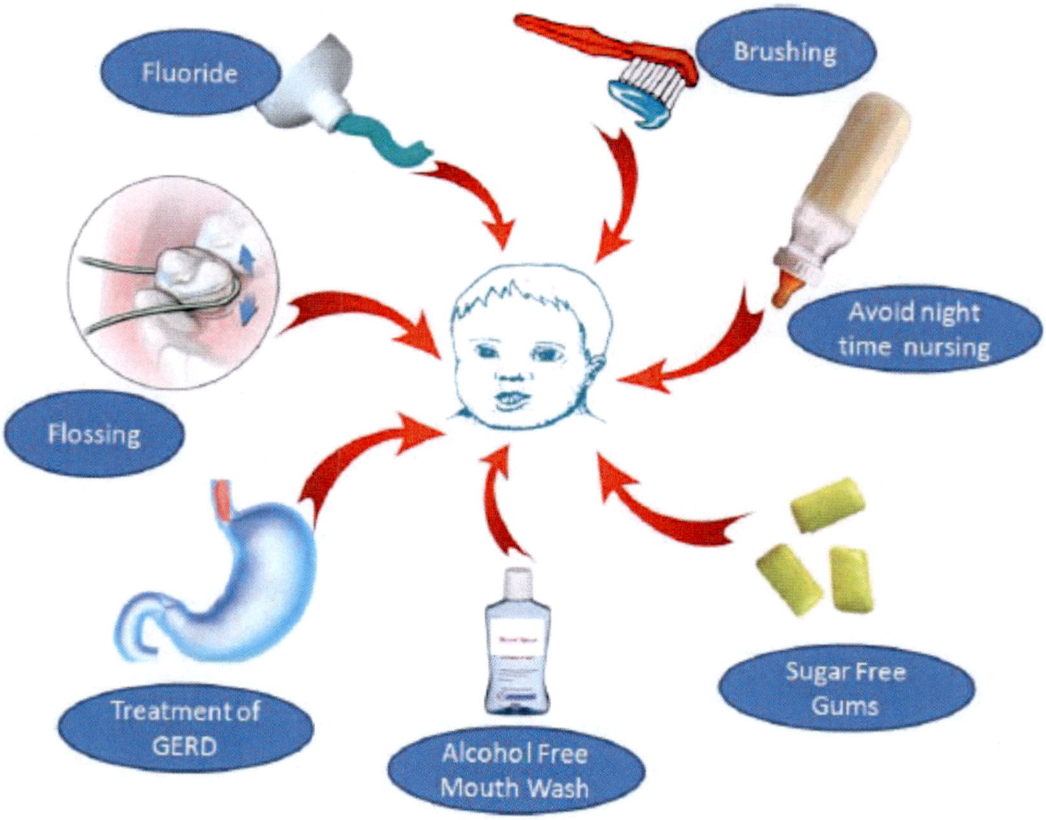

Fig. (9). Measures to prevent dental caries in children with Down syndrome include avoid night time nursing, proper brushing, use of fluoride, adequate flossing, use of sugar free gums and avoid sugary and/or sticky foods, rinse mouth with alcohol free mouth wash and treatment of associated gastroesophageal reflux.

Tooth brushing should be done in the correct way that ensures adequate cleaning of the teeth with minimal discomfort for the child. The caregivers should fix the infant's head in their lap while brushing the first teeth. The child can sit in a high seat or the corner of a sofa. The newly erupted teeth can be brushed as soon as they erupt, using a small film of fluoride toothpaste along the toothbrush. If there are more teeth; brushing can be done area by area; starting from outside of the base of the teeth from one corner of the mouth to the other in small circular movements with the brush where the teeth and gums come together with moderate pressure for chewing surfaces. Then, brushing of the inner side of the teeth is done. The same will be repeated to the upper teeth in a similar way. Tooth brushing should be done regularly twice daily, at morning and bedtime, even if only for a short period. Since many DS children have a powerful gag reflex, it may be easier to use a very tiny toothbrush with a small head. With regular brushing, the procedure becomes considerably easier. Once the child accepts brushing, flossing can be done in the same step-by-step approach as what is done in brushing. Most DS children are able to learn how to brush and floss by their selves but some kids still need some or complete support. A good standard is to brush the child's teeth till they are able to knot their shoelaces [89, 133].

The oral mucosa should be kept moist. Children with DS should drink adequate clean water regularly. Sugarless chewing gum can help to stimulate saliva flow. Children with DS should reduce the intake of refined sugary and/or sticky foods such as honey, raisins, or other similar foods that will stick to the teeth; because the reduce saliva will not be able to loosen food debris and cavities may develop much more rapidly. Medications with high sugar content or that causes dryness of the mouth are better to be avoided if possible. Using Xylitol-containing products before the use of sweetened medications will reduce the frequency of dental decay. The child is advised to use a bactericidal mouthwash to reduce the bacterial load and oral infections. It is advisable to use alcohol free mouth wash to avoid alcohol-induced dryness of the mouth. If the child has exaggerated gagging, difficulty in swallowing, or not be able to rinse with mouthwash, the caregiver can immerse a toothbrush in mouthwash and rub the bristles along the gums [134].

6.3. Preoperative Antibiotic Prophylaxis Against Infective Endocarditis

If the child with DS has structural heart lesions, antibiotic prophylaxis for infective endocarditis should be considered before certain surgical procedures. However, routine antibiotic prophylaxis before dental procedures is not recommended any more according to the most recent guidelines of National Institute for Health and Clinical Excellence except if there is real proof of ongoing infection or for routine surgical site infection (SSI) prophylaxis. However, there are number of conditions with increased risk of infective endocarditis and a consultation with a cardiologist and the decision should be tailored according to each condition. These conditions include valve replacement; congenital heart defect (except for an isolated ASD, repaired VSD or repaired PDA); and history of previous infective endocarditis. On the other hand, children with pacemaker or arrhythmia are not considered at increased risk of infective endocarditis [135].

6.4. Orthodontic Treatment

Surgical orthodontic Therapy has major indications in DS patients. Cooperative ability of the patient is very important determining factor for successful orthodontic appliance therapy. However, successful orthodontic treatment is attainable for many patients. If the child has severe mental retardation, the initial placement of limited fixed appliances or bonded/cemented bite planes can be done under general anesthesia [136].

6.5. Care During Local and General Anesthesia

In children with DS, sedation or general anesthesia is indicated in presence of lack of cooperation, or multiple morbidities. However, difficulty can arise for patients who need general anesthesia due to repeated chest infections as a result of lowered immunity; ligament laxity, particularly the atlantoaxial ligament, which preserves the appropriate position of the first and second cervical vertebrae; presence of congenital heart disease; and difficult intubation as a result of underdeveloped midface and small trachea. The difference between sedation levels and general anesthesia is not obvious. Local anesthesia and conscious sedation are favored over general anesthesia to perform dental procedures. If intravenous general anesthesia without tracheal intubation is indicated for dental management, teamwork between the dentist, dental assistant, and anesthesiologist is required. Cooperation between the dentist and healthcare provider is vital to accomplish safe and successful dental treatment under sedation or general anesthesia [137]. So; risk assessment and proper planning must be done before going to general anesthesia.

Precautionary measures should be taken for safe, successful and complete dental procedure under general anesthesia to avoid morbidity and even mortality [116]. These measures include: preoperative screening for atlanto-occipital joint instability before any treatments on a dental chair; avoid vigorous neck flexion and extension in these patients due to the likelihood of atlanto-axial instability, anticipating uneasy venous cannulation in younger children (gaseous induction with halothane or sevoflurane will be helpful); premedication with an H_2 antagonist (*e.g.* Rantidine) if gastro-oesophageal reflux is expected; small tracheal tube may be required due to sub-glottic stenosis; and incase of difficult intubation a laryngeal mask airway can be used [138, 139].

During the procedure; the child should be under proper monitoring and all the invasive procedures should be done under complete aseptic safety measures. Sensitivity to atropine has been reported in patients with DS, so caution should be given when using it. The child should be monitored intimately in the recovery room and care of hypotonia, with proper position of the child in the lateral side should be done to preserve patent airways till complete recovery from anesthesia. Use of airway options like oropharyngeal or nasopharyngeal airway can be done when suitable. Postoperative evaluation of atlanto-axial instability should be done when suspected [140].

6.6. Sleep Apnea

The dentist should be alert to the increased rate of sleep apnea in children with DS which may reach up to one third of them. It characterized by sleep fragmentation, oxygen desaturation and daytime somnolence. Untreated, sleep apnea increases the risk of craniofacial developmental delay and lead to pulmonary hypertension. When suspected, the dentist should refer the child to a sleep disorder specialist. The treatment varies from adenotonsillectomy, occlusal repositioning devices and/or positive airway pressure. Proper sleep apnea management is important in enhancing the quality of life of patients with DS [120].

CONCLUSION

Children with DS are more liable to have dental problems due to a variety of reasons. The role of the dentist is to detect and to appropriately manage these problems through an integrated team work including the family and the child primary physician. Good oral hygiene and healthy dental life are of paramount importance for an integrated health and better quality of life for such children.

CONFLICT OF INTEREST

The authors confirm that this chapter contents have no conflict of interest.

ACKNOWLEDGEMENTS

Declared none.

REFERENCES

[1] Weijerman ME, de Winter JP. Clinical practice. The care of children with Down syndrome. Eur J Pediatr 2010; 169(12): 1445-52.
[http://dx.doi.org/10.1007/s00431-010-1253-0] [PMID: 20632187]

[2] Bouvy-Berends EC, Reuland-Bosma W. ['Emily goes to the dentist'. Oral care for individuals with Down syndrome]. Ned Tijdschr Tandheelkd 2006; 113(6): 234-8.
[PMID: 16821469]

[3] Quintanilla JS, Biedma BM, Rodríguez MQ, Mora MT, Cunqueiro MM, Pazos MA. Cephalometrics in children with Down's syndrome. Pediatr Radiol 2002; 32(9): 635-43.
[http://dx.doi.org/10.1007/s00247-002-0703-x] [PMID: 12195302]

[4] Nadel L. Down's syndrome: a genetic disorder in biobehavioral perspective. Genes Brain Behav 2003; 2(3): 156-66.
[http://dx.doi.org/10.1034/j.1601-183X.2003.00026.x] [PMID: 12931789]

[5] Desai SS. Down syndrome: a review of the literature. Oral Surg Oral Med Oral Pathol Oral Radiol Endod 1997; 84(3): 279-85.
[http://dx.doi.org/10.1016/S1079-2104(97)90343-7] [PMID: 9377191]

[6] Macho V, Coelho A, Areias C, Macedo P, Andrade D. Craniofacial features and specific oral characteristics of Down syndrome children. Oral Health Dent Manag 2014; 13(2): 408-11.
[PMID: 24984656]

[7] Korayem MA, AlKofide EA. Characteristics of Down syndrome subjects in a Saudi sample. Angle Orthod 2014; 84(1): 30-7.
[http://dx.doi.org/10.2319/030813-195.1] [PMID: 23745979]

[8] Panchón-Ruiz A, Jornet-Carrillo V, Sanchez del Campo F. Palate vault morphology in Down syndrome. J Craniofac Genet Dev Biol 2000; 20(4): 198-200.
[PMID: 11354516]

[9] Bäckman B, Grevér-Sjölander AC, Holm AK, Johansson I. Children with Down Syndrome: oral development and morphology after use of palatal plates between 6 and 18 months of age. Int J Paediatr Dent 2003; 13(5): 327-35.
[http://dx.doi.org/10.1046/j.1365-263X.2003.00485.x] [PMID: 12924988]

[10] Skrinjarić T, Glavina D, Jukić J. Palatal and dental arch morphology in Down syndrome. Coll Antropol 2004; 28(2): 841-7.
[PMID: 15666619]

[11] Beriaghi S, Myers SL, Jensen SA, Kaimal S, Chan CM, Schaefer GB. Cleft lip and palate: association with other congenital malformations. J Clin Pediatr Dent 2009; 33(3): 207-10. [http://dx.doi.org/10.17796/jcpd.33.3.c244761467507721] [PMID: 19476092]

[12] Seagriff-Curtin P, Pugliese S, Romer M. Dental considerations for individuals with Down syndrome. N Y State Dent J 2006; 72(2): 33-5. [PMID: 16711590]

[13] de Moraes ME, de Moraes LC, Dotto GN, Dotto PP, dos Santos LR. Dental anomalies in patients with Down syndrome. Braz Dent J 2007; 18(4): 346-50. [http://dx.doi.org/10.1590/S0103-64402007000400014] [PMID: 18278307]

[14] Bell E, Townsend G, Wilson D, Kieser J, Hughes T. Effect of Down syndrome on the dimensions of dental crowns and tissues. Am J Hum Biol 2001; 13(5): 690-8. [http://dx.doi.org/10.1002/ajhb.1107] [PMID: 11505477]

[15] Kieser J, Townsend G, Quick A. The Down syndrome patient in dental practice, part I: Pathogenesis and general and dental features. N Z Dent J 2003; 99(1): 5-9. [PMID: 15330383]

[16] Kelsen AE, Love RM, Kieser JA, Herbison P. Root canal anatomy of anterior and premolar teeth in Down's syndrome. Int Endod J 1999; 32(3): 211-6. [http://dx.doi.org/10.1046/j.1365-2591.1999.00223.x] [PMID: 10530209]

[17] Chow KM, O'Donnell D. Concomitant occurrence of hypodontia and supernumerary teeth in a patient with Down syndrome. Spec Care Dentist 1997; 17(2): 54-7. [http://dx.doi.org/10.1111/j.1754-4505.1997.tb00867.x] [PMID: 9582700]

[18] Ondarza A, Jara L, Bertonati MI, Blanco R. Tooth malalignments in Chilean children with Down syndrome. Cleft Palate Craniofac J 1995; 32(3): 188-93. [http://dx.doi.org/10.1597/1545-1569(1995)032<0188:TMICCW>2.3.CO;2] [PMID: 7605785]

[19] Shapira J, Chaushu S, Becker A. Prevalence of tooth transposition, third molar agenesis, and maxillary canine impaction in individuals with Down syndrome. Angle Orthod 2000; 70(4): 290-6. [PMID: 10961778]

[20] Borenstein M, Persico N, Kagan KO, Gazzoni A, Nicolaides KH. Frontomaxillary facial angle in screening for trisomy 21 at 11 + 0 to 13 + 6 weeks. Ultrasound Obstet Gynecol 2008; 32(1): 5-11. [http://dx.doi.org/10.1002/uog.5334] [PMID: 18512854]

[21] Sforza C, Ferrario VF. Soft-tissue facial anthropometry in three dimensions: from anatomical landmarks to digital morphology in research, clinics and forensic anthropology. J Anthropol Sci 2006; 84: 97-124.

[22] Sforza C, Elamin F, Rosati R, Lucchini MA, Tommasi DG, Ferrario VF. Three-dimensional assessment of nose and lip morphology in North Sudanese subjects with Down syndrome. Angle Orthod 2011; 81(1): 107-14. [http://dx.doi.org/10.2319/042510-222.1] [PMID: 20936962]

[23] Faulks D, Collado V, Mazille MN, Veyrune JL, Hennequin M. Masticatory dysfunction in persons with Down's syndrome. Part 1: aetiology and incidence. J Oral Rehabil 2008; 35(11): 854-62. [http://dx.doi.org/10.1111/j.1365-2842.2008.01877.x] [PMID: 18702629]

[24] Hashimoto M, Igari K, Hanawa S, *et al.* Tongue pressure during swallowing in adults with down syndrome and its relationship with palatal morphology. Dysphagia 2014; 29(4): 509-18. [http://dx.doi.org/10.1007/s00455-014-9538-5] [PMID: 24844770]

[25] Nakazawa K, Ikeda D, Ishikawa S, Makita K. A case of difficult airway due to lingual tonsillar hypertrophy in a patient with Down's syndrome Anesth Analg 2003; 97(3): 704-5. [http://dx.doi.org/10.1213/01.ANE.0000074347.64382.A4] [PMID: 12933389]

[26] Chaushu S, Becker A, Chaushu G, Shapira J. Stimulated parotid salivary flow rate in patients with Down syndrome. Spec Care Dentist 2002; 22(1): 41-4. [http://dx.doi.org/10.1111/j.1754-4505.2002.tb01208.x] [PMID: 12014860]

[27] Siqueira WL, Nicolau J. Stimulated whole saliva components in children with Down syndrome. Spec Care Dentist 2002; 22(6): 226-30. [http://dx.doi.org/10.1111/j.1754-4505.2002.tb00276.x] [PMID: 12790231]

[28] Ferrario VF, Dellavia C, Serrao G, Sforza C. Soft tissue facial angles in Down's syndrome subjects: a three-dimensional non-invasive study. Eur J Orthod 2005; 27(4): 355-62. [http://dx.doi.org/10.1093/ejo/cji017] [PMID: 16043473]

[29] Bagić I, Verzak Z, Cuković-Cavka S, Brkić H, Susić M. Periodontal conditions in individuals with Down's syndrome. Coll Antropol 2003; 27 (Suppl. 2): 75-82. [PMID: 12971174]

[30] Al Habashneh R, Al-Jundi S, Khader Y, Nofel N. Oral health status and reasons for not attending dental care among 12- to 16-year-old children with Down syndrome in special needs centres in Jordan. Int J Dent Hyg 2012; 10(4): 259-64. [http://dx.doi.org/10.1111/j.1601-5037.2012.00545.x] [PMID: 22335361]

[31] Knoll S, Janal M, Khocht A. Radiographic assessment of periodontitis in African-Americans with Down syndrome. J Int Acad Periodontol 2008; 10(1): 16-21. [PMID: 18333596]

[32] Morgan J. Why is periodontal disease more prevalent and more severe in people with Down syndrome? Spec Care Dentist 2007 Sep-Oct; 27(5): 196-201. [http://dx.doi.org/10.1111/j.1754-4505.2007.tb00346.x] [PMID: 17990479]

[33] Brkić H, Bagić I, Vojvodić D. The prevalence of taurodontism in Croatian population. Acta Stomatol Croat 1992; 26(2): 79-84.

[34] López-Pérez R, Borges-Yáñez SA, Jiménez-García G, Maupomé G. Oral hygiene, gingivitis, and periodontitis in persons with Down syndrome. Spec Care Dentist 2002; 22(6): 214-20. [http://dx.doi.org/10.1111/j.1754-4505.2002.tb00274.x] [PMID: 12790229]

[35] Modéer T, Barr M, Dahllöf G. Periodontal disease in children with Down's syndrome. Scand J Dent Res 1990; 98(3): 228-34. [PMID: 2140909]

[36] Cichon P, Crawford L, Grimm WD. Early-onset periodontitis associated with Down's syndrome--clinical interventional study. Ann Periodontol 1998; 3(1): 370-80. [http://dx.doi.org/10.1902/annals.1998.3.1.370] [PMID: 9722720]

[37] Morinushi T, Lopatin DE, Van Poperin N. The relationship between gingivitis and the serum antibodies to the microbiota associated with periodontal disease in children with Down's syndrome. J Periodontol 1997; 68(7): 626-31.
[http://dx.doi.org/10.1902/jop.1997.68.7.626] [PMID: 9249633]

[38] Morinushi T, Lopatin DE, Nakao R, Kinjyo S. A comparison of the gingival health of children with Down syndrome to healthy children residing in an institution. Spec Care Dentist 2006; 26(1): 13-9.
[http://dx.doi.org/10.1111/j.1754-4505.2006.tb01504.x] [PMID: 16703929]

[39] Albandar JM. Aggressive and acute periodontal diseases. Periodontol 2000 2014; 65(1): 7-12.
[http://dx.doi.org/10.1111/prd.12013] [PMID: 24738583]

[40] Scully C, van Bruggen W, Diz Dios P, Casal B, Porter S, Davison MF. Down syndrome: lip lesions (angular stomatitis and fissures) and Candida albicans. Br J Dermatol 2002; 147(1): 37-40.
[http://dx.doi.org/10.1046/j.1365-2133.2002.04741.x] [PMID: 12100182]

[41] Daneshpazhooh M, Nazemi TM, Bigdeloo L, Yoosefi M. Mucocutaneous findings in 100 children with Down syndrome. Pediatr Dermatol 2007; 24(3): 317-20.
[http://dx.doi.org/10.1111/j.1525-1470.2007.00412.x] [PMID: 17542890]

[42] Fung E, Witmans M, Ghosh M, Cave D, El-Hakim H. Upper airway findings in children with Down syndrome on sleep nasopharyngoscopy: case-control study. J Otolaryngol Head Neck Surg 2012; 41(2): 138-44.
[PMID: 22569015]

[43] Sedaghat AR, Flax-Goldenberg RB, Gayler BW, Capone GT, Ishman SL. A case-control comparison of lingual tonsillar size in children with and without Down syndrome. Laryngoscope 2012; 122(5): 1165-9.
[http://dx.doi.org/10.1002/lary.22346] [PMID: 22374875]

[44] Gisel EG, Lange LJ, Niman CW. Tongue movements in 4- and 5-year-old Down's syndrome children during eating: a comparison with normal children. Am J Occup Ther 1984; 38(10): 660-5.
[http://dx.doi.org/10.5014/ajot.38.10.660] [PMID: 6238533]

[45] Carlstedt K, Krekmanova L, Dahllöf G, Ericsson B, Braathen G, Modéer T. Oral carriage of Candida species in children and adolescents with Down's syndrome. Int J Paediatr Dent 1996; 6(2): 95-100.
[http://dx.doi.org/10.1111/j.1365-263X.1996.tb00219.x] [PMID: 8957847]

[46] Shetty S, Kini U, Joy R. Isolated lingual mucormycosis in an infant with Down syndrome. Ear Nose Throat J 2008; 87(1): 34-35, 43.
[PMID: 18357944]

[47] Bauer D, Evans CA, Begole EA, Salzmann L. Severity of occlusal disharmonies in down syndrome. Int J Dent 2012. 2012:872367
[http://dx.doi.org/10.1155/2012/872367] [PMID: 22934114]

[48] Suri S, Tompson BD, Atenafu E. Prevalence and patterns of permanent tooth agenesis in Down syndrome and their association with craniofacial morphology. Angle Orthod 2011; 81(2): 260-9.
[http://dx.doi.org/10.2319/070910-391.1] [PMID: 21208078]

[49] Andersson EM, Axelsson S, Austeng ME, *et al.* Bilateral hypodontia is more common than unilateral hypodontia in children with Down syndrome: a prospective population-based study. Eur J Orthod

2014; 36(4): 414-8.
[http://dx.doi.org/10.1093/ejo/cjt063] [PMID: 24014738]

[50] Macho V, Palha M, Macedo AP, Ribeiro O, Andrade C. Comparative study between dental caries prevalence of Down syndrome children and their siblings. Spec Care Dentist 2013; 33(1): 2-7.
[http://dx.doi.org/10.1111/j.1754-4505.2012.00297.x] [PMID: 23278142]

[51] Boyd D, Quick A, Murray C. The Down syndrome patient in dental practice, Part II: clinical considerations. N Z Dent J 2004; 100(1): 4-9.
[PMID: 15346875]

[52] Davidovich E, Aframian DJ, Shapira J, Peretz B. A comparison of the sialochemistry, oral pH, and oral health status of Down syndrome children to healthy children. Int J Paediatr Dent 2010; 20(4): 235-41.
[http://dx.doi.org/10.1111/j.1365-263X.2010.01045.x] [PMID: 20536584]

[53] Lee SR, Kwon HK, Song KB, Choi YH. Dental caries and salivary immunoglobulin A in Down syndrome children. J Paediatr Child Health 2004; 40(9-10): 530-3.
[http://dx.doi.org/10.1111/j.1440-1754.2004.00457.x] [PMID: 15367146]

[54] Mathias MF, Simionato MR, Guaré RO. Some factors associated with dental caries in the primary dentition of children with Down syndrome. Eur J Paediatr Dent 2011; 12(1): 37-42.
[PMID: 21434734]

[55] Asokan S, Muthu MS, Sivakumar N. Dental caries prevalence and treatment needs of Down syndrome children in Chennai, India. Indian J Dent Res 2008; 19(3): 224-9.
[http://dx.doi.org/10.4103/0970-9290.42955] [PMID: 18797099]

[56] Oredugba FA. Oral health condition and treatment needs of a group of Nigerian individuals with Down syndrome. Downs Syndr Res Pract 2007; 12(1): 72-6.
[http://dx.doi.org/10.3104/reports.2022] [PMID: 17692192]

[57] López-Pérez R, López-Morales P, Borges-Yáñez SA, Maupomé G, Parés-Vidrio G. Prevalence of bruxism among Mexican children with Down syndrome. Downs Syndr Res Pract 2007; 12(1): 45-9.
[http://dx.doi.org/10.3104/reports.1995] [PMID: 17692187]

[58] Miamoto CB, Pereira LJ, Ramos-Jorge ML, Marques LS. Prevalence and predictive factors of sleep bruxism in children with and without cognitive impairment. Braz Oral Res 2011; 25(5): 439-45.
[http://dx.doi.org/10.1590/S1806-83242011000500011] [PMID: 22031058]

[59] Faulks D, Mazille MN, Collado V, Veyrune JL, Hennequin M. Masticatory dysfunction in persons with Down's syndrome. Part 2: management. J Oral Rehabil 2008; 35(11): 863-9.
[http://dx.doi.org/10.1111/j.1365-2842.2008.01878.x] [PMID: 18793251]

[60] Spender Q, Stein A, Dennis J, Reilly S, Percy E, Cave D. An exploration of feeding difficulties in children with Down syndrome. Dev Med Child Neurol 1996; 38(8): 681-94.
[http://dx.doi.org/10.1111/j.1469-8749.1996.tb12138.x] [PMID: 8761164]

[61] Lewis E, Kritzinger A. Parental experiences of feeding problems in their infants with Down syndrome. Downs Syndr Res Pract 2004; 9(2): 45-52. 1
[http://dx.doi.org/10.3104/reports.291] [PMID: 15332438]

[62] Gisel EG, Lange LJ, Niman CW. Chewing cycles in 4- and 5-year-old Down's syndrome children: a

comparison of eating efficacy with normals. Am J Occup Ther 1984; 38(10): 666-70. [http://dx.doi.org/10.3104/reports.291] [PMID: 6238534]

[63] Frazier JB, Friedman B. Swallow function in children with Down syndrome: a retrospective study. Dev Med Child Neurol 1996; 38(8): 695-703. [http://dx.doi.org/10.1111/j.1469-8749.1996.tb12139.x] [PMID: 8761165]

[64] Subramaniam P, Girish Babu K, Mohan Das L. Assessment of salivary total antioxidant levels and oral health status in children with Down syndrome. Spec Care Dentist 2014; 34(4): 193-200. [http://dx.doi.org/10.1111/scd.12054] [PMID: 24188359]

[65] Chaushu S, Becker A, Chaushu G, Shapira J. Stimulated parotid salivary flow rate in patients with Down syndrome. Spec Care Dentist 2002; 22(1): 41-4. [http://dx.doi.org/10.1111/j.1754-4505.2002.tb01208.x] [PMID: 12014860]

[66] Shetty PK, Pattabiraman TN. Salivary glycoproteins as indicators of oral diseases. Indian J Clin Biochem 2004; 19(1): 97-101. [http://dx.doi.org/10.1007/BF02872400] [PMID: 23105437]

[67] Komatsu T, Duckyoung Y, Ito A, *et al.* Increased oxidative stress biomarkers in the saliva of Down syndrome patients. Arch Oral Biol 2013; 58(9): 1246-50. [http://dx.doi.org/10.1016/j.archoralbio.2013.03.017] [PMID: 23714170]

[68] Komatsu T, Lee MC, Miyagi A, *et al.* Reactive oxygen species generation in gingival fibroblasts of Down syndrome patients detected by electron spin resonance spectroscopy. Redox Rep 2006; 11(2): 71-7. [http://dx.doi.org/10.1179/135100006X101039] [PMID: 16686997]

[69] Cavalcante LB, Tanaka MH, Pires JR, *et al.* Expression of the interleukin-10 signaling pathway genes in individuals with Down syndrome and periodontitis. J Periodontol 2012; 83(7): 926-35. [http://dx.doi.org/10.1902/jop.2011.110056] [PMID: 22050548]

[70] Tsilingaridis G, Yucel-Lindberg T, Modéer T. T-helper-related cytokines in gingival crevicular fluid from adolescents with Down syndrome. Clin Oral Investig 2012; 16(1): 267-73. [http://dx.doi.org/10.1007/s00784-010-0495-6] [PMID: 21221679]

[71] Siqueira WL, Siqueira MF, Mustacchi Z, de Oliveira E, Nicolau J. Salivary parameters in infants aged 12 to 60 months with Down syndrome. Spec Care Dentist 2007; 27(5): 202-5. [http://dx.doi.org/10.1111/j.1754-4505.2007.tb00347.x] [PMID: 17990480]

[72] Siqueira WL, Bermejo PR, Mustacchi Z, Nicolau J. Buffer capacity, pH, and flow rate in saliva of children aged 2-60 months with Down syndrome. Clin Oral Investig 2005; 9(1): 26-9. [http://dx.doi.org/10.1007/s00784-004-0282-3] [PMID: 15378405]

[73] Madar R, Straka S, Baska T. Detection of antibodies in saliva--an effective auxiliary method in surveillance of infectious diseases. Bratisl Lek Listy (Tlacene Vyd) 2002; 103(1): 38-41. [PMID: 12061087]

[74] Cogulu D, Sabah E, Kutukculer N, Ozkinay F. Evaluation of the relationship between caries indices and salivary secretory IgA, salivary pH, buffering capacity and flow rate in children with Down's syndrome. Arch Oral Biol 2006; 51(1): 23-8. [http://dx.doi.org/10.1016/j.archoralbio.2005.06.001] [PMID: 16039983]

[75] Barr-Agholme M, Dahllöf G, Modéer T, Engström PE, Engström GN. Periodontal conditions and salivary immunoglobulins in individuals with Down syndrome. J Periodontol 1998; 69(10): 1119-23. [http://dx.doi.org/10.1902/jop.1998.69.10.1119] [PMID: 9802710]

[76] Chaushu S, Yefenof E, Becker A, Shapira J, Chaushu G. Severe impairment of secretory Ig production in parotid saliva of Down Syndrome individuals. J Dent Res 2002; 81(5): 308-12. [http://dx.doi.org/10.1177/154405910208100504] [PMID: 12097442]

[77] Bachrach G, Chaushu G, Zigmond M, *et al.* Salivary LL-37 secretion in individuals with Down syndrome is normal. J Dent Res 2006; 85(10): 933-6. [http://dx.doi.org/10.1177/154405910608501012] [PMID: 16998135]

[78] Tsilingaridis G, Yucel-Lindberg T, Modéer T. Altered relationship between MMP-8 and TIMP-2 in gingival crevicular fluid in adolescents with Down's syndrome. J Periodontal Res 2013; 48(5): 553-62. [http://dx.doi.org/10.1111/jre.12038] [PMID: 23298307]

[79] Murakami J, Kato T, Kawai S, Akiyama S, Amano A, Morisaki I. Cellular motility of Down syndrome gingival fibroblasts is susceptible to impairment by Porphyromonas gingivalis invasion. J Periodontol 2008; 79(4): 721-7. [http://dx.doi.org/10.1902/jop.2008.070400] [PMID: 18380567]

[80] Barr-Agholme M, Modéer T, Luthman J. Immunohistological study of neuronal markers in inflamed gingiva obtained from children with Down's syndrome. J Clin Periodontol 1991; 18(8): 624-33. [http://dx.doi.org/10.1111/j.1600-051X.1991.tb00100.x] [PMID: 1839031]

[81] Dougherty MA, Slots J. Periodontal diseases in young individuals. J Calif Dent Assoc 1993; 21(1): 55-69. [PMID: 7682608]

[82] Keinan D, Smith P, Zilberman U. Microstructure and chemical composition of primary teeth in children with Down syndrome and cerebral palsy. Arch Oral Biol 2006; 51(10): 836-43. [http://dx.doi.org/10.1016/j.archoralbio.2006.04.003] [PMID: 16756941]

[83] Zilberman U, Patricia S, Kupietzky A, Mass E. The effect of hereditary disorders on tooth components: a radiographic morphometric study of two syndromes. Arch Oral Biol 2004; 49(8): 621-9. [http://dx.doi.org/10.1016/j.archoralbio.2004.02.008] [PMID: 15196980]

[84] Peretz B, Katzenel V, Shapira J. Morphometric variables of the primary second molar in children with Down syndrome. J Clin Pediatr Dent 1999; 23(4): 333-6. [PMID: 10551134]

[85] Khocht A, Yaskell T, Janal M, *et al.* Subgingival microbiota in adult Down syndrome periodontitis. J Periodontal Res 2012; 47(4): 500-7. [http://dx.doi.org/10.1111/j.1600-0765.2011.01459.x] [PMID: 22221039]

[86] Martinez-Martinez RE, Loyola-Rodriguez JP, Bonilla-Garro SE, *et al.* Characterization of periodontal biofilm in Down syndrome patients: a comparative study. J Clin Pediatr Dent 2013; 37(3): 289-95. [http://dx.doi.org/10.17796/jcpd.37.3.d70710016518p58n] [PMID: 23855174]

[87] El Housseiny AA. Aggregatibacter actinomycetemcomitans in Down's syndrome children. J Clin Pediatr Dent 2012; 36(4): 417-21.

[http://dx.doi.org/10.17796/jcpd.36.4.w805wm3r52474g24] [PMID: 23019843]

[88] Altun C, Guven G, Akgun OM, Akkurt MD, Basak F, Akbulut E. Oral health status of disabled individuals attending special schools. Eur J Dent 2010; 4(4): 361-6. [PMID: 20922154]

[89] Shyama M, Al-Mutawa SA, Honkala S, Honkala E. Supervised toothbrushing and oral health education program in Kuwait for children and young adults with Down syndrome. Spec Care Dentist 2003; 23(3): 94-. [http://dx.doi.org/10.1111/j.1754-4505.2003.tb01668.x] [PMID: 14650557]

[90] Määttä T, Kaski M, Taanila A, Keinänen-Kiukaanniemi S, Iivanainen M. Sensory impairments and health concerns related to the degree of intellectual disability in people with Down syndrome. Downs Syndr Res Pract 2006; 11(2): 78-83. [http://dx.doi.org/10.3104/reports.317] [PMID: 17048801]

[91] Bhattarai B, Kulkarni AH, Kalingarayar S, Upadya MP. Anesthetic management of a child with Down's syndrome having atlanto axial instability. JNMA J Nepal Med Assoc 2009; 48(173): 66-9. [PMID: 19529062]

[92] Ram G, Chinen J. Infections and immunodeficiency in Down syndrome. Clin Exp Immunol 2011; 164(1): 9-16. [http://dx.doi.org/10.1111/j.1365-2249.2011.04335.x] [PMID: 21352207]

[93] Izumi Y, Sugiyama S, Shinozuka O, Yamazaki T, Ohyama T, Ishikawa I. Defective neutrophil chemotaxis in Down's syndrome patients and its relationship to periodontal destruction. J Periodontol 1989; 60(5): 238-42. [http://dx.doi.org/10.1902/jop.1989.60.5.238] [PMID: 2525619]

[94] Amano A, Murakami J, Akiyama S, Morisaki I. Etiologic factors of early-onset periodontal disease in Down syndrome. Jpn Dent Sci Rev 2008; 44: 118-27. [http://dx.doi.org/10.1016/j.jdsr.2008.07.001]

[95] Coleman M. Thyroid dysfunction in Down syndrome: A review. Downs Syndr Res Pract 1994; 2(3): 112-5. [http://dx.doi.org/10.3104/reviews.40]

[96] Huber MA, Terézhalmy GT. Risk stratification and dental management of the patient with thyroid dysfunction. Quintessence Int 2008; 39(2): 139-50. [PMID: 18560652]

[97] Gupta R, Goel K, Solanki J, Gupta S. Oral manifestations of hypothyroidism: a case report. J Clin Diagn Res 2014; 8(5): ZD20-2. [http://dx.doi.org/10.7860/JCDR/2014/8905.4379] [PMID: 24995258]

[98] Pavlova TV, Peshkova EK, Goncharov IIu, Kolesnikov DA, Nesterov AV. [Impairments in the ultrastructure and macro- and microelement composition of hard tooth tissues in caries in patients with hypothyroidism and in those without thyroid disease]. Arkh Patol 2014; 76(2): 17-21. [PMID: 25051720]

[99] Aitken RJ, Mehers KL, Williams AJ, *et al.* Early-onset, coexisting autoimmunity and decreased HLA-mediated susceptibility are the characteristics of diabetes in Down syndrome. Diabetes Care 2013;

36(5): 1181-5.
[http://dx.doi.org/10.2337/dc12-1712] [PMID: 23275362]

[100] Anwar AJ, Walker JD, Frier BM. Type 1 diabetes mellitus and Down's syndrome: prevalence, management and diabetic complications. Diabet Med 1998; 15(2): 160-3.
[http://dx.doi.org/10.1002/(SICI)1096-9136(199802)15:2<160::AID-DIA537>3.0.CO;2-J] [PMID: 9507919]

[101] Ryan ME. Diagnostic and therapeutic strategies for the management of the diabetic patient Compend Contin Educ Dent 2008; 29(1): 32-8-40-4. 18361339

[102] Bruwier A, Chantrain CF. Hematological disorders and leukemia in children with Down syndrome. Eur J Pediatr 2012; 171(9): 1301-7.
[http://dx.doi.org/10.1007/s00431-011-1624-1] [PMID: 22113227]

[103] Webb D, Roberts I, Vyas P. Haematology of Down syndrome. Arch Dis Child Fetal Neonatal Ed 2007; 92(6): F503-7.
[http://dx.doi.org/10.1136/adc.2006.104638] [PMID: 17804520]

[104] Berger R. Acute lymphoblastic leukemia and chromosome 21. Cancer Genet Cytogenet 1997; 94(1): 8-12.
[http://dx.doi.org/10.1016/S0165-4608(96)00351-2] [PMID: 9078285]

[105] Genc A, Atalay T, Gedikoglu G, Zulfikar B, Kullu S. Leukemic children: clinical and histopathological gingival lesions. J Clin Pediatr Dent 1998; 22(3): 253-6.
[PMID: 9641103]

[106] Dreizen S, Menkin DJ, Keating MJ, McCredie KB, O'Neill PA. Effect of antileukemia chemotherapy on marrow, blood, and oral granulocyte counts. Oral Surg Oral Med Oral Pathol 1991; 71(1): 45-9.
[http://dx.doi.org/10.1016/0030-4220(91)90519-I] [PMID: 1994322]

[107] Macchini F, Leva E, Torricelli M, Valadè A. Treating acid reflux disease in patients with Down syndrome: pharmacological and physiological approaches. Clin Exp Gastroenterol 2011; 4: 19-22.
[http://dx.doi.org/10.2147/CEG.S15872] [PMID: 21694868]

[108] Zárate N, Mearin F, Hidalgo A, Malagelada JR. Prospective evaluation of esophageal motor dysfunction in Down's syndrome. Am J Gastroenterol 2001; 96(6): 1718-24.
[http://dx.doi.org/10.1111/j.1572-0241.2001.03864.x] [PMID: 11419820]

[109] Bell EJ, Kaidonis J, Townsend GC. Tooth wear in children with Down syndrome. Aust Dent J 2002; 47(1): 30-5.
[http://dx.doi.org/10.1111/j.1834-7819.2002.tb00300.x] [PMID: 12035955]

[110] Oliveira AC, Pordeus IA, Luz CL, Paiva SM. Mothers' perceptions concerning oral health of children and adolescents with Down syndrome: a qualitative approach. Eur J Paediatr Dent 2010; 11(1): 27-30.
[PMID: 20359278]

[111] Suvarna RM, Rai K, Hegde AM. Oral health of children with congenital heart disease following preventive treatment. J Clin Pediatr Dent 2011; 36(1): 93-8.
[http://dx.doi.org/10.17796/jcpd.36.1.h337135318140078] [PMID: 22900451]

[112] Wilson W, Taubert KA, Gewitz M, *et al.* AHA Guideline. Prevention of infective endocarditis: guidelines from the American Heart Association. Circulation 2007; 116(15): 1736-54.

[http://dx.doi.org/10.1161/CIRCULATIONAHA.106.183095] [PMID: 17446442]

[113] Abanto J, Ciamponi AL, Francischini E, Murakami C, de Rezende NP, Gallottini M. Medical problems and oral care of patients with Down syndrome: a literature review. Spec Care Dentist 2011; 31(6): 197-203.
[http://dx.doi.org/10.1111/j.1754-4505.2011.00211.x] [PMID: 22070358]

[114] Tasioula V, Balmer R, Parsons J. Dental health and treatment in a group of children with congenital heart disease. Pediatr Dent 2008; 30(4): 323-8.
[PMID: 18767512]

[115] Chung EM, Sung EC, Sakurai KL. Dental management of the Down and Eisenmenger syndrome patient. J Contemp Dent Pract 2004; 15(5(2)): 70-80.
[PMID: 15150635]

[116] Unkel JH, Edwards JS, Piscitelli WP, Tye GW. Dental surgery and anesthetic precautions of a patient with Down syndrome and juvenile rheumatoid arthritis: a case report. Pediatr Dent 2012; 34(7): 517-20.
[PMID: 23265174]

[117] Byard RW. Forensic issues in Down syndrome fatalities. J Forensic Leg Med 2007; 14(8): 475-81.
[http://dx.doi.org/10.1016/j.jflm.2007.01.001] [PMID: 17961872]

[118] Whaley WJ, Gray WD. Atlantoaxial dislocation and Down's syndrome. Can Med Assoc J 1980; 5(123(1)): 35-7.
[PMID: 6448087]

[119] American Academy of Pediatrics: Health supervision for children with Down syndrome. Pediatrics 2001; 107(2): 442-9.
[http://dx.doi.org/10.1542/peds.107.2.442] [PMID: 11158488]

[120] Waldman HB, Hasan FM, Perlman S. Down syndrome and sleep-disordered breathing: the dentist's role. J Am Dent Assoc 2009; 140(3): 307-12.
[http://dx.doi.org/10.14219/jada.archive.2009.0159] [PMID: 19255174]

[121] Butler MG, Hayes BG, Hathaway MM, Begleiter ML. Specific genetic diseases at risk for sedation/anesthesia complications. Anesth Analg 2000; 91(4): 837-55.
[http://dx.doi.org/10.1097/00000539-200010000-00014] [PMID: 11004035]

[122] Pinto A, Glick M. Management of patients with thyroid disease: oral health considerations. J Am Dent Assoc 2002; 133(7): 849-58.
[http://dx.doi.org/10.14219/jada.archive.2002.0299] [PMID: 12148678]

[123] Bjelland S, Bray P, Gupta N, Hirscht R. Dentists, diabetes and periodontitis. Aust Dent J 2002; 47(3): 202-7.
[http://dx.doi.org/10.1111/j.1834-7819.2002.tb00329.x] [PMID: 12405458]

[124] Padmini C, Bai KY. Oral and dental considerations in pediatric leukemic patient. ISRN Hematol 2014; 47(3): 202-7. eCollection 2014
[http://dx.doi.org/10.1155/2014/895721] [PMID: 24724033]

[125] Lalla RV, Sonis ST, Peterson DE. Management of oral mucositis in patients who have cancer. Dent Clin North Am 2008; 52(1): 61-77.

[http://dx.doi.org/10.1016/j.cden.2007.10.002] [PMID: 18154865]

[126] Miller MM, Donald DV, Hagemann TM. Prevention and treatment of oral mucositis in children with cancer. J Pediatr Pharmacol Ther 2012; 17(4): 340-50.
[http://dx.doi.org/10.5863/1551-6776-17.4.340] [PMID: 23413048]

[127] Barg E, Bury M, Marczyk T, Pałac K, Wirth M. [Psychosexual problem in young people with Down syndrome in parents' opinions - personal experience]. Pediatr Endocrinol Diabetes Metab 2008; 14(4): 225-30.
[PMID: 19239790]

[128] Bhowate R, Dubey A. Dentofacial changes and oral health status in mentally challenged children. J Indian Soc Pedod Prev Dent 2005; 23(2): 71-3.
[http://dx.doi.org/10.4103/0970-4388.16445] [PMID: 16012208]

[129] Grant E, Carlson G, Cullen-Erickson M. Oral health for people with intellectual disability and high support needs: positive outcomes. Spec Care Dentist 2004; 24(2): 70-9.
[http://dx.doi.org/10.1111/j.1754-4505.2004.tb01682.x] [PMID: 15200231]

[130] Pilcher ES. Treating the patient with Down syndrome. J Contemp Dent Pract 2001; 15(2(4)): 58.
[PMID: 12167922]

[131] Law CS. Management of premature primary tooth loss in the child patient. J Calif Dent Assoc 2013; 41(8): 612-8.2013; Review
[PMID: 24073500]

[132] Areias CM, Sampaio-Maia B, Guimaraes H, Melo P, Andrade D. Caries in Portuguese children with Down syndrome. Clinics (Sao Paulo) 2011; 66(7): 1183-6.
[http://dx.doi.org/10.1590/S1807-59322011000700010] [PMID: 21876971]

[133] Sandström A, Cressey J, Stecksén-Blicks C. Tooth-brushing behaviour in 6-12 year olds. Int J Paediatr Dent 2011; 21(1): 43-9.
[http://dx.doi.org/10.1111/j.1365-263X.2010.01080.x] [PMID: 20659179]

[134] Norwood KW Jr, Slayton RL. Oral health care for children with developmental disabilities. Pediatrics 2013; 131(3): 614-9.
[http://dx.doi.org/10.1542/peds.2012-3650] [PMID: 23439896]

[135] Centre for Clinical Practice at NICE (UK). Antimicrobial prophylaxis against infective endocarditis in adults and children undergoing interventional procedures 2008.London. 2008. National Institute for Health and Clinical Excellence (UK); 2008 Mar; (http://www.ncbi.nlm.nih.gov/pubmedhealth/PMH0009942/. (accessed 10 September 2014) [PMID: 21656971]

[136] Dinesh RB, Arnitha HM, Munshi AK. Malocclusion and orthodontic treatment need of handicapped individuals in South Canara, India. Int Dent J 2003; 53(1): 13-8.
[http://dx.doi.org/10.1111/j.1875-595X.2003.tb00650.x] [PMID: 12653334]

[137] Wang YC, Lin IH, Huang CH, Fan SZ. Dental anesthesia for patients with special needs. Acta Anaesthesiol Taiwan 2012; 50(3): 122-5.
[http://dx.doi.org/10.1016/j.aat.2012.08.009. 23026171]

[138] Borland LM, Colligan J, Brandom BW. Frequency of anesthesia-related complications in children with

Down syndrome under general anesthesia for noncardiac procedures. Paediatr Anaesth 2004; 14(9): 733-8.
[http://dx.doi.org/10.1111/j.1460-9592.2004.01329.x] [PMID: 15330954]

[139] Kawamata M, Omote K, Tago N, Namiki A. Anesthesia for Down's syndrome with atlantoaxial instability using laryngeal mask airway. Br J Anaesth 1994; 8: 221-3.

[140] Hata T, Todd MM. Cervical spine considerations when anesthetizing patients with Down syndrome. Anesthesiology 2005; 102(3): 680-5.
[http://dx.doi.org/10.1097/00000542-200503000-00030] [PMID: 15731610]

SUBJECT INDEX

D

E

F

G

H

I

J

L

M

N

O

P

Q

R

S

T

U

V

Made in the USA
Las Vegas, NV
10 November 2024

11349647R10290